Comprehensive Management of Swallowing Disorders

Comprehensive Management of Swallowing Disorders

Edited By

Ricardo L. Carrau, M.D., F.A.C.S.
Professor
Department of Otolaryngology
University of Pittsburgh, School of Medicine
Pittsburgh, Pennsylvania

and

Thomas Murry, Ph.D.
Professor
Speech-Language Pathology
Department of Otolaryngology–Head and Neck Surgery
College of Physicians and Surgerons
Columbia University
New York, New York

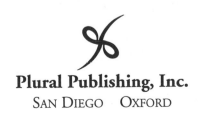

Plural Publishing, Inc.
SAN DIEGO   OXFORD

Plural Publishing, Inc

5521 Ruffin Road
San Diego, CA 92123

e-mail: info@pluralpublishing.com
Web site: http://www.pluralpublishing.com

49 Bath Street
Abingdon, Oxfordshire OX14 1EA
United Kingdom

Original printing 1999.

Typeset in 10/12 Palatino Light by So Cal Graphics
Printed in the United States of America by Bang Printing

ISBN-13: 978-1-59756-099-3
ISBN-10: 1-59756-099-5

Library of Congress Cataloging-in-Publication Data

Comprehensive management of swallowing disorders / edited by Ricardo
    L. Carrau and Thomas Murry.
        p. ; cm.
    Originally published: San Diego : Singular Pub. Group, c1999, in series:
Dysphagia series.
    Includes bibliographical references and index.
    ISBN-13: 978-1-59756-099-3 (softcover)
    ISBN-10: 1-59756-099-5 (softcover)
    1. Deglutition disorders. I. Carrau, Ricardo L. II. Murry, Thomas, 1943- .
[DNLM: 1. Deglutition Disorders. WI 250 C737 1999a] RC815.2.C65
2006 616.3'23--dc22

2006007757

Contents

Foreword

Scientific and clinical activities in dysphagia are among the fastest growing in health care. Speech-language pathologists, physicians, surgeons, nurses, dietitians, dentists, occupational and physical therapists, physiologists, and social workers are among the professionals doing the work. The highest levels of research and clinical productivity in dysphagia require responsible scholarship, the ability to cope with ambiguity, respect for interdisciplinary cooperation, and a recognition that dysphagia's effects on people extend well beyond mealtime.

Comprehensive Management of Swallowing Disorders edited by Ricardo L. Carrau, M.D., and Thomas Murry, Ph.D., is as perfect a contribution to the field as can be imagined. It contains 55 chapters; authors are drawn from all the major professions presently involved in dysphagia, and each profession's perspective is clearly outlined. The field's entire content is represented: normal and abnormal swallowing; child and adult; oropharynx and esophagus; structural and functional etiologies; prognosis; evaluation and treatment; surgical, medical, and behavioral management; rehabilitation and compensation.

General books risk being a mile wide and a foot deep. Not so this book. The reader is not limited to wading; immersion is possible even for the experienced practitioner. Myotomy, vocal fold augmentation and medialization, Nissen fundoplication, Zenker's diverticulectomy, and gastrostomy are among the surgical procedures included in chapter-length discussions. The array of etiologies and medical and behavioral evaluations and treatments are equally grand. Dysphagic patients are usually not well served by a practitioner with only one or a severely limited number of explanatory, evaluation, or treatment approaches. The contributors to this book obviously serve their patients well. Careful readers will be able to do the same. And there is enough new information in this book so that even the most experienced can come away with more alternatives.

John C. Rosenbek, Ph.D.
Professor and Chair
Department of Communicative Disorders
University of Florida

Preface

Not long ago, there was scarce literature addressing the diagnosis and management of swallowing disorders. A dramatic change ensued during the late 1980s when we saw the development of journals, conferences, and discussion groups devoted primarily to swallowing. Increased interest and subsequent research led to a plethora of new treatments and management strategies for swallowing problems. Even more important is the increased awareness of the prevalence and importance of swallowing disorders among various medical and rehabilitation specialists. Clinicians now take courses in swallowing; multi-disciplinary conferences are now offered and the functional needs of patients with swallowing problems are being considered when planning their rehabilitation. Needs ranging from construction of special spoons and cups for eating and drinking to surgical correction of anatomical problems to manage dysphagia and prevent aspiration are now being addressed.

Clinicians who pioneered work in all of these areas are the impetus for this text. From the time when swallowing was taken for granted to the present day, research in every aspect of eating, chewing, swallowing, and nutrition has advanced the rehabilitation of patients with swallowing problems. The treatment of swallowing disorders is not yet a science, but it is no longer overlooked in the overall management of patients suffering from disorders such as a stroke, cancer, and other acute or chronic catastrophic diseases. We have seen the changes in clinical pathways that have occurred in major medical centers to improve the rehabilitation of patients through the efforts of those who treat swallowing.

It is because of the ever-evolving changes in the management of swallowing disorders and the inevitable and necessary interaction with all the many specialists who treat swallowing disorders that we undertook this book. Our experience, gained after a number of years working in a multi-disciplinary environment, studying swallowing both in the normal and disordered populations, is that swallowing problems are complex even when the diagnosis is known. Moreover, our philosophical approach is that swallowing is not the domain of only the speech pathologists or the medical or surgical specialists. Rather, it is in the best interest of the patients suffering from a swallowing disorder that all clinicians involved in their care are active participants in their rehabilitation.

Thus, this text addresses the swallowing problems from the point of view of all those specialists in medical, surgical, and rehabilitative medicine who are involved in the management of these patients. We feel that each discipline must understand each other's role in the management of swallowing disorders. Central to that notion is the understanding of the normal swallow. We have devoted a considerable number of pages to the normal pediatric and adult swallow, including a detailed discussion of the anatomy, physiology, and pathophysiology of swallowing. The clinician who understands the anatomy, physiology, and neurology of normal swallowing will better understand the effects of diseases, disorders, and functional changes that present as swallowing disorders.

This text is divided into seven sections. In the first, an introduction to the myriad of swallowing disorders is presented. A vast array of conditions that are associated with swallowing disorders and their epidemiology are introduced.

Part II describes the anatomy and physiology of swallowing. Both the organs of swallowing and the normal swallow are reviewed in detail.

Part III addresses the evaluation of swallowing from seven perspectives: otolaryngology, speech pathology, pediatrics, gastroenterology, neurology, physical and rehabilitative medicine, and nutrition. Each specialist describes the clinical evaluation and procedures that he or she uses when first evaluating a patient with a swallowing problem. Although some of these techniques are similar among all and, therefore, the text may appear to be repetitive, each discipline provides a unique perspective to the aspects important for making a diagnosis and planning treatment. Part III also includes four chapters on various tests of swallowing function. These include the various radiographic examinations, endoscopic tests of swallowing, gastroenterologic tests, and electromyography. The benefits and disadvantages, along with the complications of each test are described.

Part IV contains 19 chapters that cover all aspects of the pathophysiology of swallowing disorders. This section or the text is a "tour de force" of medical, surgical, and neurological problems that lead to swallowing disorders; the identifying signs and the disorders; and, in some chapters, case studies of management. The detail with which this section of the book is assembled reflects the strong multi-disciplinary nature of the entire text.

Part V is devoted to the nonsurgical treatment of swallowing disorders. Four chapters are devoted to diet modification, behavioral techniques, prosthodontics, and swallowing management of adults with tracheotomies. Each chapter includes methods and procedures for each stage of swallow rehabilitation.

Part VI reviews the surgical treatment of swallowing disorders. Twelve chapters are devoted to the various surgical procedures that are both temporary and permanent treatments for laryngeal, pharyngeal, esophageal, and gastric disorders.

Part VII addresses swallowing problems in special populations. Special problems of the pediatric population are addressed, as well as problems of critical care patients, aging patients, terminally ill patients, and patients with intractable aspiration pneumonia. The authors also address the organization of a multi-disciplinary dysphagia team.

We are indebted to the many specialists who have taken time to address swallowing from a multi-disciplinary perspective. Their commitment to this text reflects the commitment that they profess to the diagnosis and treatment of swallowing disorders. Each contributor has kept the focus of this text in mind when addressing his or her specific topic.

Acknowledgments

To my wife, Janet, my daughters, Diana D. and Janet L., for their patience, understanding, and support during this endeavor; to the faculty of the Departments of Otolaryngology—Head and Neck Surgery at the University of Puerto Rico and the University of Pittsburgh, which provided me with the fund of knowledge and skills to continue my professional growth; and to my patients for the continual lessons about both the frailties and strengths of the human body and who have to endure my efforts to help them.

Ricardo L. Carrau

To Marie-Pierre, who through her love and understanding has supported my professional goals, and to Nicholas, whose energy, enthusiasm, and challenges make the journey worthwhile.

Thomas Murry

Infinite thanks to Maggi Dadisman for her manuscript processing and management—we could not have completed this project without her assistance. We are grateful to all our authors for their commitment to this enterprise, at the cost of great effort and personal time—a rare commodity in the present health care environment.

Contributors

Sanjiv S. Agarwala, M.D.
Assistant Professor of Medicine
Co-Director, Head and Neck Cancer Program
Department of Medicine
Division of Medical Oncology
Montefiore University Hospital
Pittsburgh, Pennsylvania

Aijaz Alvi, M.D.
Director, Head and Neck Surgery
Department of Otolaryngology and
  Bronchoesophagology
Temple University School of Medicine
Philadelphia, Pennsylvania

Robert J. Andrews, M.D.
Department of Otolaryngology
Vanderbilt University Medical Center
Nashville, Tennessee

Jonathan E. Aviv, M.D., F.A.C.S.
Director, Division of Head and Neck Surgery
Department of Otolaryngology—Head and Neck
  Surgery
Columbia-Presbyterian Medical Center
College of Physicians and Surgeons, Columbia
  University

Sanjeev Bahri, M.D.
Radiation Oncology
Assistant Professor
University of Pittsburgh Medical Center
Pittsburgh, Pennsylvania

Susan M. Baser, M.D.
Allegheny Neurological Associates
Allegheny General Hospital
Pittsburgh, Pennsylvania

Farrel J. Buchinsky, M.D.
Department of Otolaryngology and
  Bronchoesophagology
Temple University School of Medicine
Philadelphia, Pennsylvania

Elmer Cano, M.D.
Department of Radiation Oncology
University of Pittsburgh Medical Center
Pittsburgh, Pennsylvania

Ricardo L. Carrau, M.D.
Department of Otolaryngology
University of Pittsburgh Medical Center
Pittsburgh, Pennsylvania

Kimberly A. Chignell, M.S.
Clinical and Research Speech Pathologist
VA Medical Center
Madison, Wisconsin

James L. Coyle, M.A.
Instructor, Senior Clinical and Research Speech
  Pathologist
University of Wisconsin, Madison
University of Wisconsin Hospitals and Clinics
  Swallowing Service
Department of Communicative Disorders
Madison, Wisconsin

Kristin Drennen, M.D.
Department of Otolaryngology
University of Pittsburgh Medical Center
Pittsburgh, Pennsylvania

David E. Eibling, M.D.
Professor
Department of Otolaryngology
University of Pittsburgh School of Medicine
Pittsburgh, Pennsylvania

Johannes J. Fagan, M.B., Ch.B., F.C.S.(SA), M.Med(Otol)
Senior Specialist and Lecturer
Department of Otolaryngology
University of Cape Town School of Medicine
Groote Schuur Hospital Observatory
Cape Town, South Africa

Magdy N. Falestiny, M.D.
James A. Haley VA Medical Center
Tampa, Florida

Peter F. Ferson, M.D.
Department of Cardiothoracic Surgery
Professor of Surgery
University of Pittsburgh Medical Center
Pittsburgh, Pennsylvania

Margaret M. Forbes, M.A., CCC-SLP
Coordinator of Speech Language Pathology
UPMC Health System
Montefiore Hospital Rehab Unit
Pittsburgh, Pennsylvania

Lisa T. Galati, M.D.
Assistant Professor
Division of Otolaryngology
Albany Medical College
Albany, New York

Andrew N. Goldberg, M.D.
Assistant Professor
Department of Otorhinolaryngology—Head and Neck
  Surgery
University of Pennsylvania School of Medicine
Philadelphia, Pennsylvania

Jennifer Rubin Grandis, M.D., F.A.C.S.
Otolaryngology
University of Pittsburgh School of Medicine
Pittsburgh, Pennsylvania

Roxann Diez Gross, M.A.
University of Pittsburgh Medical Center
Pittsburgh, Pennsylvania

Jonas T. Johnson, M.D.
Professor
Departments of Otolaryngology and Radiation
  Oncology
University of Pittsburgh School of Medicine
Pittsburgh, Pennsylvania

Robert J. Keenan, M.D., F.R.C.S.(C.)
Assistant Professor of Surgery
University of Pittsburgh
Vice-Chief, Cardiothoracic Surgery
University of Pittsburgh Medical Center
Pittsburgh, Pennsylvania

Karen M. Kost, M.D., F.R.C.S.(C)
Assistant Professor of Otolaryngology
McGill University
Montreal, Canada

Rodney J. Landreneau, M.D.
Professor of Surgery
Allegheny University of the Health Sciences
Director, Thoracic Surgery
Allegheny General Hospital
Pittsburgh, Pennsylvania

Brendan Levy, M.D.
Carl T. Hayden VA Medical Center
Phoenix, Arizona

James D. Luketich, M.D.
Section of Thoracic Surgery
University of Pittsburgh Medical Center
Pittsburgh, Pennsylvania

Richard Maley, M.D.
Section of Thoracic Surgery
Department of Surgery
University of Pittsburgh Medical Center
Pittsburgh, Pennsylvania

Albert L. Mercati, M.D.
Assistant Professor
Director, Laryngeal Laboratory
Kansas University Medical Center
Kansas City, Kansas

Laura Molseed, M.S., R.D.
Nutrition Coordinator
The University of Pittsburgh Medical Center
Pittsburgh, Pennsylvania

Michael C. Munin, M.D.
Assistant Professor
Division of Medicine and Rehabilitation
University of Pittsburgh Medical Center
Pittsburgh, PA

Thomas Murry, Ph.D.
Professor, Speech-Language Pathology
Department of Otolaryngology-Head and Neck Surgery
College of Physicians and Surgeons
Columbia University
New York, New York

Eugene N. Myers, M.D.
Professor and Chairman
Department of Otolaryngology
University of Pittsburgh School of Medicine
Pittsburgh, Pennsylvania

James L. Netterville, M.D.
Department of Otolaryngology
Vanderbilt University Medical Center
Nashville, Tennessee

Lisa A. Newman, Sc.D.
University of Tennessee, College of Medicine
Department of Otolaryngology—Head and Neck
  Surgery
Director, Speech, Voice and Swallowing Service
Co-Director, Feeding Team, LeBonheur Children's
  Medical Center
Memphis, Tennessee

Ninh T. Nguyen, M.D.
Section of Thoracic Surgery
Department of Surgery
University of Pittsburgh Medical Center
Pittsburgh, Pennsylvania

Sukhdeep Padda, M.D.
Section of Gastroenterology
Carl T. Hayden VA Medical Center
Phoenix, Arizona

Andrew B. Peitzman, M.D.
Professor of Surgery
University of Pittsburgh School of Medicine
Presbyterian University Hospital
Pittsburgh, Pennsylvania

Mario Petersen, M.D., M.S.
University of Tennessee, College of Medicine
Department of Pediatrics
Division of Developmental Pediatrics
Co-Director, Feeding Team, LeBonheur Children's
  Medical Center
Memphis, Tennessee

Anna M. Pou, M.D.
Assistant Professor—Department of Otolaryngology
University of Texas Medical Branch, Galveston
Galveston, Texas

Michael Rainer, M.D.
Resident Physician
Physical Medicine and Rehabilitation
UPMC Health System
Pittsburgh, Pennsylvania

Clark A. Rosen, M.D.
Director, University of Pittsburgh Voice Center
Assistant Professor
Department of Otolaryngology
University of Pittsburgh
Pittsburgh, Pennsylvania

John C. Rosenbek, Ph.D.
Chief, Audiology and Speech Pathology
VA Medical Center
Madison, Wisconsin

Robert T. Sataloff, M.D., D.M.A.
Professor of Otolaryngology
Department of Otolaryngology—Head and Neck
  Surgery
Thomas Jefferson University
Chairman Department of Otolaryngology—
  Head and Neck Surgery
Allegheny University Hospitals, Graduate,
Philadelphia, Pennsylvania

Ibraham Sbeitan, M.D.
Division of Medical Oncology
University of Pittsburgh Medical Center
Pittsburgh, Pennsylvania

Jesse Selber, B.A.
University of Rochester
Rochester, New York

Melissa A. Simonian, M.Ed., CCC-SLP
Senior Speech-Language Pathologist
Department of Pennsylvania Medical Center
Philadelphia, Pennsylvania

Carl H. Snyderman, M.D.
Associate Professor
Department of Otolaryngology
University of Pittsburgh Medical Center
  Eye & Ear Hospital
Pittsburgh, Pennsylvania

Ahmed M. S. Soliman, M.D.
Department of Otolaryngology and
  Bronchoesophagology
Temple University School of Medicine
Philadelphia, Pennsylvania

Joseph R. Spiegel, M.D., F.A.C.S
Associate Professor of Otolaryngology,
Department of Otolaryngology—Head and Neck Surgery
Thomas Jefferson University, Vice Chairman
Department of Otolaryngology—Head and Neck
  Surgery
Allegheny University Hospitals, Graduate,
Philadelphia, Pennsylvania

Erica R. Thaler, M.D.
Assistant Professor
Department of Otolaryngology
University of Pennsylvania
Philadelphia, Pennsylvania

Jane L. Weissman, M.D.
Associate Professor of Radiology and Otolaryngology
Director of Head and Neck Imaging
University of Pittsburgh Medical Center
Pittsburgh, Pennsylvania

William Welch, M.D., F.A.C.S.
Department of Neurosurgery
Department of Orthopedic Surgery
University of Pittsburgh, School of Rehabilitative
  Sciences
Pittsburgh, Pennsylvania

Randy T. Woods, M.D.
Fellow: Trauma/Critical Care
University of Pittsburgh Medical Center—Presbyterian
  Hospital
Pittsburgh, Pennsylvania

Gayle E. Woodson, M.D.
Department of Otolaryngology
University of Tennessee Health Science Center
Memphis, Tennessee

Michele A. Young, M.D.
Chief, Gastrointestinal Motility
Carl T. Hayden VA Medical Center
Assistant Professor of Clinical Medicine
University of Arizona
Phoenix, Arizona

Victor L. Yu, M.D.
Infectious Diseases Section
Pittsburgh VA Medical Center
Pittsburgh, Pennsyslvania

Hussein S. Zaki, D.D.S., M.Sc.
Director, Maxillofacial Department
Montefiore University Hospital
University of Pittsburgh
Pittsburgh, Pennsylvania

PART I

INTRODUCTION

The Introduction offers a brief summary of the current literature regarding the incidence and prevalence of swallowing disorders in various patient populations. Data regarding swallowing disorders is evolving rapidly. As more disciplines are becoming aware of the significance of swallowing disorders, it may be expected that epidemiology studies will continually change our concepts on these issues. Factors affecting the different populations most commonly afflicted by swallowing disorders are highlighted in this section.

CHAPTER 1

∎ ∎ ∎

Epidemiology of Swallowing Disorders

Thomas Murry, Ph.D.
Ricardo L. Carrau, M.D.
David E. Eibling, M.D.

"The consequences of inhaling various substances into the bronchi and lungs provide a subject for interesting study and vital importance for many patients. Bronchopneumonia is one of these consequences."

J. B. Amberson, 1937

I. INTRODUCTION

The preceding quote introduced Amberson's landmark treatise on aspiration. The statement is still as relevant today. Amberson clearly saw the importance and significance of aspiration in most aspects of a medical practice and rehabilitation since aspiration bronchopneumonia may turn the tide unfavorably, when otherwise recovery would be expected.[1]

The evaluation and management of patients with swallowing dysfunction has evolved into a major clinical activity for many disciplines in the medical community. Despite the prolific scientific and clinical findings presented in the past 10 years, the study of dysphagia remains an inexact science. We are still pursuing the goals that Amberson eloquently outlined more than 60 years ago, namely, the circumstances under which dysphagia occurs, the management of the case after it does occur, and, especially, the possibilities and means of prevention.

Although the true incidence of swallowing disorders may not be known, it is apparent that this problem is widespread and its consequences may be severe. The true incidence of dysphagia in the general population remains unknown, as many cases come to light only after an acute or significant medical incident that might not otherwise call attention to dysphagia. In this chapter, the epidemiology of dysphagia is presented. Although epidemiology refers to both prevalence and cause, this chapter focuses primarily on prevalence as causes are covered throughout the text.

II. PREVALENCE OF DYSPHAGIA AND ASPIRATION

Dysphagia is a common comorbidity associated with a wide variety of disease states, and is often associated with illnesses that result in anatomic abnormalities or neuromuscular dysfunction of the oral cavity, pharynx, larynx, and esophagus. Dysphagia due to primary esophageal disease is not rare, but is not encountered as frequently as is oropharyngeal dysphagia.[2,3] Any illness that results in weakness, either from specific neurologic or muscular pathology or from generalized debilitation, is likely to have dysphagia related to it.

A. Stroke Patients

Brain injury due to stroke is one of the most common causes of dysphagia. Stroke is the third most common cause of death in the U.S. each year, with approximately 500,000 new cases reported annually with an estimated 150,000 individuals dying from stroke each year. Between 30% to 40% percent of stroke victims will demonstrate symptoms of significant dysphagia, and as many as 20% will die from aspiration pneumonia in the first year.[4] A prospective study of stroke victims suggests that there is a 50% incidence of aspiration in this group of patients.[5] Moreover, half of those patients who aspirate do so silently, eg, without obvious symptoms or clinical findings.[6] As a result, the quoted figure of 30% may be a low estimate due to the frequency with which aspiration occurs without clinical signs in many stroke patients.

Although the correlation of site and size of a stroke with subsequent dysphagia is variable, the trend is that the larger the area of infarction, the greater the impairment of swallowing. In general, brainstem strokes produce dysphagia more frequently and more severely than cortical strokes. Robbins et al suggest that the severity of dysphagia in patients with left hemisphere strokes seems to correlate with the presence of apraxia and the reported deficits are more significant during the oral stage of swallowing.[7] Patients with strokes affecting the right hemisphere have more pharyngeal dysfunction, including aspiration and pharyngeal pooling.

Although recovery of neuromotor functions following stroke is unpredictable, dysphagia, with its attendant risk of aspiration, decreases over time in most patients. Unfortunately, many patients do not recover sufficient neuromuscular function to safely tolerate a regular diet, placing them at risk for the potentially fatal consequences of aspiration. Thus, in addition to the 20% of stroke victims who die of aspiration pneumonia in the first year following a stroke, approximately 10% to 15% of stroke victims die of aspiration pneumonia in the years following the stroke.[6]

B. Nursing Home Residents

The population residing in nursing homes is increasing. In 1985, 5% of the U.S. population over the age of 65, and 22% of the population over the age of 85 years, resided in nursing homes.[8] Studies carried out in nursing homes have demonstrated that 30% to 40% of the residents have clinical evidence of dysphagia and the prevalence of pneumonia has been estimated to be 2%.[9] Moreover, autopsy studies have demonstrated that there is a failure to diagnose pneumonia in this population in as many as 27% of cases.[10]

A prospective study of 152 nursing home patients followed for 3 years by Feinberg and coworkers revealed 55 episodes of pneumonia, defined as a new infiltrate persisting for more than five days.[11] During the first year, one third of these 55 patients were found to dem-

onstrate major aspiration of clinical significance, one third minor aspiration of no significance, and one third did not aspirate on initial examination with videofluoroscopy. After 3 years, a total of 90 of the 152 patients developed pneumonia and 41 expired over the 3-year period of the study. Pneumonia was considered to be the cause of death in 27 of those who expired, or 18% of the original 152 patients.

In another surveillance study following the population of 13 nursing homes, with a total of 1754 residents, Beck-Sague et al found an incidence of pneumonia of 27% during a 6-month period.[12] Although it is not clear how many of these infections were secondary to aspiration, the data obtained from other studies suggest that the incidence is extremely high.

Pneumonia in the nursing home population is associated with a higher mortality than community acquired pneumonia or any other infection.[13] The mortality rate for patients admitted to acute care hospitals from nursing homes with pneumonia has been reported to be 40%, as compared to patients with community acquired pneumonia, which was 28%. Patients with pneumonia admitted from nursing homes constituted 14% of all cases admitted with the diagnosis of pneumonia.[14] Although it is unknown how many of these patients developed pneumonia as a result of aspiration, there is general consensus that as many as 70% to 90% of elderly patients, even those without known neurologic disease, have some degree of swallowing dysfunction, if not true dysphagia.

One can assume, therefore, that due to the large number of patients with dysphagia residing in nursing homes, the total number of admissions of nursing home patients to acute care hospitals for aspiration-induced pneumonia is significant. It is estimated that a typical nursing home of 120 beds can expect to transfer one patient per month to an acute care hospital for the treatment of pneumonia. Therefore, each year in the United States approximately 150000 nursing home patients require hospitalization for pneumonia. The cost of acute care hospitalization for management of these patients with pneumonia had been estimated to be about $20000 per patient. The cost of the treatment of this complication, in most cases probably due to aspiration, is estimated to exceed $3 billion each year in the U.S. alone.[13] The actual costs are probably even higher, considering treatment for patients who are not admitted or for the isolation of patients who develop infections with resistant organisms from the antibiotic therapy required for the management of pneumonia.

C. Dementia And Dysphagia Patients

Dysphagia is common in elderly patients with dementia. Feinberg demonstrated normal swallowing function in only 9 of 131 (7%) patients with dementia studied with videofluoroscopy.[15] Nearly one third of the patients (30%) were restaged following examination, demonstrating the inaccuracies of routine history and physical in this patient population. His study demonstrated not only the high percentage of clinically significant dysphagia in this population, but also pointed out the difficulties in assessing this group of patients because of their dementia, as well as the ineffectiveness of therapeutic maneuvers that require patient cooperation.

D. Hospitalized Patients

Nosocomial pneumonia occurs in a significant percentage of Medicare patients hospitalized for other, unrelated illnesses. Mortality is estimated at between 20% to 50% of these patients, and the average increase in hospital cost due to nosocomial infection was estimated to be $5800 per hospitalization in 1991.[13] In many instances, this increase in hospitalization costs raised the costs significantly above the reimbursement received from Medicare for the care given. It can be safely assumed that this cost differential has increased in the years since this study; hence, it is likely that the cost of treating nosocomial pneumonia, many cases of which are probably due to aspiration, is a significant factor in health care costs and ultimately, profitability, for hospitals and managed health care plans. Despite the significant costs of medical care generated by patients with aspiration, there is remarkably little emphasis on the evaluation and management of these patients, and reimbursement for the time required for evaluation and treatment is so low as to discourage physician involvement in all but a few major institutions with an academic commitment to the study and management of dysphagia.

The incidence of swallowing disorders in patients admitted to critical care units is increased by the need for endotracheal and nasogastric intubation, tracheotomy, and use of sedatives, along with impaired consciousness and the debilitated status of many of the patients requiring critical care. These and many other factors predispose these patients to aspiration of oral secretions, food, and gastric refluxate. The incidence of pneumonia in the ICU, however, is not necessarily higher than in the general hospital population, perhaps due to the skill and intensity of nursing care,[16] which can obviously alter the outcome in patients with swallowing disorders.

Valles et al[17] prospectively followed 77 patients requiring mechanical ventilation. The incidence of ventilation pneumonia episodes was 39.6/1000 ventilator days. He found that in another group of 76 patients whose subglottis was being continuously aspirated, the incidence was 19.9/1000 ventilation days, demonstrating the importance of aspiration as an etiology for pneumonia and the therapeutic implications of suctioning the aspirate.

E. Normal Elderly Population

Many apparently normal elderly patients suffer chronic dysphagia. As many as 50% of elderly patients have difficulty eating that leads to nutritional deficiencies with associated weight loss, increased risk of falling, poor healing, and increased susceptibility to other illnesses associated with weakness.[18] Sarcopenia, or "loss of flesh," is considered the major challenge of the geriatric population[19] and is undoubtedly related to decreased caloric intake. Multiple factors are thought to be responsible for this reduced oral intake, including loss of teeth, reduced oral sensitivity, changes in taste and smell, decreased hand-eye coordination, vision loss, solitary eating, and depression.[20] Difficulties with mobility lead to a reduced ability to live independently, limiting going out to buy groceries or even selecting a proper diet. It has been demonstrated that the degree of sarcopenia correlates well with serum albumin levels, which is strongly correlated with nutritional status.[21] Recent studies also have demonstrated that caloric requirements for the elderly are surprisingly high, and often not met by dietary intake.[22] Therefore, it is intuitive that a major cause of sarcopenia is related to inadequate caloric intake from self-imposed dietary restriction related to chronic dysphagia.

Although much of the recent literature has addressed exercise and activity levels, there has been surprisingly little emphasis on nutritional factors and the role of dysphagia. Moreover, the weakness associated with muscle atrophy further increases the degree of dysphagia due to further reduction in effectiveness of swallowing function.

F. Head And Neck Oncology Patients

Head and neck squamous cell carcinoma represents 4% of all malignancies, and comprises 95% of all the malignant tumors arising within the upper aerodigestive tract. Forty- to sixty-thousand new cases are diagnosed every year, accounting for 10000 deaths a year. The presence of tumor in the upper aerodigestive tract may affect swallowing by mechanical obstruction due to bulk or extraluminal compression, decreased pliability of the soft tissue because of neoplastic infiltration, direct invasion of nerves leading to paralysis of important pharyngeal or laryngeal muscles, or pain.

Virtually all treatments for head and neck cancer result in a temporary or permanent swallowing problem. Treatment for squamous cell carcinoma, namely surgery and radiation therapy, produces disabilities that are usually proportional to the volume of the resection and/or the radiation field. Surgery produces division and fibrosis of muscles and produces anesthetic areas due to the transection or extirpation of afferent neural fibers and/or receptors. This is most evident in patients who require resection of large oropharyngeal tumors in which the swallowing reflex or the "trigger" of the pharyngeal swallow will be delayed or absent or in patients who undergo a supraglottic laryngectomy, in whom the loss of supraglottic and pharyngeal sensation almost invariably leads to aspiration. Radiation therapy leads to xerostomia, which, in many cases, is permanent and a primary source of patient complaints. Irradiation produces fibrosis of the oropharyngeal and laryngeal musculature. Furthermore, many patients presenting with large tumors will require combination therapy using both surgery and radiation therapy, which results in severe restriction of motion due to the consequences already mentioned. Recent trends toward the use of conservation protocols using chemotherapy and radiation seem to yield similar problems, with even more fibrosis of the soft tissues. D'Antonio reported the quality of life and functional status measurements of patients with squamous cancer of the head and neck demonstrated that 69% of these patients have some problem associated with swallowing.[23]

Murry et al reported on acute and chronic changes in swallowing and quality of life following an intra-arterial chemoradiation protocol.[24] They found that quality of life and swallowing are related during the acute phase of treatment and early posttreatment. However, the strongest relationship between swallowing and quality of life was found at 6 months postchemoradiation, pointing out the importance of swallowing function following chemoradiation. Swallowing function was most severely degraded in patients with oropharyngeal tumors. The researchers also found that swallowing improved significantly 6 months after chemoradiation, compared to pretreatment values. Swallowing function appears to be related to both site and stage of disease.

In general, patients with so-called anterior tumors, such as floor of the mouth or oral tongue, have better posttreatment outcome regarding swallowing than patients with so-called posterior tumors, such as oropharynx or hypopharynx. This is not to say that patients with oral tumors have no problem swallowing, as the oral phase is definitely affected.[25] These patients usually compensate by exhibiting piecemeal swallowing or clearing swallows.

As stated before, the greater the extent of resection, the greater the ensuing disability, especially if the resection involves areas with motor or sensory function that are critical for swallowing. Patients undergoing hemilaryngectomies have been found to recover their swallowing function sooner than patients undergoing supraglottic laryngectomies, who, in turn, recover much more quickly than patients undergoing extended supraglottic laryngectomies (extended to the base of the tongue).[26]

List et al reported a prospective study following patients with carcinoma of the larynx.[27] Those patients with T-1 tumors were treated with radiation therapy, while other patients were treated with either a hemilaryngectomy or a total laryngectomy, according to the extent of the tumor. At 6 months follow-up, both the postirradiation patients and patients who underwent hemilaryngectomy were consuming a normal diet, with only 50–60% of the total laryngectomy patients consuming a normal diet. The postradiation patients recovered their swallowing function more quickly than the postsurgical patients. Sixty percent of patients at 6 weeks follow-up, and 80% at 12 weeks follow-up, demonstrated normal swallowing. This has been demonstrated in other studies, which have shown that patients who undergo a total laryngectomy have decreased function of the pharyngeal constrictors, therefore diminished driving pressure, needing to compensate by increasing their tongue pump.

A study by Naudo et al of patients after supracricoid laryngectomy with cricohyoidoepiglottopexy (CHP) demonstrated that 98.4% of their patients had what they describe as "normal swallowing."[28] These patients recovered in a manner similar to postradiation patients, described by List, 68% of whom demonstrated a normal diet after the first month. Nonetheless, Naudo describes that 23% of these patients had Grade 1-2 aspiration during this first month. At 1 year follow-up, 8.5% of these patients suffered aspiration pneumonia, and 0.5% required a total laryngectomy.

The method of reconstruction has also been implied in swallowing problems. Logeman et al found that patients with reconstruction by primary closure have the least problem swallowing.[29] This has not been the case in other series. Martini et al, in a study of patients with T-3 and T-4 tumors, demonstrated no difference in postoperative function between patients undergoing reconstruction with primary closure and patients undergoing reconstruction with regional vascularized flaps.[30] This series, however, also demonstrates that patients with larger tumors required obliteration of more function and tissue and therefore suffer greater postoperative deficits.

Finally, swallowing therapy can alter the rehabilitation progress and swallowing outcome. Pauloski et al have demonstrated that patients undergoing oropharyngeal cancer surgery do not improve progressively between 1 and 12 months.[31] The postoperative swallowing status at 3 months reflected their swallowing status at a follow-up of 1 year after surgery. These authors suggested that this may be related to the relative lack of therapy that patients receive during the postoperative period between 3 to 12 months. In fact, these authors reported that some parameters of the swallowing function had a reversal at the 6-month evaluation point. The authors suggest that this may be due to the postradiation effects, such as fibrosis of the tissue or reduced salivary flow. Patients who were irradiated had a delay in their swallowing recovery.

References

1. Amberson JB. Aspiration bronchopneumonia. *International Clinics*, 1937:126-138.
2. Kahrilas PJ. Esophageal motor activity and acid clearance. *Gastroenterol Clin N Am*. 1990;19:537-550.
3. Jacob P, Kahrilas PJ, Vanagunas A. Peristaltic dysfunction associated with nonobstructive dysphagia in reflux disease. *Dig Dis Sci*. 1990;38:939-942.
4. Schmidt EV, Smirnov VE, Ryabova US. Results of the seven-year prospective study of stroke patients. *Stroke*. 1988;19:1942-1949.
5. Alberts MJ, Horner J, Gray L, Brazer SR. Aspiration after stroke: lesion analysis by brain MRI. *Dysphagia*. 1992;7: 170-173.
6. Horner J, Massey EW, Riski JE, Lathrop DL, Chase KN. Aspiration following stroke: clinical correlates and outcome. *Neurology*. 1988;38:1359-1362.
7. Robbins J, Levine RL. Swallowing after unilateral stroke of the cerebral cortex: preliminary experience. *Dysphagia*. 1988;3:11-17.
8. Smith PW. Infections in long-term care facilities. *Infect Control* [editorial]. 1985;6:435-436.
9. Garibaldi RA, Brodine S, Matsumiya S. Infections among patients in nursing homes. *N Engl J Med*. 1981;305:731-735.
10. Gross JS, Neufeld RR, Libow LS, Rodstein M. Autopsy study of the elderly institutionalized patient-review of 234 autopsies. *Arch Intern Med*. 1988;148:173-174.
11. Feinberg MJ, Knebl J, Tully J. Prandial aspiration and pneumonia in an elderly population followed over 3 years. *Dysphagia*. 1996;11:104-109.
12. Beck-Sague C, Villarino E, Giuliano D, Welbel S, Latts L, Manangan LM, Sinkowitz RL, Jarvis WR. Infectious disease and death among nursing home residents: results of surveillance in 13 nursing homes. *Infect Control Hosp Epidemiol*. 1994;15:494-496.
13. Boyce TM, Potter-Boyne G, Dziobed L, Solomon SL. Nosocomial pneumonia in Medicare patients: hospital costs and reimbursement patterns under the prospective payment system. *Arch Intern Med*. 1991;151:1109-1114.
14. Marrie TJ, Durant H, Kwan C. Nursing home-acquired pneumonia: a case-control study. *J Am Geriatr Soc*. 1986;34: 697-702.
15. Feinberg MJ, Ekberg O, Segall L, Tully J. Deglutition in elderly patients with dementia: findings of videofluorographic evaluation and impact on staging and management. *Radiology*. 1992;183:811-814.
16. Mullan H, Roubenhoff RA, Roubenoff R. Risk of pulmonary aspiration among patients receiving enteral nutrition support. *J Parenter Enteral Nutr*. 1993;16:160-164.
17. Valles J, Artigas A, Rello J, Bonsoms N, Fontanals D, Blanch L, Fernandez R, Baigorri F, Mestre J. Continuous aspiration of subglottic secretions in preventing ventilator-associated pneumonia. *Ann Intern Med*. 1995;122:179-186.
18. Schroeder PL, Richter JE. Swallowing disorders in the elderly. *Practical Gastroenterol*. 1996;18(2):19-41.
19. Dutta C. Significance of sarcopenia in the elderly. *J Nutrition*. 1997;127:992S-993S.
20. Ship JA, Duffy V, Jones JA, Langmore S. Geriatric oral health and its impact on eating. *J Am Geriatr Soc*. 1996;44: 456-464.
21. Baumgarten RN, Koehler KM, Romero L, Garry PJ. Serum albumin is associated with skeletal muscle in elderly men and women. *Am J Clin Nutrition*. 1996;64(4):553-558.
22. Roberts SB. Effects of aging on energy requirements and the control of food intake in men. *J Gerontol*. 1995;50 spec:101-106.
23. D'Antonio LL, Zimmerman GJ, Cella DF, Long SA. Quality of life and functional status measures in patients with head and neck cancer. *Arch Otolaryngol Head Neck Surg*. 1996;122:482-487.
24. Murry T, Madasu R, Martin A, Robbins KT. Acute and chronic changes in swallowing and quality of life following intraarterial chemoradiation for organ preservation in patients with advanced head and neck cancer. *Head Neck*. 1998;20:31-37.
25. Stachler RJ, Hamlet SL, Mathog RH, Jones L, Heilbrun LK, Manov J, O'Campo JM. Swallowing of bolus types by postsurgical head and neck cancer patients. *Head Neck*. 1994;16:413-419.
26. Rademaker AW, Logemann JA, Pauloski BR, Bowman JB, Lazarus CL, Sisson GA, Milianti FJ, Graner D, Cook BS, Collins SL, Stein DW, Beery QC, Johnson JT, Baker TM. Recovery of postoperative swallowing patients undergoing partial laryngectomy. *Head Neck*. 1993;15:325-334.
27. List MA, Ritter-Sterr CA, Baker TM, Colangelo LA, Matz G, Pouloski BA, Logemann JA. Longitudinal assessment of quality of life in laryngeal cancer patients. *Head Neck*. 1996;8:1-10.
28. Naudo P, Laccourreye O, Weinstein G, Jouffre V, Laccourreye H, Brasnu D. Complications and functional outcome after supracricoid partial laryngectomy with cricohyoidoepiglottopexy. *Otolaryngol Head Neck Surg*. 1998;118:129.
29. Logemann JA, Pauloski BR, Rademaker AW, Colangelo LA. Speech and swallowing rehabilitation for head and neck cancer patients. *Oncology*. 1997;11:651-663.
30. Martini DV, Har-El G, Lucente FE, Slavit DH. Swallowing and pharyngeal function in postoperative pharyngeal cancer patients. *Ear Nose Throat J*. 1997;76:450-456.
31. Pauloski BR, Logemann JA, Rademaker Aw, McConnel FMS, Stein D, Beery Q, Johnson JT, Heiser MA, Cardinale S, Shedd D, Graner D, Cook B, Milanti F, Collins S, Baker T. Speech and swallowing function after oral and oropharyngeal resection: one-year follow-up. *Head Neck*. 1994;16: 313-322.

PART II

ANATOMY AND PHYSIOLOGY OF SWALLOWING

An understanding of the anatomy and physiology of swallowing is critical for the accurate diagnosis and treatment of patients with swallowing disorders. Although different specialists involved with the management of dysphagic patients have different perspectives based on their experience and patient populations, the fund of knowledge regarding the anatomy and physiology of swallowing should be common to every specialist. With the formation of multidisciplinary teams, contributions to the understanding of the anatomy and physiology of swallowing made by different healthcare disciplines have been integrated into a common fund of knowledge to be used as the foundation to clinical pathways.

CHAPTER 2

■ ■ ■

Organs of Swallowing

David E. Eibling, M.D.

I. INTRODUCTION

Ingestion of nutritional substances to provide energy and raw materials for sustenance is one of the most basic of all requirements for life. The greater the complexity of the organism to be sustained, the greater the complexity of the organ systems required to provide adequate nutrition. In higher animals the basic alimentary tract found in lower organisms such as the earthworm is much longer to enhance nutrient absorption, as well as expanded to include provision for gas exchange. In mammals this arrangement requires the sharing of the cephalad end of the tract (pharynx) for both food and air. In humans this region has further developed the ability to close the respiratory tract from the alimentary tract and to provide communication with specialization of the laryngeal glottis for airway protection and speech. The multiple functions of the larynx and pharynx require extensive central neural control to assure that respiration and ingestion of food can be maximized without undue adverse effect on the other.

The basic requirements for functional "time sharing" of the laryngopharynx are intact sensory receptors, muscle effectors, and central control with appropriate "wiring" to assure adequate sensory input and muscular control. The majority of the sensory input is through the touch and proprioreceptors of the oral cavity, oropharynx, pharynx, and larynx. Nonetheless, the effect of other sensory input such as chemosensory input and visual input, and even the sound of food preparation, are readily apparent. It is evident, then, that feeding is a basic need of all of life, and that it is increasingly diffi-cult to isolate particular functions as our knowledge of the process increases. Examples of the effect of various other types of sensory input are readily encountered in our daily lives, and undoubtedly have a significant sensitizing (or inhibitory) effect on swallowing function per se. One example of the degree of peripheral inhibition or excitation on central control of swallowing is the ability of mastication to inhibit swallowing function. (Try to swallow while chewing.) Recognition of the wide range of sensory input that in one fashion or another affects eating and swallowing function is key to an understanding of the wide variability encountered in studies of swallowing function, even in the same subject.

II. NEURAL SYSTEM

A. Central Nervous System

Swallowing is a basic function and the central control processors are located in the brainstem in the same area as those controlling respiration, blood pressure, temperature, etc. Eating, on the other hand, requires more global contributions, including the ability to recognize, seek out, procure, place the food in the mouth and masticate it to prepare it for swallowing. Patients who have suffered significant cognitive dysfunction from any of a wide range of disease processes may be unable to *eat* even if reflexive swallowing function is unaffected.

The swallowing center is positioned in the brainstem adjacent to the sensory and motor nuclei of the vagus nerve. Some measure of the basic level of the reflexes that drive the pharyngeal swallow is the rapidity of the glottic closure reflex, which has a latency of less than 25 milliseconds (one fortieth of a second). The quickest hand-eye reflex, by comparison, is about 4 times that much (100 milliseconds) and the entire pharyngeal swallow is timed at about 750 milliseconds (three quarters of a second). A reflex of this short duration must occur at lower brainstem level, without requiring higher contributions.

The reflex activities do not function in isolation, however. Sasaki has demonstrated dramatic alterations in laryngeal reflexes by any number of physiologic changes such as hypercapnia, hypoxia, sedation, etc.[1] Changes in swallowing due to subtle alterations in pharyngeal reflexes will often result in symptoms that can be quantified by radiographic or other means of study.

Changes in swallow function in association with normal aging are perhaps the best studied of the various disorders of swallowing. Increases in reflex latency are well documented in the elderly, and account in part for the absence of septuagenarians in the ranks of racquetball champions. In a similar manner, physiologic changes in swallowing functions occur with aging including decreased mucosal sensitivity, increased reflex latency, and slower and weaker muscle activity.

B. Cranial Nerves

1. Vagus Nerve

The "nerve" of the upper aerodigestive tract is the vagus nerve which provides motor and sensory innervation to the palate, pharynx, larynx, esophagus and stomach. Not only does the nerve provide sensory and motor innervation to the alimentary tract, but also the respiratory tract and is intimately involved in the regulation of blood pressure and cardiac output by direct effects on vasculature as well as cardiac rate and contractility. Sectioning of the vagus nerve at the skull base has significant effect on the regulatory function of blood pressure, gastric emptying and esophageal function, but the greatest effect is on swallowing function. Kirchner in 1958 demonstrated dramatic effects on cricopharyngeal function in a canine model after bilateral section of the vagus nerve at the level of the skull base. His landmark contribution demonstrates the significance of vagus nerve integrity in that the dogs were unable to eat following nerve section.[2]

The term "vagus" is a derivation of *vagabond*, or wanderer, and describes the course of the vagus nerve through the neck, chest, and torso, innervating the various structures as it passes. Central contributions include motor innervation from the nucleus ambiguous and sensory innervation from the nucleus solitarius. There are a vast number of brainstem ramifications of the

vagus nerve and nearly all brainstem functions appear to be affected in some way by its manipulation or stimulation. It is reported that 80% of the fibers within the vagus nerve are sensory. The nerve conveys the majority of the visceral preganglionic parasympathetic nerve fibers to the pharynx, heart, thoracic contents, and gastrointestinal tract

The vagus nerve leaves the skull through the jugular foramen in direct proximity to the internal jugular vein, the glossopharyngeal (IXth) cranial nerve, and the accessory (XIth) cranial nerve. Immediately adjacent to the jugular foramen is the hypoglossal canal from which exits the hypoglossal (XIIth) cranial nerve. The syndromes of lower cranial neuropathies caused by disease processes carry with them eponyms to describe the various combinations of the functional loss associated with nerve dysfunction. Immediately inferior to the jugular foramen the nerve widens to contain a ganglion, the nodose ganglion. In direct approximation to this ganglion are nests of chemoreceptor cells which monitor the levels of carbon dioxide within peripheral blood. These chemoreceptor bodies are termed "paraganglioma," or "glomus," bodies and may occasionally give rise to histologically benign tumors. Because of their location these tumors can result in devastating effects, despite their benign histologic appearance, due to the effect of their growth on adjacent structures. Hoarseness due to vocal fold paralysis and neck mass is a common presentation of these benign tumors.

The vagus nerve travels immediately adjacent to the internal and then common carotid artery moving generally in a posterior medial to an anterolateral position as the nerve moves from superior to inferior. It is at-risk for surgical trauma during carotid procedures as it lies juxtaposed to the artery itself. As it travels inferiorly, it gives off several branches, the most significant of which are the superior and the recurrent laryngeal nerves (Fig 2-1). The superior laryngeal nerve (SLN) passes deep to the carotid system and provides sensory innervation to the supraglottis and anterior portion of the hypopharynx. The recurrent laryngeal nerve (RLN) innervates the majority of the intrinsic laryngeal muscles. Hence, lesions of the vagus nerve cranial to the branch point of the superior laryngeal nerve are particularly devastating in that they result in both paralysis and anesthesia of the ipsilateral pharynx and larynx (Fig 2-2).

A number of branches leave the vagus nerve in the midportion of the neck to innervate the pharyngeal musculature. These branches arborize and intercommunicate with branches of the glossopharyngeal nerve (IXth cranial nerve) to form a plexus enveloping the constrictor musculature of the pharynx. This plexus, along with additional contributions from the vagus nerve, continues along the esophagus and into remainder of the alimentary tract. Disruption of this plexus or its contribu-

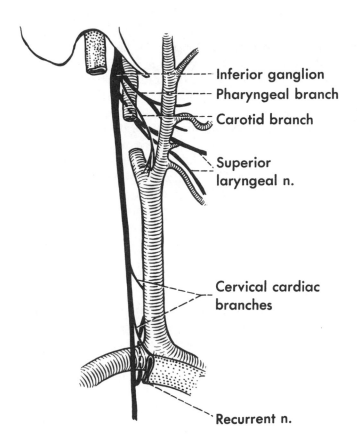

Inferior ganglion

Pharyngeal branch

Carotid branch

Superior laryngeal n.

Cervical cardiac branches

Recurrent n.

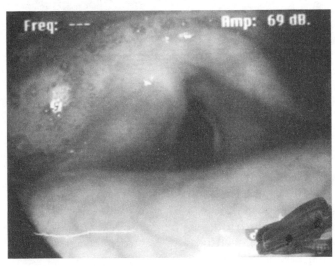

FIG 2-2. A photograph of a larynx in a patient with a high vagal paralysis due to a glomus tumor involving the vagus nerve at the skull base. The right vocal fold is paralyzed as is the right hypopharynx. This patient is experiencing significant dysphagia due not only to the paralysis, but the sensory loss of the supraglottis and hypopharynx. Note the pooling of secretions in the paralyzed right pyriform sinus.

FIG 2-1. Path of right recurrent laryngeal nerve in the neck. Note the pharyngeal branch, one of several contributions to the pharyngeal plexus. The superior laryngeal nerve passes deep to the carotid before entering the larynx to supply sensation to the mucosa of the supraglottis as well as motor intervation to the cricothyroid muscle. The recurrent laryngeal nerve loops the right subclavian artery before ascending along the tracheoesophageal groove to innervate the remaining intrinsic laryngeal muscles. The left recurrent laryngeal nerve (not shown) loops the arch of the aorta just distal to the ligamentum arteriosum. (From Hollingshead, *Anatomy for Surgeons*, Lippincott-Raven, Philadelphia, 1982. Used with permission.)

tions from the vagus nerve has deleterious effect on the constrictor activity of the pharyngeal musculature and will hinder swallowing function. Surgical procedures on the cervical spine often require that the vagal contributions to the pharyngeal plexus be interrupted, as the pharynx is dissected away from the spine and carotid system. This may play a role in the dysphagia commonly encountered in these patients postoperatively.

The vagus also gives contributions to the baroreceptors located in the adventitia of the carotid artery near the carotid bulb. Stimulation of these baroreceptors provides a vagal mediated inhibitory effect on cardiac rate and blood pressure that can be so severe as to result in syncope. This effect can be blocked by anesthesia of the vagal nerve or its contributions from the baroreceptors. Additional paraganglia are also located in these regions

and may give rise to carotid body tumors that are histologically indistinguishable from tumors arising adjacent to the vagus nerve at the skull base.

Following the branch point from the recurrent laryngeal nerve low in the neck, the vagus nerve continues in a caudal direction and provides parasympathetic innervation for the heart and great vessels and innervates the esophageal musculature as well as mucosal sensory and stretch receptors within the esophageal walls. The vagus then innervates the stomach muscles as well as the secretory glands of the gastric mucosa. Bilateral vagotomy will reduce gastric acid production, but results in gastric atony. The resultant gastroparesis will result in inability to empty the stomach unless the pyloric sphincter is surgically sectioned to permit gastric emptying. Hence, traditional gastric surgery for peptic ulcer disease includes not only vagotomy (to decrease acid production), but also a pyloroplasty to compensate for the lack of gastric motility accompanying the vagotomy.

2. Superior Laryngeal Nerve

The SLN branches from the vagus high in the neck, passes medial to the carotid artery and its branches, and comes to lie roughly parallel to the superior laryngeal branches of the superior thyroid artery. As it approaches the superior lobe of the thyroid, it may pass between the arborizing branches of the artery, placing it at-risk when the artery or its branches are divided during thyroidectomy. The SLN bifurcates into two major divisions, an internal and an external division. The external division innervates the cricothyroid muscle, which distracts the posterior cricoid lamina from the thyroid lamina, effectively opening the airway by lengthening the anterior to posterior dimension of the glottis. The muscle is active during respiration, and also during speech, when its activity serves to tighten the vocal fold and increase the pitch (Fig 2-3). The internal branch of the SLN provides mucosal touch and proprioceptive sensory input from the supraglottic larynx, cricoarytenoid joints, posterior aspect of the larynx, and the pharyngeal mucosa in the pyriform sinuses. Interruption of the external branch during thyroid lobectomy is not uncommon and is well tolerated by most patients, with minimal loss of higher vocal pitch. For professional vocalists, however, injury to this nerve is devastating due to the inability to lengthen the vocal folds with resultant loss of range. Loss of the internal branch results in anesthesia of the supraglottis and pyriform sinuses with resistant dysphagia and aspiration. Recent innovations by Aviv and co-workers in sensory testing of the larynx have improved our ability to map the regions innervated by the superior laryngeal nerve and will undoubtedly continue to provide additional information to enhance the appreciation of the role of sensory feedback in swallowing function.[3]

3. Recurrent Laryngeal Nerve

The RLN derives its unusual path by the embryologic development of the mammal and the ascent of the pharyngeal structures (or descent of the vascular structures), which results in looping of the recurrent laryngeal nerves around the vascular structures derived from the fourth branchial arch. The fourth branchial arch becomes the arch of the aorta and the right subclavian artery. Hence, the left RLN passes around the arch of the aorta (in an anterior to posterior direction), passing immediately caudal to the ligamentum arteriosum. This arrangement is found in all mammals and results in an extremely long left RLN in giraffes. The right RLN passes around the subclavian artery. On occasion, the right fourth arch fails to develop into the right subclavian artery, so the recurrent nerve does not loop, resulting in the so-called *nonrecurrent* recurrent laryngeal nerve. Both nerves ascend in the tracheoesophageal groove, with the right being significantly shorter than the left and approaching the larynx and trachea from a somewhat more lateral position. This has significant implications for laryngeal retraction during spine surgery, in that moving the larynx toward the left during surgical approaches to the cervical spine places more tension on the right recurrent laryngeal nerve than moving the larynx to the right does on the left recurrent laryngeal nerve.

All the intrinsic muscles of the larynx, with the exception of the cricothyroid muscle, are innervated by the recurrent laryngeal nerve. The most significant muscle for respiration is the posterior cricoarytenoid muscle, which is the only abductor of the glottis (Fig 2-4). Bilateral interruption of the recurrent laryngeal nerves results in inability to abduct the vocal cords. This will frequently result in an inadequate glottic airway for supporting respiration and often will require a tracheotomy. The recurrent laryngeal nerves enter the larynx immediately posterior to the cricothyroid joint and arborize within the larynx to its various intrinsic muscles (Fig 2-5). The anterior branch supplies the lateral cricoarytenoid muscle and the thyroarytenoid muscle (adduction/tension), whereas the posterior branch supplies the posterior cricoarytenoid muscle, the sole abductor of the glottis.

4. Glossopharyngeal Nerve

The glossopharyngeal nerve (cranial nerve IX) provides sensory innervation to the oropharynx, base of tongue, and conveys taste fibers to the tongue base. It provides motor innervation to a single muscle, the stylopharyngeus. Although it clearly provides significant contributions to swallowing function, both through its motor branch as well as its sensory distribution, it is not clear to what extent its loss disrupts this function as isolated glossopharyngeal nerve loss is extremely uncommon. In most instances, the nerve is lost in association with loss of the vagus, which by itself results in dramatic physiologic changes.

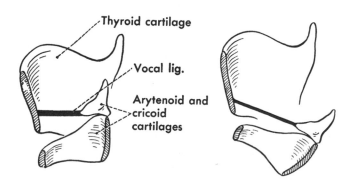

Thyroid cartilage

Vocal lig.

Arytenoid and cricoid cartilages

FIG 2-3. The cricothyroid muscle is the only muscle innervated by the superior laryngeal nerve. Activation of this muscle increases the distance between the posterior aspect of the thyroid cartilage and the posterior lamina of the cricoid cartilage by both translation and rotation of the cricoid. This action serves to lengthen the vocal folds resulting in a longer glottic aperture as well as raised vocal pitch due to increasing vocal fold tension. (From Hollingshead, *Anatomy for Surgeons*, Lippincott-Raven, Philadelphia, 1982. Used with permission.)

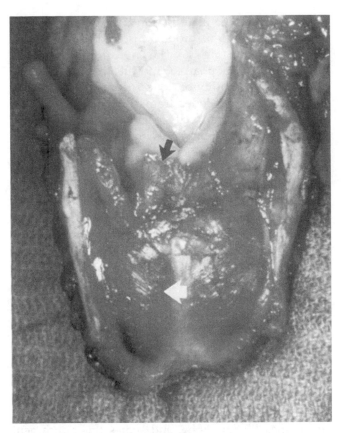

FIG 2-4. A photograph of the larynx viewed posteriorly after removal of the mucosa overlying the posterior lamina of the cricoid cartilage and the posterior cricoarytenoid muscles. The arytenoid cartilages can be visualized (small black arrow). Contraction of the posterior cricoarytenoid muscles (large white arrow) serves to rotate the arytenoid laterally, widening the posterior glottic gap. The medial aspect of the muscle also serves to maintain the arytenoid in an upright position. Vocal fold paralysis therefore results not only in inability to abduct or adduct the vocal fold, but frequently the arytenoid is tipped anteriorly due to the loss of this activity.

5. Trigeminal Nerve

Sensation within the oral cavity is transmitted to the brainstem via branches of the trigeminal nerve (Vth cranial nerve), the nerve of the face. Of the three divisions of the Vth cranial nerve, the second and third divisions are most intimately involved with swallowing and speaking function. Both pass through the gasserian ganglion, which is located on the posterior aspect of the temporal bone in a shallow depression termed Meckel's cave. Sensory branches arborize to the Vth cranial nucleus that extends from the most cranial portion of the brainstem down into the spinal cord as the spinal tract of V. The wide anatomic ramifications of this cranial nerve gives some indication of its significance to maintenance of life for an organism.

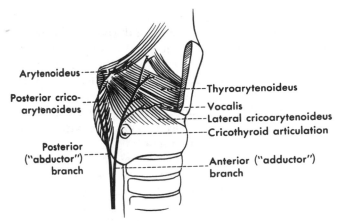

FIG 2-5. The recurrent laryngeal nerve innervates all the intrinsic muscles of the larynx with the exception of the cricothyroid muscle. The nerve enters the larynx just posterior to the cricothyroid joint. The posterior branch innervates the posterior cricoarytenoid, the only vocal fold abductor, whereas the anterior branch innervates the vocal fold adductors and tensors. (From Hollingshead, *Anatomy for Surgeons*, Lippincott-Raven, Philadelphia, 1982. Used with permission.)

In addition to providing sensation of the mucosal and proprioceptive receptors of the oral cavity, the Vth cranial nerve also provides motor function to the muscles of mastication. A separate motor root leaves the brainstem and passes through the gasserian ganglion, accompanying the second division to innervate the muscles of mastication.

The second division of the Vth cranial nerve provides innervation to palate, both hard and soft, as well as the upper alveolus, teeth, lips, and gingivobuccal sulcus. The nerve exits the middle cranial fossa through the foramen rotundum and then arborizes within the pterygopalatine fossa to innervate the mucosa, skin, teeth, and palate. Branches to the nasal mucosa pass through the sphenopalatine foramen along with postganglionic fibers to the nasal mucosal vasculature and glands. Branches to the palate pass through the descending palatine canal and exit via the greater and accessory palatine foramina. The branches to the sinus mucosa and teeth pass through the bone of the posterior maxilla and innervate the respective structures. The cheek, nasal skin, and upper lip are innervated by the infraorbital nerve, which passes through a groove on the floor of the orbit prior to exiting the maxilla through the infraorbital foramen, which is just inferior to the orbital rim. Injury to this nerve is commonly encountered in facial trauma or surgery and results in sensory disorder of the upper lip. Injury of the main trunk of V-2 or to the branches innervating the palate is rare, and therefore unlikely to be a cause of disordered swallowing.

The third division of the trigeminal nerve supplies innervation to the tongue (lingual nerve) and to the inferior alveolus, buccal mucosa, and the lower lip (inferior alveolar nerve). Sensation of the base of the tongue is supplied through the cranial nerve IX (glossopharyngeal nerve), whereas innervation of the oral tongue is conferred via the lingual nerve, which leaves V-3 just after it exits the skull base through the foramen ovale. It passes medial to the mandible and the submandibular gland and immediately adjacent to Wharton's duct, which passes just under the mucosa of the floor of the mouth. Injury or sacrifice of this nerve is common during extirpative head and neck surgery and will result in an anesthetic ipsilateral oral tongue that may lead to frequent accidental "tongue biting," difficulty in forming a bolus, and initiating swallow. This difficulty in forming a bolus is actually quite common following cardiovascular accident (CVA), especially right hemisphere CVA, which may result in significant neglect, leading to loss of food into the buccal-gingival and gingival-lingual sulci, termed "pocketing." This lack of control can lead to aspiration should this material pass into the pharynx when the patient is unaware of its presence.

Recent investigators have demonstrated the adverse affect of defective oral sensation on swallowing function. Moreover, there is evidence that these changes are physiologic components of aging and progressive with increasing age.[4]

III. LARYNX AND PHARYNX

The mammalian pharynx and larynx has been tasked with the dual roles of providing access for both ingestion of food and respiration. Both functions require that the ingested or inhaled substances be diverted to specific organs, hence the pharyngolarynx must effectively switch between food and air as required by the organism. Moreover, lung tissue required for absorption of oxygen and discharge of carbon dioxide requires a specific surfactant coating for function and is intolerant of soilage by liquid or solids. Hence, highly specialized protective mechanisms have evolved to prevent contamination of airways and lung tissues with food and liquid during deglutition. Sasaki has pointed out that the most basic form of larynx is a simple sphincter that serves to protect the airway from soilage.[5]

The effective function of this anatomic region is dependent on intact specific mobile structures, as well as precise timing during the various functions for which it is responsible.

A. Anatomy of the Pharynx

The pharynx begins at the posterior aspect of the nasal and oral cavities and extends caudally to connect with the esophagus. The pharynx can be easily subdivided into the nasopharynx, oropharynx, and hypopharynx, based on location (Fig 2-6). The larynx forms the anterior wall of the hypopharynx and fills the lumen at rest because of the rigidity of the cartilageous framework. The pharynx is suspended from the skull base and contiguous with the oral cavity, palate, tongue, nasal cavity, and eustachian tube. It lies immediately anterior to the clivus of the sphenoid bone and cervical vertebrae, separated only by a dense fibrous ligament and anterior paraspinal muscles. A loose areolar tissue plane lies between the constrictor muscles and the fascia overlying the prevertebral muscles. This loose areolar tissue permits unimpeded motion of the pharynx during swallowing, and scarring following surgical dissection in this plane during procedures on the cervical spine may adversely affect swallow function.

1. Pharyngeal Constrictor Muscles

The muscles of the pharynx are positioned to close the lumen and raise the pharynx (Fig 2-7). The superior constrictor attaches to the skull base and the eustachian tube, passing anterior and inferiorly to insert on the sphenomandibular raphe, and shares this attachment with the buccinator muscle, which maintains oral cavity integrity. The inferior constrictor inserts on the larynx, on the oblique line, and constricts the pharynx and elevates the larynx with contraction (Fig 2-8).

2. Cricopharyngeus Muscle

The most inferior component of the pharyngeal constrictors is the cricopharyngeus muscle, which inserts on the cricoid cartilage and encircles the pharynx more or less in an axial plane, in contradistinction to the angulated posterior-to-anterior direction of the other constrictors. Moreover, the cricopharyngeus does not have a posterior midline raphe. The midline gap between the inferior edge of the inferior constrictor and the superior edge of the cricopharyngeus creates a posterior dehiscence in the muscular pharyngeal wall, termed *Killian's triangle*. The cricopharyngeus muscle is the major component of the upper esophageal sphincter and maintains a constant level of contraction, essentially closing the lumen by approximating the pharynx to the posterior lamina of the cricoid cartilage. During swallowing, the muscular sphincter relaxes to permit laryngeal elevation and opening of the esophagus to permit passage of the bolus into the esophagus. There is considerable debate regarding cricopharyngeal dysfunction and its role in the pathophysiology of dysphagia, and particularly, the generation of upper esophageal diverticula.

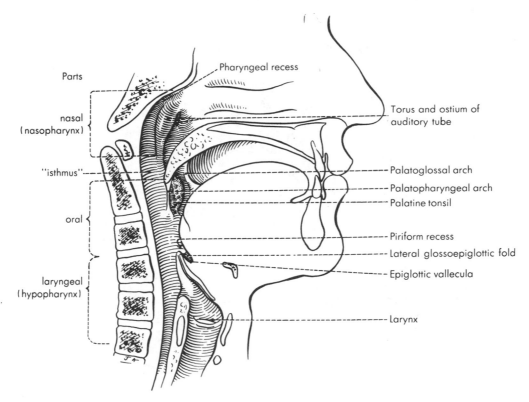

Fig 2-6. Anatomy of the pharynx. The oral pharynx is actually the mid portion of the pharynx as the nasal pharynx is the superior extension and communicates with the nasal airway. The hypopharynx includes the base of tongue, piriform sinuses, larynx and extends down to the level of the cricopharyngeus muscle. (From Hollingshead, *Anatomy for Surgeons*, Lippincott-Raven, Philadelphia, 1982. Used with permission.)

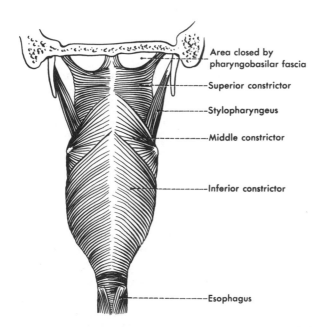

Fig 2-7. Posterior view of the pharyngeal constrictor muscles. Note that the middle and inferior constrictors not only narrow the lumen, but also assist in elevating the hyoid and laryngeal complex. The most inferior portion of the inferior constrictor is the cricopharyngeus muscle which functions as the upper esophageal sphincter. (From Hollingshead, *Anatomy for Surgeons*, Lippincott-Raven, Philadelphia, 1982. Used with permission.)

B. Anatomy of the Larynx

1. Comparative

The role of the larynx in swallowing dysfunction has been well documented by many anatomists and physiologists. Comparative anatomic studies demonstrate that the most basic laryngeal function is airway protection. The primitive air exchange sac of the lungfish has no protection, but a rudimentary laryngeal sphincter is required for protection of the air exchange system for fish that spend greater periods of time out of the water. Active dilatation of the airway is encountered in reptiles that must run to capture food or escape becoming food, themselves. Adaptation for laryngeal phonation occurs only in higher reptiles and mammals and is most highly developed in man. The relative length of the membranous vocal folds is greatest in humans, permitting increased modulation of vibratory characteristics needed for highly developed social requirements.

Sharing of the upper aerodigestive tract for both airway and deglutive functions requires specific anatomic and physiologic adaptation. The most basic of these adaptations is that of "time sharing" in which the aerodigestive tract is utilized alternatively for the passage of either air or food and liquid. This strategy requires effective

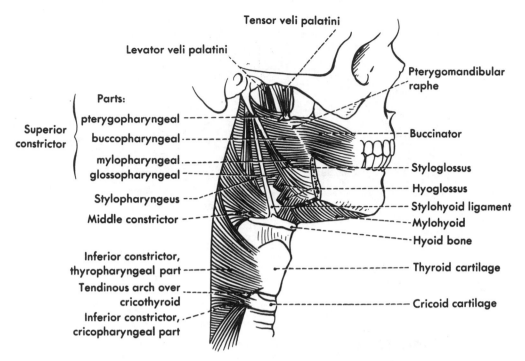

FIG 2-8. Lateral view of pharyngeal constrictor muscles and mandibular-hyoid complex. Note that a portion of the superior constrictor muscle inserts on the pterygo-mandibular sphenomandibular raphe, which is continuous with the buccinator muscle anteriorly. The middle constrictor inserts onto the hyoid complex whereas the inferior constrictor muscle inserts onto the thyroid cartilage. The cricopharyngeal muscle, the most inferior portion of the inferior constrictor, inserts on the cricoid cartilage and functions as the superior esophageal sphincter. (From Hollingshead, *Anatomy for Surgeons*, Lippincott-Raven, Philadelphia, 1982. Used with permission.)

closure of the airway and then motion of the food and liquid bolus into the esophagus when the airway is closed. In certain vertebrates, adaptations exist that permit respiratory and deglutive functions to occur simultaneously. In the alligator, this adaptation consists of a double palate that interdigitates with the epiglottis, effectively separating the upper aerodigestive tract into a naso-laryngeal tract and two lateral oro-esophageal tracts. This permits the alligator to hold its mouth underwater to drown a victim, while continuing to breathe through nostrils above water. The snake continues to breathe during the tediously slow process of ingesting large objects (often larger than its diameter), by evaginating its larynx out of the mouth, effectively separating the upper aerodigestive tract into dedicated compartments for the two functions.[6] Certain herbivores are able to continue to breathe while feeding by interdigitating the epiglottis behind the palate. It has been postulated that this strategy permits these animals to continue to sample the air for the scent of predators while grazing. Human infants can also feed and breathe simultaneously via separation of the naso-laryngeal and oro-pharyngeal tracts through positioning of the tip of the epiglottis in the nasopharynx.[7] Adult humans and most mammals, however, must cease respiration and effect glottic closure prior to deglutition.

2. Physiology

Laryngeal function for airway protection, respiration, vocalization, and deglutition depends on a mobile, flexible mucosal-lined tube that is altered in configuration by complex interaction of cartilages, ligaments, and muscles. Laryngeal anatomy and vocal fold function is well known by all students of the health care disciplines. The glottis opens for inspiration, both by lengthening as well as widening the aperture. Glottic lengthening occurs because of distraction of the posterior lamina of the cricoid (with the attached arytenoid cartilages and vocal folds) from the thyroid through contraction of the cricothyroid muscle, innervated by the external branch of the SLN. Widening of the posterior glottic aperture occurs from both rotation and lateral displacement of the arytenoid cartilages on the superior edge of the cricoid lamina and is dependent on the posterior cricoarytenoid muscles, innervated by the RLN.

a. Arytenoid Motion

Vocal fold motion is dependent on functional cricoarytenoid joints, which are true synovial joints and subject to the same disorders that affect synovial joints elsewhere. The arytenoids do not merely "swivel" on the cricoid lamina, but also slide in a multidimensional plane. During phonation, the vocal folds are approximated by *rotation* of the arytenoids medially, and *medial displacement* through the action of the interarytenoid muscle. Rotation without medial displacement results in excessive air escape during phonation and occurs during whispering, as well in various forms of laryngeal dysfunction, particularly hyperfunctional disorders. Inappropriate arytenoid positioning for phonation, as well as dystonic thyroarytenoid muscle hyperfunction, results in the various forms of spasmodic dysphonia.

Pitch is regulated by cricothyroid action to distract the posterior lamina of the cricoid as well as anterior and posterior displacement of the arytenoid to adjust membranous vocal fold tension. The medial portion of the posterior cricoarytenoid muscle thus serves to "right" the arytenoid in its position on the posterior lamina of the cricoid and is necessary not only for pitch modulation, but also to maintain the arytenoids in position during inspiration when the action of the cricothyroid muscle lengthens the glottic aperture. Loss of this function is readily apparent by the anterior displacement of the arytenoid encountered in vocal fold paralysis.

b. Glottic Closure

Vocal fold closure is the key intrinsic laryngeal function required for airway protection, and is effected by rapid contraction of the thyroarytenoid and lateral cricoarytenoid muscles. Thyroarytenoid muscle activity is mediated by the recurrent laryngeal nerves, and occurs very rapidly. The glottic closure reflex has a latency of less than 25 milliseconds, which establishes it as one of the fastest reflexes in the body. Studies by Sasaki have demonstrated that a wide range of stimuli can produce reflex glottic closure, including (in the cat model) stimulation of essentially every cranial nerve.[1] Glottic closure occurs in a sequential fashion, with approximation of the true vocal folds preceding false vocal fold approximation, and finally approximation of the arytenoids to the petiole of the epiglottis. Glottic closure follows cessation of respiration, which is typically interrupted during expiration and precedes laryngeal elevation.

There are a variety of conditions that can disrupt glottic closure, including structural abnormalities such as prior partial laryngeal surgery or atrophy of the vocal folds ("bowing," or presbylarynx) or neurologic abnormalities, the most common of which is vocal fold paralysis. Interestingly, there is convincing evidence that glottic closure is disrupted by the loss of subglottic air pressure that accompanies tracheotomy.

c. Supraglottic Structures

It is widely supposed by the lay public that the epiglottis is the major component of glottic closure. It seems logical that this "flapper valve" will fall over the glottic aperture during swallowing and seal the opening. The infrahyoid portion of the epiglottis is approximated to the arytenoids during glottic closure, but the suprahyoid portion of the epiglottis does not effectively "seal" the larynx. In fact, the epiglottis does play a role, but it is more akin to the prow of a boat, deflecting the bolus stream laterally into the pyriform sinuses. The cartilage of the epiglottis is elastic, resulting in significantly more flexibility than the rigid hyaline cartilages that constitute the structural support of the larynx. Epiglottic "rotation" (actually more like *folding*) occurs as a result of laryngeal elevation (shortening the distance between the hyoid bone and thyroid cartilages, relaxing the hyoepiglottic ligament), increased pressure in the preepiglottic fat space, and the weight of the bolus, itself. In actuality, observations of ineffective epiglottic rotation serve to indicate swallow dysfunction and do not indicate the primary pathology.

The laryngeal vestibule is defined as the area of the larynx superior to the vocal cords. This region is defined not only by the epiglottis, but also by the arytenoid and corniculate cartilages, the interarytenoideus muscle, and the aryepiglottic folds that connect them with the epiglottis. The result is a mucosal-lined tube above the vocal folds that stands as a "vertical pipe" in the anterior portion of the hypopharynx. The significance of this anatomic relationship can be appreciated by endoscopically observing a swallow of liquid in an elderly individual or one with a pathologically mildly slowed swallow. The liquid will be seen to flow around the aryepiglottic folds into the pyriform sinuses and not enter (or "penetrate") the laryngeal vestibule, although the level of the vocal folds is significantly lower than the level of the liquid (something like a cofferdam). This function is lost following supraglottic laryngectomy, in which not only the epiglottis is resected, but the aryepiglottic folds as well, resulting in exposure of the true vocal folds to all liquid or other bolus material that is ingested. (Essentially 100% "penetration.")

d. Laryngeal Elevation (and Depression)

Key to swallowing function is the ability to move the larynx in a vertical plane during swallowing. Not only does this superior and anterior displacement of the larynx result in movement of the glottis out of the direct path of the bolus, but it also shortens the distance the bolus must move to pass the laryngeal inlet. One way of thinking of it is to view the larynx as sliding up the bolus simultaneously with its caudad peristaltic-driven motion. One manifestation of the significance of this laryngeal motion is to examine the extent and complexity of the extrinsic laryngeal muscles. The larynx is firmly suspended from the skull base at both the mastoid (posterior belly of the digastric muscle) as well as the styloid process via the stylohyoid ligament and muscle. The hyoid bone is further suspended from the mandible by the geniohyoid, mylohyoid, the intrinsic tongue muscles, and the anterior belly of the digastric (see Fig 2-8). The hyoid bone is further secured inferiorly to the sternum as well as the scapula by the sternohyoid and omohyoid muscles. The relationship of the thyroid cartilage to the hyoid and the sternum is active as well through the action of the thyrohyoid and sternothyroid muscles. All of these strap muscles are rather substantial and are preserved across species, found in all mammals. Some indication of their significance can be deduced by the level of redundancy found in the muscles themselves and the dual innervation pattern of the ansa cervicalis nerve. It should be recognized that the larynx not only rises during swallowing, (and the thyroid cartilage is approximated to the hyoid as well) but rapidly returns to its "resting" position for respiration.

C. Esophagus

The esophagus is a muscular, mucosal-lined tube that is considered to begin at the caudal end of the pharynx inferior to the cricopharyngeus sphincter and extend through the thoracic cavity through the diaphragm and into the peritoneal cavity, emptying into the stomach. The esophagus permits the separation of the vertebrate body into respiratory and alimentary segments, the former of which is rigid and maintained at negative atmospheric pressure through rib positioning and diaphragmatic muscles. The esophagus serves as a conduit to pass food through the thoracic cavity into the abdominal cavity for digestion and absorption. The esophagus passes through the posterior mediastinum, dorsal to the tracheobronchial tree, the heart, and most of the great vessels. It is located adjacent to the vertebral column, and anterior-medial to the aorta and azygos venous system. In contradistinction to the remainder of the digestive system, there is no enveloping fascia around the esophagus, hence disease (or trauma) involving the muscular wall has direct access to the mediastinal contents.

The muscular wall of the esophagus consists of both striated and smooth muscle, mimicking its location between the striated muscle of the pharynx and the smooth muscle of the remainder of the alimentary tract. The muscles are arranged in circular and longitudinal bundles, with the longitudinal muscles located on the exterior surface. The peristaltic wave travels at a relatively constant velocity and is due to the combination of constricting forces behind the bolus mediated by contraction of the circular muscles and shortening of the esophagus from contraction of the longitudinal muscle groups. A wide variety of disease processes may affect the muscles of the esophagus, with scleroderma representing the prototype.

The coordinated muscular activity is mediated by an integral myoneural plexus that receives contributions from the vagus nerves, the parasympathetic nervous system, and the somatic segmental nerves. Sensory innervation is via the somatic segmental nerves, hence, pain in the esophagus is referred to the corresponding dermatome, experienced by the patient as substernal pain.

Disorders of muscular coordination are manifested by failure of peristalsis (weak peristalsis or even atony) or uncoordinated contractions that fail to move the bolus into the stomach (tertiary contractions). Diseases such as diabetes mellitus that are associated with peripheral neuropathy are frequently associated with esophageal dysfunction due to loss of an intact coordinating function.

1. Lower Esophageal Sphincter

The body of the esophagus lies within the thoracic cavity, which is maintained at a subatmospheric pressure to facilitate respiration, while the distal esophagus and stomach lie within the peritoneal cavity, which is of higher-than-atmospheric pressure. Maintenance of swallowed food within the stomach, therefore, requires a functional sphincter that will open to permit passage of food and liquid into the stomach, but maintain a resting tone to prevent regurgitation. The normal resting tone of this lower esophageal sphincter (LES) is maintained in part by the sphincteric function of the circular muscular fibers of the esophagus and in part by its position within the crural folds in the diaphragmatic muscle. This arrangement provides for a constant resting pressure that falls to subatomospheric just prior to the arrival of the bolus. Failure of this sphincter to relax results in inability of the bolus to move through into the stomach and is termed *achalasia*. If the ligamentous attachments that maintain the distal esophagus within the crura of the diaphragm fail or weaken, then the distal esophagus and stomach may prolapse into the thoracic cavity, probably because of the relative pressure gradient across the diaphragm. This disorder, termed *hiatus hernia*, disrupts the normal physiologic position and function of the lower esophageal sphincter, permitting regurgitation of gastric contents into the esophagus.

The mucosal lining of the esophagus is nonkeratinizing squamous mucosa from the upper sphincter to the gastric mucosa at the cardia of the stomach. The demarcation line is clearly evident during esophagoscopy, as the pale squamous mucosa of the normal esophagus changes to the hypertrophic, rich pink gastric mucosa. Dramatic changes can occur at this location, primarily because of exposure of the esophageal lining to gastric acid. These changes may include ulceration, inflammation, dysplastic maturation, or metaplasia of the normal squamous mucosa to an intestinal columnar epithelium termed *Barrett's esophagitis*. This entity is recognized as a premalignant condition and is currently the focus of much investigation, especially in light of the increasing prevalence of both this premalignant condition as well as esophageal cancer in the Western population.

2. Other Processes

A wide variety of other pathologic processes can affect the esophagus, either mucosal or neuromuscular. For example, an esophageal motility disorder develops in some alcoholics. This condition is characterized by tertiary waves on manometry and contrast studies. The polyneuropathy that accompanies diabetes is also associated with esophageal motility disorders. The presence of a nasogastric tube can disrupt swallowing function due to mucosal irritation of the esophagus, pain in the pharynx, and incompetence of gastroesophageal sphincter.

IV. CONCLUSIONS

The organs of swallowing are responsible for conveying ingested food to the alimentary tract, where digestion and absorption of nutrients can occur. The process is complex because of the sharing of the gas exchange function and, therefore, significant anatomic and functional adaptations are required. These adaptations are very sensitive to relatively minor changes in structural, muscular, or sensory integrity. Alterations in any or all of these may lead to dysphagia.

References

1. Sasaki CT, Suzuki M. Laryngeal reflexes in cat, dog, and man. *Arch Otolaryngol.* 1976;102:400.
2. Kirchner, JA. The Motor activity of the cricopharyngeus muscle. *Laryngoscope.* 1958;68:1119-1159.
3. Aviv J, Martin JH, Keen MS, Debell M, Blitzer A. Air pulse quantification of supraglottic and pharyngeal sensation: a new technique. *Ann Rhinol Laryngol.* 1993;102:777-780.
4. Capra NF. Mechanisms of oral sensation. *Dysphagia.* 1995; 10:235-247.
5. Sasaki CT, Isaacson G. Functional anatomy of the larynx. *Otolaryngol Clini North Am.* 1988;21:595-612.
6. Kirchner JA. The vertebrate larynx: adaptions and aberrations. *Laryngoscope.* 1993;103:1197-1201.
7. Sasaki CT, Levine PA, Laitman JT, et al. Postnatal descent of the epiglottis in man: a preliminary report. *Arch Otolaryngol.* 1977;103:169.

CHAPTER 3

■ ■ ■

The Normal Swallow

Jonathan E. Aviv, M.D., F.A.C.S.

I. INTRODUCTION

The purpose of swallowing is to safely transport food from the mouth to the stomach. A myriad of diseases and conditions affect this basic purpose. Therefore, understanding the normal swallow is one of the keys to developing a therapeutic plan for the patient with impaired deglutition. One would not spend effort attempting to change something about a swallow that may well be within the normal range of deglutition. This chapter details the normal swallow. Emphasis is placed on correlating the normal physiology of swallowing with the relevant anatomy of the head and neck. The stages of swallowing can be divided into three phases: oral, pharyngeal, and esophageal, with the oral phase under voluntary neuromuscular control and the latter two phases under involuntary neuromuscular control.

II. SWALLOW

A. Oral Phase

The oral phase of swallowing can be further subdivided into the oral preparatory and the oral transport phase. In the oral preparatory phase, the lips, tongue, mandible, palate, and cheeks act in concert with salivary flow to grind and manipulate the presented food into a consistency and position so that the subsequent phases of swallowing can take place safely and appro-

priately. The afferent and efferent contributions of the cranial nerves which are essential for carrying out the oral phase are listed in Table 3-1. Once the food bolus is prepared, the oral transport phase occurs as the musculature of the lips and cheeks contract followed by tongue contraction against the hard palate.[1] As tongue-hard palate contact occurs, the soft palate elevates as the tensor veli palatini, levator veli palatini and palatophayrngeus muscles contract, drawing the velum superiorly and posteriorly against the nasopharyngeal mucosa and musculature.[2]

Normal movement of the anterior two thirds of the tongue is essential for carrying out the tasks of the oral stage of swallowing. Tongue musculature can be broadly divided into extrinsic and intrinsic muscles. The extrinsic muscles are the genioglossus, hyoglossus, styloglossus, and palatoglossus muscles. These muscles have their origin along the mental spine, hyoid bone, styloid process, and soft palate, respectively and insert either into the hyoid bone or into the other extrinsic or intrinsic tongue muscles. The primary actions of the extrinsic tongue muscles are to pull the tongue forward, backward, upward, and downward.[3]

The intrinsic tongue muscles are bundles of interlacing fibers containing connective tissue septae. These muscles originate in the tongue submucosa and insert into each other and into the extrinsic tongue muscles in various locations throughout the tongue. The primary action of the intrinsic muscles is to produce changes in the shape of the tongue during articulation and deglutition.

Because of the complex variety of origins and insertions of the tongue muscles, to physiologically repro-

Table 3-1. *Oral Phase of Deglutition—Contributions of Cranial Nerves*

Structure	Afferent	Efferent
Lips	V2 (maxillary) V3 (lingual)	VII
Tongue	V3 (lingual)	XII
Mandible	V3 (mandibular)	V (muscles of mastication), VII
Palate	V, IX, X	IX, X
Buccal region/Cheeks	V	V (muscles of mastication), VII

duce the intertwining muscular actions of the tongue is daunting and inefficient. Hence, there is a disparate range of swallowing difficulties necessarily encountered after ablative cancer surgery of the tongue, no matter how sophisticated the reconstruction.[4]

While a functioning oral tongue (anterior two thirds) is critical to normal functioning of the oral phase of deglutition, the base of tongue (posterior one third), also plays an important role in the generation of forces that propel a food bolus posteriorly toward the pharynx. Without a functioning base of tongue, tongue-soft palate contact cannot be made. With impaired tongue-soft palate contact during the oral phase of swallowing, the nasopharynx cannot be sealed from the oral cavity, so insufficient negative pressure is generated when the hyomandibular complex elevates away from the posterior pharyngeal wall during the pharyngeal phase of swallowing.[5] As a result, bolus propulsion becomes significantly impaired.

For normal tongue function to take place, both the motor and sensory systems of the tongue must be intact. To assess tongue motor function, the tongue should first be examined while at rest along the floor of the mouth with the mouth open. A physical examination demonstrating tongue fasciculation can be the first clue to impaired neurological function in general and impaired neurological function in the tongue, specifically.[6] To further assess tongue motor function, one can assess tongue mobility by having the patient move his or her tongue superiorly, inferiorly, and laterally on command. Tongue strength can be assessed by having the patient press the tongue against a tongue blade or against his or her buccal mucosa.

Assessment of tongue sensation is also critical to the assessment of the swallow. Using two-point discrimination testing, it has been shown that the tongue tip is the most sensitive area of the tongue surface, followed by the lateral dorsal tongue, lateral ventral tongue, and floor of mouth.[7] Impairment of tongue sensation has been shown to result in major disturbances in oral function, both in healthy controls and in patients with oral cavity cancer.[8,9]

There are age-related changes in sensory discrimination of the tongue, with people over 60 years of age hav-

ing a statistically significant less sensitive two-point discrimination level in the anterior two thirds of the tongue than people less than 40 years old.[10] There are also age-related changes in normal tongue motor function, with oral transit time in individuals over 60 years of age prolonged when compared to people less than 60.[11] Diminished tongue sensory and motor functions coupled with increasing age might contribute to the increased prevalence of dysphagia, aspiration, and pneumonia seen in the elderly.[12,13]

In healthy individuals, the oral phase of swallowing is generally completed in approximately 1 second.[14]

B. Pharyngeal Phase

Once the food bolus encroaches on the palatoglossal folds, or anterior tonsilar pillars, the pharyngeal phase of swallowing reflexively begins. Factors other than the food bolus coming in contact with the anterior faucial arches are thought responsible for the initiation of swallowing, such as posterior tongue movement and stimulation of the pharynx.[15,16] Furthermore, it has been shown in several studies that the swallowing reflex can be initiated entirely by peripheral stimulation of the internal branch of the superior laryngeal nerve.[17-20] The afferent and efferent contributions of the cranial nerves essential for carrying out the pharyngeal phase of deglutition are listed in Table 3-2.

What actually takes place as the swallowing reflex is initiated is as follows:

1. Velopharyngeal closure to prevent reflux of material into the posterior choana.
2. Closure of the larynx in a specific sequence to prevent aspiration.
3. Contraction of the pharyngeal constrictor muscles in a superior to inferior direction.
4. Elevation of the larynx and hyoid bone toward the base of tongue.
5. Relaxation of the tonically contracted cricopharyngeus to allow passage of the food bolus into the esophagus.

Table 3-2. *Pharyngeal Phase of Deglutition—Contributions of Cranial Nerves*

Structure	Afferent	Efferent
Tongue Base	IX	XII
Epiglottis (lingual surface)	IX	X
Epiglottis (laryngeal surface)	X (internal branch of superior laryngeal nerve)	X
Larynx (to level of true vocal folds)	X (internal branch of superior laryngeal nerve)	X
Larynx (below true vocal folds)	X (recurrent laryngeal nerve)	X
Pharynx (naso- and oro-)	IX	X (except for stylopharyngeus which is innervated by IX)
Pharynx (hypopharynx)	X (internal branch of superior laryngeal nerve)	X

Velopharyngeal closure is effected by contraction of the levator veli palatini muscles, which elevate the soft palate against the posterior nasopharyngeal wall. Medial contraction of the lateral pharyngeal wall musculature in combination with slight anterior movement of the posterior pharyngeal wall creates Passavant's ridge, which is a ridge of tissue against which the velum is approximated during the first portion of the pharyngeal phase of swallowing.[21,22]

Following velopharyngeal closure, the first event in the normal swallow sequence, preceding even genioglossus electromyography activity that signals elevation of the hyoid-laryngeal complex, is true vocal fold adduction.[23,24] It is true vocal fold closure that provides the primary laryngopharyngeal protective mechanism to prevent aspiration during the swallow.[24] Subsequently, false vocal fold adduction, adduction of the aryepiglottic folds, and retroversion of the epiglottis take place.[25] Retroversion of the epiglottis, while not the primary mechanism of protecting the airway from laryngeal penetration and aspiration, acts to anatomically direct the food bolus laterally towards the pyriform sinuses. As the true vocal folds adduct during the swallow, a finite period of apnea must necessarily take place with each swallow. When relating deglutition to respiration, it has been demonstrated that deglutition occurs most often during expiration and includes a period of apnea ranging from 0.3 sec to 2.5 seconds.[26,27] The clinical significance of this finding is that patients with a baseline of compromised lung function will, over a period of time, develop respiratory distress as a meal progresses. This will lead to fatigue during the meal and the consequent risks of laryngeal penetration and aspiration.[27] This underscores the importance of having a swallowing evaluation technique available that permits observation of patient fatigue.

Following closure of the larynx, pharyngeal peristalsis then takes place by sequential contraction of the superior, middle, and inferior pharyngeal constrictor muscles.[28] With contraction of the superior pharyngeal constrictor muscle, laryngeal elevation takes place. The larynx elevates because of the hyoid bone and tongue base moving anteriorly secondary to contraction of the mylohyoid, geniohyoid, stylohyoid, and anterior digastric muscles.[5] This anterior movement of the larynx, combined with the contraction of the middle and inferior constrictor muscles, strips the food bolus inferiorly, ushering in the final portion of the pharyngeal phase, which is entry of the food bolus into the cervical esophagus.

The duration of the pharyngeal phase of swallowing is about 1 second. Increasing bolus viscosity has been shown to delay pharyngeal transit, increase the duration of pharyngeal peristaltic waves, and prolong and increase upper esophageal sphincter (UES) opening. Increasing bolus volume results in earlier onset of tongue base movement, superior palatal movement, anterior laryngeal movement, and UES opening.[29] Earlier UES opening results in increased duration of sphincter opening as well as increasing sphincter diameter. Pharyngeal transit time also increases slightly with advancing age. The peristaltic wave sweeping down the pharynx moves along at a rate of approximately 12 cm/second.[29]

Although the oral and pharyngeal phases of swallowing are presented sequentially, the physiologic reality is that these phases are integrally related. McConnel described swallowing as a pressure-generation mechanism powered by a two-pump system. He called these pumps the oropharyngeal propulsion pump (OPP) and the hypopharyngeal suction pump (HSP).[30] The OPP is the pressure generated as the anterior two thirds of the tongue propels the food into the oropharynx accompanied by contraction of the pharyngeal constrictor muscles. The HSP is the negative pressure generated as the hyoid-laryngeal complex is elevated away from the posterior pharyngeal wall, effectively drawing the food bolus towards the UES. Underscoring the importance of normal tongue mobility for normal deglutition to take place is that any condition that affects the anterior two thirds of the tongue will necessarily affect the OPP and that any problems affecting the base of tongue will alter the HSP.

The UES provides a high pressure zone between the pharynx and esophagus, remaining closed at rest so as to separate the laryngopharynx from the esophagus. Three muscles contribute to the formation of the UES, the cricopharyngeus muscle, the most inferior muscle fibers of the inferior constrictor muscle, and the most superior portion of the longitudinal esophageal muscular fibers.[31] These three muscles attach to the posterior lamina of the cricoid cartilage. Just deep to the UES, also along the posterior lamina of the cricoid cartilage, is the posterior cricoarytenoid muscle, the primary abductor of the vocal folds.

At rest, the posterior aspect of the cricoid cartilage is in contact with the posterior hypopharyngeal wall. On elevation of the larynx away from the posterior pharyngeal wall, the postcricoid region separates from the posterior hypopharyngeal wall, thereby creating a stretching effect upon the UES.[32]

The cricopharyngeus has a continual basal tone that relaxes during the swallow.[33,34] Studies have shown that UES relaxation takes place during elevation of the hyoid and larynx and reaches its most complete relaxation at the apex of hyoid and laryngeal elevation.[35] What is anatomically taking place is that the cricoid cartilage is pulled forward by the motion of the hyoid bone and by contraction of the thyrohyoid muscle. This forward motion of the cricoid snaps open the UES.[36] The UES then closes while the larynx is descending to its resting position.[37] Of note, the UES exhibits a sustained contraction prior to resuming its basal tone, presumed to assist in preventing immediate regurgitation once the food bolus enters the esophagus.[38]

Most information about motor and sensory innervation of the cricopharyngeus has been obtained from nonhuman subjects, thereby creating significant controversy when applying animal subject findings to human physiology. Recent investigations in humans have led to a consensus that the cricopharyngeus receives its motor innervation primarily from the vagus nerve and, to a lesser extent, from the glossopharyngeal nerve and from sympathetic nerves through the cranial nerve ganglia.[39,40] The significant sensory contributions to the cricopharyngeus are from the cranial nerve IX with additional contributions from the vagus nerve (cranial nerve X).[40-42]

C. Esophageal Phase

Like the pharyngeal phase of swallowing, the esophageal phase of swallowing is under involuntary neuromuscular control. However, propagation of the food bolus is significantly slower than in the pharynx with transit time decreasing to 3-4 cm/second.[29]

The esophagus connects the pharynx to the stomach and can be divided into three zones.[43] The upper zone of the esophagus contains striated muscle beginning at the UES and continuing inferiorly for approximately 6-8 cm, where the striated muscle of this zone begins to interdigitate with the smooth muscle of the middle zone, which represents the main portion of the esophagus. The outer fibers of the upper zone are arranged longitudinally, with the inner fibers having a circular configuration. Subsequent to relaxation of the cricopharyngeus, the primary peristaltic wave of esophageal propagation begins to be manifested by contraction of the longitudinal muscles, followed immediately by contraction of the circular muscle.[43] Recent work has demonstrated that the primary peristaltic wave is actually two waves, with the first wave dissipating at the end of the upper zone of the esophagus simultaneous with the generation of a second wave, which continues to the distal portion of the esophagus.[44] This physiologic second wave is likely what has been called secondary esophageal peristalsis, which is defined as a reflex response to esophageal distention alone.[45]

The middle zone begins where the striated and smooth muscle regions join and extends to within 4 cm of the lower esophageal sphincter (LES). Although the upper zone peristaltic wave is under direct central neural control, the middle zone peristaltic wave is controlled primarily by the nerves of the myenteric plexus which are located between the outer longitudinal and inner circular muscle layers.[46]

The lower zone of the esophagus contains a short segment of smooth muscle esophagus terminating into the LES. The LES is an actual anatomic sphincter with localized muscle changes in the circular muscle.[47] Like the UES, the LES is tonically contracted; however, unlike the UES, there is no constant EMG activity in the LES.[43] Anatomically contributing to the LES are the diaphragmatic crura, which have a sphincteric action during inspiration or straining, which is normally superimposed on the LES.[48]

III. AIRWAY PROTECTIVE MECHANISMS AGAINST ASPIRATION

The airway protective mechanisms that prevent aspiration of refluxate can be divided into two groups, basal mechanisms and response mechanisms.[49] The basal mechanisms operate constantly, typically without need for stimulation, with the LES and UES being the two best examples. The response mechanisms are a series of reflexes that generally require either distension of the esophagus or mechanical stimulation of the pharynx. These reflexes include the esophago-UES reflex,[50] the pharyngo-UES reflex, the esophagoglottal closure reflex, and the pharyngoglottal closure reflex.

The esophago-UES reflex is a vagally mediated reflex in which distention of the esophagus causes increased UES pressure or increased cricopharyngeal EMG activity. Distention of the proximal esophagus is a stronger stimulus for eliciting this reflex than distention of the distal esophagus.[50,51] The afferent nerve supply to this reflex is from vagal afferents and slow adapting fibers of the muscular wall of the esophagus.

The pharyngo-UES reflex is an experimentally induced reflex resulting in an increase in resting tone of the UES with water stimulation of the pharynx.[42] The superior laryngeal nerve (SLN) branch of the vagus is the afferent nerve supply to this reflex with the efferent source the somatomotor nerves from the vagus.

Abrupt distention of esophagus results in the vocal fold adduction of the esophagoglottal closure reflex.[52] The afferent supply is the vagus nerve carrying sensory fibers to the brainstem in response to stimulation of stretch receptors in the body of the esophagus. This reflex is evoked during spontaneous gastroesophageal reflux (GER) episodes.[53]

Finally, the pharyngoglottal closure reflex is a presumed airway protective reflex that results in brief vocal fold closure on stimulation of the pharynx with water.[54] The afferent and efferent nerve supply is similar to that of the laryngeal adductor reflex, with afferent innervation via the internal branch of the superior laryngeal nerve and motor action from the recurrent laryngeal nerve branch of the vagus.

IV. NEURAL CONTROL OF SWALLOWING

Swallowing is a centrally mediated phenomenon that can be divided into supratentorial and infratentorial regions of control. The supratentorial area of control is located in the frontal cortex anterior to the sensorimotor cortex.[55] The infratentorial, or brainstem, areas involved in control of swallowing are located in the dorsal region within and subjacent to the nucleus of the tractus solitarius as well as in the ventral region around the nucleus ambiguus.[56] In both brainstem sites, the neurons surrounding the adjacent medullary reticular formation are also involved.[57]

In general, the cortical and subcortical regions of the brain are important pathways in the voluntary initiation of swallowing.[58,59] Studies using transcranial magneto-electric stimulation to identify corticofugal projections to the muscles of swallowing have demonstrated that oral muscles, such as the mylohyoid, are represented symmetrically between the two cortical hemispheres, with laryngopharyngeal and esophageal muscles represented asymmetrically and most people having a dominant swallowing hemisphere.[60] The clinical implication of these findings is that one could expect oropharyngeal dysphagia to result from a unilateral cortical stroke.[61]

The brainstem is responsible for the involuntary (pharyngeal and esophageal) phases of swallowing. The dorsal and ventral medullary regions controlling swallowing are represented on both sides of the brainstem and are interconnected. Either side can coordinate the pharyngeal and esophageal stages of deglutition; however because they are interconnected, normal motor and sensory functioning on each side of the laryngopharynx depends on adequate function of both sides of the medulla.[62,63] The clinical implication is that a unilateral medullary lesion after an embolic stroke, for example, can result in bilateral pharyngeal motor and sensory dysfunction.[64,65]

References

1. Flowers C, Morris H. Oral-pharyngeal movement during swallowing and speech. *Cleft Palate J*. 1973;10:181-191.
2. Hrycyshyn AW, Basmajian JV. EMG of the oral stage of swallowing in man. *Am J Anatomy*. 1972;133:333-340.
3. Hollinshead WH: *Anatomy for Surgeons: Volume 1. The Head and Neck*. 3rd ed. Philadelphia: Harper & Row; 1982: 367-371.
4. Hirano M, Kuroiwa Y, Tanaka S, Matsuoka H, Sato K, Yoshida T. Dysphagia following various degrees of surgical resection for oral cancer. *Ann Otol Rhinol Laryngol*. 1992;101:138-141.
5. McConnel FMS. Analysis of pressure generation and bolus transit during pharyngeal swallowing. *Laryngoscope*. 1988;98:71-78.
6. Kent RD, Kent JF, Weismer G, Sufit RL, Rosenbeck JC, Martin RE, Brooks BR. Impairment of speech intelligibility in men with amyotrophic lateral sclerosis. *J Speech Hearing Disord*. 1990;55:721-728.
7. Aviv JE, Hecht CS, Weinberg H, Dalton JF, Urken ML. Surface sensibility of the floor of mouth and tongue in healthy controls and in radiated patients. *Otolaryngol Head Neck Surg*. 1992;107: 418-423.
8. Kapur KK, Garrett NR, Fischer E. Effects of anesthesia of human oral structures on masticatory performance and food particle size distribution. *Arch Oral Biol*. 1990;35:397-403.
9. Teichgraeber J, Bowman J, Goepfert H. Functional analysis of treatment of oral cavity cancer. *Arch Otolaryngol Head Neck Surg*. 1986;112:959-965.
10. Aviv JE, Martin JH, Jones ME, Wee TA, Diamond B, Keen MS, Blitzer, A. Age-related changes in pharyngeal and supraglottic sensation. *Ann Otol Rhinol Laryngol*. 1994;103: 749-752.
11. Sonies BC, Parent LJ, Morrish K, Baum BJ. Durational aspects of the oral-pharyngeal phase of swallow in normal adults. *Dysphagia*. 1988;3:1-10.
12. Ward PH, Colton R, McConnel FMS, Malmgren L, Kashima H, Woodson G. Aging of the voice and swallowing. *Otolaryngol Head Neck Surg*. 1989;100:283-286.
13. Niederman MS, Fein AM. Pneumonia in the elderly. *Clin Geriatr Med*. 1986;2:241-268.

14. Blonsky E, Logemann J, Boshes B, Fisher HB. Comparison of speech and swallowing function in patients with tremor disorders and in normal geriatric patients: a cinefluorographic study. *J Gerontol.* 1975;30:299-303.

15. Ali GN, Laundl TM, Wallace KL, deCarle DJ, Cook IJS. Influence of cold stimulation on the normal pharyngeal swallow response. *Dysphagia.* 1996;11:2-8.

16. Palmer J, Rudin N, Lara G, Crompton A. Coordination of mastication and swallowing. *Dysphagia.* 1992;7:187-200.

17. Ludlow CL, Van Pelt F, Koda J. Characteristics of late responses to superior laryngeal nerve stimulation in humans. *Ann Otol Rhinol Laryngol.* 1992;101:127-134.

18. Aviv JE, Martin J, Kim T, Thomson JE, Sacco RL, Diamond B, Close LG. The laryngeal adductor reflex and laryngopharyngeal sensation. *Ann Otol Rhinol Laryngol.* 1999; in press.

19. Sinclair W. Initiation of reflex swallowing from the naso- and oropharynx. *Am J Physiol.* 1970;218:956-959.

20. Storey A. Laryngeal initiation of swallowing. *Exp Neurol.* 1968;20:359-365.

21. Miller JL, Watkin KL. Lateral pharyngeal wall motion during swallowing using real time ultrasound. *Dysphagia.* 1997;12:125-132.

22. Ekberg O, Nylander G. Cineradiography of the pharyngeal stage of deglutition in 150 individuals without dysphagia. *Br J Radiol.* 1982;55:253-257.

23. Shaker R, Dodds WJ, Dantas RO, Hogan WJ, Arndorfer RC. Coordination of deglutitive glottic closure with oropharyngeal swallowing. *Gastroenterology.* 1990;98: 1478-1484.

24. Wilson JA, Pryde A, White A, Maher L, Maran AGD. Swallowing performance in patients with vocal fold motion impairment. *Dysphagia.* 1995;10:149-154.

25. Adran G, Kemp F. The mechanism of the larynx. II. The epiglottis and closure of the larynx. *Br J Radiol.* 1967;40: 372-389.

26. Selley WG, Ellis RE, Flack FC, Bayliss CR, Pearce VR. The synchronization of respiration and swallow sounds with videofluoroscopy during swallowing. *Dysphagia.* 1994;9: 162-167.

27. Smith J, Wolkove N, Colacone A, Kreisman H. Coordination of eating, drinking and breathing in adults. *Chest.* 1989; 96:578-582.

28. Olsson R, Nilsson H, Ekberg O. Simultaneous videoradiography and pharyngeal solid state manometry (videomanometry) in 25 nondysphagic volunteers. *Dysphagia.* 1995;10:36-41.

29. Dantas RO, Kern MK, Massey BT, Dodds WJ, Kahrilas PJ, Brasseur JG, Cook IJ, Lang IM. Effect of swallowed bolus variables on the oral and pharyngeal phases of swallowing. *Am J Physiol.* 1990;258:G675-G681.

30. McConnel FMS, Cerenko D, Mendelsohn MS. Manofluorographic analysis of swallowing. *Otolaryngol Clin North Am.* 1988;21:625-635.

31. Lang IM, Shaker R. Anatomy and physiology of the upper esophageal sphincter. *Am J Med.* 1997;103:50S-55S.

32. Brasseur JG, Dodds WJ. Interpretation of intraluminal manometric measurements in terms of swallowing mechanics. *Dysphagia.* 1991;6:100-119.

33. Lang IM, Shaker R. Anatomy and physiology of the upper esophageal sphincter. *Am J Med.*1997; 103:50S-55S.

34. Elidan J, Shochina M, Gonen B, Gay I. Electromyography of the inferior constrictor and cricopharyngeal muscles during swallowing. *Ann Otol Rhinol Laryngol.* 1990;99(6 Pt 1):46-49.

35. Kahrilas PJ, Dodds WJ, Dent J, Logemann JA, Shaker R. Upper esophageal sphincter function during deglutition. *Gastroenterology.* 1988;95:52-62.

36. Jacob P, Kahrilas P, Logemann JA, Shah V, Ha T. Upper esophageal sphincter opening and modulation during swallowing. *Gastroenterology.* 1989;97:1469-1478.

37. Kahrilas PJ, Logemann JA, Lin S, Ergun GA. Pharyngeal clearance during swallowing: a combined manometric and videofluoroscopic study. *Gastroenterology.* 1992;103: 128-136.

38. Kahrilas PJ. Upper esophageal sphincter function during antegrade and retrograde transit. *Am J Med.* 1997;103:56S-60S.

39. Murakami Y, Fukuda H, Kirchner JA. The cricopharyngeus muscle. An electrophysiological and neuropharmacological study. *Acta Otolaryngol Suppl (Stockh).* 1972;311: 1-19.

40. Mu L, Sanders I. The innervation of the human upper esophageal sphincter. *Dysphagia.* 1996;11:234-238.

41. Medda BK, Lang IM, Layman R, Hogan WJ, Dodds WJ, Shaker R. Characterization and quantification of a pharyngo-UES contractile reflex in cats. *Am J Physiol.* 1994; 167:(Gastrointest Liver Physiol 30) G972-G983.

42. Ren J, Shaker R, Lang I, Sui Z. Effect of volume, temperature and anesthesia on the pharyngo-UES contractile reflex in humans. *Gastroenterology.* 1995;108:A677.

43. Pope CE. The esophagus for the nonesophagologist. *Am J Med.* 1997;103:19S-22S.

44. Li M, Brasseur JG, Dodds WJ. Analyses of normal and abnormal esophageal transport using computer simulations. *Am J Physiol.* 1994;266:G525-G543.

45. Christensen J. Mechanisms of secondary esophageal peristalsis. *Am J Med.* 1997;103:44S-46S.

46. Christensen J. The forms of argyrophilic ganglion cells in the myenteric plexus throughout the gastrointestinal tract of the opossum. *J Auton Nerv Syst.* 1988;24:251-260.

47. Stein HJ, Liebermann-Meffert D, DeMeester TR, Siewert JR. Three-dimensional pressure image and muscular structure of the human lower esophageal sphincter. *Surgery.* 1995;117:692-698.

48. Dent J. Patterns of lower esophageal sphincter function associated with gastroesophageal reflux. *Am J Med.* 1997; 103:19S-22S.

49. Dua K, Bardan E, Ren J, Hogan WJ, Arndorfer RC. Effect of cigarette smoking on pharyngo-upper esophageal sphincter (UES) contractile reflex. *Gastroenterology.* 1997; 112:A72.

50. Enzmann DR, Harell GS, Zboralske FF. Upper esophageal responses to intraluminal distension in man. *Gastroenterology.* 1977;72:1292-1298.

51. Gerhardt DC, Shuck TJ, Bordeaux RA, Winship DH. Human upper esophageal sphincter response to volume, osmotic, and acid stimuli. *Gastroenterology.* 1978;75:268-274.

52. Shaker R, Dodds WJ, Ren J, Hogan WJ, Arndorfer RC. Esophagolottal closure reflex: a mechanism of airway protection. *Gastroenterology.* 1992;102:857-861.

53. Shaker R, Ren J, Hogan WJ, Liu J, Podvrsan B, Sui Z. Glottal function during postprandial gastroesophageal reflux. *Gastroenterology.* 1993;104:A581.

54. Ren J, Shaker R, Dua K, Trifan A, Podvrsan B, Sui Z. Glottal adduction response to pharyngeal water stimulation stimulation: evidence for a pharyngoglottal closure reflex. *Gastroenterology.* 1994;106:A558.

55. Jean A, Car A. Inputs to the swallowing medullary neurons from the peripheral afferent fibers and the swallowing cortical area. *Brain Res.* 1979;178:567-572.

56. Jean A. Brainstem organization of the swallowing network. *Brain Behav Evol.* 1984;25:109-116.

57. Martin JH. The somatic sensory system. In: Martin JH, *Neuroanatomy: Text and Atlas.* New York: Elsevier; 1989: 122-123.

58. Miller AJ, Bowman JP. Precentral cortical modulation of mastication and swallowing. *J Dent Res.* 1977;56:1154.

59. Martin RE, Sessle BJ. The role of the cerebral cortex in swallowing. *Dysphagia.* 1993;8:195-202.

60. Hamdy S, Aziz Q, Rothwell JC, Singh KD, Barlow J, Hughes DG, et al. The cortical topography of human swallowing musculature in health and disease. *Nat Med.* 1996;2:1217-1224.

61. Hamdy S, Aziz Q, Rothwell JC, Crone R, Hughes DG, et al. Explaining oropharyngeal dysphagia after unilateral hemispheric stroke. *Lancet.* 1997;350:686-692.

62. Doty RW, Richmond WH, Storey AT. Effect of medullary lesions on coordination of deglutition. *Exp Neurol.* 1967; 17:91-106.

63. Neumann S, Buchholz D, Jones B, Palmer J. Pharyngeal dysfunction after lateral medullary infarction is bilateral: review of 15 additional cases (Abstract). *Dysphagia.* 1995; 10:136.

64. Aviv JE, Mohr JP, Blitzer A, Thomson JE, Close LG. Restoration of laryngopharyngeal sensation by neural anastomosis. *Arch Otolaryngol Head Neck Surg.* 1997;123: 154-160.

65. Buchholz DW, Neumann S. Comments on selected recent dysphagia literature. *Dysphagia.* 1998;13:66-67.

PART III

EVALUATION

A. Clinical Evaluation

The clinical evaluation of swallowing by various specialists follows similar paths at the outset of the evaluation. However, each specialist ultimately examines the nature of the swallowing disorder in his or her unique manner. In this section, seven distinct specialists offer their respective views of the clinical evaluation of patients presenting with swallowing disorders. Inevitably, there is overlap and repetition in the discussion of their respective diagnostic algorithms. We have elected to preserve the redundancy as it provides the reader with an overview of the philosophy and techniques followed by each specialist.

CHAPTER 4

■ ■ ■

The Otolaryngologist's Perspective

Ricardo L. Carrau, M.D.

I. INTRODUCTION

The average human swallows more than 2000 times in a day and even swallows while asleep; thus, it is not surprising that a disordered swallowing mechanism produces a significant disability. The spectrum of symptomatology produced by swallowing disorders is broad and parallels the variety of etiologies for the deficit. Thus, the evaluation of patients presenting with a swallowing disorder can be a complex and challenging endeavor. Furthermore, the presence of a swallowing disorder most often represents just one symptom or the sequelae of a primary problem, which may occur distant from the organs of swallowing or at a systemic level. Although not specific for the evaluation of the swallowing mechanism, the otolaryngologist's clinical examination provides clues that guide him or her to select tests to provide the data required to complete an assessment and initiate the treatment of patients with swallowing disorders.

II. CLINICAL EVALUATION

A. History

When a patient complains of a swallowing disorder, a thorough clinical evaluation is essential to formulate an initial differential diagnosis (Table 4-1) and to better choose which tests would be most accurate and cost effective to corroborate the clinical impression. In many instances, the history cannot be fully obtained from a

Table 4-1. *Differential Diagnosis*

Congenital	Dysphagia lusoria
	Tracheoesophageal fistula
	Laryngeal clefts
	Other foregut abnormalities
Inflammatory	GERD
Infections	Lyme disease, neuropathies/encephalitis
	Chagas' disease
Trauma	CNS
	Upper aerodigestive tract
Endocrine	Goiter
	Hypothyroid
	Diabetic neuropathy
Neoplasia	Upper aerodigestive tract
	Thyroid
	Central nervous system
Systemic	Autoimmune
	Dermatomyositis
	Scleroderma
	Sjögren's syndrome
	Amyloidosis
	Sarcoidosis
Iatrogenic	Surgery
	Chemotherapy
	Other medications
	Radiation

patient and will require that the physician review all available medical charts and interview the patient's family and/or caregivers.

Once the demographic data (age, gender, and so forth) is noted, the taking of the history should commence with questions to define the nature and the severity of the swallowing problem[1-9] (Table 4-2). "Difficulty swallowing" does not mean the same thing for every patient or even every clinician. Frequently, what the patient initially describes as "difficulty swallowing" turns out to be a sensation of globus, fatigue, or even the need to frequently clear his or her throat. After the nature of the swallowing problem has been defined, its onset, duration, and progression should be established. Equally important is the site at which the patient feels that the problem is occurring and the time at which the problem appears after the initiation of swallowing. Although the former piece of information is most frequently offered spontaneously by the patient, the latter requires specific queries by the clinician.

Associated symptoms, such as pain, fever, weight loss, lumps in the neck, drooling, nasal regurgitation, episodes of coughing, frequent clearing of the throat, cyanosis, shortness of breath, heartburn, or gastropharyngeal reflux, should be noted. Changes in the patient's ability to communicate or changes in voice or speech, such as slur, hoarseness, or a wet, gurgly quality, are also important, as they reflect the status of the glottis and/or tongue functions.

A complete review of systems may reveal symptoms that suggest a systemic disorder such as neurologic degenerative disease, autoimmune disease, or cardiopulmonary problems that may impact on the patient's ability to swallow. The otolaryngologist should also address the intake of medications, as many prescription-only and over-the-counter medications influence a patient's ability to swallow.[1]

Habits, diet, and lifestyle, such as smoking and/or drinking, may place a patient at a high risk for cancer of the upper aerodigestive tract, and/or gastroesophageal reflux. Although controversial, the use of recreational, albeit illegal drugs, such as marijuana, have also been implicated in the etiology of head and neck carcinomas, especially in the younger population (less than 40 years of age). Patients with a history of cocaine freebasing often suffer pharyngeal burns that may go unnoticed when the individuals are under the influence of the drug, but who later have atypical swallowing complaints and findings.

A complete history on past and present illnesses, as well as previous surgical interventions, irradiation, or trauma are also important. This is especially relevant for those conditions that may affect the neurological system or upper aerodigestive tract, such as CVA, diabetes, cancer, immunosuppression, sarcoidosis, amyloidosis, multiple sclerosis (MS), myasthenia gravis, trauma, or surgery to the head and neck or esophagus.

From a simplistic standpoint, a swallowing problem can be classified as either obstructive, due to the narrowing by intrinsic or extrinsic space-occupying lesions, or functional, which can be of neural, neuromuscular, or muscular origin. A clinical history by itself may help to place a patient's problem in one of those categories of swallowing disorders. For example, an obstructive problem, such as a slow-growing neoplasm or a stricture, usually is evidenced by progressive dysphagia to solids, while neurogenic dysphagia in many cases initially presents with dysphagia to liquids, a motility problem usually includes dysphagia to both solids and liquids, and a degenerative neurologic disease may be accompanied by swallowing fatigue and changes in speech.

The onset at which the patient perceives the swallowing problem after the initiation of the swallow may help to elucidate whether the patient has a pharyngeal or an esophageal problem. The pharyngeal swallow is extremely fast, usually lasting less than 1 second; thus, patients with pharyngeal swallowing have symptoms less than 2 seconds after initiation of the swallow and often require multiple swallows. Conversely, the esophageal phase usually lasts 3-4 seconds, and may extend up to 20 seconds after initiation of the swallow; thus, the presence of problems that begin 2 seconds after the initiation of swallowing suggests an esophageal disorder. As a general rule, the longer the elapsed time between initiation of the swallow and the onset of symptoms, the more distal the site of lesion. The presence of associated symptoms, such as reflux or heartburn, also suggests an esophageal disorder. However, it should be noted that esophageal disease, even at the area of the lower esophageal sphincter, may refer pain, discomfort, or a sensation of a globus to the pharyngeal region. In fact, one third of patients with lesions at this area will have referred pharyngeal symptoms.[2]

Table 4-2. *Critical Components of the Clinical History*

- Define the problem
- Onset, progression
- Time elapsed from initiation of swallow to symptoms
- Associated symptoms
- Present and past:
    Illnesses
    Surgery
    Trauma
- Medications
- Social history/habits
- Family history
- Review of systems

B. Physical Examination

The physical examination should be complete and should include a basic neurological examination with assessment of gait, balance, sensory and motor function of the extremities; deep tendon reflexes; and full assessment of the cranial nerves (Table 4-3). As an otolaryngologist, however, my emphasis is in the upper aerodigestive tract. Assessment of speech/voice, oral continence, facial symmetry, tongue strength, and range of motion, as well as sensation of the face, oral cavity, oropharynx, and larynx are important. A fiberoptic examination of the pharynx and larynx is critical. The presence of the wet, gurgly voice suggests the pooling of secretions caused by an incomplete swallow, with a breathy or whispery voice suggesting a glottic insufficiency (e.g., paralysis, weakness, or atrophy of the vocal folds). Inability to form the sound /k/, as in "Coca-Cola," suggests a velopharyngeal insufficiency. Both of these problems are suspected by listening to the patient and/or corroborated with direct visualization, using a fiberoptic endoscope. Palpation of the thyroid notch on swallowing provides an estimate of laryngeal elevation and coordination of the pharyngeal swallow and may suggest laryngotracheal deviation due to displacement by a tumor. Palpation of the neck may suggest the presence of a paraganglioma, a primary or metastatic neoplasm that may explain the presence of dysphagia or a cranial neuropathy. Of significance, is the presence of neck spasticity or rigidity with limited range of motion, seen in severe degenerative kyphosis or patients with cerebral palsy (CP).

During the flexible laryngoscopy, the anatomy of the pharynx and larynx is observed during quiet and forced respiration, coughing, speaking, and swallowing. Attention is also given to the motion of the base of tongue, pharyngeal walls, arytenoids, and other endolaryngeal structures. Symmetry, coordination, and range of movement between the two sides of the upper aerodigestive tract are also noted. Pooling of secretions or food residue in the vallecula or piriform sinuses is noted. The laryngeal closure reflex can be tested by gentle touch of the epiglottis or aryepiglottic folds with the tip of the endoscope. This maneuver requires some experience and should be as gentle as possible to avoid eliciting a gag reflex or laryngospasm. I often defer this test until all other information is obtained. Sensation of the vallecula and lateral pharyngeal walls also can be tested using this technique.

Table 4-3. *Clinical Examination*

Neurological
Gait/balance
Cranial nerves
Motor function/fine skills
Deep tendon reflexes

Oral
Oral continence
  Lip pursing
  "Trumpeter" maneuvers
  Drooling
Tongue range of motion
  Extends beyond lower lip
  Approximates gingivo-buccal areas
  Can push against tongue blade
  Tongue sensation

Oropharynx
Motion of soft palate:
Sensation
  Tongue blade/swab
  Cold laryngeal mirror
  Gag reflex
  Swallow reflex

F/L
Anatomy of base of tongue, vallecula, hypopharynx, endolarynx
Retention of secretions
Penetration/aspiration of secretions
Motion (symmetry, range) of base of tongue, arytenoid, epiglottis, false vocal cords, true vocal cords (fixation vs. paralysis)
Velopharyngeal closure
  Lateral walls
  Velum

Neck
Laryngeal elevation
Adenopathy
Thyroid
Other masses

III. OTHER TESTS

Once the evaluation has been completed, the otolaryngologist can decide whether or not the patient requires tests that would demonstrate an anatomical abnormality or mechanical obstruction, such as a barium swallow, CT (computed tomography) scan, MRI (magnetic resonance imaging), or direct laryngoscopy/esophagoscopy. These tests delineate the anatomy of the upper aerodigestive tract. Alternatively, the patient may require functional tests of swallowing, such as a flexible fiberoptic evaluation of swallowing, modified barium swallow, and scintigraphy, which should be performed with the assistance of a speech pathologist. Immediate consultation with other specialists, especially neurologists, physical medicine and rehabilitation specialists, or gastroenterologists, is advised, if specific conditions are suggested from the clinical evaluation.

A. Functional Evaluation of Swallowing

Functional evaluation of swallowing is recommended for patients who are suspected of having neurogenic or muscular deficits of the oral, pharyngeal, or laryngeal areas. These tests include the modified barium swallow (MBS), the fiberoptic evaluation of swallowing (with or without sensory testing), scintigraphy, ultrasound, and, recently, rapid sequence magnetic resonance imaging. (See Chapters 11 and 12, Appendixes A and B.) These tests, especially the modified barium swallow and the fiberoptic evaluation of swallowing, provide diagnostic information as they assess the swallowing of the patient under a variety of circumstances employing boluses with different consistencies and positions of the neck. These tests help in the planning of a therapeutic protocol, as compensatory maneuvers, as well as diet modifications, can be initiated during a test to ascertain the influence on a patient's swallowing.

B. Barium Swallow and CT Scan

Imaging techniques, such as the barium swallow esophagogram, the CT scan, and MRI, are recommended when alterations of the anatomy of a patient, caused by previous surgery and/or space occupying lesions, are suspected. The esophagogram provides an evaluation of the endoluminal anatomy, suggests extraluminal compression, and demonstrates the motility of the pharyngeal and esophageal tract. The barium swallow esophagogram detects obstruction, such as that caused by neoplasms, strictures, webs, or achalasia, with high accuracy. (See Chapter 11.) A CT scan or MRI provide exquisite definition of the anatomy within the head and neck area and chest. They are usually reserved to detect neoplasms, vascular abnormalities/strokes, or even the presence of some degenerative neurological conditions, such as multiple sclerosis (MS).

C. Electromyography

Electromyography is recommended to ascertain the presence of specific nerve or neuromuscular unit deficit, such as that accompanying vocal fold paralysis or to elucidate or corroborate the presence of a systemic myopathy or degenerative neuromuscular disease. When used for the diagnosis of vocal fold paralysis, it may also provide information regarding the prognosis for spontaneous recovery. Electromyography is also used as a guide to inject botulinum toxin to hyperkinetic muscles of the larynx, pharynx, or neck. (See Chapter 14.)

D. Direct Laryngoscopy/Esophagoscopy

Endoscopy of the upper aerodigestive tract is recommended to rule out or biopsy a neoplasm that may be suspected to be the cause of dysphagia or odynophagia. I have a low threshold when recommending a direct endoscopy for patients at high risk to develop a cancer, such as smokers and heavy drinkers. Occasionally, the endoscopy may be part of the treatment, as in those patients requiring injection of a paralyzed vocal fold, injection of botulinum toxin, or dilation of the esophagus for the treatment of cricopharyngeal achalasia or strictures.

E. Flexible Endoscopy, 24-hour pH-metry, or Manometry

These tests are utilized for patients in whom neoplasms, motility disorders, or gastroesophageal reflux are suspected. (See Chapter 13.) Whether any of these tests are initially ordered after the clinical evaluation or after a consultation with other specialists is highly variable. It depends on the particular clinical findings, the availability of other consultants and tests, as well as socioeconomic factors. In general, obstructive dysphagia is relatively easy to diagnose and treat, requiring few physicians and tests. Conversely, functional dysphagia requires a multi-disciplinary approach, with early intervention of a speech-language pathologist and nutritionist to optimize remaining compensatory mechanisms in the patient and consultation with other specialists as needed.

References

1. Stoschus B, Allescher HD. Drug-induced dysphagia. *Dysphagia*. 1993;8:154-159.

2. Edwards DA, Discriminatory value of symptoms in the differential diagnosis of dysphagia. *Clin Gastroenterol.* 1976; 5:49-57.

3. Halama AR. Clinical approach to the dysphagic patient. *Acta Oto-Rhino-Laryngol Belg.* 1994;48:119-126.

4. Eibling DE, Boyd EM. Rehabilitation of lower cranial nerve deficits. *Otolaryngol Clin North Am.* 1997;30:865-875. *Am J Otolaryngol.* 1992;13:133-138.

5. Marshall JB. Dysphagia: diagnostic pitfalls and how to avoid them. *Postgrad Med.* 1989;85:243-260.

6. Buchholz D. Neurologic causes of dysphagia. *Dysphagia,* 1987;1:152-156.

7. Mathog RH, Fleming SM. A clinical approach to dysphagia. *Am J Otlaryngol.* 1992;13:133-138.

8. Hendrix TR. Art and science of history taking in the patient with difficulty swallowing. *Dysphagia.* 1993;8:69-73.

9. Horner J, Massey EW. Managing dysphagia: special problems in patients with neurologic disease. *Postgrad Med.* 1991;89:203-213.

CHAPTER 5

■ ■ ■

Speech-Language Pathology: The Clinical Swallow Examination

Thomas Murry, Ph.D.

I. INTRODUCTION

The bedside swallow examination, sometimes called the clinical examination of swallowing, is the speech-language pathologist's first step in assessing a dysphagic patient. This test provides information that influences the diagnostic and treatment planning of a patient presenting with a swallowing disorder. It focuses on information gathering before further objective testing. Table 5-1 describes the critical elements of this assessment.

The bedside clinical examination is done by the speech-language pathologist when first consulted to evaluate and treat a patient presenting with a swal-

lowing disorder. It may also be used to assess a patient who is already eating but who requires diet modification or to assess a patient who is recovering from a significant dysphagia-related problem, such as aspiration pneumonia, and thus requires further assessment to develop compensatory techniques to increase oral nutrition.

An important decision often required of the speech-language pathologist after conducting the bedside clinical examination is whether to keep a patient on nonoral feeding (NPO) or to proceed with testing that may require oral intake. In cases where definitive testing is not immediately possible, the patient should remain NPO until a diagnostic test of swallowing is

Table 5-1. *Critical Elements of the Bedside Swallow Examination*

- History of the disorder.
- Medical status including nutritional support.
- Examination of sensory and motor functions of the swallowing mechanism:

  Lips

  Tongue

  Palate

  Vocal folds

- Presence, type, and length of time of tracheostomy.
- The patient's ability to follow instructions for more definitive testing of swallowing.

conducted. If several days have passed between the bedside examination and the scheduled diagnostic examination (eg, modified barium swallow or fiberoptic evaluation of swallowing), a follow-up bedside clinical examination may be warranted.

II. History of the Disorder

Prior to any swallowing trials, the medical chart is reviewed and a thorough case history is taken from the patient and caregivers, if they are available. Kazandjian, Dikeman, and Adams have outlined the critical aspects of the clinical presentation of the swallowing disorder.[1] These include the conditions surrounding the onset of the problem, current symptoms, whether the problem is stable or changing, current nutrition and oral intake, whether the swallowing problem varies with food consistencies, medications or posture, type and size of tracheotomy tube (if present), and patient awareness of the problem. The clinician also needs to know if there is a history of unpredictable behavior, such as seizure activity or laryngospasm, that would prevent further evaluation.

The best way to begin is to review the patient's medical record to identify previous surgeries, medical complications, or comorbidities and neurological status. Current medications should be noted and the clinician should consult the physician or *Physician's Desk Reference* (PDR) to evaluate the possible impact that medications could have on the patient's ability to swallow or cooperate during an examination. The medical record should also be reviewed for incidents of pain, choking, or nasal regurgitation associated with swallowing, as well as history of respiratory problems, such as chronic cough, pneumonia, bronchitis, and cyanosis.

Once the medical record has been reviewed, the clinician should directly ask the patient about any pain associated with swallowing, if food gets "caught" in one place or another, are some foods or liquids easier to swallow than others, and what happens when the patient tries to swallow. If the patient is on a nonoral diet at the time of the examination, the clinician should not encourage the patient to demonstrate swallowing then, but wait until other aspects of the bedside swallow are completed.

III. ORAL-PERIPHERAL SENSORY MOTOR EXAMINATION

A. Oral Structures

An examination of the patient's anatomy is done during the bedside swallow assessment.[2] This usually begins with lip seal and tongue movement. The oral phase of swallowing depends on good proprioceptive ability. Thus, lip control (rounding, spreading, and sealing) should be evaluated. Of importance is evaluation of oromandibular movements during chewing, with the clinician noting symmetry of motion, labial closure, and control of saliva during fixed expression and chewing. Tongue range of motion (lateral, anteroposterior, and vertical) and strength should be noted, along with tongue elevation anteriorly and posteriorly. Tongue-palate contact is evaluated by having the patient say /k/ or /ka/ both rapidly and with increased effort.

B. Reflex Testing

Testing certain reflexes, especially the gag reflex, is important in understanding the nature of the disorder but results may also be misleading.[3] For example, pseudobulbar paralysis is usually accompanied by a hyperactive gag reflex, but the patient may have significant oral dysphagia. Conversely, the gag reflex may be absent in patients with no swallowing problem. Rapid repetition of the /a/ vowel allows the clinician to observe the elevation and retraction of the soft palate. Touching a cold mirror to the anterior edge of the soft palate stimulates palatal movement; touching the mirror to the base of the tongue or posterior pharyngeal wall elicits the gag reflex in normal individuals. While testing these reflexes, the clinician may want to assess overall oral sensitivity by lightly touching areas in the oral cavity, such as various areas of the tongue, the anterior faucial arches, and various areas of the oral mucosa.

C. Vocal Folds and Larynx

At bedside, a flexible fiberoptic endoscope may be used to examine laryngeal function during phonation as well as swallowing.[4] However, when this is not feasible, the clinician should assess voice quality, noting any evidence of retained secretions ("wet" or "gurgly" voice), and assess the ability to produce a loud voice and a strong cough. Evaluation of pitch variation and ability to change the loudness of the voice, plus measurement of the maximum phonation time provide information about vocal fold closure and stability.[5] Table 5-2 presents mean fundamental frequency, frequency range, and ranges of maximum phonation times for normal adults. When a patient produces voice out of these ranges, the clinician should request consultation with an otolaryngologist to determine adequacy of vocal fold closure. In addition, during trial swallowing, the clinician should feel the larynx at

Table 5-2. *Normal Mean Fundamental Frequency, Frequency Range, and Maximum Phonation Times for Adult Males and Females*

	Mean Fundamental Frequency (H2)	Frequency Range (H2)	Maximum Phonation Time (sec)
Males	120	95-140	18-22
Females	210	190-240	14-18

the thyroid notch to determine if the patient demonstrates laryngeal elevation. Laryngeal elevation is an important contribution to airway closure and cricopharyngeal opening.

The patient with a tracheotomy presents with specific problems with regard to laryngeal function. No laryngeal function can be tested with an inflated cuff. When a cuffless tracheotomy tube is present, the airflow is diverted (ie, the patient cannot generate subglottic pressure) and cough may not be possible. Patients with long-term tracheotomy often present with a weak cough or throat clearing, despite the ability to close the vocal folds.

IV. TESTING THE SWALLOW

Special tests for patients with a tracheotomy, such as the blue dye test or the glucose dipstick, may be carried out.[6] These tests are discussed in another part of this text. For the patient without a tracheotomy tube, the clinician assesses the actual swallow and determines the best posture, food, or liquid consistency and amount of material to be swallowed, based on case history and diagnosis. In addition, the clinician should discuss the procedures and expectations with the patient so that the patient is aware that coughing may occur. The clinician talks the patient through the procedure several times before trying the swallow with liquid or food. If necessary, a written protocol can be used and step-by-step trial swallows are practiced. Thus, the cognitive status of the patient is important, as their cooperation is essential.

When the patient is ready to swallow liquids or other food consistencies, the clinician assesses which posture, consistency, and compensatory maneuver may be helpful during swallowing. Coughing is encouraged and poor performance is expected on the first or second swallow, especially if the patient has not swallowed for several days.

The results of the bedside swallow assessment are reported to the dysphagia management team, with recommendations made based on the results of the examination. The clinician must, however, always inter-

pret the bedside assessment with caution. Interpretation of the oral motor examination, assessment of cognitive status, and observations of actual swallows are products of clinical experience. Rarely is the bedside swallow assessment the final procedure for determining if a patient can safely begin oral nutrition. Rather, it should be considered the first step in advancing the patient to the next step of oral nutrition.

V. RISKS ASSOCIATED WITH THE CLINICAL SWALLOW EXAMINATION

The single most important risk of the bedside clinical assessment is to allow a patient to swallow when there is no definitive evidence that swallowing is safe. The bedside assessment relies on the clinician's observation skills and is highly subjective. The ability to feel laryngeal elevation during the practice swallows, the accurate assessment of vocal fold closure, and the ability to maintain good communication with the patient regarding his or her perceptions of how the food or liquid was passed are skills that a clinician develops with experience. Conservative interpretation of the clinician's subjective impressions is important to the patient's safety. Furthermore, objective testing of the swallow is guided by a bedside evaluation. As there is no way to definitively assess aspiration during a bedside swallow assessment, the patient who has been NPO and is deemed ready for oral intake requires a modified barium swallow or other functional test of swallowing. (See Chapters 11 and 12.)

References

1. Kazandjian MS, Dikeman KJ, Adams E. Communication management of the ventilator-dependent and tracheotomized patient. Paper presented at: Annual Convention of the American Speech-Language-Hearing Association; November 1991; Atlanta, Ga.

2. Logemann JA. *Evaluation and Treatment of Swallowing Disorders*, San Diego, Calif: College-Hill Press; 1983: 108-109.

3. Logemann JA. Management of tracheostomy tubes, intubation, ventilators during swallowing assessment and

treatment. Paper presented at: Special Consultations in Dysphagia. Northern Speech Services, April 1993; Chicago, Ill.

4. Carrau RL, Pou A, Eibling DE, Murry T, Ferguson BJ. Laryngeal framework surgery for the management of aspiration *Head and Neck*. 1998: In press.

5. Pou A, Carrau RL, Eibling DE, Murry T. Laryngeal framework surgery for the management of aspiration in high vagal lesions. *Am J Otolaryngol*, 1998;19:1-7.

6. Dikeman KJ, Kazanjian MS. *Communication and Swallowing Management of Tracheotomized and Ventilator-Dependent Adults*. San Diego, Calif: Singular Publishing Group; 1995.

CHAPTER 6

■ ■ ■

Clinical Evaluation of Swallowing Disorders: The Pediatric Perspective

Lisa A. Newman, Sc.D.
Mario Petersen, M.D., M.S.

I. INTRODUCTION

Information gleaned from clinical research concerning physiological parameters of the normal and abnormal swallow in adults is not always applicable to infants or children. The parameters used to examine infant and pediatric swallowing must be specific to these populations. This chapter reviews the clinical examination and objective tests of infants and young children with swallowing disorders.

II. THE CLINICAL EXAMINATION

The evaluation of swallowing disorders must begin with a good history. The history should include birth history; medical history including illnesses, hospitalizations, diagnostic tests; surgical history; medications; eating/nutrition history; and family support system. The history can be obtained by interviewing the parents or caregivers and reviewing all medical records. After a complete history, the child should be clinically examined. The child must be assessed for level of alertness and interaction. The clinician should observe general motor ability, including head control, trunk support for seating, and the need for or appropriateness of assistive seating devices. The child's ability to cooperate and participate in any therapeutic program must be deter-

mined. Thus, assessment of behavior and communication skills is a necessity. A good oral motor examination should include assessment of structure, symmetry, tone, and function of the lips, tongue, palate, jaw, and vocal function. If the child has been eating, the clinician must ascertain how food has been administered, the position of the child during feeding, utensils, adaptive feeding devices, textures of foods, whether the child can manage secretions, how the child responds to strange feeding situations, and whether the child self-feeds. In addition to information gleaned from the clinical examination, the clinician also determines how to adapt the instrumental assessment to most effectively obtain diagnostic information and assesses therapeutic strategies.

III. INSTRUMENTAL ASSESSMENT

A. Overview

The swallowing process and its disorders are extremely complex and cannot be visualized by clinical observation. Furthermore, anatomic or neurologic deficits may affect any or all stages of swallowing. Therefore, dysphagia must be diagnosed accurately and effectively. Swallowing is a rapid moving process that is best assessed with a dynamic instrumental technique.

Several methods have been used to examine the oropharyngeal stages of swallowing, the most frequent being videofluoroscopy. Additional dynamic methods include fiberoptic endoscopic examination of swallowing (FEES) and ultrasound. Other methods have been proposed to assess a specific aspect of swallowing or as a screening technique to determine if there are swallowing problems, with the methods including air pulse quantification, radionuclide milk scanning, and cervical auscultation.[1] (See Chapter 12.) This section briefly describes the advantages and disadvantages of each method of pediatric swallowing evaluation and focuses on the radiographic technique of videofluoroscopy.

Endoscopic examination of the anatomy and vocal fold function is invaluable in assessing a child with swallowing disorders. However, most children have difficulty cooperating during a swallowing examination with an endoscope in place. Furthermore, FEES does not allow visualization of the sucking and/or the oral phase of swallowing. The deflection of the epiglottis covers the laryngeal introitus and obstructs visualization of the pharyngeal response and there is no visualization of the cervical esophageal stage of swallowing. Thus, it may be difficult to diagnose the parameters which cause dysphagia, eg, the underlying cause of aspiration.

Air pulse quantification is designed to assess supraglottic and pharyngeal sensation by delivering an air puff of controlled pressure and duration to the anterior wall of the pyriform sinus. (See Chapter 12.) This technique has not been widely applied for use with children. However, the issue of sensory function in the pediatric dysphagia patient is a constant question for the clinician. Further research into sensory function may help in the management of pediatric swallowing disorders.

Ultrasound is most effective for the study of oral preparatory (including sucking) and oral stages of swallowing. However, ultrasound does not allow for a complete understanding of the dynamics of pharyngeal and cervical esophageal swallowing. It has been used effectively to examine tongue function in infants.[2,3]

Radionuclide milk scanning, a nuclear medicine procedure, is a more sensitive method for detecting aspiration. It involves feeding a child formula to which a radioactive isotope has been added. A gamma camera is used to determine the presence of any of the radioactive isotope in the lung. This technique, known as scintigraphy, is far more sensitive to aspiration than the barium swallow; however, it does not distinguish between aspiration from oral and pharyngeal swallowing dysfunction or gastroesophageal reflux (GER). Furthermore, scintigraphic studies do not identify the physiologic reason for aspiration. Radionuclide milk scanning may be a useful addition to a modified barium swallow in documenting delayed aspiration.

Cervical auscultation has been proposed as a clinical bedside technique to identify patients who aspirate. In older children, a contact microphone, or accelerometer, is placed on the lateral border of the trachea immediately inferior to the cricoid cartilage or midpoint between the center of the cricoid cartilage and the site immediately superior to the jugular notch.[1] With smaller infants, the accelerometer is placed at the level of the larynx.[4] The ability to detect aspiration or swallowing disorders in the pediatric population has not been documented. In the adult population, there was 76% agreement (statistically significant) between patients who aspirated during clinical examination using cervical auscultation and a separate modified barium swallow. Agreement was not statistically significant for identifying other pharyngeal disorders, such as pharyngeal delay and pharyngeal residue.[5] Both pharyngeal delay and pharyngeal residue are swallowing disorders that may result in aspiration of material and should be diagnosed in determining the potential for aspiration. Cervical auscultation does not diagnose swallowing disorders and its value in bedside screening has not yet been documented for use in the pediatric population.

B. Videofluoroscopic Evaluation of Swallowing: Modified Barium Swallow

Videofluoroscopy has been cited as the best available method to assess the dynamic process of swallowing. It is the only procedure designed to study the anatomy and physiology of all four stages of swallowing: oral preparatory, oral stage, pharyngeal stage, and cervical esophageal stage. For infants and children, videofluoroscopy provides a systematic and objective method for analyzing the entire swallowing mechanism. It is not used merely as a study to rule out aspiration or a pass/fail study. The modified barium swallow (MBS) examines the anatomy and physiology of the oropharyngeal cavities during swallowing, thus identifying abnormalities that can cause laryngeal penetration, aspiration, naso-pharyngeal backflow, or pharyngeal residue. As in adults, it is also imperative that potential management strategies to improve swallowing be assessed during the radiographic procedure. The swallowing clinician must be highly trained and competent in assessing the parameters of the swallowing mechanism that lead to a diagnosis and determination of treatment strategies. The protocols used for the MBS must be age-appropriate with regard to viscosity, presentation, and position.

The clinician must pay particular attention to equipment used for the MBS. Necessary equipment includes a fluoroscope, videorecorder, monitor, an optional (but desirable) timing device, and seating adaptations. The resolution of the fluoroscope has been steadily improving. The recent addition of digital fluoroscopy with 1024-line resolution gives the best image to date. When digital fluoroscopy is calibrated and subdued for use in children, there is a 40% reduction in patient radiation exposure as compared to currently available nondigital fluoroscopic unit.[6]

The fluoroscopic examination must be recorded for later review and analysis. In addition, the MBS can be archived so that repeat MBS studies can be compared to earlier studies to assess progressive changes over time. Recording devices most compatible with digital fluoroscopy include direct image storage in a digital form (to a computer hard drive, tape drive, disk, etc.) and high-definition videorecorders and monitors. These recording devices are very expensive, which may limit replay capacity, as some facilities may not have the equipment. If digital storage or high-definition recording equipment is not available, then the image must be altered to allow for recording on Super-VHS or 3/4" U-matic equipment. Also, the image must be converted from digital to analog by a D/A converter. It must be stressed that high quality recording equipment allows for good resolution during slow motion and frame-by-frame analysis of the examination. For example, the pediatric pharyngeal swallow occurs more frequently and with greater speed that of the adult.[7,8] The parameters of the oral and pharyngeal stages, which occur in less than 1 second, cannot be visualized in real time and can only be observed in slow motion. The timing counter superimposes a time code onto the videotape and displays minutes, seconds, and 1/100 seconds. This allows for the analysis of temporal measures throughout the swallow.

Infants and children are best viewed in the lateral and/or anterior-posterior projections for examination of the swallowing function. Seating adaptations present a particular problem for the pediatric facility and must accommodate the range from a premature infant through a fully grown adolescent with neurologic difficulties and fit in the narrow space of the fluoroscopic setup. Premature or young infants need head and trunk support while placed in a semireclining position that can be altered, if necessary. Children of varying sizes and motor skills also need to be accommodated, with special adaptations available for head and/or trunk control. Adult size seating is required for evaluation of fully grown adolescents who experience dysphagia following head trauma, neurosurgical procedures, or cancer treatment. Furthermore, patients with developmental disabilities and skeletal abnormalities require special seating adaptations that may not fit between the tube and X-ray table. The pediatric facility must provide a range of seating devices and adaptations to facilitate the fluoroscopic examination of swallowing for this diverse population.

A standard protocol to begin the MBS is recommended; however it must be appropriate for age, skill, and developmental level. For example, sucking should be examined in a 2-month-old infant and he or she should not be presented with semisolids or solid materials on a spoon. Protocols give the clinician a starting point and allow for the collection of baseline data and comparison between repeated MBS studies. One may begin with a protocol and then individualize how and what materials are administered, according to the skills and swallowing disorders presented by the infant or child. The following two protocols are suggested for infants and children. Protocols differ by facility and should be designed to answer specific diagnostic questions and assess therapeutic options. It is extremely important that the child be alert and clinically stable during the MBS.

The infant protocol up to 12-18 months should assess sucking from a bottle. For example, 40 wt/wt liquid barium suspension is administered by 2-ounce bottle and nipple. The barium, which is thicker than formula, needs a slightly larger than typical hole in the nipple. A standard cross-cut nipple provides an easy way to enlarge the nipple opening. The clinician can cut a slit with a scalpel connecting the hole and the cross cut for a 3-mm cut. The infant is given the bottle and nipple (preferably by the parent) while placed in the lateral projection with proper seating support. The first few swallows are visualized on fluoroscopy. If the infant can suck well, then the infant is allowed to finish the 2 ounces, with intermittent viewing of a swallow every 30 to 60 seconds to reduce radiation exposure while assessing the effects of fatigue. If the infant is unable to suck, then 1-ml volumes of barium are administered via small syringe. An infant 6 months or older may be given pudding mixed with barium if he or she is taking baby food.

For the older child, adaptation of the Logemann protocol for MBS is recommended. (See Chapter 11.) Measured liquid boluses are administered: 1- and 3-ml volumes given by spoon, 5-ml volumes given by syringe, and 10-ml volume is optional depending on the age and skills of the child. Drinking from a sippy cup or a cup may also be attempted, depending on the age and ability of the child. Beginning the examination with a small volume minimizes the risk for aspiration and allows the clinician to visualize the oral, pharyngeal, and cervical esophageal structures. A barium pudding mixture of two parts chocolate pudding and one part barium paste is administered in 1-ml and 3-ml volumes. Barium paste mixed with any other baby food may also be attempted. Mastication and bolus formation in an adult protocol is accomplished by coating a piece of cookie with the barium pudding mixture. Children, however, usually will swallow the pudding, leaving minimal contrast for observation of mastication of the cookie. Therefore, coating the piece of cookie on all sides with barium pudding or barium powder is most effective for a child fluoroscopic examination. Any other food textures mixed with barium may also be administered. Therapeutic interventions need to be individualized for the patient.

It should be emphasized that it is desirable to have a parent or caregiver help with the MBS in infants, toddlers, and children with developmental disabilities. Otherwise, the behavior of the child can make the examination extremely difficult or nonrepresentative of baseline swallowing function.

IV. MULTIDISCIPLINARY MANAGEMENT OF PEDIATRIC DYSPHAGIA

Given the heterogeneity of diagnosis and complexity of dysphagia in the pediatric population, the diagnostic team must be prepared to adapt to a child's needs. Rigid systems do not work well with a diverse population of infants and children. There are many types of teams composed of representatives of different disciplines. The team should have, as a minimum, a core that includes a physician, a feeding/swallowing specialist (usually a speech-language pathologist), and a nutritionist. The specialty of the physician (gastroenterology, developmental or general pediatrics, otorhinolaryngology, or pulmonology) is not as important as the skills to work in a team and ability to evaluate all the areas involved in the process of feeding. It is the responsibility of the physician to integrate the medical information and consider the need for further medical tests and referrals to other specialists. It is extremely important that the medical etiology, underlying disease processes, and complications be considered in the diagnosis and management of an infant or child with dysphagia.

Another key member of the team is the feeding/swallow specialist (usually a speech-language pathologist or sometimes an occupational therapist) who is responsible for the evaluation of feeding and for the instrumental assessment. The evaluation should include a clinical examination, observation of feeding, and evaluation of the intrinsic mechanisms of swallowing by an MBS. The nutritionist is responsible for evaluating the nutritional status of the patient, determining appropriateness of the diet, and monitoring the patient's progress.

Depending on the specific place and population, the team may need to include other professionals. A social worker can be instrumental obtaining community resources and providing counseling to the child and/or parent. The psychologist has a fundamental role in the cognitive and behavioral evaluation and can play a major role in the treatment of children with behavioral problems. For example, some children with mental retardation may display behaviors that are not related to the swallowing disorder and are intended to avoid certain situations or obtain attention. The physical therapist may be required for some children, particularly children with cerebral palsy (CP) who need adaptive seating with specific postures for feeding. Occupational therapists can help in the decision of appropriate utensils and can also provide input on positioning. As mentioned previously, the occupational therapist may be the swallowing expert. The speech-language pathologist can compliment the occupational therapist in the assessment or treatment of swallowing. The speech-language pathologist also has a major role in the assessment of language and communication.

Acknowledgment

Supported in part by Grant 90-DD-0364-03 from the U.S. Department of Health and Human Services, Administration for Children and Families and by Grant MCJ-479158-06 from the Health Resources and Services Administration's Maternal and Child Health Bureau.

References

1. Takashashi J, Groher M, Michi K. Methodology for detecting swallowing sounds. *Dysphagia*, 1994;9:54-62.
2. Weber F, Woolridge M, Baum, J. A ultrasonographic study of the organization of sucking and swallowing by newborn infants. *Dev Med Child Neurol.* 1986;28:19-24.
3. Bu'Lock F, Woolridge MW, Baum, JD. Development of coordination of sucking, swallowing and breathing: ultrasound study of term and preterm infants. *Dev Med Child Neurol.* 1990;32:669-678.
4. Vice FL, Bamford O, Heinz JM, Bosma JF. Correlation of cervical auscultation with physiological recording during suckle-feeding in newborn infants. *Dev Med Child Neurol.* 1995;37:167-179.
5. Zenner PM, Losinski DS, Mills RH. Using cervical auscultation in the clinical dysphagia examination in long-term care. *Dysphagia.* 1995;10:27-31.
6. Cleveland R, Constantinou C, Blickman J, Jaramillo D, Webster E. Voiding cystourethography in children: value of digital fluoroscopy in reducing radiation dose. *Am J Radiol.* 1992;137:142.
7. Kramer S. Special swallowing problems in children. *Gastrointest Radiol.* 1985;10:241-250.
8. Newman LA, Cleveland RH, Blickman, JG, Hillman RE, Jaramillo D. Videofluoroscopic analysis of the infant swallow. *Inves Radiol.* 1991;10:870-873.

CHAPTER 7

■ ■ ■

Evaluation of Swallowing:
The Gastroenterologist's Perspective

Sukhdeep Padda, M.D.
Michele A. Young, M.D.

I. INTRODUCTION

Swallowing is the process whereby oral contents are transferred into the stomach. It integrates a complicated mechanism, principally because the pharynx frequently serves several other functions. For a brief interval, the pharynx is converted into a tract responsible for the propulsion of food. In general, we may divide swallowing into (1) the *voluntary stage*, which initiates the swallowing process; (2) the *pharyngeal stage*, which is a brief highly coordinated involuntary event: the nasopharynx closes as the soft palate contracts and elevates to become opposed to the hard palate, and the tongue moves posteriorly in response to contraction of the styloglossus and hyoglossus muscles, with the epiglottis then closing and the inferior pharyngeal constrictors propelling the food bolus into a receptive esophagus with a relaxed upper esophageal sphincter[1-3]; (3) the *esophageal stage*[4] is another involuntary phase that promotes passage of food through the esophagus into the stomach.

The oropharyngeal swallowing mechanism is followed by primary and secondary peristaltic contractions of the esophageal body. This usually transports solid and liquid boluses from the mouth to the stomach within 10 seconds. When these orderly contractions fail to develop or progress, an ingested bolus may not clear the esophagus resulting in intraluminal distention and discomfort. These symptoms associated with difficulty swallowing are known collectively as dysphagia. Dysphagia may result from disruption of any of the mechanisms involved in swallowing or

from mechanical obstruction. Several modalities are used to evaluate swallowing. An integrated approach between the primary care physician, radiologist, speech-language pathologist, otolaryngologist, and gastroenterologist is required. This chapter describes the modalities used to evaluate the swallowing process.

II. HISTORY

Taking a careful and thorough patient history is the first step in the diagnosis of dysphagia. As diagnostic tests become more available, complex, and expensive, the importance of the patient history cannot be overemphasized. Specific clues to the diagnosis will be apparent from the patient's history. First, it is important to note if the patient has any coexisting medical illnesses. An excellent example of this is in CREST syndrome. In this illness, dysphagia is a part of the diagnostic syndrome, which is described as a variant of progressive systemic sclerosis with coexisting calcinosis, Raynaud's phenomenon, esophageal dysmotility, sclerodactyly, and telangiectasias. If the patient has had a recent cerebral vascular accident (CVA), the likely etiology of the dysphagia is neurologic, and symptoms of bolus transfer or oropharyngeal dysphagia should be elicited.

It is critical to assess the nature of the food boluses that the patient has difficulty with. Patients with only solid food dysphagia are more likely to have esophageal dysphagia from an obstructing lesion. On the other hand, more difficulty with liquids is likely to indicate transfer dysphagia. Functional esophageal dysphagia is typically intermittent and similar for both solids and liquids. Evaluation of the frequency of dysphagia should differentiate between those disorders that present intermittently from those that are constant. The progression of the illness will also provide clues as to the etiology of the symptoms.

A comprehensive assessment of a patient's prescribed and over-the-counter medications provides critical information to the diagnostic process. A cost-effective evaluation of a patient presenting with dysphagia begins with taking a complete medical, drug, and swallowing history. A comprehensive physical examination should always be an inherent part of the evaluation process. It should include a thorough evaluation of the oral cavity, head and neck, supraclavicular structures, and abdomen. It should also include a thorough neurologic examination, particularly of the cranial nerves. In patients with suspected neurogenic dysphagia, the clinical neurologic examination should distinguish abnormalities at the upper motor neuron level from those due to lower motor neuron disease or myopathies.

III. RADIOLOGICAL TESTS

Normal swallowing requires the coordination of very rapid sequential neuromuscular events[3]; therefore, a specialized approach to the evaluation is required. Because of the dynamic nature of swallowing, static studies are of limited value in the diagnostic process. In addition to barium fluoroscopy, videoradiography, radionucleotide imaging as well as endoscopic ultrasound (EUS) are used to evaluate the oropharynx and the esophagus during swallowing (Table 7-1).

Visual inspection of the oropharynx is inadequate for the evaluation of swallowing function. Recent advances in radiological techniques allow for a comprehensive evaluation of the mechanisms involved in swallowing. Standard techniques used for the routine multiphasic examination of the esophagus include

Table 7-1. *Diagnostic Tests of Dysphagia and Gastroesophageal Reflux*

Test	Indication
Barium esophagram	Structural lesions
Videoradiography	Pharyngeal function
Scintigraphy	Aspiration
Endoscopic ultrasound	Submucosal lesions
Endoscopy	Structural and mucosal lesions
Esophageal manometry	Motility disorders
24-Hour ambulatory pH	Gastroesophageal reflux (GER)

double contrast, full column, mucosal relief, and fluoroscopic observation with motion recording.[5,6] Double contrast films are obtained by coating the esophagus with a dense barium suspension followed by air inflation. The full column method requires rapid filling of the esophagus with barium and is done with the patient in the prone position. Mucosal relief films are taken with the esophagus collapsed and coated with a dense barium suspension.[7] These routine studies allow one to identify gross structural abnormalities of the esophagus and to a lesser degree the pharynx. These studies are inadequate to identify subtle structural defects and more importantly to identify esophageal motility disorders[7]

A. Barium Swallow and Modified Barium Swallow

A barium swallow is regarded by many as the best initial examination for most esophageal diseases associated with symptomatic dysphagia. A radiographic assessment of esophageal motility includes an examination of the esophageal body and both sphincters.[7] Videofluorography permits the evaluation of rapid motor sequences by slow motion picture analysis.[5-9] This is important in the oropharyngeal phase of swallowing because of the speed with which the bolus travels through this region. Major structural abnormalities, including webs, rings, and diverticula, that may affect swallowing in the pharyngeal phase can be seen with barium esophagography, especially if special attention is given to the cervical region. Barium esophagograms, however, provide little information regarding the presence, extent, and volume of reflux material and correlate poorly with more sophisticated measures of GER disease. Esophageal transit times—that is, the amount of time for a bolus to navigate the esophagus and enter the stomach—can be calculated with fluoroscopic imaging. The importance of this measure is unclear and it is not widely used in clinical practice.

Recently, a multidisciplinary approach to the patient with oropharyngeal dysphagia utilizing the skills and cooperation of several medical specialists has improved the accuracy of diagnosis with radiographic studies. A modified barium swallow (MBS) examination, when performed under the direction of a speech-language pathologist, is extremely useful in the diagnosis and management of oropharyngeal, or transfer, dysphagia.[9,10] In this examination, the patient is given barium-labeled food and liquids of different consistencies. Using this technique, the speech-language pathologist can determine which consistency of bolus preparation can be safely swallowed by a patient. Laryngeal penetration and tracheal aspiration can also be closely monitored. Rings and webs not seen by a standard barium swallow can often be detected through the use of barium-impregnated solid food or capsules.

1. Procedure

The patient is usually given a suspension of barium sulfate in water to swallow. The patient may also be asked to swallow a barium tablet. The pharynx is outlined by the barium very briefly as the patient swallows. The bolus moves so rapidly that fluoroscopy is not a satisfactory method of evaluating the process of oropharyngeal swallowing. Review of the video images, sequence by sequence, provides a more accurate measure of these dynamic pharyngeal movements. Thick barium is used to coat the mucosa after the bolus has passed into the esophagus. Lateral and frontal views are obtained for further review. Because of the increased risk of aspiration, thick barium should be avoided or used with caution in patients whose history is suggestive of oropharyngeal swallowing difficulty.

The technique of examination may vary to some degree depending on the presenting problem and the radiologist performing the procedure. Generally, the esophagus is examined by fluoroscopy with the patient in the upright and recumbent positions. The Trendelenburg position (a supine position which is angled so that the pelvis is higher than the head) may be employed, if necessary to keep the esophageal lumen dilated. Different variations in the methods used in the double contrast examination can enhance delineation of the mucosal integrity and the esophageal outline. A mouthful of barium followed by water is a frequently used technique. In this examination the barium coats the mucosa and the water dilates the esophagus. Another technique involves administering a gas-forming substance such as Seidlitz powders along with the barium. Regardless of the technical aspect of the examination, at least 5 barium swallows are required for an adequate evaluation of esophageal motility and LES relaxation.[7] Single swallows must be observed to allow for recovery from the first swallow. A second swallow taken during the refractory period of the initial swallow would inhibit the peristalsis induced by the first swallow. This can cause confusion during the analysis of the examination and it could be interpreted as esophageal dysmotility. Rapid swallowing does not allow for assessment of esophageal motility, but this process does distend the esophagus, which improves the accuracy of the structural evaluation.[7] Therefore, a more complete examination is done when both slow and rapid swallows are elicited from the patient.

As barium is propelled through a relaxed UES, a normal primary peristaltic wave is seen progressing in caudal direction. The peristaltic wave usually obliterates the esophageal lumen and strips the barium bolus from the esophagus. In young individuals, the peristaltic wave is occlusive to the lumen, preventing proximal escape of the swallowed contents. However with age, increasing proximal escape may be seen that may be interpreted as a weakness in peristalsis.[11,12]

2. Videoradiography

Videoradiography has essentially replaced cineradiography, the older method of photographing these fluoroscopic images. A film recording of these images allows for repeat, slow, and fast motion viewing of the fluoroscopic images. This technique is of great value in evaluating motility disorders of the esophagus as well as oropharyngeal causes of dysphagia.

B. Radionuclide Imaging

Radionuclide imaging has been used for studying functional disorders of the oropharynx, esophagus, and stomach. These techniques are helpful in determining esophageal transit time and emptying. In this technique the patient is given a technetium-99 radiolabeled solid or mixed liquid and solid meal. Clearance of a ^{99}Tc radiolabeled meal from the esophagus is then documented by scintigraphy. The patient undergoes immediate scanning to document esophageal reflux of labeled material. Scanning the following morning to document pulmonary aspiration may follow this initial study. Radionuclide scanning is a very specific test in demonstrating GER or pulmonary aspiration; however, it is not sensitive to the cause of aspiration and it is expensive. In a recent study comparing scintigraphy to other modes of diagnosis, a sensitivity of only 36% was seen; however, the specificity was greater than 88%.[13] Other studies have found similar values.[6,14] The sensitivity of radionuclide scanning for the diagnosis of GER disease in otolaryngology patients was reported to be only 11%.[15] This may be due in part to the intermittent nature of GER disease or the short duration of scintigraphic studies.

References

1. Ardan GM, Kemp FH. A radiographic study of movements of the tongue in swallowing. *Dent Practitioner.* 1955; 5:252-261.
2. Kahrilas PJ, Dodds WJ, Dent J, Logemann JA, Shaker RO. Upper esophageal sphincter function during deglutition. *Gastroenterol.* 1988;95:52-62.
3. Logemann JA. Swallowing physiology and pathophysiology. *Otolaryngol Clin North Am.* 1988;21:613-623.

4. Silbiger ML, Pikielney R, Donner MW. Neuromuscular disorders affecting the pharynx. *Invest Rad.* 1967;2:442-448.

5. Ott DJ, Gelfand DW, Wu WC. Reflux esophagitis: radiographic and endoscopic correlation. *Radiology.* 1979; 130:583-588.

6. Ott DJ. Radiological diagnosis of esophageal dysphagia. *Cur Probl Diagn Radiol.* 1988;17:1-33.

7. Ott DJ. Motility disorders. In: Gore RM, Levine MS, Laufer I. eds. *Textbook of Gastrointestinal Radiology.* Philadelphia, Pa: WB Saunders Co; 1994:346-352.

8. Ott DJ, Chen YM, Hewson EG, Richter JE, Dalton CB, Gelfand DW, et al. Esophageal motility: assessment with synchronous videofluroscopy and manometry. *Radiology.* 1989;173:419-422.

9. Ramsey GH, Watson JS, Gramiak R, Weinberg SA. Cinefluororscopic analysis of the mechanism of swallowing. *Radiology.* 1955;64:498-518.

10. Bastian RW. Videoendoscopic evaluation of patients with dysphagia: an adjuct to the modified barrow swallow. *Otolaryngol Head Neck Surg.* 1991;104:339-350.

11. Margulis AR, Koehler RE. Radiological diagnosis of esophageal disordered motility. *Radiological Clin N Am.* 1976;14:429-439.

12. Robbins J. Normal swallowing and aging. *Semin Neurol.* 1996;16:309-317.

13. Shay SS, Abreu SH, Tsuchida A. Scintigraphy in gastroesophageal reflux disease: a comparison to endoscopy, LESp, and 24-H pH score, as well as to simultaneous pH monitoring. *Am J Gastroenterol.* 1992;87:1094-1101.

14. Chernow B, Johnson LF, Janowitz WR, Castell DO. Pulmonary aspiration as a consequence of gastroesophageal reflux: a diagnostic approach. *Dig Dis Sci.* 1979;24: 839-844.

15. Kuriloff DB, Golfarb R, Chodosh P, Ongseng F. Detection of gastroesophageal reflux in head and neck: the role of scintigraphy. *Ann Otol Rhinol Laryngol.* 1989;98(1 Pt 1):74-80.

CHAPTER 8

■ ■ ■

The Neurologist's Perspective

Susan M. Baser, M.D.

I. INTRODUCTION

Dysphagia is best defined clinically as the sensation of delay in the passage of a food bolus from the mouth into the stomach within 10 seconds of initiation of a swallow. Neurogenic dysphagia results from sensorimotor impairment of the oral and pharyngeal phases of swallowing because of a neurologic disorder. The symptoms of neurogenic dysphagia include drooling, difficulty initiating swallowing, nasal regurgitation, difficulty managing secretions, choking/coughing episodes while feeding, and food sticking in the throat. If unrecognized and untreated, neurogenic dysphagia can lead to dehydration, malnutrition, and respiratory complications. The symptoms of neurogenic dysphagia may be relatively inapparent because of both compensation for swallowing impairment and diminution of the laryngeal cough reflex due to a variety of factors.

Treatment of neurogenic dysphagia involves treatment of the underlying neurologic disorder whenever possible, swallowing therapy if oral feeding is reasonably safe to attempt, and gastrostomy if oral feeding is unsafe or inadequate.[1]

The three major types of dysphagia may be categorized as transfer, transit, and obstructive. Transfer dysphagia represents a pathologic alteration in the neuromotor mechanism of the oropharyngeal phase of swallowing. Transit dysphagia is classically represented by achalasia, a disorder characterized by absent primary and secondary peristalsis in the body of the esophagus and increased pressure with incomplete relaxation of the lower esophageal sphincter in most cases. Obstructive dysphagia is caused by mechanical narrowing, or stenosis, in the pharynx or esophagus or at the esophagogastric junction.

The patient with a neuromotor disorder affecting the pharynx and hypopharynx (transfer dysphagia) will have a history of first experiencing dysphagia with liquids and solids passing with minimal or no significant difficulty. The most common cause of this particular condition is cerebral vascular disease that results in a stroke; other disorders, such as myasthenia gravis, amyotrophic lateral sclerosis (ALS), polymyositis, and botulism, may have transfer dysphagia as the major symptom.[2]

II. NEUROPHYSIOLOGY OF SWALLOWING

Normal swallowing is divided into four stages, the oral preparatory stage, the oral stage, the pharyngeal stage, and the esophageal stage.[3] (See Chapter 3.) The first two stages are mechanical and under voluntary control, with the last two stages reflexive.

The *oral preparatory stage* is essentially chewing. It involves the coordination of lip, buccal, jaw, tongue, and soft palate movements to prepare food for swallowing. At the end of this phase, the tongue pulls the food into a bolus and holds it against the hard palate. The most important neuromuscular function in this phase is the lateral rolling motion of the tongue, as persons without normal tongue mobility have great difficulty chewing.

The *oral stage* is the second stage of swallowing. It lasts about 1 second, and it moves food from the front of the oral cavity to the anterior faucial arches. Again, tongue movement is the most important aspect of this phase of swallowing, as it shapes, lifts, and squeezes the bolus upward and backward along the hard palate, triggering reflex stages.

The *pharyngeal stage* begins when the bolus reaches the anterior faucial arches. Food in the pharynx stimulates receptors with afferents in cranial nerves V and IX leading to the medulla. This swallowing reflex results in neuromuscular functions, including velopharyngeal closure to prevent nasopharyngeal reflux, closure of the larynx, and pharyngeal peristalsis.

The swallow reflex may also be triggered by the superior laryngeal nerve (SLN) at the laryngeal inlet.[4] When a swallow reflex occurs late in this second mechanism, the patient is said to have a delayed swallow reflex. The swallow reflex is mediated in the reticular formation of the brainstem, adjacent to the respiratory center. It is modulated by input from the respiratory center and cortical areas.

Reflex efferent signals travel via cranial nerves V, IX, X, and XII to elevate the soft palate to seal off the nasopharynx, move palatopharyngeal walls medially, and close the glottis while depressing the epiglottis. The larynx moves superiorly and anteriorly under the base of the tongue to shield the larynx and widen the hypopharynx, the cricopharyngeus relaxes, and the superior constrictor closes as the bolus passes into esophagus. The pharyngeal stage lasts a maximum of 1 second.

The fourth and final stage of swallowing is the *esophageal stage*, innervated by vagi and myenteric plexus. The esophageal stage is involuntary, with liquids usually falling by gravity and peristaltic wave pushes of solids. It is more variable and prolonged than the other phases of swallowing, lasting from between 8 and 20 seconds. Esophageal transit time significantly increases with age.

III. NEUROLOGIC EXAM

The diagnosis of the cause of dysphagia relies heavily on an accurate history and physical examination. Endoscopy and biopsies, as well as radiographic examinations, are confirmatory. Functional alterations in swallowing may be evaluated with modified barium swallow (MBS), fiberoptic evaluation of swallowing, scintigraphy, or pharyngeal manometry with fluoroscopy. (See Chapters 11-13.) Treatment is based on the etiology of the dysphagia. Treatment is also aimed at compensation or an alteration in swallowing, especially if the etiology is unknown or the effect is irreversible. Table 8-1 presents an outline that provides a guide to the diagnosis of neurogenic dysphagia.

Initially, it is important to determine whether dysphagia or odynophagia is the chief complaint. If odynophagia is the chief complaint, the location, timing, and duration of the pain, as well as any associated ear pain, change in pain with swallowing, weight loss, change in voice, or bloody sputum should be documented. If dysphagia is present, then the onset, duration, severity and timing of the dysphagia should be sought. In addition, dysphagia for solids versus liquids is important, and the perceived level of obstruction should be sought. Regurgitation may be oral or nasal and may fluctuate in severity. The patient should be questioned about weight loss and the presence or absence of hoarseness. Other symptoms such as arthritis, skin rash, or muscular complaints may point to the etiology of dysphagia.

Chronic cough may indicate aspiration. Aspiration is the entry of material into the airway below the true vocal folds. It is important because it may lead to acute and chronic pulmonary complications. However, the timing of aspiration in relation to swallowing can help elucidate the cause of a swallowing disorder. For example, aspiration that occurs prior to the reflexive swallow is due to either reduced tongue control or a delayed or absent swallow reflex. Aspiration during swallowing is due to inadequate airway closure. Aspiration after swallowing occurs because of retained pharyngeal residue, due to either reduced laryngeal elevation, reduced pharyngeal peristalsis, unilateral pharyngeal paralysis, or pharyngoesophageal dysfunction.

A great deal can be learned about a patient's swallowing difficulty during the neurological examination. The patient should be observed chewing and swallowing, with special attention paid to the degree of oral control, mastication ability, and the presence or absence of coughing. Examination of motor strength is a critical portion of the dysphagia examination. The presence of fluctuating motor strength, fatigue, and weakness of neck extensors and/or proximal muscles may give invaluable clues as to the underlying neuromuscular condition contributing to dysphagia.

The function of cranial nerves VII, IX, X, and XII should be closely examined as part of the dysphagia workup.[5] The facial nerve (VII) is evaluated with a complete head and neck and cranial nerve examination. Peripheral facial weakness is evidenced by fewer prominent wrinkles on the forehead of the affected side, (than on the other side), an eyebrow droop, a flattened nasolabial fold, and a turning down of the corner of the mouth. A patient with peripheral facial weakness is unable to wrinkle the forehead, raise the eyebrow, wrinkle the nasolabial fold, purse lips, show teeth, or completely close an eye, and shows the Bell phenomenon (visible vertical rotation of globe on closing the affected eye) on the affected side. With central facial paralysis, uncrossed contributions from ipsilateral supranuclear areas tend to spare movements of the frontal and upper orbicularis oculi. There may be facial movement on the affected side during emotional expression.

The neurological evaluation of dysphagia includes examination of the glossopharyngeal (IX) and vagus (X) nerves. Symmetry of upward palatal movement should

Table 8-1. *Neurological Differential Diagnosis of Neurogenic Dysphagia*

1. Involuntary phase of swallowing
   a. *Mechanical obstruction*
   Cancer of pharynx or base of tongue
   Neurogenic tumors and glomus tumors
   b. *Disordered function*
   Velopharyngeal insufficiency. Nasal regurgitation, choking, hypernasal voice. Cleft palate, stroke, ALS, bulbar palsy, myasthenia gravis. Palatal lift prosthesis or obturator mechanically maintains closure.
   c. *Inadequate pharyngeal wall mobility*
   Barium swallow shows incoordination, atonic pharyngeal walls, pooling in pyriform sinuses. Scleroderma, Duchenne muscular dystrophy (DMD), inflammatory myopathy, spinal muscular dystrophy (SMA), limb girdle muscular dystrophy (LGMD). Treatment includes pureed diet.
   d. *Laryngeal incompetence*
   Choking, coughing, and aspiration. Seen in laryngeal paralysis, sensory deficit, or incoordination due to neurologic disease. If aspiration significant, with infection or risk of infection, consider tracheotomy for pulmonary toilet and/or Teflon injection of vocal fold. Severe aspiration may require laryngeal closure.
   e. *Cricopharyngeal dysfunction*
   "Sticking" of food at level of cricoid cartilage. Liquids affected as well as solids. May have aspiration. Oculopharyngeal dystrophy, limb girdle muscular dystrophy (LGMD).

2. Voluntary phase of swallowing
   Mechanical obstruction
   Macroglossia—Duchenne muscular dystrophy (DMD) and a variety of storage disorders
   Cricopharyngeal spasm due to hypertrophy or dysfunction. Oculopharngeal dystrophy, limb girdle muscular dystrophy (LGMD), myotonic dystrophy.
   Zenker's diverticulum

3. Esophageal phase of swallowing
   a. *Mechanical obstruction*
   Esophageal cancer
   Benign esophageal tumors
   Esophagitis
   Esophageal rings, webs, or strictures
   Foreign body
   b. *Extrinsic compression*
   Thyroid, thymus, parathyroid, mediastinal nodes, atrial enlargement, vascular malformation, and so on
   c. *Diffuse esophageal spasm*
   Dermatomyositis, scleroderma, achalasia

be checked during a gag reflex. Furthermore, the patient may be asked to repeat sounds such as hard G's, which require rapid palatal elevation and relaxation, to check for a spastic palate, in which case those sounds cannot be produced rapidly because of delayed palatal relaxation. But the presence of a gag reflex does not necessarily mean the patient can swallow without risk of aspiration. In the setting of dysarthria, a swallowing evaluation may be necessary to rule out the risk of aspiration.

Evaluation of hypoglossal nerve (cranial nerve XII) includes inspection and testing of tongue function. The tongue should be checked for atrophy, midline protrusion, and strength of tongue movement to the left and right. Prominent atrophy and fasciculation of the tongue should raise the possibility of amyotrophic lateral sclerosis (ALS). Deviation of the tongue on attempted midline protrusion suggests weakness of the genioglossus muscle on the side to which the tongue is deviated because of a contralateral upper motor neuron lesion or an ipsilat-

eral lower motor neuron lesion. Inserting the examining finger into the mouth and having the patient press his or her tongue against the hard palate gives one an appreciation of any lingual muscular weakness. Asking the patient to repeatedly say the phrase "putaka putaka putaka" allows an estimate of fine motor coordination mediated by the cranial nerves VII and XII.

Supranuclear connections of cranial nerves VII and XII influence swallowing. Dysarthria and dysphagia, when associated with emotional lability, is suggestive of pseudobulbar palsy, a condition characterized by weakness of muscles innervated by the medulla (palate, pharynx, and larynx) because of interruption of corticobulbar fibers, as may be seen with multiple bilateral strokes. Motor neuron disease producing bulbar palsy, pseudobulbar palsy, or a combination of the two can present as gradually progressive dysphagia and dysarthria. Degenerative disorders such as dementias can present with swallowing apraxia.[6]

IV. LABORATORY EVALUATION OF NEUROGENIC DYSPHAGIA

A. Barium Swallow and Modified-Barium Swallow

Barium swallow and modified barium swallow (MBS) are commonly ordered to evaluate a patient's complaint of dysphagia (see Chapter 11). Barium contrast radiography is quite reliable for the diagnosis of neuromotor disorders that produce transfer and transit dysphagia. Videofluoroscopic recording permits slow motion and stop-frame analysis of the oropharyngeal stage of swallowing. Swallow function, using small and large boluses, including both liquids and solids, are evaluated during the modified barium swallow. It is the method of choice to evaluate suspected aspiration, and is helpful in diagnosing and planning the treatment of functional deficits such as those caused by neurologic disorders.[7]

The etiology of the swallowing dysfunction can often be found during the modified barium swallow and recommendations can be made regarding compensatory maneuvers and facilitating postures to permit swallowing without aspiration. Compensatory maneuvers should be tested during the MBS to rule out silent aspiration and to plan treatment strategies. The MBS provides radiographic support of the swallow dysfunction, when procedures such as vocal fold medialization or cricopharyngeal myotomy may be indicated.

Patients with neurogenic dysphagia typically have impairment of oropharyngeal motor performance and/or laryngeal protection. The functional evaluation of the oropharyngeal swallow can be accomplished by a videofluoroscopic swallowing study that assesses efficacy of functional elements within the swallow: nasopharyngeal closure, upper esophageal sphincter, airway protection, tongue loading, tongue propulsion, and pharyngeal clearance.[9]

During videofluoroscopy, management techniques are tailored for the particular impairment. For example, if aspiration occurs before the initiation of the pharyngeal phase because of weakness of the base of the tongue, the patient may be instructed and helped to flex the neck. Information is also obtained regarding pharyngeal peristalsis and cricopharyngeal malfunctioning. Because videofluoroscopy captures swallowing function for only a short finite period, it may underestimate swallowing impairment. False negative examinations can also be caused by poor patient concentration, anxiety, or fatigue. Because videofluoroscopy involves X ray exposure to the patient, all possible treatment techniques cannot be attempted during X ray. The clinician should select those techniques that are most appropriate for each patient's anatomy and swallow physiology prior to the study to limit exposure time. When effective techniques are identified, the videotape of the diagnostic procedure can be used as an educational tool with the patient and his or her family, nurses, physicians, and others to educate and counsel them regarding the rationale for use of particular procedures with the patient, including introduction of particular posture and diets. This type of visual evidence often improves patient and family compliance with therapy recommendations.[10]

Traditional barium swallow esophagogram is recommended for transit or obstructive symptoms. Conditions like achalasia or other dismotility disorders, webs, strictures, and neoplasms are well demonstrated by this study.

B. Endoscopy

Esophagoscopy is recommended for every patient with dysphagia because of the need to rule out or precisely define the location and nature of the obstructing lesion and to detect any lesion of significance whose presence may greatly influence therapeutic decisions. Videopharyngoesophagoscopy provides superb detail and permits biopsy and cytologic examination under direct vision. These methods offer a high diagnostic accuracy for carcinoma and strictures. Frequent tertiary contractions, aperistalsis, and hypertensive lower esophageal sphincter (LES) may be recognized endoscopically. Esophagoscopy is of value in the diagnosis of neuromotor disorders to evaluate for any associated disease contributing to the presence of dysphagia.[8]

C. Manometry and Manofluorography

Pharyngeal function involves rapid changes in pressure and motion; therefore, accurate measurement requires simultaneous fluoroscopy and solid state manometry or manofluorography. During swallowing, pharyngeal pressure is generated by the tongue, palate, larynx, and the pharyngeal walls. Manofluorography quantifies the pressure applied to the bolus from each of these structures. Therefore, the structure(s) responsible for the swallowing dysfunction may be identified. Disorders that cause transfer or transit types of dysphagia are best defined by careful study of motility patterns.

Manofluorography has been used to study the abnormal swallowing characteristics of neurogenic disorders. Examples include Wallenberg's syndrome, dermatomyositis, Guillian-Barré syndrome, and oculopharyngeal muscular dystrophy.[11]

V. MANAGEMENT OF NEUROGENIC DYSPHAGIA

A. Swallowing Therapy

In most cases, the introduction of therapy procedures into the diagnostic evaluation can immediately enable the patient to begin eating. In other cases, therapy procedures can be used with a patient to build neuromuscular control necessary to return to oral intake. Patients with neurological deficits of the oral or pharyngeal phases of swallowing may benefit from swallowing therapy. Swallowing therapy techniques may include strengthening and coordination exercises, or compensatory maneuvers to aid in swallowing. These techniques are presented in greater detail in Chapter 35.

The supraglottic swallow, Mendelsohn maneuver, and neck turning with swallowing are examples of compensatory maneuvers and are also reviewed in Chapter 35. Patients with unilateral pharyngeal paralysis can turn their head toward the paralyzed side, which diverts the bolus down the functioning side of the pharynx. Using these techniques, achievement of oral feeding is not associated with undue risk of pneumonia.[13]

Not all therapy procedures can be introduced into the diagnostic setting, however, as they do not all result in immediate effects. For example, range of motion exercises for the lips, tongue, and/or jaw do not have an immediate effect, but typically show an effect after 2 to 3 weeks. However, the clinician can still quantify the effects of range of motion exercises by measuring the patient's structural movement at each therapy session.

When a second assessment is completed, change in range of motion of the target structure can be assessed by comparing the first and second studies. Introducing treatment techniques into the diagnostic swallowing assessment requires the clinician to read the results of the radiographic study or other imaging procedure immediately and identify the physiologic dysfunction so that appropriate therapy procedures can be selected and introduced.

B. Surgery

Surgical treatment for dysphagia includes dilation, cricopharyngeal myotomy, laryngeal framework surgery, laryngotracheal separation, and gastrostomy. Dilation is the most common surgical procedure performed for dysphagia. Strictures, webs, and achalasia are often treated with dilation. The next most common procedure performed for dysphagia is cricopharyngeal myotomy.

The indications for cricopharyngeal myotomy are controversial. Cricopharyngeal myotomy will improve only those disorders with PE segment relaxation problems. Cricopharyngeal myotomy should be considered for disorders in which there is incomplete PE segment relaxation (pressure greater than 0 mm Hg) or abnormal muscular contractions during the relaxation period. Lower esophageal sphincter (LES) incompetence with reflux is a contraindication to cricopharyngeal myotomy, because this procedure may lead to worsening reflux with significant aspiration. Aspiration may

require surgical management if chronic in duration and unresponsive to swallowing therapy.[14]

Surgery can sometimes completely correct aspiration. Examples are aspiration due to a paralyzed abducted vocal fold and aspiration caused by Zenker's diverticulum. A paralyzed abducted vocal fold can be corrected with injection of Teflon, Gelfoam, fat, or surgical medialization (see Chapters 40 and 41). In patients with unremitting chronic aspiration, a tracheostomy may be indicated. However, tracheostomy does not prevent aspiration and may actually increase it. If patients with this severe form of aspiration wish to resume oral feeding, some type of laryngeal closure procedure may be required. These include supraglottic or glottic closure, laryngeal stints, cricoid resection, laryngoplasty, laryngotracheal diversion, or laryngectomy. None of the procedures is appropriate in all cases of refractory aspiration and treatment must be individualized.[15]

Oral feeding should be discontinued if aspiration is significant and a feeding tube should be put into place. If the feeding tube is required for more than 2 months, a percutaneous or open gastrostomy tube should be considered.

References

1. Buchholz DW. Dysphagia associated with neurological disorders. *Acta Otorhinolaryngol Belg.* 1994;48:143-155.
2. Groher ME. Dysphagic patients with progressive neurologic disease. *Semin Neurol.* 1996;16:355-363.
3. Logemann JA. Swallowing physiology and pathophysiology. *Otolaryngol Clin North Am.* 1988;21:613-623.
4. Logemann JA. Physiology. In: Cummings CW, Fredrickson JM, Harker LE, Krause CJ, Schuller DE, eds. *Otolaryngology—Head and Neck Surgery.* 2nd ed. St. Louis, Mo: Mosby; 1993:1704-1711.
5. Brazis PW, Masdeu JC, Biller J. *Localization in Clinical Neurology.* 2nd ed. Boston, Ma: Little, Brown; 1990.
6. Buchholz DW. Neurogenic dysphagia: what is the cause when the cause is not obvious? *Dysphagia.* 1994;9:245-255.
7. Castell DO. Approach to the patient with dysphagia. In: Yamada T, ed. *Textbook of gastroenterology.* New York, NY: JB Lippincott; 1991:562-572.
8. Ott DJ, Chen YM, Wu WC, Gelfand DW, Muniz HA. Radiographic and endoscopic sensitivity in detecting lower esophageal mucosal ring. *Am J Roentgenol.* 1986;147:261-265.
9. Kahrilas PJ. Current investigation of swallowing disorders. *Baillieres Clin Gastroenterol.* 1994;8:651-664.
10. Logemann JA. The dysphagia diagnostic procedure as a treatment efficacy trial. *Clin Commun Disord.* 1993;3:1-10.
11. McConnel FMS, Cerenko D, Mendelsohn MS. Manofluorographic analysis of swallowing. *Otolaryngol Clin North Am.* 1988;21:625-636.
12. Logemann JA. Screening, diagnosis, and management of neurogenic dysphagia. *Semin Neurol.* 1996;16:319-327.
13. Neumann S, Bartolome G, Buchholz D, Prosiegel M. Swallowing therapy of neurologic patients: correlation of

outcome with pretreatment variables and therapeutic methods. *Dysphagia*. 1995;10:1-5.

14. Wilson J, Pryde A, Allan P, Maran AG. Cricopharyngeal dysfunction. *Otolaryngol Head Neck Surg*. 1992;106:163-168.

15. McConnel FMS. Dysphagia. In: Gates GA, ed. *Current Therapy in Otolaryngology—Head and Neck Surgery*. 5th ed. St. Louis, Mo: Mosby; 1994:491-498.

CHAPTER 9

■ ■ ■

Evaluation of Swallowing Disorders: Rehabilitation in the Multidisciplinary Unit

Michael C. Munin, M.D.
Margaret M. Forbes, M.A.

I. INTRODUCTION

A rehabilitation unit is an interdisciplinary setting comprising dietitians, nurses, occupational and physical therapists, physicians, psychologists, and speech-language pathologists. This setting lends itself quite naturally to a team approach the diagnosis and treatment of dysphagia. Although each of these professionals has particular specialties and concerns in caring for patients, the group works as a team, discussing and formulating an overall plan for the maximum rehabilitation of each patient.

II. EVALUATION

A. History

Evaluation of dysphagia begins prior to a patient's admission to the rehabilitation unit. In most large acute-care hospitals, a speech-language pathologist assesses swallowing prior to entry. Usually, the speech-language pathologist in the rehabilitation unit can obtain information about a patient's swallowing history, either from the speech-language pathologist, the acute care unit staff, or from the patient's medical records. The records often include important information such as reports of previous videofluoroscopy examinations

(modified barium swallow [MBS]) or a history of aspiration pneumonia. As swallowing problems tend to have an impact on a patient's daily life, they are addressed early. The patient or the family can frequently provide useful information about the swallowing history. Although such information can be helpful, it is, of course, no substitute for an objective clinical evaluation of swallowing, as the ability to swallow can change rapidly.

B. Rehabilitation Unit

On a rehabilitation unit, physicians are usually the first to enquire about swallowing problems. If the patient reports problems or gives some indication that he or she is at-risk for aspiration, the physician consults the speech-language pathologist for an evaluation. On many rehabilitation units, all patients with diagnoses that affect the brainstem, motor centers, peripheral muscles, or the larynx are referred for evaluation. Patients with neurological or psychiatric disorders may deny that they have a problem, although a clinical swallow evaluation often makes it clear that swallowing is disordered.

The basic clinical examination is essentially the same as that conducted on an acute care unit. It includes a review of the patient's medical status, an oral examination, an assessment of cognitive and behavioral status, and observation of the patient swallowing a variety of consistencies of food and liquid. (See Chapter 5.) If the patient demonstrates clinical signs of aspiration, such as decreased volitional cough, coughing, choking, or voice change during the swallow, the speech-language pathologist recommends a modified barium swallow (MBS), which is ordered by the physician and conducted by a team consisting of a speech-language pathologist and a radiologist.

III. TREATMENT

Treatment is aimed at ascertaining safe swallowing of the quality and quantity of food needed to maintain or re-establish good nutritional status. The inability to do this may be caused by one or a combination of factors. The oral and pharyngeal swallowing mechanisms may be affected, and the problem can be compounded by factors such as decreased cognition, paralysis or paresis, deconditioning, or compromised gastrointestinal status. Each discipline provides input regarding the medical perspective on the swallowing problem. The speech-language pathologist works with the patient on self-monitoring and awareness of the difficulty and recommends food consistencies, posture modifications, and the appropriate level of supervision. The occupational therapist provides assistive eating devices and helps to train the patient in independent eating. The psychologist addresses the patient's emotional response to the swallowing difficulty, loss of, taste and the importance of nutritional needs.

IV. CASE EXAMPLE

A patient with a right hemisphere stroke serves to illustrate the rehabilitation team approach to dysphagia. Typically, these individuals have oropharyngeal dysphagia resulting from weakness and incoordination. The problem may be magnified by the patient's impulsivity in eating and drinking, and because of anosagnosia, the patient may deny that a problem exists. The otolaryngologist addresses the anatomical and functional status of the pharyngeal and laryngeal tract. The speech-language pathologist recommends a certain consistency for the patient's diet and works with the dietitian to make sure the patient's diet is nutritious and meets all dietary restrictions. The speech-language pathologist also instructs the patient regarding bolus size, safe neck and body positioning, and provides individualized swallowing precautions for the patient. The occupational therapist helps to incorporate dietary precautions during motor re-education of muscles required for food preparation. The occupational therapist can also suggest adaptive equipment such as built-up utensils to minimize effects of hand weakness from the

stroke. The psychologist helps the patient to recognize the left hemibody to minimize neglect and inattention. The rehabilitation unit physician recommends modifications, such as intravenous fluids or temporary use of alternate feeding methods, to maintain nutrition. Nurses or nurse aides supervise eating at meals, following the aspiration precautions posted at bedside for each dysphagic patient. The patient and family are also part of the team and are kept fully informed about the swallowing status of the patient.

Recent literature indicates that dysphagia teams are becoming more common.[1-4] A 1995 survey in Kentucky, for example, reported that 29% of that state's hospitals had interdisciplinary dysphagia teams.[4] Many practitioners advocate a multidisciplinary approach to the diagnosis and management of dysphagia.[1,2,4] These authors all believe a multidisciplinary approach improves patient outcome, but they do not report data to support these anecdotal impressions. The report published by Martens and colleagues[5] is the exception. Their group of 16 patients treated by a team showed significantly greater weight gain and increase in calorie intake than the comparison group of 15 patients treated by "existing ward routine."

V. SUMMARY

The goal of dysphagia treatment on a rehabilitation unit is to ensure that patients swallow safely a diet that is as normal as possible in consistency and variety. Achieving this goal involves the participation of practitioners from a number of disciplines. The multidisciplinary nature of a rehabilitation unit lends itself to this team approach, which many clinicians believe improves patient outcomes. Research is clearly needed to support the efficacy of an interdisciplinary team approach to swallowing in the rehabilitation setting.

References

1. Bach DB, Pouget S, Belle K, Kilfoil M, Alfieri M, et al. An integrated team approach to the management of patients with oropharyngeal dysphagia. *J Allied Health*. 1989;18:459-468.
2. Logemann JA. Multidisciplinary management of dysphagia. *Acta Otorhinolaryngol Belg*. 1994;48:235-238.
3. Atchison JW, Bryan D, Lumm S, Morgan M, Nickerson N, Niehaus A, et al. Dysphagia: diagnosis and treatment of Kentucky. *J Ky Med Assoc*. 1995;93:203-210.
4. Singh V, Brockbank MJ, Frost RA, Tyler S. Multidisciplinary management of dysphagia: the first 100 cases. *J Laryngol Otol*. 1995;109:419-424.
5. Martens L, Cameron T, Simonsen M. Effects of a multidisciplinary management program on neurologically impaired patients with dysphagia. *Dysphagia*. 1990;5:147-151.

CHAPTER 10

■ ■ ■

Clinical Evaluation of Swallowing: the Nutritionist's Perspective

Laura Molseed, M.S., R.D.

I. INTRODUCTION

Dysphagia, or difficulty swallowing, can have a significant impact on nutritional status, respiratory status, quality of life, and self-esteem.[1] Undiagnosed or untreated swallowing disorders may result in an array of macronutrient and micronutrient deficiencies and protein-calorie malnutrition.[1,2]

The importance of adequate nutrition care cannot be underestimated in this population. Early nutrition intervention can diminish the risk of aspiration, maintain strength and functional status, maintain immune function, and improve nutritional status.[1,2,3]

II. NUTRITION SCREENING

Early identification of swallowing disorders and potential nutritional deficiencies can minimize the complications often associated with malnutrition. One of the first signs of dysphagia is weight loss or changes in diet.[1,3] Nutrition screening is a method of early identification of potential nutrition problems and the prioritization of nutrition care. Nutrition screening incorporates both subjective and objective data. Recent changes in weight, chewing and swallowing difficulties, changes in appetite, and gastrointestinal (GI) problems are commonly noted. Mealtime observations and client/family interviews can also elicit nutrition and swallowing problems or dysphagia "triggers"[4] (Table 10–1). If any "triggers" are identified, the nutritionist should request assistance from a speech-language pathologist to assess the individual's safety and swallowing function.[4]

III. NUTRITION ASSESSMENT

When the nutrition screening identifies an individual to be at-risk for malnutrition or dysphagia, a nutrition evaluation should be completed. The primary goals for nu-

Table 10-1. *Dysphagia Triggers*

• Unintentional, recent, progressive weight loss	• Wet, "gurgly" voice
• Choking or coughing with eating/swallowing	• Complaints of food "sticking" in throat
• Complaints of pain with swallowing	• Unexplained aversion to particular foods
• Drooling	• Nasal regurgitation
• Poor lip closure	• Pocketing of food in cheek
• Excessive chewing	• Poor head control
• Poor body positioning	• Reduced attention span

trition professionals working with individuals with swallowing disorders are to:

■ Evaluate nutritional status
■ Establish nutrition goals in collaboration with the medical team
■ Determine the most appropriate method of meeting these goals
■ Monitor tolerance to the established nutrition plan
■ Assist the individual and/or caregiver in safely meeting these goals

Evaluating nutritional status involves a thorough review of a variety of medical, biochemical and nutrition factors[5] (see Table 10–2).

III. NUTRITIONAL REQUIREMENTS

Nutrition goals are established based on the findings of the nutrition assessment and a review of the swallowing plan. Calorie, protein, and fluid requirements should be estimated (Table 10–3) and the most appropriate method of meeting these requirements should be determined.[4,6] Oral feedings, enteral nutrition, or a combination of the two is often used to attain nutrition goals.

IV. MONITORING

Once the nutrition goals are established and a plan is implemented, the individual should be monitored routinely to determine his or her tolerance to the plan and the effectiveness of the nutritional therapy. Working with the individual and his or her family assures compliance with the developed plan and alerts the nutritionist to further swallowing complications.[7]

References

1. Baker DM. Assessment and management of impairments in swallowing. *Nur Clin North Am.* 1993;28:793-805.
2. Sitzman JV. Nutritional support of the dysphagic patient: methods, risks and complications of therapy. *JPEN.* 1990; 14:60-63.
3. Tripp F, Cordero O. Dysphagia and nutrition in the acute care geriatric patient. *Top Clin Nutr.* 1991;6:60-69.
4. Lewis MM, Kidder JA *Nutrition Clinical Practice Guidelines for Dysphagia.* Chicago, Ill: The American Dietetic Association; 1996.
5. Hammond, K. Nutrition focused physical assessment. *Support Line.* 1996;18:1-4.
6. Page CP, Hardin TC, Melnick G. *Nutritional Assessment and Support: A Primer.* 2nd ed. Baltimore, Md: Williams and Wilkins; 1994.
7. Mead Johnson Nutritionals. *Perspectives on Dysphagia: A Study Guide.* Evansville, Ind: Bristol-Myers, Squibb; 1990.

Table 10-2. *Components of a Nutrition Assessment*

Physical Exam

- Muscle and fat stores
- Coordination skills
- Presence of decubitus
- Skin turgor
- Ascites
- Feeding skills
- Dentition
- Edema
- Anthropometrics

Medical History

- Recent surgical history
- History of medical comorbidity
- Gastrointestinal history
- Review swallowing function
- Alterations of gastrointestinal tract
- Planned medical procedures
- Neuromuscular conditions
- Cognitive status

Nutrition History

- Diet history
- Food intolerances or aversions
- Complaints of anorexia
- Use of vitamin supplements
- History of pica eating
- Previous or current diet modifications
- Use of nutrition supplements
- Normal eating patterns
- Alcohol intake
- Ability to use utensils

Medication Review

- Drug/Nutrient interactions
- Administration schedule
- Impact on feeding schedule and ability to eat and cognitive status

Biochemical Data

- Visceral protein store measures (albumin, transferrin, prealbumin)
- Electrolytes
- Glucose
- Blood Urea Nitrogen/Creatinine
- Hemoglobin/Hematocrit
- Total lymphocyte count

Table 10-3. *Determining Nutritional Requirements*

Energy Requirements

Harris Benedict Equation:
   Men: $66 + 13.7 \text{ (wt)} + 5 \text{ (ht)} - 6.7 \text{ (A)} = \text{REE}$
   Women: $655 = 9.6 \text{ (wt)} + 1.8 \text{ (ht)} - 4.8 \text{ (A)} = \text{REE}$
wt = Weight in kg   ht = height in cm   A = Age

Calories per Kilogram: 25 kcal/kg = weight maintenance
                        25–30 kcal/kg = mild stress
                        30–35 kcal/kg = moderate stress
                        35–40 kcal/kg = severe stress

Protein Requirements

1.0 to 1.2 grams per kilogram for mild to moderate stress
1.2 to 1.5 grams per kilogram for moderate to severe stress

Fluid Requirements

1.0 cc/kcal or 30–35 cc/kg for most adults. Fluid requirements are increased in individuals with a fever, diarrhea, fistula, or tracheostomy. Fluid requirements are decreased in congestive heart failure, edema, renal failure, or liver failure and for geriatric patients.

PART III

EVALUATION

B. Functional Tests

The final four chapters of this section offer complementary information regarding functional tests of swallowing. Each of these tests offers specific and objective information used by each of the specialists who offer treatment for swallowing disorders.

CHAPTER 11

■ ■ ■

The Radiographic Evaluation of Dysphagia: The Barium Swallow (Pharyngoesophagram) and the Modified Barium Swallow

Jane L. Weissman, M.D.

I. INTRODUCTION

Barium studies play an important role in the evaluation of dysphagia.[1] There are two distinctly different barium studies available, the "traditional" barium swallow or pharyngoesophagram,[2,3] and the modified barium swallow (MBS)[3-5] (triphasic study, cookie swallow). These names are confusing, and there is no standardized terminology. It is therefore important that referring clinicians and radiologists "speak the same language" so that the appropriate examination is requested and performed.

II. TERMINOLOGY AND TECHNIQUES

A. Diagnostic Barium Swallow

A barium swallow ("traditional," or diagnostic barium swallow, pharyngoesophagram) evaluates the upper aerodigestive tract between the oral cavity or oropharynx and the gastric fundus or cardia. The names "esophagram" and "upper GI series" are inaccurate, as more than the esophagus is included and often the stomach and duodenum are not studied.

The subjective location of dysphagia does not always correspond to the anatomic location of pathology.[6] Therefore, the barium study to evaluate dysphagia should extend as low as the gastric fundus or cardia.[2] When the examination includes the entire stomach and duodenum, the name upper gastrointestinal series may be used.

Two techniques are available for performing a diagnostic barium swallow. The single contrast study fills and distends the lumen with thin liquid barium. Intrinsic mural irregularities and masses and extrinsic impressions are visible. An air-contrast study provides the same information and also allows a more detailed view of the mucosa.[6] For an air-contrast barium study, the patient ingests effervescent crystals followed by thick barium. The crystals dissolve and release gas that distends the lumen; dense barium then coats the mucosa of the distended lumen. A barium swallow has both dynamic and static components. The dynamic portion, fluoroscopy, can be recorded on tape (videofluoroscopy, cineradiography) for later review.[2] Frontal (anteroposterior) and lateral views of the hypopharynx are routinely obtained to evaluate morphology[6] and may be supplemented by oblique views, as indicated. The esophagus is best evaluated with oblique views so that the barium column is not superimposed on the spine.

The barium swallow can identify intrinsic and extrinsic pathology. Intrinsic abnormalities include tumors, cricopharyngeal dysfunction, aspiration of barium into the airway or reflux into the nasopharynx, diverticula, webs, and esophageal dysmotility. Extrinsic masses such as cervical osteophytes and an enlarged thyroid gland may be visualized directly or suspected by their effect on the barium column.

B. Modified Barium Swallow

The modified barium swallow is also called a videofluorographic swallowing study and a "cookie swallow."[3-5] The modified barium swallow is a multidisciplinary evaluation of the swallowing mechanism,[3] a collaboration between a radiologist and a speech-language pathologist (SLP). This examination is best suited for patients with the subjective complaint of dysphagia after a normal barium swallow has been obtained, for patients with postoperative swallowing dysfunction (after supraglottic laryngectomy, for example), and for patients with neuromuscular problems including stroke and other disorders of the central nervous system.[3-5]

Under fluoroscopic observation controlled by the radiologist, the patient ingests barium of varying consistencies offered to him or her at the discretion of the speech-language pathologist. The study usually starts with a thin liquid barium preparation and, if the patient is able, proceeds to barium the consistency of thick liquid, pudding, and solid (usually pieces of cookie or a marshmallow coated with barium). These consistencies are chosen to approximate the consistencies of food that a patient is likely to encounter in his or her daily diet. Some investigators use other preparations, such as deviled chicken and beef stew, to test the patient's ability to handle different consistencies of food.[4]

Frontal and lateral views are obtained during the modified-barium swallow with the patient standing or sitting. Unlike the diagnostic barium swallow, the modified barium swallow (MBS) is purely dynamic; the study is recorded on videotape, but static film images are usually not made.

The modified swallow concentrates on the oral, oropharyngeal, and hypopharyngeal phases of deglutition. This purely dynamic study evaluates formation of the bolus in the mouth; tongue motion; coordination, timing, and completeness of swallowing; movement of the epiglottis; elevation of the larynx; and cricopharyngeal contraction.[3]

III. PATHOLOGY

A. Diagnostic Barium Swallow

The development of sophisticated cross-sectional imaging, computed tomography (CT), and magnetic resonance imaging (MRI), when combined with the physical examination, has largely replaced barium evaluation of the oral cavity and oropharynx. Therefore, the diagnostic barium swallow usually commences with the hypopharynx.

The postcricoid region is seen best on lateral views (Fig 11-1a). Irregularity of the anterior wall of the hypopharynx at this level has been attributed to redundant mucosa[7] and a submucosal venous plexus.[7] This irregularity tends to be pliable and not fixed, as tumor would be. This is best appreciated on lateral dynamic (fluoroscopic) views and can be confirmed by endoscopy or CT scanning (Fig 11-1b), if necessary.

Lateral pharyngeal diverticula and pouches are probably of no clinical significance. Some authors make a distinction between pouches or pseudodiverticula (which are transient) and diverticula (which persist).[2]

The cricopharyngeus muscle is part of the upper esophageal sphincter.[2] Cricopharyngeal dyssynergy is abnormal coordination or timing of contraction of the cricopharyngeal muscle. The muscle should not indent the barium column when the bolus passes (Fig 11-2). A prominent cricopharyngeus has been reported in a small number of otherwise normal patients who are presumed to have gastroesophageal reflux (GER).[2] In these patients, the cricopharyngeus may protect the airway from the reflux.[2]

Cricopharyngeal dyssynergy appears as indentation by the contracted muscle on the posterior wall of the barium column at the level of the larynx (Fig 11-2). The muscle may fail to relax as the bolus arrives or contract too soon while the bolus is still present. Fibrosis of the cricopharyngeal muscle has also been documented by histological inspection.[8] Fibrosis may cause constant impression of the cricopharyngeus on the barium column. Static films may not be able to make the distinction between transient and constant cricopharyngeal dysfunction; dynamic videofluoroscopy provides the necessary information.

Longstanding cricopharyngeal dyssynergy presumably leads to formation of a Zenker's diverticulum (Fig 11-3). This is readily apparent on barium studies. Barium may collect in the diverticulum and stay there or the diverticulum may fill and empty over the course of the study. Carcinoma arising in a Zenker's diverticulum is exceedingly rare and may be suspected if the walls of the diverticulum are irregular or ulcerated. It is important not to mistake barium collecting around residual food within the diverticulum for ulceration of the wall.

Nasopharyngeal reflux (Fig 11-4) may be an isolated abnormality, but often accompanies other manifestations of neuromuscular incoordination, including tracheal aspiration of barium (Fig 11-4). Sometimes, cricopharyngeal dysfunction is associated with aspiration of barium. An impacted bolus of food causes acute dysphagia. The diagnosis is usually apparent from the history, but a barium swallow demonstrates the location of the bolus (Fig 11-5). The acute impaction usually causes mucosal edema. Therefore, a diagnostic barium swallow to identify the cause of the obstruction (tumor, stricture) should be deferred for days or weeks after removal of the impacted bolus until the mucosal edema subsides.

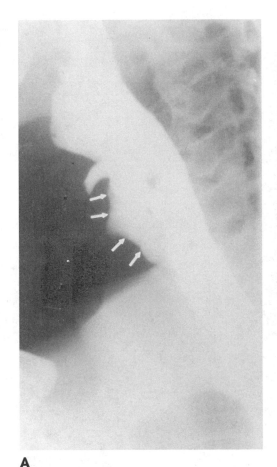

A

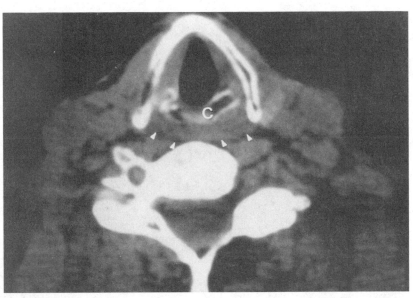

B

Fig 11-1. Normal postcricoid irregularity. **A.** Lateral view from a barium swallow shows an irregular postcricoid region (*arrows*). This appeared pliable on fluoroscopy and normal at endoscopy. This is the normal appearance of the postcricoid region. **B.** Axial CT scan of the same patient at the level of the cricoid cartilage (*c*) shows a normal post-cricoid hypopharynx (*arrowheads*).

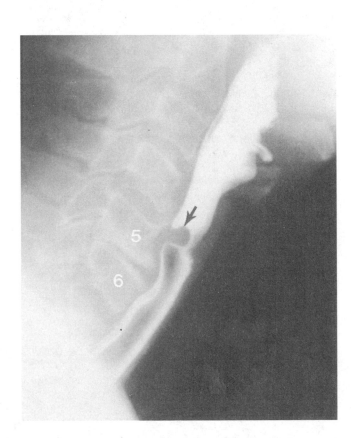

Fig 11-2. Cricopharyngeal dyssynergy. Lateral view of a barium swallow shows the impression of a prominent cricopharyngeus muscle (*arrow*) on the barium column. An osteophyte at C5-6 (5, 6) causes a smaller impression.

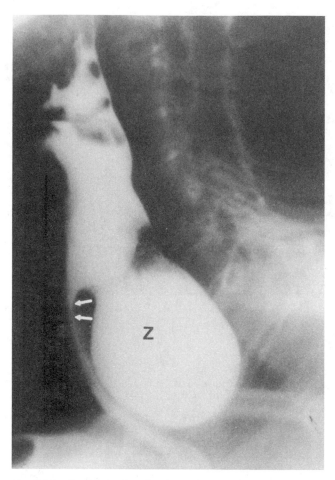

FIG 11-3. Zenker's diverticulum. Oblique view of the cervicothoracic junction shows a large Zenker's diverticulum (Z) that arises above a prominent cricopharyngeus muscle that narrows the barium column (*arrows*). The diverticulum fills completely and its walls are smooth.

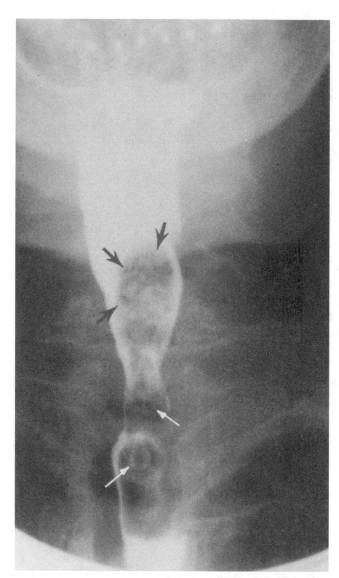

FIG 11-5. Impacted foreign body. Frontal view shows an irregular filling defect in the barium column at the level of the hypopharynx (*black arrows*). This was a shrimp the patient had been eating. Swallowed air is more lucent (*white arrows*).

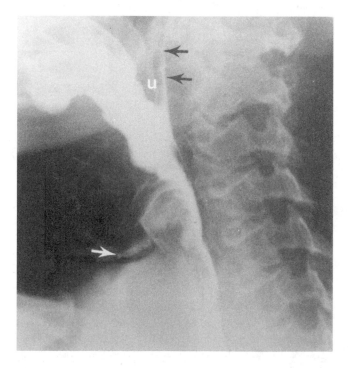

FIG 11-4. Nasopharyngeal reflux and tracheal aspiration. Lateral view from a barium swallow shows barium (*black arrows*) extending above the uvula (*u*) and soft palate. This is nasopharyngeal reflux. There is also barium in the trachea (*white arrow*), indicating that the patient aspirated.

Webs are thin, linear lucencies in the barium column (Fig 11-6). Webs usually arise from the anterior wall of the upper cervical esophagus.[9] They may be concentric and cause symptoms but are rarely obstructive.

Degenerative changes of the cervical spine that may cause dysphagia include osteophytes ("spurs") (Fig 11-7), and intervertebral disks that bulge anteriorly (Fig 11-7). Typical degenerative changes occur most often at C5-6; osteophytes at other levels, in the absence of disease at C5-6, suggest prior trauma may have caused (premature) degeneration.

An enlarged thyroid lobe may cause dysphagia by compressing the esophagus. The diagnosis can be suspected when there is a smooth, extrinsic impression on the barium column at the level of the thyroid gland and the mucosa is intact. Clinical examination, ultrasonography, or a CT scan can confirm the diagnosis.

In the thorax, extrinsic impressions on the esophagus are rare. Tortuous mediastinal vessels and mediastinal lymphadenopathy can be suspected by their location. Dysphagia lusoria is the dysphagia produced by an aberrant retroesophageal right subclavian artery pressing on the esophagus.[10] This congenital anomaly is not rare, being reported in approximately 1 in 200.[10] An aberrant retroesophageal left subclavian artery arising from a right aortic arch is much more rare. Symptoms are probably attributable to progressive compression of the esophagus by an atherosclerotic tortuous or dilated artery.[10] The location of the impression on the posterior thoracic esophagus just superior to the aortic arch is

characteristic (Fig 11-8a), and pulsation can sometimes be seen on fluoroscopy. A CT scan (Fig 11-8b) confirms the diagnosis.

Barium studies remain one of the most sensitive tests to detect carcinoma of the hypopharynx[2] and esophagus.[11] Although CT and MRI studies delineate bulky or deeply infiltrating tumors in great detail, superficial mucosal tumors may not be detected by CT or MRI. Irregularity of a wall on a barium study suggests an ulcerated tumor (Fig 11-9, a-c, Fig 11-10). Flattening (on static images) and abnormal motility (on videofluoroscopy) of a wall raises the possibility of submucosal spread of tumor, especially if the overlying mucosa appears to be intact on barium study and clinical examination. An exophytic tumor is a mass extending into (and displacing) the barium (Fig 11-9, a,c). Another presentation of a tumor is a small, persistent filling defect (Fig 11-11). Unlike an air bubble, which is mobile and transient, a tumor is seen in the same location on all images. In addition, a tumor is less lucent (less black) than an air bubble (Fig 11-11).

Esophageal dysmotility is frequently seen in elderly patients.[8,12] In this population, some dysmotility is probably to be considered normal.[8] Dysmotility may also be

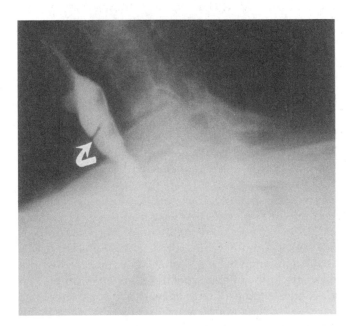

Fig 11-6. Esophageal web. Lateral view of the hypopharynx and cervical esophagus shows the thin, smooth, linear web arising from the anterior wall of the cervical esophagus (*arrow*). There is no obstruction to the flow of barium.

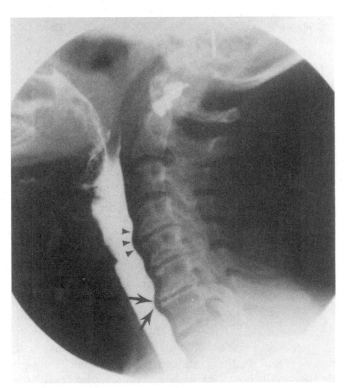

Fig 11-7. Osteophytes ("spurs"). Lateral view of a barium swallow shows anterior cervical osteophytes indenting the posterior wall of the barium-filled cervical esophagus at C6-7 (*arrows*). Anterior disk bulges or nonmineralized osteophytes also deform the barium column (*arrowheads*).

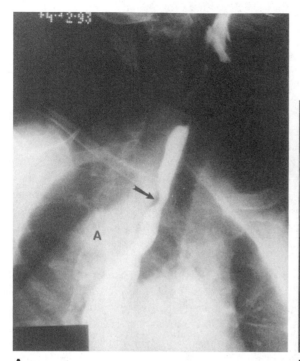

A

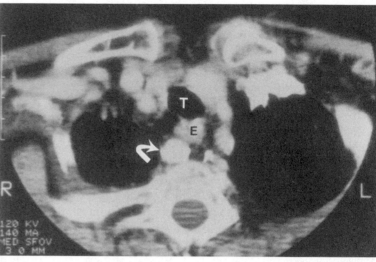

B

Fig 11-8. Aberrant retroesophageal right subclavian artery (dysphagia lusoria). **A.** Oblique view of the thoracic esophagus shows a smooth indentation (*arrow*) on the posterolateral wall of the esophagus just above the aortic arch (*A*). Under fluoroscopic observation, this indentation by the aberrant retroesophageal right subclavian artery pulsated. **B.** Axial CT scan shows an aberrant retroesophageal right subclavian artery (*arrow*) passing behind the esophagus (*E*) and trachea (*T*).

more pronounced in persons with diabetes, and, possibly, in patients with peripheral vascular disease. A diminished primary peristaltic wave, diffuse esophageal spasm,[11,12] and delayed, ineffective tertiary contractions can be seen both on dynamic and on static (Fig 11-12) components of the barium swallow.

A hiatal hernia is protrusion of stomach above the diaphragmatic hiatus for the esophagus (Fig 11-13). A lower esophageal ring is an indentation on the distal esophagus at the junction of the squamous mucosa of the esophagus and the columnar mucosa of the stomach.[13] When dysphagia or other symptoms are present, this ring is termed a Schatzki ring.[13]

Gastroesophageal reflux (GER) can occur whether a hiatal hernia is present or not. Reflux may be spontaneous or elicited. The Valsalva maneuver is one way to elicit reflux. Positioning the patient supine may also reveal reflux, as this position facilitates reflux through the normally posterior gastroesophageal junction—the level to which barium refluxes should be recorded. It is important that the esophagus be completely cleared of swallowed barium before looking for reflux, as swallowed barium (moving down) can be mistaken for reflux barium. The diagnosis of reflux must be made on the dynamic portion of the study. On static films, it is impossible to determine if barium in the esophagus is

going down (as part of a normal swallow) or up (reflux). Failure to observe spontaneous reflux or to elicit reflux with maneuvers during a barium study does not mean that gastroesophageal reflux (GER) does not occur at other times.

Chronic GER may cause a long, smooth, tapered stricture of the lower thoracic esophagus.[9] Reflux may also cause esophagitis, which can be diagnosed on barium studies. The etiology (reflux) of the esophagitis can be suspected because of the lower thoracic esophageal location, even if reflux is not elicited.

In immunosuppressed patients, candida esophagitis can be seen on air-contrast barium studies as small ulcerations or as plaques that vary from small and granular plaques to large and confluent.[9,11] Herpes esophagitis causes innumerable small ulcerations[9,11]; CMV esophagitis may have a similar appearance.[11] Because these are mucosal abnormalities, they are seen best on air-contrast studies. Graft-versus-host disease after bone marrow transplantation tends to cause cervical esophagitis and strictures.[9]

Tumors of the gastric fundus or cardia can present with hypopharyngeal or cervical dysphagia.[6] For this reason, a complete barium evaluation of the patient with dysphagia should include single- or double-contrast views of the gastric fundus and cardia, preferably after

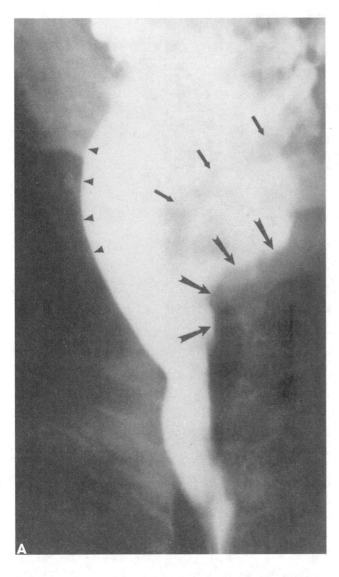

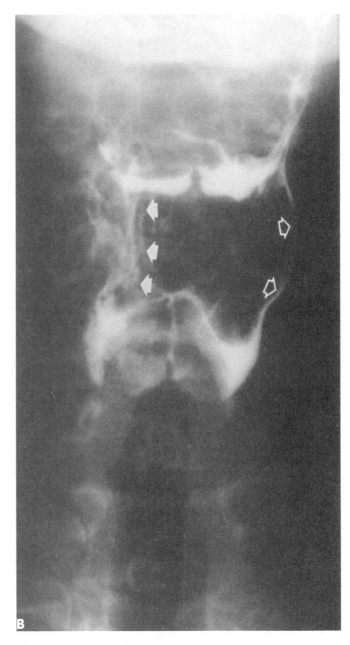

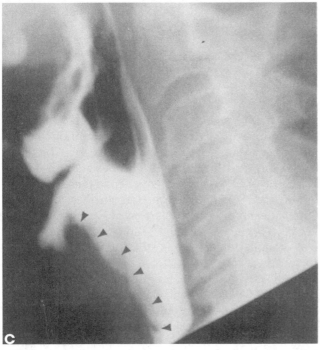

Fig 11-9. Hypopharyngeal carcinoma. **A.** Frontal view from a single-contrast barium swallow shows an ulcerated squamous cell carcinoma as a pronounced irregularity of the lateral wall of the left pyriform sinus (*large arrows*), and a mass within the lumen (*small arrows*). The right pyriform sinus is normal (*arrowheads*). **B.** Frontal view of another patient's double-contrast barium swallow shows barium coating the bulky, irregular mucosal tumor of the right pyriform sinus (*solid arrows*). Barium also coats the smooth, normal mucosa of the left pyriform sinus (*open arrows*). **C.** Lateral view of the hypopharynx shows irregularity of the postcricoid region (*arrowheads*), which is more pronounced than the normal postcricoid irregularity (see A), and was not pliable at fluoroscopy. This was postcricoid (hypopharyngeal) invasion by a laryngeal squamous cell carcinoma.

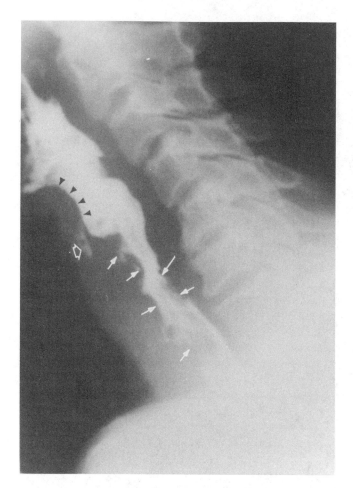

FIG 11-10. Cervical esophageal carcinoma. Lateral view of the cervical esophagus shows the ulcerated tumor (*solid arrows*) replacing the mucosa along the anterior and posterior walls of the cervical esophagus. This tumor is lower and more extensive than the normal postcricoid irregularity (*arrowheads*), and was fixed, not pliable, under fluoroscopic observation. The patient aspirated a small amount of barium (*open arrow*).

the patient has fasted so that the stomach no longer contains food.

B. Modified Barium Swallow

The modified swallow is the best way to evaluate the oral and pharyngeal phase of swallowing. Pathology that may cause dysphagia includes abnormal movements of the tongue in forming the bolus and initiating deglutition, residual barium that pools in the valleculae or pyriform sinuses, and aspiration of barium into the airway.[3-5] Because the entire fluoroscopic study is recorded on videotape, the study can provide a highly detailed analysis of the coordination and timing of swallowing.

It is never normal for barium to enter the airway. Aspiration of barium into the airway may be the most

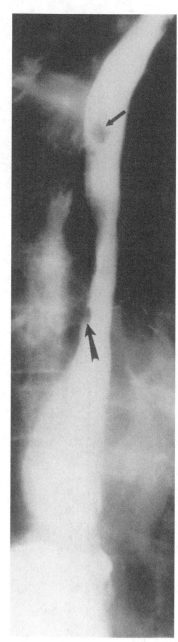

FIG 11-11. Thoracic esophageal carcinoma. Oblique view of the thoracic esophagus shows a small mass (*large arrow*) that was present on all views. This represented a second primary squamous cell carcinoma in a patient with a known squamous cell carcinoma of the floor of the mouth. The lucency just above the tumor (*small arrow*) was an air bubble, and disappeared on subsequent views.

important observation the team performing the modified barium swallow can make.[5] The location and extent of aspiration should be defined clearly. The terms "aspiration" and "penetration" are not standardized and have been used by authors who define these terms differently.[3,5] To complicate matters further, the terms "glottic penetration" and "laryngeal penetration" have also been used.[4] As with the "traditional" barium swallow, nasopharyngeal reflux of barium should also be documented.

The clearest and most clinically useful solution to the problem of terminology to describe barium in the airway is to state the location of the barium that extends lowest into the airway. This may be as subtle as coating of the laryngeal surface of the epiglottis or as obvious

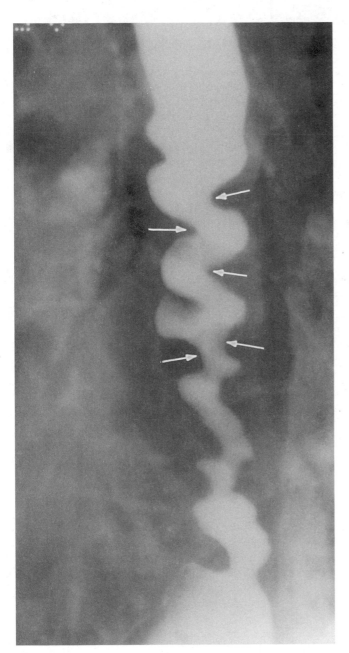

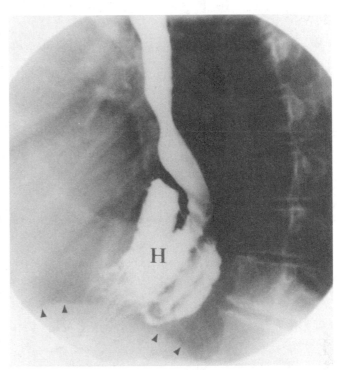

FIG 11-13. Hiatal hernia. Oblique view of the gastroesophageal junction shows a moderately large hiatal hernia (*H*) above the diaphragm (*arrowheads*).

FIG 11-12. "Corkscrew esophagus" (tertiary contractions). Oblique view of the thoracic esophagus shows irregularly spaced contractions (*arrows*) causing indentations of the thoracic esophagus. At fluoroscopy, this was transient but recurred and the bolus was ineffectively propelled through the thoracic esophagus. This elderly woman complained of substernal dysphagia.

gross aspiration of barium into the lower tracheobronchial tree.

The modified barium swallow can often identify the cause of aspiration. Abnormal motion of the epiglottis, diminished contractions of the pharyngeal constrictor muscles, abnormal laryngeal "rise" can all be identified on the modified barium swallow. "Silent" aspiration is aspiration into the tracheobronchial tree that fails to

elicit a normal cough response to clear the barium. Silent aspiration is evidence of underlying neurological dysfunction. Silent aspiration may remain undetected on clinical (bedside) swallowing examination, but is readily apparent on the modified barium swallow.[5]

If barium enters the airway, the effectiveness of "airway-protective maneuvers" and varying the consistency of the barium bolus can be assessed directly by viewing under fluoroscopy. Fluoroscopic examination has been shown to be far more sensitive to even small amounts of aspiration than a bedside swallowing study.[3] Maneuvers include prompted coughing if the patient does not cough spontaneously (silent aspiration), repeated swallowing to clear retained barium,[4] neck flexion to propel the bolus into the esophagus or neck extension to allow gravity to assist in swallowing,[4] various tilting and turning positions of the head,[4,5] and the "supraglottic swallow" to close the larynx before swallowing.[4]

VI. SUMMARY

Both the barium swallow and modified barium swallow evaluate deglutition and the upper aerodigestive tract. The two studies provide different information, which may be complementary. Understanding the strengths and weaknesses of each makes it easier to obtain the best study for each patient.

References

1. Goyal RK. Diseases of the esophagus. In: Isselbacher KJ, Braunwald E, Wilson JD, Martin JB, Fauci AS, Kasper DL, eds. *Harrison's Principles of Internal Medicine*. 13th ed. New York, NY: McGraw-Hill, Inc; 1994:1355-1363.
2. Rubesin SE. Oral and pharyngeal dysphagia. *Gastroenterol Clin North Am.* 1995;24:331-352.
3. Gustafson-Yoshida N, Maglinte DDT, Hamaker RC, Kelvin FM. Evaluation of swallowing disorders: the modified barium swallow. *Indiana Med.* 1990;83:892-895.
4. Palmer JB, Kuhlemeier KV, Tippett DC, Lynch C. A protocol for the videofluorographic swallowing study. *Dysphagia.* 1993;8:209-214.
5. Dodds WJ, Logemann JA, Stewart ET. Radiologic assessment of abnormal oral and pharyngeal phases of swallowing. *Am J Roentgenol.* 1990;154:965-974.
6. Levine MS, Rubesin SE. Radiologic investigation of dysphagia. *Am J Roentgenol.* 1990;154:1157-1163.
7. Pitman RG, Dodds WJ. The postcricoid impression on the esophagus [letter and reply]. *Am J Roentgenol.* 1992;158: 690-691.
8. Ekberg O, Feinberg MJ. Altered swallowing function in elderly patients without dysphagia: radiologic findings in 56 cases. *Am J Roentgenol.* 1991;156:1181-1184.
9. Karasick S, Lev-Toaff AS. Esophageal strictures: findings on barium radiographs. *Am J Roentgenol.* 1995;165:561-565.
10. Nguyen P, Gideon RM, Castell DO. Dysphagia lusoria in the adult: associated esophageal manometric findings and diagnostic use of scanning techniques. *Am J Gastroenterol.* 1994;89:620-623.
11. Levine MS, Rubesin SE, Ott DJ. Update on esophageal radiology. *Am J Roentgenol.* 1990;155:933-941.
12. Weissman JL. Corkscrew esophagus. *Am J Otolaryngol.* 1993; 14:53-54.
13. Rohrmann CA. When is a Schatzki ring clinically significant? [letter]. *Am J Roentgenol.* 1994;163:215.

CHAPTER 12

■ ■ ■

Functional Tests of Swallowing

Thomas Murry, Ph.D.
Ricardo L. Carrau, M.D., F.A.C.S.

I. INTRODUCTION

The functional assessment of dysphagia has seen a proliferation of techniques and methods since the introduction of the modified barium swallow examination.[1] Some of these techniques may not be unique to swallow assessment, but nonetheless offer specific functional information to identify the causes of dysphagia and suggest treatments (see Table 12-1). In each of these tests, the emphasis is on swallow function rather than on simply identifying the presence or absence of aspiration. By identifying the phase of swallowing that is dysfunctional, rehabilitation specialists can offer strategies targeted to the specific problems seen in each phase of swallowing.

II. TESTS

A. FEES (Fiberoptic Endoscopic Evaluation of Swallowing)

The FEES assessment was first described by Langmore, Shatz, and Olson.[2] The assessment of swallowing using this technique requires the passage of a fiberoptic nasendoscope into the nares, over the velum to a position above the epiglottis. Specific amounts of liquids and food consistencies treated with food dye are viewed as they pass the pharynx and larynx. During the time of airway closure, the swallow cannot be visualized, as the pharyngeal walls contract over the bolus, collapsing the lumen over the endoscope ("whiteout

Table 12-1. *Functional Information Provided by Techniques Used to Assess Swallow Function*

	Defines Anatomy	Detects Aspiration	Quantifies Aspiration	Detects Etiology	Availability	Cost*
MBS	+	++	+	+	+	3
FEES	++	+	2	+	++	2
U/S	±	2	2	2	±	4
Bedside Evaluation	2	+†	2	±	++	1
Scintigraphy	2	++	++	2	±	5

*Order from least to most expensive
† Can detect actual aspiration in patients with tracheotomies

phase"). Monitoring of the bolus is only possible before and after the pharyngeal swallow. However, the bolus can be monitored as it enters into view from the oral cavity to the pharynx. The speed of the pharyngeal swallow, premature flow of food or liquid into the pharyngeal and laryngeal areas, and residual amounts of the bolus can all be seen during this examination. The endoscope may remain in place for long periods, to monitor the residual bolus and examine anatomical structures. Swallowing, using compensatory strategies and changes in neck position, is easily accomplished while the endoscope is in place. FEES is more sensitive than MBS in detecting subtle abnormalities of the palate, pharynx, and larynx and provides better anatomical information than the MBS. It does not completely assess the oral phase and does not evaluate the esophageal phase of swallowing.

The examination should be performed by an individual trained in the proper and safe use of the endoscope as well as trained to understand the normal anatomy and physiology of swallowing. This test is often performed by an otolaryngologist and speech-language pathologist. A video camera and recorder coupled to the endoscope provide a permanent record of the examination for later review by clinicians and patient and to serve as a baseline to monitor the patient's progress. In selected cases, FEES can provide a patient with visual feedback that may aid the rehabilitation process.

1. Indications

A FEES examination is indicated if the clinical examination and/or bedside swallow assessment suggest the presence of swallowing dysfunction. This examination may be particularly useful when a patient cannot be easily transported to a radiology unit, has a significant voice quality change, has limited ability to follow directions, and/or is on a ventilator. The equipment needed for the FEES examination is portable and, thus, the test can be easily performed in either the outpatient office setting or at the bedside.

2. Procedure

The FEES is done following a clinical interview and examination (bedside swallow examination). The nasal cavity is decongested and topical anesthesia is applied using cotton tip applicators to avoid anesthetizing the pharynx. Before liquid or food is offered to the patient, the endoscope is placed and the examiner notes the anatomic structures and observes the functions of the velum (sustained phonation, repeating "coca cola"), epiglottis, and larynx. Trial "dry" swallows to observe laryngeal elevation are prompted and phonation to ob-

serve vocal fold closure is elicited. The amount of retained secretions present in the vallecula and hypopharynx is also noted. Pharyngeal and laryngeal functions should be documented with different bolus consistencies and amounts, along with various positional changes of the head. The supraglottic swallow and chin tuck strategies may also be used to identify the possible causes of dysphagia. Figure 12-1 shows a frame from a FEES exam in which the patient has residual amounts of liquid in the piriform sinus and laryngeal inlet.

3. Contraindications

The FEES may not be indicated for patients with extreme movement disorders, those who cannot tolerate the endoscope, or those who have a history of bronchospasm or laryngospasm.

B. FEES ST (fiberoptic endoscopic evaluation of swallowing with sensory testing)

This procedure employs the standard FEES testing with the addition of sensory testing of the supraglottic mucosa to determine the presence of a sensory dysfunction in dysphagic patients. To do the test, an air pulse generator is used to send a pulse of air through a port in a specially designed flexible endoscope. Air

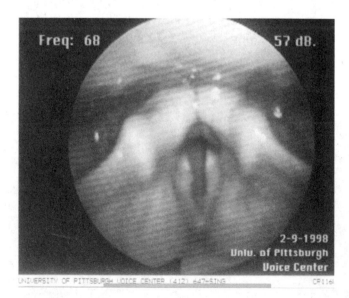

FIG 12-1. FEES Procedure: View of larynx following swallow of liquid by a 58-year-old male with bilateral vocal fold paresis and atrophy. Note the presence of liquid on the right vocal fold and a drop of liquid between the vocal folds, anteriorly.

pulses can be delivered to the supraglottic larynx and pharynx areas. Sensory thresholds can then be determined using one of the psychophysical testing methods. This procedure was first described by Aviv et al in 1993.[3]

FEES ST can be added to any FEES examination once the examiner has the stimulator, a method for delivery of air pulse and a method to record the response. Testing of sensory function is rather new, although silent aspiration in patients with sensory loss has been reported for some time.[4,5] Although FEES ST is not yet a standard office protocol, its value has been demonstrated and its use will continue to grow as the system for performing the test becomes easier to use and less expensive to obtain. FEES ST is especially useful in aging patients who progressively lose sensory discrimination ability in the oral cavity and pharynx.[6]

C. Scintigraphy

Scintigraphy is a procedure used to track movement of the bolus and quantify the residual bolus in the oropharynx, pharynx, larynx, and trachea. This is done by having the patient swallow a small amount of a radionuclide material (such as Technetium 99m) combined with liquid or food. A special camera (gamma camera) records images of the organs of interest over time to obtain a quantitative image of the transit and metabolic aspects.

1. Indications

The indications for scintigraphic assessment of swallowing are a history of swallowing disorders, airway penetration of foods or liquids, cough associated with swallowing, aspiration, delayed cough after swallowing, pneumonia, or possibly pulmonary aspiration from gastric sources.[7] As there is no time limit for the testing, scintigraphy can be used to identify trace aspiration and quantify the aspiration over short or long time periods. Scintigraphy can also be used to calculate the transit time and residual "pooling" of a bolus in patients suffering degenerative neuromuscular diseases, before and after treatment.[8] Perhaps the strongest indication for scintigraphy is to identify patients who, despite limited aspiration, have the ability to clear the aspirate quickly or those on whom the aspirate does not reach the distal airways—thus identifying a subset of patients who may be fed by mouth

2. Procedure

Scintigraphy is typically performed in the nuclear medicine test suite by trained personnel. Cobalt markers are fixed to the skin at the angle of the mandible and anterior cricoid to identify oral and pharyngeal regions. Patients are then given a bolus mixed with a radionuclide. The camera with its collimator is triggered and the patient swallows the bolus. Data acquisition may be continuous at frame rates of up to 25/sec. Acquisition of data from the oral cavity to the thoracic and even upper abdominal cavities may be dynamic during the swallow and then followed by static images over longer time periods ranging from several minutes to several hours. The results are generally reported in time-activity curves.[9]

The precise amount of aspiration or residual bolus may be identified through computer analysis of the scans made at various time intervals. With the use of scintigraphy, the amount of aspirate in each region may be quantified. Moreover, as the examination can be followed over a longer time than with fluoroscopy and as swallowing water can identify regions where the bolus is cleared or reduced, scintigraphy offers a valuable tool to identify and quantify aspiration and to ascertain the ability of the patient to clear the aspirate (ie, tracheobronchial clearance) without the prolonged radiation exposure required by fluoroscopy.[9] Scintigraphy may be more sensitive than barium swallow studies for long-term assessment of bolus location and it has the added advantage of permitting the use of common food as the bolus.

Despite its objective quantitative analysis of aspiration, scintigraphy does not provide an adequate definition of the anatomy of the upper aerodigestive tract. Currently, scintigraphy is more costly than videofluorography or FEES.

3. Contraindications

As this test requires cooperation from the patient, not all patients are candidates for this test. Patients with known movement disorders, severe cognitive disorders, and the inability to remain standing or sitting in front of the gamma camera may not be candidates for this test.

D. Ultrasound

This technique uses high frequency sounds (>2 MHz) from a transducer held or fixed in contact with skin to obtain a dynamic image of soft tissues. As ultrasound does not penetrate bone, its use is limited to the soft tissues of the oral cavity and parts of the oropharynx. The ultrasound transducer is usually placed beneath the chin. By rotating it, one can get sagittal and coronal images. This technique is completely noninvasive; therefore, repeated studies can be done without risk. Because it is noninvasive, it is highly useful for children or when multiple swallows are required to make a diagnosis. The swallowing functions of the upper surface of the tongue, the intrinsic tongue muscles, and the soft tissue anatomy of the mouth are within the "view" of the transducer. The motion of the hyoid can be tracked, as it casts a shadow on the sonogram to note the termination of the oral and pharyngeal phases of the swallow.[10]

1. Procedure

In ultrasound studies of swallowing, a hand-held transducer is placed submentally and is rotated 90°. Peng and colleagues describe a cushion scanning technique that reduces movement of the scanner and compression of the submental region during the swallow.[11]

Ultrasonography provides a method to study tongue morphology and identify lingual tumors, as well as a method to study tongue movement and control of bolus in the oral preparation and oral phases of swallowing. Ultrasonography does not require the use of any special bolus or contrast (real food can be used). As the technique is noninvasive and does not require exposure to radiation, it is a completely safe way to study infant tongue patterns for speech as well as swallowing.

The introduction of intraluminal ultrasound probes has allowed the evaluation of the esophageal wall thickness. Endoluminal ultrasonography has been used for the study of esophageal and cricopharyngeal diseases, including esophagitis, strictures, and motility disorders.[12] (See Chapter 13.)

2. Contraindications

If dysphagia due to pharyngeal or laryngeal dysfunction is suspected, this technique offers little diagnostic or treatment information. Ultrasound waves cannot penetrate the hyoid bone. Also, as there is a need to maintain consistent contact on the soft tissue with the transducer, any extreme movement disorder may induce artifacts that would make it difficult to interpret tongue movement associated with bolus control with this method.

Intraluminal probes are invasive and thus are not tolerated by all patients. The use of ultrasound intraluminal probes requires a high degree of experience and sometimes the probe cannot be passed through a tight stricture.

E. Magnetic Resonance Imaging

High speed magnetic resonance imaging (MRI), such as fast low angle shot (FAST) or echoplanar imaging, has allowed a dynamic analysis of the pharyngeal phase of swallowing that was impossible using conventional MRI.[13,14] The pharyngeal cavity, oral cavity, laryngeal lumen, and musculature can be evaluated during motion, allowing the assessment of the swallowing mechanism.

During a FAST MRI, intravenous contrast is injected into the patient and the patient is given an oral contrast containing ferric ammonium sulphate as a food bolus substitute. Images are obtained as the bolus is moved from the oral cavity to the esophagus. This technique, however, can only assess the activity of the oral cavity and pharynx during short periods of time.

MRI has the advantage of not involving exposure to radiation. However, temporal and spatial resolution of MRI is inferior to videofluoroscopy, producing images with poor resolution. Thus, the need for both intravenous and oral contrast, which highlights the tissue and tissue-air/liquid interfaces, improving the resolution of images.[13]

MRI is costly and swallowing in the supine position may not reflect the true physiologic mechanism of swallowing. Similarly, patient acceptance is reduced, despite its noninvasive nature, because the narrow gantry induces claustrophobia in many patients. In addition, if aspiration occurs in the gantry of the MRI machine, it cannot be easily treated and usually requires aborting the study.

At present, this technique is considered experimental, although technological advances may soon lead to more affordable MRI with better imaging quality.

References

1. Logemann J. *Evaluation and treatment of swallowing disorders.* San Diego, Calif: College-Hill Press; 1983.
2. Langmore S, Shatz K, Olsen N. Fiberoptic endoscopic examination of swallowing safety in a new procedure. *Dysphagia*, 1988;2:216-219.
3. Aviv J, Martin JH, Keen MS, Debell M, Blitzer A. Air pulse quantification of supraglottic and pharyngeal sensation: a new technique. *Ann Otol Rhinol Laryngol.* 1993;102:777-780.
4. Zavala DC. The threat of aspiration pneumonia in the aged. *Geriatrics,* 1997;32:46-51.
5. Horner J, Massey E, Riski J, Lathrop D, Chase K. Aspiration following stroke: clinical correlates and outcome. *Neurology,* 1988;38:1359-1362.
6. Aviv J, Martin JH, Sacco RL, et al. Supraglottic and pharyngeal sensory abnormalities in stroke patients with dysphagia. *Ann Otol Rhinol Laryngol.* 1996;105:92-97.
7. Horsely JR, Sproule BJ. Radio-isotope evaluation of nocturnal aspiration in patients with chronic obstructive pulmonary disease. *Postgrad Med J.* 1986;62:69-70.
8. Wang S-J, Chia L-G, Hsu C-Y, Lin W-Y, Kao CH, Yeh S-H. Dysphagia in Parkinson's disease: assessment by solid phase radionuclide scintigraphy. *Clin Nucl Med.* 1994;19: 405-407.

9. Hamlet S, Choi J, Kumpuris T, Holiday J, Stackler R. Quantifying aspiration in scintigraphic deglutiton testing: tissue attenuation effects. *J Nucl Med*. 1994;35:1007-1013.

10. Shawker T, Sonies B, Stone MN, Baum B. Real-time ultrasound visualization of tongue movement during swallowing. *J Clin Ultrasound*, 1983;11:485-490.

11. Peng CL, Jost-Brinkmann P, Miethke R. The cushion scanning technique: a method of dynamic tongue sonography and its comparison with the transducer-skin coupling scanning technique during swallowing. *Acad Radiol*. 1996;3:239-244.

12. Sobin J, Nathanson A, Engstrom CF. Endoluminal ultrasonography: a new method to evaluate dysphagia. *J Otorhinolaryngol*. 1996;58:105-109.

13. Suto Y, Kamba M, Kato T. Dynamic analysis of the pharynx during swallowing using Turbo-FLASH magnetic resonance imaging combined with an oral positive contrast agent—a preliminary study [technical note]. *Br J Radiol*. 1995;68:1099-1102.

14. Gilbert RJ, Daftary S, Woo P, Seltzer S, Shapshay SM, Weisskoff RM. Echo-planar magnetic resonance imaging of deglutitive vocal fold closure: normal and pathologic patterns of displacement. *Laryngoscope*, 1996;106:568-572.

CHAPTER 13

■ ■ ■

Gastroenterologic Evaluation of Swallowing

Sukhdeep Padda, M.D.
Michele A. Young, M.D.

I. INTRODUCTION

This chapter is a discussion of invasive techniques that complement the clinical and radiological evaluation presented in Chapter 7.

II. ENDOSCOPIC TESTS

A. Fiberoptic Endoscopic Examination

Fiberoptic endoscopic examination of swallowing (FEES) is a relatively new procedure performed by otolaryngologists in the assessment of the pharyngeal phase of swallowing in patients with dysphagia. The pharyngeal area is intubated with a very narrow diameter flexible nasopharyngolaryngoscope in patients for whom traditional videofluoroscopic evaluation may be difficult or impossible to perform.[1] This procedure can often be done at the bedside with minimal discomfort to the patient. This technique is used to detect aspiration and to determine the safety of oral feeding in patients with probable oropharyngeal dysphagia. A clear and direct view of the hypopharynx and larynx can be obtained and studied without interfering with the function of the other structures.

B. Endoscopic Ultrasound

Endoscopic ultrasound (EUS) is a recently developed method that combines the benefits of endoscopy and ultrasound into one radiographic imaging instrument. EUS is helpful in evaluating both mucosal and intramural abnormalities, which may result in dysphagia.[2,3] It is especially important in the evaluation of submucosal lesions, which cannot be adequately assessed with standard endoscopic techniques. Ultrasound imaging systems consist of a probe (ultrasonic transducer), an electronic processor for activating the transducer and processing the echo, an imaging device, and accessories (balloon, water). Two types of ultrasound endoscopes have been developed and are commercially available: the mechanically rotating radial imaging transducer and the convex phased array electronic transducer. Both of these instruments have oblique viewing optics and standard endoscopic capabilities, which allow optically guided advancement and positioning of the ultrasound transducer. The primary difference between the two types of ultrasound endoscopes is the direction of scanning. A mechanically rotated transducer at the tip of the radial scanning instrument produces a 360° circular image in a plane perpendicular to the shaft of the endoscope. Radial scanning instruments produce a radial 360° image, which is easier to orient and therefore has wider appeal for gastroenterologists.

1. Procedure

The esophagus is intubated with the endoluminal ultrasound instrument to the level of the lesion to be examined, at which point a water-filled balloon is inflated and the images are recorded. If the lesion is suspected to be a malignancy, then the scope will be advanced into the stomach to obtain images of the celiac nodes. Throughout the GI tract, the wall layer echo structure is examined endosonographically. The layer in closest proximity to the transducer is an echo-rich layer that offers a border echo as the ultrasound waves exit the water surrounding the transducer, pass through the surrounding balloon, and enter the gut wall. The second layer is an echo-poor layer, which roughly corresponds to the mucosa. The third layer is an echo-rich layer, which roughly corresponds to the submucosa. The fourth layer is an echo-poor layer, which represents the muscularis propria. The fifth layer is an echo-rich layer, which corresponds to a border echo with surrounding fat in the esophagus and corresponds to the serosa and subserosa in the stomach.[2] Normally, the wall layers are in continuity, an abnormality may be present when a disruption of any of the wall layers is noted. Figure 13-1 is an example of an endoluminal ultrasound photograph, which details the esophageal layering.

C. Upper GI Endoscopy

In recent years, esophagoscopy has become a primary diagnostic procedure for many esophageal disorders, including evaluation of dysphagia. Esophagoscopy is performed as a part of a standard upper GI endoscopy. Dysphagia and odynophagia are common indications for upper GI endoscopy and may be performed as the initial test in the evaluation of these disorders.

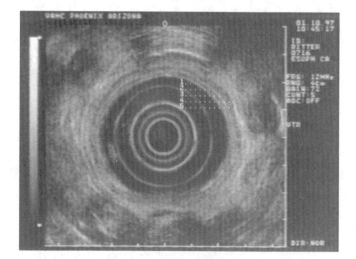

Fig 13-1. A photograph of an endoscopic ultrasound image taken in the esophagus. Layer 1 depicts the superficial mucosa, layer 2 is the deep mucosa, layer 3 corresponds to the submucosa, layer 4 corresponds to the muscularis propria, and layer 5 corresponds to surrounding fat in the esophagus, as there is no serosa in the esophagus.

1. Procedure

Following an overnight fast, the patient is taken to the GI lab, where the procedural nurses meet and assess the patient. The procedure is performed under conscious sedation while the patient's vital signs are monitored. The esophagus is intubated under direct visualization of the posterior hypopharynx. The endoscope is usually advanced through the UES, which appears as a slit-like opening in the cricopharyngeus muscle at about 20 cm from the incisor teeth. The entire length of the esophagus is in direct view of the endoscope until its termination at the gastroesophageal junction, which lies at the diaphragmatic hiatus. The location of the diaphragmatic hiatus can be noted by asking the patient to sniff, which pinches the hiatus. The longitudinal esophageal folds, which appear as a rosettelike structure in a nondistended organ, are obliterated when air is insufflated. The esophagus is usually closed at the gastroesophageal junction, but this is easily distended with air insufflation. This allows the endoscope to easily advance through the LES into the stomach. The entire esophagus is lined by squamous epithelium, which appears endoscopically as a whitish pink mucosa. The squamocolumnar junction, Z-line, which marks the transition of the esophageal to gastric mucosa that in contrast to the esophagus is reddish pink in appearance. In adults the Z-line normally lies at about 40 cm from the incisor teeth.

2. Contraindications

Absolute contraindications for endoscopy include suspected perforation of the GI tract, lack of adequately trained personnel, and lack of informed consent. There are many situations in which endoscopy is relatively contraindicated and clinical judgment should be exercised to ascertain the risk-benefit ratio for an individual patient. Relative contraindications are the same as for any procedure that uses conscious sedation and has minor stresses to the patient.

3. Indications

Upper endoscopy is the most specific test for identifying esophageal complications of gastroesophageal reflux (GER), esophageal ulcers, infectious disorders, and benign and malignant neoplasms. Esophagitis may be seen in up to 40% of reflux patients and Barrett's metaplasia may be found in approximately 15% of patients endoscoped for GER disease. Esophagoscopy has limited usefulness in demonstrating a relationship between GER disease and atypical symptoms. It is, however, more useful in defining the cause of disease in patients with solid-food dysphagia. Benign masses can be differentiated from malignant processes with endoscopically obtained biopsy specimens. Similarly, benign clean, smooth appearing peptic strictures can easily be differentiated from malignant strictures with endoscopic brushings and biopsies. Cervical webs and distal esophageal rings, such as a Schatzki's ring, may be apparent during an endoscopy; however, diagnosis is best made with a barium pill study. Although some abnormalities in esophageal motility may be detected during a routine endoscopy, most findings are nonspecific and diagnosis is best accomplished with manometric studies.

III. PHYSIOLOGICAL TESTS

A. Esophageal Manometry

Esophageal motility studies examine the static and dynamic functions of the pharyngeal and esophageal mechanisms responsible for swallowing. Pharyngeal manometry can be performed in conjunction with esophageal motility studies. Normally, the response of the oropharynx to swallowing has two components: (1) Compression of the catheter against the pharyngeal wall by the tongue, which results in a high, sharp-peaked amplitude pressure wave; and (2) a low amplitude, long duration wave, which reflects the initiation of pharyngeal peristalsis. A rapid, high-amplitude pressure upstroke ending in a single, sharp peak, followed by a rapid return to baseline is produced by the contraction of the middle and inferior pharyngeal constrictor muscles to provide the mid pharyngeal response to swallowing.[4] Esophageal manometry provides a qualitative as well as quantitative assessment of esophageal motility, pressures, and coordination. Accurate measurement of esophageal pressures can be performed with low-pressure perfusion or solid state systems. Pharyngeal manometry can also be done at the same time, although it is more difficult to evaluate. Pharyngeal measurements are best obtained with the solid state system because of the speed and fidelity inherent in this sophisticated system. The advent of computer technology has simplified the technique, while providing more accuracy in measurements.

Manometry is rarely the initial study in evaluating dysphagic patients. Standard manometry is of limited usefulness in the evaluation of oropharyngeal dysphagia. These structures are not radially symmetrical and, therefore, the measurements obtained will vary with the catheter placement. Further, water-perfused catheter systems do not respond rapidly enough to adequately follow the motor events produced in the striated muscle regions of the pharynx and UES. There is some evidence, however, to suggest that measurements of intrabolus pressures during the pharyngeal phase of swallowing may be used to predict which patients will respond to a

surgical myotomy. Therefore, pharyngeal manometry may have some role in the evaluation of oropharyngeal dysphagia. Esophageal dysmotility can cause dysphagia, therefore, esophageal motility studies are frequently performed in the etiologic work up of dysphagia. It is important, however, for the physician to understand the low probability of identifying a motor abnormality that could explain a patient's symptoms of dysphagia. Manometry is used in the evaluation of esophageal motility disorders including achalasia and diffuse esophageal spasm. It is also important in the identification of motor abnormalities associated with other systemic diseases, such as scleroderma, diabetes mellitus, and chronic intestinal pseudo-obstruction. Although the role of manometry in the evaluation of GER disease is limited, it is done to locate the LES for proper placement of a pH probe. It is an important part of the preoperative evaluation prior to any antireflux procedure. Although evidence regarding the force of peristalsis and the success of a Nissen fundoplication is lacking, patients with very poor peristalsis will likely suffer from postoperative dysphagia following a standard antireflux procedure. Therefore, the results of a preoperative manometry study can be used to select which patients may benefit from an antireflux procedure.

1. Procedure

The equipment consists of the manometry catheter system, transducers, and the physiograph or computer. A polyvinyl catheter with multiple pressure sensors is passed transnasally, and the patient is instructed to perform a series of wet and dry swallows. LES pressure is measured at baseline and in response to a swallow. LES pressure is measured as a step up in pressure from the gastric baseline referenced as atmospheric. Complete LES relaxation with a swallow is demonstrated by a decrease in pressure to gastric baseline for approximately 6 seconds. The catheter is then pulled into the esophagus in the oral direction in 0.5-1.0 cm steps every 15 seconds (station pull through) or it is withdrawn at a continuous speed of 0.5-1.0 cm/s while respiration is suspended (rapid pull through). Regardless of the manner in which the catheter is withdrawn, it is important for each sensor port to transverse the esophagus. A negative baseline pressure, reflecting intrathoracic pressure indicates location of the catheter within the esophagus, and positive pressure waves should be present on swallowing. Peristaltic waves are analyzed with respect to the amplitude, duration, and morphology of the waveform (Fig 13-2). Once esophageal body measurements have been obtained, the catheter is further withdrawn in the oral direction to obtain measurements of the UES. Basal UES sphincter pressures can be identified as a rise in pressure above the esophageal baseline. Because of the asymmetry of the UES, this is normally 50-100 mm Hg, depending on the direction of the pressure sensor,

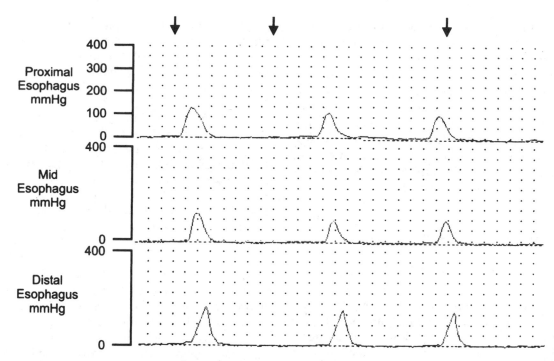

FIG 13-2. Intraluminal pressure recordings during an esophageal manometric study of a normal patient. The arrows represent 3 wet swallows taken by the patient. Normal peristaltic activity is shown for each of the 3 swallows.

whether lateral or anterior/posterior. Evaluation of UES relaxation and correlation of sphincter relaxation with pharyngeal contraction is obtained by instructing the patient to perform a series of wet swallows. A normal UES response to a swallow is a U-shaped drop to esophageal baseline, which is followed by a rise in pressure higher than the original pressure, followed by a return to UES pressure.

2. Contraindications

This examination is minimally invasive, causing only transient mild discomfort to the patient, complications are rare, and it is widely used in clinical practice, with well-established reference values.

B. 24-Hour Ambulatory pH Monitoring

Prolonged esophageal pH monitoring is the most reliable test for diagnosing GER. It is especially important in the diagnostic evaluation of patients with atypical presentations of GER disease.[4,5] The sensitivity of the test in diagnosing GER disease is approximately 90%. In addition, ambulatory monitoring devices permit evaluation of the temporal relationship between reflux episodes and atypical symptoms. Although this is the most reliable test, it is relatively expensive, not available at all institutions, and it may be uncomfortable to some pa-

tients. The addition of a pharyngeal probe to the traditional single distal esophageal pH studies has improved the diagnostic accuracy of atypical reflux symptoms. Placement of the distal pH probe in both the standard and dual pH monitoring systems is 5 cm above the LES. Placement of the proximal probe has been less standardized. An electrode placed in the hypopharynx may be affected by the intermittent variations in moisture and dryness, normally seen in the hypopharynx. This may affect the impedance of the electrode resulting in recordings of pseudoreflux events. Therefore, placement of the proximal probe below the UES may provide more accurate recordings.[4]

2. Procedure

Following an overnight fast, the pH catheter is inserted transnasally into the esophagus. The standard placement of the distal probe is 5 cm above the proximal border of the LES. This position can be determined in two ways. Most often, esophageal manometry is performed to determine the location and length of the LES. Recently, pH catheters with built in LES identifiers have become available. The advantage of this latter catheter is that only one catheter is used to intubate the esophagus. Thus, it is more comfortable for the patient and the amount of time to place the pH catheter is reduced. The main disadvantage of this combined system is that the catheter that needs to be worn for 24 hours is of a greater diameter to accommodate both pressure and pH sensors. Regardless of the manner in which the pH catheter is placed, it is ultimately attached to a recording device. Patients are asked to record in a diary the times that they eat, sleep, or perform any other activities. More importantly, patients will be asked to record any type of discomfort that they have, including heartburn, chest pain, wheezing, and coughing and to record the time that these symptoms occurr. In addition to recording these activities and symptoms in their diaries patients can push event buttons on the display of the recording devices. Depressing the buttons records any of the previously mentioned events. This information can be used to correlate the pH at the time a symptom or activity took place and a symptom index can be calculated.

Several parameters may be considered in the diagnosis of pathologic GER. Table 13-1 summarizes the various measurements that can be generated from a 24-hour ambulatory pH recording. The most valuable discriminator between physiologic and pathologic reflux is the percentage of total time that the pH is less than 4. Many studies in normal populations suggest an upper limit of

normal of 4.5%-7%, with most people using 5% of total recording time with pH less than 4 from the distal pH recording site.[6] Normal values for the proximal probe have not yet been established. Several investigators, however, have used 1.1% of the total recording that the pH is less than 4 as the upper limit of normal for the proximal probe.[7] Similar to obtaining the percentage of total time the pH is less than 4, percentage values can also be obtained for the percentage of reflux time in both the supine and upright positions. This can be important to identify the nocturnal refluxers as they frequently have atypical presentations of GER disease. The number of reflux episodes (below pH 4) lasting longer than 5 minutes during a 24-hour study can be determined and may indicate the severity of the problem. A symptom index can be calculated by determining the number of times a symptom is reported and is associated with a reflux event compared to the total number of times the symptom is reported regardless of its association with a reflux event. This is a statistical attempt to define the correlation between intermittent, atypical symptoms and reflux. This method statistically compares esophageal pH data temporally related to symptoms with pH data recorded during symptom free episodes.[8] DeMeester et al[9] devised a scoring system for the distal pH probe that is composed of 6 measures of reflux used determine the degree to which the patient's reflux pattern differs from the norm. Included in this score are: % time < pH 4 total; % time < pH 4 upright; % time < pH4 supine; # reflux episodes < pH4; # of episodes >5 minutes; longest reflux episode in minutes.[9] Figure 13-3 is an example of a pH tracing from a patient with gastroesophageal reflux. The arrows indicate times when pH dropped below 4.0.

Table 13-1. *pH Measurements Obtained During 24-hour Monitoring*

Percentage of the total time that reflux occurred
Percentage of time in the upright position that reflux occurred
Percentage of time in the supine position that reflux occurred
Number of episodes of reflux lasting greater than 5 minutes
Longest episode of reflux in minutes
Total number of reflux episodes occurring in 24 hours
DeMeester score
Symptom index

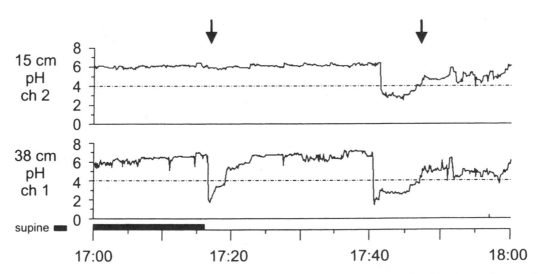

Fig 13-3. One hour of a 24-hour ambulatory pH recording from the distal and proximal esophagus shows 2 episodes of reflux. The normal intraesophageal pH of 6.5-7.5 is maintained by swallowed saliva and, to a lesser extent, esophageal secretions. Intermittent relaxation of the lower esophageal sphincter or stress reflux results in a sudden fall in pH from this normal level to the pH of gastric juice (1.5-2.5). Each reflux episode is labeled with an arrow. In the second reflux episode, acid reflux in the distal esophagus reaches the proximal esophagus or higher.

IV. SUMMARY

The evaluation of swallowing may require several specialized tests to determine the cause or causes of the swallowing disorder. No single test can provide all the information needed to initiate treatment. Rather, the case history and symptoms should be used to direct the test selection. The gastroenterologist provides an important link in the evaluation of swallowing, especially for those problems related to the esophageal stage of swallowing.

References

1. Langmore SE, Schatz K, Olsen N. Fiberoptic endoscopic examination of swallowing safety: a new procedure. *Dysphagia* 1988;2:216-219.
2. Murata Y, Muroi ML, Yoshida M, Ide H, Hanyu F. Endoscopic ultrasonography in the diagnosis of esophageal carcinoma. *Surg Endosc.* 1987;1:11-16.
3. Deschner WK, Benjamin SB. Extraesophageal manifestations of gastroesophageal reflux disease. *Am J Gastroenterol.* 1989;84:1-5.
4. Jacob P, Kahrilas PJ, Herzon G. Proximal esophageal pH-metry in patients with "reflux laryngitis." *Gastroenterol.* 1991;100:305-310.
5. Koufman JA. The otolaryngologic manifestations of gastroesophageal reflux disease (GERD): a clinical investigation of 225 patients using ambulatory pH monitoring and an experimental investigation of the role of acid and pepsin in the development of laryngeal injury. *Laryngoscope.* 1991;101:1-78.
6. DeMeester TR. Prolonged oesophageal pH monitoring. In: DeMeester TR, Matthews HR, eds. *International Trends in General Thoracic Surgery.* St. Louis, Mo: Mosby; 1989:99-127.
7. Harding SM, Richter, JE, Guzzo MR, Schan CA, Alexander RW, Bradley LA. Asthma and gastroesophageal reflux: acid suppressive therapy improves asthma outcome. *Am J Med.* 1996;100:395-405.
8. Wiener GJ, Richter JE, Copper JB, Wu WC, Castell DO. The symptom index: a clinically important parameter of ambulatory 24-hour esophageal pH monitoring. *Am J Gastroenterol.* 1988;83:358-361.
9. DemeesterTR, Stein HJ, Fuchs KH. Diagnostic studies in the evaluation of the esophagus; physiologic diagnostic studies. In: Orringer MB, ed. *Shackelford's Surgery of the Alimentary Tract.* 3rd ed., Philadelphia, Pa: WB Saunders; 1991:94-126.

CHAPTER 14

■ ■ ■

Laryngeal Electromyography

Michael C. Munin, M.D.
Michael Rainer, M.D.

I. INTRODUCTION

The first descriptions of laryngeal electromyography were done by Weddell et al[1] in 1944. Disorders of movement of the larynx traditionally had been diagnosed using endoscopic laryngoscopy or indirect mirror examinations. Laryngeal electromyography has now become an important procedure in providing a more accurate description of laryngeal nerve dysfunction.[2-5]

Laryngeal electromyography is used in the diagnosis and management of laryngeal nerve disorders, swallowing disorders, spasmodic dysphonia, and laryngeal joint injuries after intubation. The detection of viable recurrent laryngeal nerve innervation to the thyroarytenoid (vocalis) muscle and the superior laryngeal nerve innervation to the cricothyroid muscle aids the investigator in understanding neurologic motor function.

The goals of laryngeal electromyography are to distinguish normal from abnormal activity and localize and assess the severity of a focal lesion by determining whether there is neuropraxia (physiologic nerve block or focal injury, with intact nerve fibers) or axonotmesis (damage to nerve fibers leading to complete peripheral degeneration). The assessment can also evaluate prognosis, which provides valuable information to either proceed to definitive surgical correction or implement temporary measures if spontaneous recovery is likely. Laryngeal electromyography can also provide localization information for botulinum toxin injections in spasmodic dysphonia.

The investigator should be aware of the limitations of laryngeal EMG. The precise site of the lesion cannot be determined, except whether it involves the vagus nerve or brainstem, the superior laryngeal nerve or the recurrent laryngeal nerve. The posterior cricoarytenoid, which is the main abductor muscle, can be technically difficult to localize. Systemic neuromuscular diseases cannot be differentiated from focal lesions without full neurologic evaluation in conjunction with EMG studies of other muscles and nerves. Finally, studies performed 6 months postinjury have a poor correlation with prognosis secondary to vocal cord fixation or synkinesis with co-activation of antagonist muscles.[2-4]

II. DETECTION OF NORMAL ELECTRICAL ACTIVITY

Normal electrical activity in laryngeal muscles is characterized by a predictable pattern of increased motor unit activation corresponding to the force of vocalization. The techniques of needle insertion have been described and reported by Blair and colleagues, Hiroto et al, Simpson and coworkers, and Rodriguez et al.[5-8] Briefly, the patient is supine with neck extended. Routine local anesthesia is unnecessary. The thyroarytenoid muscle is approached by insertion of a monopolar or concentric electrode through the cricothryoid ligament midline 0.5-1.0 cm then angled superiorly 45° and laterally 20° for a total depth of 2 cm. The cricothryoid muscle is reached by inserting the electrode 0.5 cm off the midline then angling superiorly and laterally 20° toward the inferior border of the thyroid cartilage.

Having the patient vocalize from a low pitch to high pitch, either using a musical scale or a variable [ee], activates the cricothyroid muscle. A sustained [ee] or the Valsalva maneuver, which adducts the vocal cords, activates the thyroarytenoid muscle. The normal patterns of laryngeal electromyography include quiet insertional activity at rest, baseline activity during deep respiration, and increased motor unit recruitment with active phonation that should produce a full interference pattern. Figure 14-1 shows a normal recruitment pattern.

III. DETECTION OF ABNORMAL ACTIVITY

Reduced motor unit recruitment is observed with focal demyelinating (neuropraxic) lesions such as found after intubation injuries. This is demonstrated by observing 1 or 2 motor units firing rapidly (>20 Hz) as the patient phonates. Motor unit configuration should be normal; see Fig 14-2. Patients with axon loss (axonotmesis or neurometsis) lesions, such as partial nerve transection after surgical procedures, will also exhibit decreased motor unit recruitment with normal configuration within the first 6 weeks after injury. However, axonal injuries will exhibit positive waves and fibrillation potentials at rest, which begin 3 to 4 weeks postinjury. Laryngeal nerve regeneration following axon-loss lesions can be observed between 6 weeks to 12 months postinjury and

is characterized by polyphasic motor unit potentials with wide duration; see Fig 14-3. As re-innervation occurs, fibrillations should diminish in both size and number. Table 14-1 summarizes the electrodiagnostic findings of vocal cord paralysis from focal lesions, especially as they relate to prognosis.

Patients with spasmodic dysphonia most often exhibit action-induced spasms with motor units firing in groups. This makes analysis of individual units difficult. The burst of activity is often irregular.

Patients with conversion disorders and malingering are often difficult to assess without direct evidence of functional impairment. Laryngeal electromyography is a useful aid in determining true neurologic dysfunction. Studies in these patients should provide normal results and other evidence would give direct information to the site and severity of a lesion.

Vocal fold immobility can be caused by laryngeal joint injuries after intubation trauma, blunt neck trauma, or thyroid surgical procedures. Delayed management of laryngeal joint injuries can lead to joint ankylosis. Laryngeal electromyography is useful in differentiating neurologic vocal fold paralysis from laryngeal joint injury. Laryngeal EMG may confirm the diagnosis of joint dislocation when a normal recruitment pattern is seen with vocal fold immobility. Patients with normal recruitment patterns and laryngeal joint dislocation should be considered for reduction of the joint. If nerve injury is present on EMG evaluation, computed tomography has been reported to be useful to evaluate superimposed joint dislocation.[9]

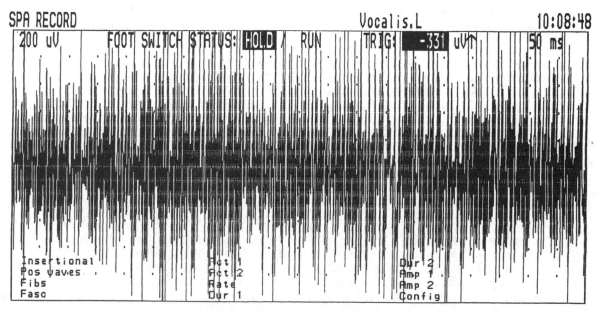

FIG 14-1. Normal voluntary motor unit recruitment of the vocalis muscle using the Valsalva maneuver. Note the full interference pattern that obliterates individual motor unit analysis when the sweep speed is set at 50 ms per division.

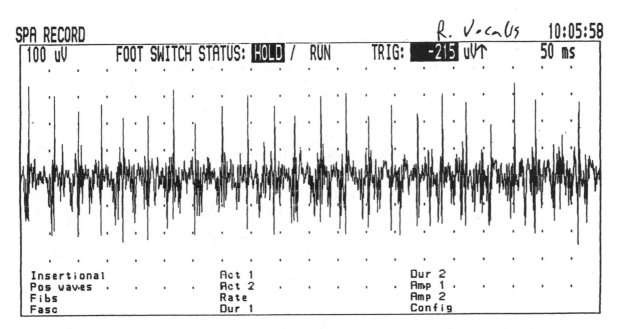

FIG 14-2. Decreased motor unit recruitment with the primary unit firing at 24 Hz. Note that there is a decreased interference pattern with the Valsalva maneuver. The sweep speed is 50 ms/division.

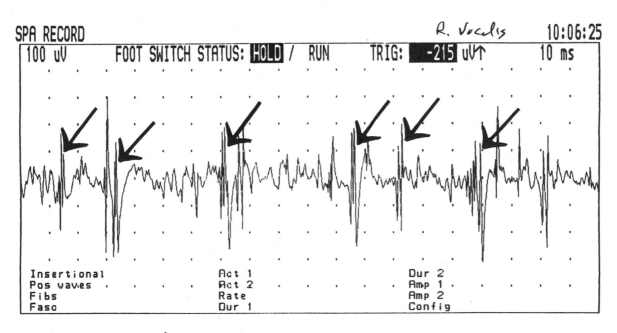

↙ = polyphasic unit

FIG 14-3. Polyphasic motor units are indicated by the arrows. These units do not exhibit typical triphasic configuration and indicate that reinnervation following an axon-loss lesion has occurred. The sweep speed is 10 ms/division.

Table 14-1. *Summary of Electrodiagnostic Findings with Vocal Cord Paralysis*

EMG FINDINGS	SEVERITY OF INJURY					
	Mild		Moderate		Severe	
	>21 days	6 months	>21 days	6 months	>21 days	6 months
Motor Unit Recruitment	↓/↓↓	NL	↓↓/NF	↓/↓↓	NF	NF
Motor Unit Configuration	NL	NL	NL	NL or Poly	0	0
Fibrillations	0	0	+	+	++/+++	CRDs +/++
Prognosis for Recovery	Excellent		Favorable		Poor	
Surgical Recommendation	No surgery		No permanent surgery Consider gelfoam injection Voice therapy		Perform permanent corrective surgery by 6 months	

Key: Recruitment ranges from normal (NL), mildly decreased (↓), moderately decreased with repetitive firing (↓↓), and non-firing motor units (NF). Configuration includes normal (NL), polyphasic potentials with increased duration (Poly), and none (0). Fibrillations range from none (0) to abundant (+++). CRDs = complex repetitive discharges and signify chronic denervation. >21 days describes an EMG evaluation performed on or after 21 days post-paralysis. 6 months refers to an EMG study performed no later than 6 months post-paralysis. Surgical recommendations assume appropriate work-up has been performed.

The three areas of interest for electrodiagnostic evaluation of swallowing are the laryngeal sphincters, the sensory ability of the supraglottic larynx and pharynx, and the cricopharyngeal sphincter.[10] The laryngeal sphincter is important in maintaining glottic closure for protection of the airway. The innervation to the primary adductors of the larynx is the recurrent laryngeal nerve and can be tested by EMG examination of the thyroarytenoid muscle. Laryngeal EMG does not evaluate sensory information, but can infer the condition of the sensory component of the superior laryngeal nerve via the motor branch that innervates the cricothyroid muscle. Denervation to the cricothyroid muscle is indirect evidence of a lesion affecting the sensory component of the superior laryngeal nerve. The cricopharyngeus muscle is unusual, in that it is active at rest and relaxes during activation of swallowing. The cricopharyngeus has been localized by placing an electrode via the lateral transcutaneous approach into the posterior aspect of the lower part of the cricoid cartilage. This technique has also been useful in delivering botulinum toxin in cases of cricopharyngeal spasm.[10]

References

1. Weddell G, Feinstein B, Pattle RE. The electrical activity of voluntary muscles in man under normal and pathologic conditions. *Brain.* 1994;67:178-256.

2. Minn Y, Finnegan E, Hoffman H, Luschei ES, McCulloch TM. A preliminary study of the prognostic role of electromyography in laryngeal paralysis. *Otolaryngol Head Neck Surg.* 1994;111:770-775.

3. Yin S, Qui W, Stucker F. Major patterns of laryngeal electromyography and their clinical applications. *Laryngoscope.* 1997;107:126-136.

4. Thumfart WF. Electrodiagnosis of laryngeal nerve disorders. *Ear Nose Throat J.* 1988;67:380-383.

5. Simpson D, Graves-Wright J, Sanders I. Vocal cord paralysis: clinical and electrophysiologic features. *Muscle and Nerve.* 1993;16:952-957.

6. Blair RL, Berry H, Briant, TD. Laryngeal electromyography—techniques, applications, and a review of personal experience. *J Otolaryngol.* 1977;6:496-504.

7. Hiroto I, Hirano M, Toyozumi Y, Shin T. A new method of placement of a needle electrode in the intrinsic laryngeal muscles for electromyography. *Oto-rhini-laryngeal Clinic Kyoto.* 1962;55:499-504.

8. Rodriguez A, Myers B, Ford C. Laryngeal electromyography in the diagnosis of laryngeal nerve injuries. *Arch Phys Med Rehab.* 1990;71:587-590.

9. Yin S, Qui W, Strucker F. Value of electromyography in differential diagnosis of laryngeal joint injuries after intubation. *Ann Otol Rhinol Laryngol.* 1996;105:446-450.

10. Hillel A, Robinson L, Waugh P. Laryngeal electromyography for the diagnosis and management of swallowing disorders. *Otolaryngol Head Neck Surgery.* 1997;116:344-8.

PART IV

PATHOPHYSIOLOGY OF SWALLOWING DISORDERS

This section is a fully integrated discussion of the diagnosis and management of swallowing disorders that range from sequellae associated with life-threatening diseases, such as cerebral vascular accidents, neuromuscular disorders, cardiopulmonary disorders, to the more insidious and benign, such as gastroesophageal reflux. The interpretation of objective swallowing tests is the basis for advising the patients of a treatment that is customized to each specific condition. Therefore, aspects of the functional tests of swallowing are reviewed in context with specific diseases and disorders. This section also addresses iatrogenic disorders caused by surgery, radiotherapy, or medications. Treatment protocols based on accurate testing and proper interpretation are emphasized. Each chapter recalls specific observations of the standard tests of swallowing when planning treatments.

CHAPTER 15

■ ■ ■

Pathophysiology of Neurogenic Oropharyngeal Dysphagia

James L. Coyle, M.A.
John C. Rosenbek, Ph.D.
Kimberly A. Chignell, M.S.

I. INTRODUCTION

Neurological injuries and diseases can suddenly or insidiously degrade or destroy the range of human abilities and behaviors including thinking, walking, talking, and swallowing. All such outcomes are deleterious to the duration and quality of a person's life. Impaired swallowing can be especially devastating because of the implications for nutrition, hydration, pulmonary health, and social interaction. Dysphagia is sometimes permanent, even in conditions such as cerebrovascular accidents for which some physiological recovery is the norm; and it may be progressive when associated with degenerative diseases such as amyotrophic lateral sclerosis (ALS).

Rehabilitative efforts targeting damaged system components, and compensatory efforts targeting the remaining intact mechanisms of swallowing are increasingly common. Rehabilitation depends, in part, on patient determination and compliance and clinician skills and judgment. The critical ingredients supplied by clinicians are (1) a strong conceptual understanding of normal oral, pharyngeal, laryngeal, and upper esophageal sphincter functions; (2) an appreciation of the pathophysiology of disordered swallowing and its response to treatment; and (3) recognition of and accomodation to the clinical presentation of dysphagia,

effects of the causative disease, and cognitive, affective, and other potentially idiosyncratic patient variables that can confound maximum effectiveness in evaluation and treatment planning and execution. This chapter describes the pathophysiology of dysphagia in various neurological conditions. The treatment implications are illustrated with case reviews. The approach in this chapter is to review data when they are available, describe our clinical experience where relevant, and consider the relationship of disease and site of lesion to normal and abnormal functioning.

Predictably, there are dangers in this approach, because the data are sometimes inconsistent and our experiences are only as orderly and precise as busy clinical practices allow. In addition, attempts to discuss neuropathophysiology of dysphagia in such disorders as stroke are inherently risky, particularly when attributing deficits to lesion sites. Some patients with clinically diagnosed cerebrovascular accident (CVA) are found on imaging to have not only one specific lesion site, but multiple foci of subclinical central nervous system damage believed to be the result of prior subclinical disease or the cumulative effect of these combined with changes associated with aging. In such cases, clinical knowledge of the "lesion site" can blind clinicians to alternative explanations for performance deficits, sometimes leading to disastrous treatment planning and prognostication.

Even reliable verification of the number and site of lesions does not establish the physiologic explanation for signs and symptoms of dysphagia. Unless the appropriate studies are done to establish the contribution of certain brain areas to swallowing performance, the current explanations are no more than speculations based on the assumed functions of various brain regions.

Appropriate basic science studies have been slow to appear. Limited pathophysiological data is common to other conditions reviewed in this chapter, including traumatic brain injury, multiple sclerosis (MS), and Parkinson's disease (PD). The exception may be amyotrophic lateral sclerosis (ALS), but even in this condition the data to explain signs and symptoms are limited. And as we have been reminded since the 19th century: To find a lesion is different from finding a function. Despite these limitations, cautious statements can be helpful as guides to further research and clinical practice.

Studies describing normal and abnormal human functions resulting from brain and brainstem and cranial nerve damage arise from observations of patients with known events such as CVA, neurodegenerative diseases, and discrete nerve lesions. Loss of blood flow to specific structures because of embolic, thrombotic, or hemorrhagic disease results in tissue death in the brain and brainstem and associated sensorimotor deficits. Neurodegenerative diseases attack the neural pathways to and from specific organs such as sensory receptors, muscles, and salivary glands. Discrete damage to cranial nerves may occur secondary to trauma or by iatrogenic means such as surgery. All of these classes of neurogenic disorders are known to affect numerous functions, including swallowing.

Patients with vascular lesions are the predominant members of a clinician's neurogenic dysphagia caseload.[1] Given the frequency with which a practitioner encounters swallowing disorders in patients with stroke and other injuries to the central and peripheral nervous systems, a review of the organization of these systems is imperative. We employ a stepwise approach by first considering occlusive vascular disease and reviewing blood supply to regions of the brain and brainstem that have been implicated in the control of the swallowing mechanism. Next, we review the functional organization of these regions to enable readers to understand the effects of specific local and regional cerebrovascular events. Parkinson's disease and dementia, also commonly encountered central nervous system disorders, are discussed this section. Finally, diseases and damage of the peripheral nervous system are briefly discussed. The reader should refer to an adequate neurology text for a summary of the overall effects of these diseases and disorders on other body systems, and should have a working understanding of anatomic terminology.

II. BRAIN AND BRAINSTEM ARTERIAL SUPPLY AND CLINICAL IMPLICATIONS

Cerebrovascular disease is perhaps the most common clinical entity producing primary neurogenic oral and pharyngeal dysphagia.[1] Major occlusive or hemorrhagic events, small vessel disease secondary to chronic hypertension and diabetes, and tiny, elusive brainstem infarcts are common etiologies of central neurogenic dysphagia.[2] The specific sites of lesion in the brain and brainstem are often undetected by our current diagnostic technology. Peripheral nerve damage, however, can be more readily identified.

The extent of CNS territory affected by circulatory deprivation, and the resultant infarct size and distribution, defines the clinical presentation of a CVA and is dependent on the degree and site of interrupted arterial supply. Obviously, larger thrombi or emboli produce occlusion of larger vessels (ie, proximal) and affect a larger territory downstream. Hence, the presentation of dysphagia in a patient with larger or multiple infarcts may be quite variable and more difficult to manage because of the influences of damage to adjacent brain structures.

There are two primary sources of arterial supply to the brain: (1) the vertebral-basilar complex, which nourishes posterior regions such as brainstem and cerebellum, and (2) the bilateral internal carotid complexes, which give rise to the main arterial vessels supplying most of the brain. The tributaries of these supply routes are interconnected, allowing a degree of collateral flow and overlap within the following model.

The internal carotid arteries give rise to the majority of the anterior and deep cerebral blood supply. Each gives rise to three main vessels: an anterior cerebral artery (ACA), a middle cerebral artery (MCA), and a posterior communicating artery that joins the anterior circulation to the posterior cerebral artery (PCA), the main branch of the basilar artery. The paired anterior cerebral arteries join via an anterior communicating artery, closing this network in a loop known as the circle of Willis. Each anterior cerebral artery supplies the ipsilateral orbital and medial frontal lobe and the medial parietal lobe. Each middle cerebral artery supplies the ipsilateral temporal lobe and the remainder of the parietal and frontal lobes, and gives off branches that join laterally with branches of the anterior cerebral artery and posterior cerebral artery. Other middle cerebral artery branches penetrate the brain and supply the ipsilateral basal nuclei, internal capsule region, and most of the thalamus and adjacent structures. Each posterior cerebral artery supplies portions of the ipsilateral brainstem and cerebellum, inferior temporal and medial occipital lobes. Caudal to the origin of the basilar artery, the paired vertebral arteries, and, to a lesser extent, the anterior and posterior spinal arteries supply branches to the medulla.

Certain lesions in the left middle cerebral artery territory are known to produce aphasia, or motor and verbal apraxia. Patients with damage to either structures within either MCA territory may present with dysarthria, hemiparesis, and dysphagia. The association between speech and swallowing disorders following stroke has been reported.[3] These deficits are associated with damage to cortical and subcortical centers associated with motor programming and execution, nearby regions of the motor and supplemental motor cortices associated with integrative sensorimotor processing, and to association cortices and tracts conveying information to and from these regions. Attempts to localize specific cortical lesion sites associated with dysphagia continue to emerge in the literature.

Posterior cerebrovascular events, with their resulting brainstem lesions and subsequent oropharyngeal swallowing deficits, have been more successfully linked. Critical components of this posterior network are the paired vertebral arteries and their important tributaries to the medulla, the posterior inferior cerebellar arteries (PICA). Lesions caused by occlusion along the posterior inferior cerebellar arteries produce damage to the posterolateral medulla and a Wallenberg's or lateral medullary syndrome (LMS). Interestingly, studies have shown that vertebral occlusion is more likely to be responsible for a lateral medullary syndrome than discrete occlusion of the posterior inferior cerebellar artery.[4]

Tables 15-1A and 15-1B summarize brainstem arterial supply, structures affected by vascular lesions, and common vascular syndromes associated with specific arterial occlusions.

III. LEVELS OF NEUROMOTOR INTEGRITY

Interruption of circulation within the preceding framework produces specific patterns of neuromuscular deficit. Although the brain remains somewhat of a magic box in that its circuitry relative to deglutition is not well understood, a firm grasp of neuromuscular organization can give the clinician a point from which to launch effective management. Unfortunately studies of central neurogenic dysphagia in humans have focused on deficits following acute insult to the brain within the vascular framework described above, and have not provided consensus regarding the pathophysiology producing observed swallowing patterns. They have also failed to adequately take into account individual variability and recovery patterns in their descriptions of post-CVA functional deficits. We encourage the reader to observe individual patient function and to consider recovery in the context of this discussion.

As discussed in an earlier chapter, there are both voluntary and involuntary components of swallowing, yet the bond between these is not well understood. (See Chapter 3.) Oropharyngeal swallowing is largely a patterned sequence of sensorimotor events, initiated by volitional intent or by reflexive response to stimuli.[5] The former is seen during eating and drinking and the latter in coma and sleep. Given the ability to initiate a swallow either consciously or unconsciously, the circuitry reviewed in Chapter 3 is understandably complex and not quite fully understood. Understanding the effects of damage at different levels of nervous system organization gives the reader insight into patterns of observed deficits.

Upper motor neurons (UMN) supplying the muscles involved in voluntary movement course from the cortex through subcortical integrating centers to brainstem nuclei or spinal nerve cell bodies. Lower motor neurons (LMN) originate at these terminal sites and provide the final common pathway for all motor output transmitted to the effector muscles. Upper motor neuron lesions may occur at any level above or rostral to the origin of the lower motor neurons, disconnecting motor input that originated above the lesion site. Pure upper motor neuron lesions produce weakness by disconnecting cortical or supranuclear input from the final common motor pathway; however, they do not produce disconnection of motor influences initiated at levels below or caudal to the lesion site. For example, high subcortical lesions to corticobulbar UMN pathways do not disconnect oral, facial, or pharyngeal muscles from motor signals that originate in the brainstem. Such upper motor neuron damage produces weakness that is soon accompanied by some degree of spasticity and hyperreflexia because of disconnection of higher level inhibitory input, but alone will not disconnect other lower level motor influences to the target muscles. Similarly, supranuclear lesions produce sensory deficits based on the level of ascending pathway damage. Hyperreflexia and spasticity are examples of disconnection from higher level influences, as muscles' responses to stretch occur without monitoring and input from above. Pure and complete lower motor neuron lesions, on the other hand, disconnect muscles from their entire motor supply, producing paralysis and, eventually, atrophy and fasciculation, which is the muscle tissues' response to the lack of motor input. Absence of stretch reflexes is seen primarily because of disconnection of the muscle's afferent sensory communication to higher levels of the nervous system.

IV. BRAINSTEM NUCLEI AND SWALLOWING

Lesions of the brainstem produce specific deficits, although some are not fully understood. The discussion of brainstem lesions is organized by major nuclei mediating sensorimotor function within the oropharyngeal complex. Motor activities during oropha-

Table 15-1. *Vascular Lesions.* **A.** *Vascular Lesions of the Medulla Affecting Swallowing*

Lesion Syndrome	Involved Vessels	Structures Affected	Deficits Related to Dysphagia
Medial medullary syndrome	Anterior spinal artery	Hypoglossal roots (LMN)	• Ipsilateral flaccid lingual paralysis
Lateral medullary syndrome (Wallenberg's)	Posterior inferior cerebellar artery (PICA) Ipsilateral vertebral artery	Nucleus ambiguus of IX, X, XI	• Ipsilateral flaccid laryngeal, pharyngeal, palatal paralysis • Loss of gag reflex (efferent limb) • Dysphagia, dysphonia, dysarthria
		Glossopharyngeal (IX) nerve roots	• Loss of gag reflex (afferent limb)
		Vagal (X) roots	• Same effects as those under Nucleus ambiguus
		Spinal trigeminal nucleus and tract	• Loss of ipsilateral facial temperature and pain sensation
		Nucleus and tractus solitarius	• Loss of taste sensation • Interruption of input to nucleus ambiguus
		Dorsal motor nucleus of vagus (X)	• Reduced bronchial smooth muscle activity (cough in response to aspiration)

B. *Vascular Lesions of the Pons Producing Dysphagia*

Lesion Syndrome	Involved Vessels	Structures Affected	Deficits Related to Dysphagia
Lateral inferior pontine syndrome	Anterior inferior cerebellar artery (AICA)	Facial nuclei and motor projections	• Ipsilateral flaccid facial paralysis • Ipsilateral loss of taste anterior 2/3 tongue
Lateral midpontine syndrome	short branches of basilar artery	Trigeminal motor and sensory nuclei and roots	• Ipsilateral paralysis of mastication muscles • Jaw deviation toward affected side • Ipsilateral facial anesthesia
Medial inferior pontine syndrome	paramedian basilar artery branches	Corticobulbar tracts	• Spastic paresis of contralateral face

ryngeal swallowing are performed by muscles that are supplied by lower motor neurons from cranial nerves V (trigeminal), VII (facial), IX (glossopharyngeal), X (vagus), XI (accessory), and XII (hypoglossal). Many of these nerves carry proprioceptive and sensory information from the musculature and associated joints, skin, mucosa, and other related receptors.

The functions of cranial nerves have been discussed in an earlier chapter. There are various degrees of "built-in redundancy" in corticobulbar motor supply to the brainstem, which is fortuitous in terms of supporting survival. The organization and effects on swallowing of lesions within the major brainstem nuclei are summarized in the next sections. Specific syndromes resulting from selected vascular lesions of medullary and pontine structures important to intact oropharyngeal swallowing are summarized in Tables 15-1A and 15-1B.

A. Trigeminal Motor Nucleus

Corticobulbar projections from the precentral gyri to the motor nuclei of cranial nerve V exert bilateral motor output influences on the muscles of mastication (V) via direct and indirect (via interneurons) input to the trigeminal nucleus. Lesions involving unilateral corticobulbar UMN fibers rostral to the trigeminal motor nucleus produce undetectable to mild bilateral weakness without atrophy because of this built-in motor redundancy. Lesions at or caudal to the trigeminal motor nuclei produce detectable ipsilateral weakness, atrophy, and fasciculations. This lower motor neuron lesion is expressed as deviation of jaw closure toward the side of the lesion because of unopposed action of the pterygoid, masseter, and temporalis muscles. Again, this patient will have some degree of symptomatology, relating difficulty with mastication and possibly a mild dysarthria resulting from loss of lingual stabilization within the mandible.

B. Facial Motor Nucleus

Bilateral corticobulbar fibers project to the motor nuclei of cranial nerve VII. However, fibers projecting to the upper face from the rostral ends of these nuclei are supplied by both direct and indirect (via interneurons) upper motor neuron tracts from both right and left cortices. Hence, a unilateral supranuclear or cortical lesion will not produce detectable asymmetry of facial muscle function, atrophy, or fasciculations. The caudal portion of the facial motor nucleus innervates the remaining muscles of expression and the posterior digastric and stylohyoid muscles, which assist in elevation of the hyoid-laryngeal complex during the pharyngeal response. Its efferent supply to the lower face is primarily via contralateral direct fibers, allowing a unilateral lesion to produce contralateral lower facial weakness. Clinical observation is not likely to reveal asymmetry in hyoid-laryngeal elevation. Lower motor lesions at or caudal to the motor nuclei of VII result in ipsilateral facial paresis, difficulty maintaining labial and buccal tension, and salivary deficits. These latter deficits may manifest as drooling, pocketing of food in the affected buccal cavity, and reduced ability to maintain intrabolus pressure during oral propulsion and, subsequently, incomplete or disordered transfer of food to the pharynx.

C. Nucleus Ambiguus

The nucleus ambiguus distributes motor output through cranial nerves IX, X, and XI to the muscles of the ipsilateral larynx, pharynx, and palate plus the rostral striated portion of the esophagus. Corticobulbar tracts project to each nucleus ambiguus (NA) from both right and left cortices. This bilateral input is transmitted to the nucleus ambiguus via interneurons (indirect pathway). Hence, unilateral supranuclear or cortical lesions alone do not produce asymmetric motor output, but rather absent-to-mild bilateral laryngeal, pharyngeal, and soft palate weakness without clinically detectable atrophy. Lesions of nucleus ambiguus or the fibers of cranial nerves IX, X, and XI which exit the nucleus produce ipsilateral lower motor neuron effects (atrophy, paresis) within innervated structures of the larynx, pharynx, soft palate, or upper esophagus. Deficits produced by this lesion may include hypernasal speech, dysphonia, and dysphagia. Clinical assessment may detect asymmetry of soft palate elevation to the contralateral (unaffected) side as the contralateral musculature performs unopposed. Within the brainstem, the nucleus ambiguus receives afferent signals from the spinal trigeminal nucleus (facial pain, temperature) and the nucleus of the tractus solitarius (taste and other input via cranial nerves VII, IX, and X). The nucleus of the tractus solitarius, the nucleus ambiguus, and other structures described in an earlier chapter are hypothesized to comprise a "swallowing center," which mediates activity related to deglutition. Although there seem to be many similarities between this region and motor outflow from a "central pattern generator," the apparent need for afferent input to evoke the patterned responses seen in the pharyngeal swallow suggests that "pattern generator" is a more accurate descriptor. Animal and human clinical studies have shown disruption in pharyngeal activity related to discrete lesions in this region of the medulla.[6]

D. Hypoglossal Motor Nucleus

The hypoglossal nuclei supply motor output to intrinsic and all extrinsic lingual musculature except the palatoglossus. Each is supplied predominantly by contralateral corticobulbar (upper motor neuron) fibers. High supranuclear lesions, such as cortical infarcts, to fibers projecting to the hypoglossal motor nuclei produce mild to clinically undetectable contralateral deficits in lingual function, such as spastic paresis. Isolated supranuclear hypoglossal lesions are rare, but have been reported along with hemiplegia in stroke and multiple sclerosis. In contrast, lesions at or caudal to the hypoglossal nuclei (lower motor neuron) produce ipsilateral lingual weakness, along with atrophy and eventually fasciculations. Since the paired nuclei are situated nearly together at the midline of the lower medulla, they may be concurrently damaged, producing profound dysphagia. This form of nuclear lingual paralysis may be seen in amyotrophic lateral sclerosis (ALS).

Unilateral hypoglossal lower motor neuron deficits can be grossly demonstrated by deviation of lingual protrusion to the side of lesion because of unopposed contralateral genioglossus contraction. This form of lower motor neuron injury is associated with skull base trauma, surgery, disease, and late effects of curative head and neck radiation therapy. Isolated hypoglossal nerve lesions produce deficits in oral preparatory and propulsive functions and ipsilateral weakness in the suprahyoid muscles responsible for hyolaryngeal excursion. This deficit is likely to result in inadequate oral bolus control, with portions of the bolus flowing erroneously into anterior or lateral oral sulci or spilling posteriorly into the pharynx prior to intentional propulsion. Postswallow pooling of residue can be detected in the valleculae and buccal cavity because of reduced intrabolus pressure, and the tongue base may be coated with residue. Laryngeal penetration during the swallow because of incomplete closure of the laryngeal inlet is another common observation with this lesion. The patient would likely present with some form of articulatory dysarthria, and may comment that his or her tongue "feels thick." Food residue often remains in the affected side of the mouth after swallowing. Patients with an isolated unilateral hypoglossal paresis and resultant dysphagia are quite physically amenable to behavioral intervention designed to direct the bolus away from the impaired side of the tongue. Prosthodontic augmentation may also be an option.

E. Afferent Processing Centers

The deficits observed during errant performance in a patient with neurologic injury or disease should not be presumed to be of purely motor origin. Motor output is largely dependent on sensory input. Afferent fibers from the reticular formation, the nucleus of the tractus solitarius, the midbrain, and the trigeminal nuclei are components of a subsystem mediating swallowing, mastication, and sucking.

Lesions of the cranial nerves, medulla, or pons may affect sensory processing centers crucial to oropharyngeal swallowing. Within the brainstem, these include the roots of the glossopharyngeal nerve (afferent limb of gag reflex); the spinal trigeminal, spinothalamic, or trigeminothalamic tracts (pain and temperature sensation from ipsilateral face); and trigeminal sensory nuclei (pressure and touch sensation from ipsilateral face).

V. CENTRAL NEUROGENIC DYSPHAGIA

Individual and isolated lesions such as those described in this section are rare. Careful assessment and deficit inventory is the only reliable method of assessing and monitoring patient function. Elderly patients with acute central nervous system damage may likely possess multiple foci of previously undocumented cerebral damage or change.[2,7] The literature is divided with regard to conclusions relating to localization of cortical and subcortical lesion and presumed characteristics of dysphagia. Clinicians must rely primarily on careful and thoughtful diagnostic assessment. Dysphagia among patients with various sites of stroke, Parkinson's disease, and dementia are summarized next. The left brain will be assumed the "dominant" hemisphere, the right "nondominant."

A. Left CVA

The literature often repeats the theme that the site-of-lesion has been inconclusively correlated with specific swallowing disorders. There is evidence, however, that delayed pharyngeal response, impaired oral transit, and apraxia are prevalent in patients with discrete lesions in the lateral precentral gyrus and posterior inferior frontal gyrus.[8] Left-sided cortical lesions tend to produce a greater degree of oral dysfunction than is seen in other lesion sites.[9,10] This pattern predisposes the patient to aspiration because of loss of adequate oral control or containment of the bolus. The impact of these deficits may be magnified by the degree of auditory and/or visual comprehension deficit exhibited by the patient. Patients with unilateral cortical stroke may exhibit facial, oral, and/or pharyngeal functional deficits as previously outlined. In attempting to eat or drink, a bolus may spill passively from the oral cavity posteriorly into the pharynx prior to initiation of a pharyngeal response and its critical airway closure component. This occurrence should not be confused with delayed initiation of a pharyngeal response following volitional oral propulsion, as the rationale for selection of management techniques for of each entity may be quite different.

Patients with a CVA of the dominant hemisphere may exhibit other oral deficits such as drooling and poor anterior oral containment because of facial paresis and reduced sensation. Unilateral stroke in this region has been reported to produce a type of "swallow apraxia" involving the tongue, lips, and facial muscles.[5] If oral and/or verbal apraxia are present, a patient may exhibit similar programming errors while introducing food or liquids to the mouth or in oral activities preceding pharyngeal swallowing, resulting in misdirection of the bolus and aspiration. The apraxic individual may attempt to imitate an examiner's cues, producing erroneous or incorrect sequential execution of discrete acts. Outwardly, these individuals may appear to be completely unable to swallow or self-feed. They often perform quite well in the absence of the examiner's cues or attempts to assist. For this reason, it is important that assessment of swallowing in brain-injured patients include observation of performance in the "automatic" mode. As is seen in performance of selected language and self-care tasks, aphasic and apraxic patients often perform over-learned tasks accurately in the absence of distracting input, despite its intentional or seemingly contextual nature.

B. Right CVA

Right-sided cortical lesions tend to produce swallowing deficits characterized by apparently accurate and volitional oral propulsion followed by a pause in initiation of the pharyngeal response and subsequent arrival of the bolus into the pharynx prior to airway closure.[9] Aspiration resulting from this pattern of swallowing in patients with a right CVA is often silent, presenting without awareness of or response to airway compromise from the patient. The patient with a right CVA is more likely to exhibit signs of hemispatial inattention, a phenomenon often described as a focal visuospatial entity. Hemispatial inattention produces extinction of input not only from visual pathways, but also from other modalities of afferent input from areas on the affected side of the patient's body, such as tactile and auditory data. This is particularly evident when simultaneous input from the unaffected side of the body is presented. While eating, this syndrome may result in accumulation of oral or pharyngeal residue on the affected side, greater than what might otherwise be expected by the degree of primary sensorimotor involvement of facial and oral structures. The patient indeed may eat only the food on the right side of his or her plate or chew food in the right side of the mouth because of this "neglect" of half of his or her "space." This attentional component of a nondominant stroke patient's profile has not been quantitatively shown to directly contribute to the observed dysphagia. However, it should not be ignored in the workup and subsequent treatment planning.

C. Brainstem CVA

The lateral medullary syndrome (LMS) or Wallenberg's syndrome, provides a rare and dramatic example of dysphagia associated with a known lesion site. Oropharyngeal swallowing in patients presenting with a lateral medullary syndrome is often characterized by essentially normal oral function, apparently intact propulsion of the bolus into the pharynx, timely attempts at airway protection, awareness of aspiration often accompanied by a vigorous and immediate cough or other protective response, and an absent or incomplete pharyngeal response. The upper esophageal sphincter may either fail to distend throughout the swallow event, or the clinician may identify a segment (a cricopharyngeal prominence or bar) of the upper esophageal sphincter that fails to distend completely

during the sphincter's opening phase, separating or occluding the bolus. This finding is illustrated in the videoprint accompanying the presented Case 15-1. The patient may be seen struggling with and usually vigorously striving to clear or prevent aspiration while attempting to swallow. Following therapeutic intervention, some patients have been effectively trained to produce great effort, apparently generating sufficient intrabolus pressure to drive the bolus into and through the sphincter. In isolated lateral medullary syndrome (a rare event), cognitive status is often unaffected by the stroke, and as a result the patient may be an excellent candidate for therapy. Unfortunately, unless significant recovery restores some degree of normal activity within the upper esophageal sphincter, behavioral intervention may not succeed without more aggressive intervention, such as cricopharyngeal myotomy, which is described in the Treatment section of this chapter.

Case 15-1 is a dramatic example of a patient with a lateral medullary syndrome, who had significant recovery.

D. Traumatic Brain Injury (TBI)

Traumatic brain injury may produce a variety of oropharyngeal deficits related to swallowing because of primary central and peripheral lesions. Any number of combinations of deficits listed in the preceding sections may be observed. Oropharyngeal swallowing deficits within this population have been reported. However, these deficits have not been linked to specific sensorimotor impairments, with the exception of cranial nerve injury attributable to trauma, including acceleration/deceleration injury of the brain and brainstem. Delayed or absent pharyngeal response, reduced lingual control, reduced pharyngeal clearance, and aspiration at various points before, during, or following the swallow event have been reported. Patients with traumatic brain injury often exhibit varying degrees of fluctuating cognitive deficits that compound assessment and management. The extent to which these deficits produce the observed and reported swallowing errors has only been hypothesized. Among the cognitive deficits in this population that may influence safe oral intake are disorders of attention, including impulsivity and agitation, memory deficits, and reduced higher level reasoning skills.[11] Patients with severe attention deficits are often quite affected by distraction. This type of patient may place food into the mouth, then begin to speak or perform an unrelated task cued by an internal and/or external distractor, and risk aspiration. The impulsive patient is not likely to accurately perform head posturing or volitional throat clearing after the swallow. Thus, impulsivity may also increase aspiration risk in brain-injured patients with

CASE 15-1. Brainstem Cerebrovascular Accident

The patient is a 65-year-old male who sustained anterolateral PICA medullary embolic cerebrovascular accident in 11/96.

For 3 weeks, the patient was obtunded and required mechanical ventilation via orotracheal intubation, after which he underwent tracheostomy. During hospitalization, he contracted nosocomial pneumonia, and a modified barium swallow study demonstrated an absent pharyngeal response with profound silent aspiration. A gastrostomy was subsequently placed. He regained limited gait and ADL function with assistance due to residual balance and equilibrium deficits, including ataxia, nystagmus, and dysphagia. He was discharged to his home with a continuous gastrostomy infusion pump and tracheostomy with inflated cuff. He used an electrolarynx for speech.

Five months later, because of his wishes to resume oral feeding without aspiration, he was referred to the University Hospital Otolaryngology Service for evaluation of his candidacy for laryngotracheal diversion. He had remained dependent on tracheostomy and gastrostomy with no changes in regimen since discharge from hospital. He had been advised to use oral suction to prevent aspiration of secretions, with which his wife assisted every 2-3 minutes. On assessment, he exhibited left vocal fold paralysis with fixation in the paramedian position, and reduced right vocal fold mobility. He was referred to the Swallowing Service for assessment to rule out nonsurgical options for resumed oral intake.

A careful history was taken. The condition of the oral mucosa suggested that salivary flow was adequate. Initial clinical assessment revealed absent movement of the left soft palate, normal functional symmetry of the facial, lingual, and jaw musculature. The examiner then queried the patient as to whether he drooled while sleeping. Both he and his wife denied drooling, indicating some degree of intactness of nonconscious swallowing of secretions. On command, the patient then apparently swallowed a saliva bolus, producing palpable hyolaryngeal excursion suggestive of a pharyngeal response. Audible turbulence was heard by the examiner during this swallow, which can be expected given the inflated tracheostomy cuff and likelihood of UES dysfunction in this population. Three small sips of water tinged with blue food coloring followed, with similar results. The patient (and his wife) immediately assumed a surprised facial expression after the first and each subsequent trial, as he had voluntarily avoided swallowing for 5 months.

Videofluoroscopic assessment revealed consistent laryngeal penetration with inability to clear residue due to tracheostomy airflow diversion. The pharyngeal response was consistently delayed, with pooling in the pharyngeal recesses. A cricopharyngeal bar was observed with good distension of the UES superior and inferior to the segment (Fig 15-1).

Systematic rehabilitation ensued, with successful and rapid weaning from the tracheostomy. During this period, the tracheostomy device was downsized, fenestrated, and uncuffed. He was trained to perform 10 to 20 small (3-5cc) water swallows each hour while occluding the tracheostomy tube during practice and clearing his throat after swallowing. He was also encouraged to speak while the tube was occluded.

Over the next 6 weeks, he progressed to occlusion and then decannulation from tracheostomy. Vocal fold movement improved bilaterally on fiberoptic exam, as did vocal quality. The patient developed no upper respiratory infections, progressed to an oral diet, and began to gain weight. The gastrostomy was weaned and removed, and owing to the duration of the tracheostomy, surgical closure was performed. He remained independent in the use of airway protection and throat-clearing maneuvers. He was discharged from formal care.

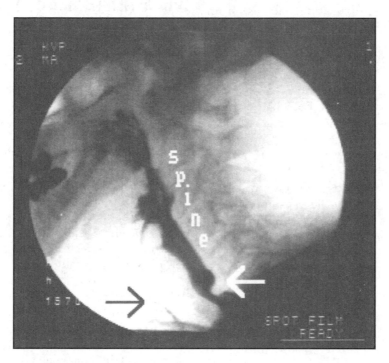

FIG 15-1. White arrow points to cricopharyngeal bar; black arrow points to aspiration during the swallow. Recording made with tracheostomy in place. Patient successfully resumed safe oral intake after decannulation and training.

concomitant oropharyngeal sensorimotor deficits that ordinarily respond to behavioral interventions.

E. Parkinson's Disease (PD)

Parkinson's disease and dysphagia are also discussed in Chapter 16. Pneumonia is one of the most prevalent primary causes of death in patients with Parkinson's disease.[12] The disease is characterized by a release of subcortical inhibitory centers within the indirect (extrapyramidal) motor system that modulate motor function. This is thought to occur because of degeneration and depigmentation of dopamine-containing neurons found in the substantia nigra and its connections to the basal nuclei. The result is depletion of dopamine in the caudate nucleus and putamen, causing a motor disturbance that includes, among other signs, rigidity and resting tremor. Rigidity is seen as reduced (hypokinetic) or slowed (bradykinetic) motion caused by simultaneous contraction of agonist and antagonist muscle groups, which are normally coordinated to produce refined movements. Oropharyngeal deficits attributable to Parkinson's disease include oral and pharyngeal phase disorders.[13,14] Oral disorders common in Parkinson's disease include excessive lingual rocking, or pumping; incomplete transfer of a bolus from oral to pharyngeal cavity; preswallow loss of bolus containment with spillage into the pharynx and/or larynx; and swallow hesitancy. Deficits during the pharyngeal phase include pooling of residue within the pharyngeal recesses and delayed onset of the pharyngeal response, predisposing the patient to aspiration before the swallow.[13,14] As one would expect, reduced lingual range of motion and generalized rigidity result in diminished hyolaryngeal excursion, producing inadequate distension of the upper esophageal sphincter and incomplete airway closure, with aspiration. Incomplete distension of the upper esophageal sphincter and esophageal motor abnormalities are also commonly detected in patients with Parkinson's.[13,15]

F. Dementia

Dementia is present in up to 20% of patients age 80 or older.[16] Dementia may result from the cumulative brain damage of multiple small cerebral infarcts as seen in chronic hypertension and diabetes, from syndromes such as Alzheimer's disease, or in the advanced stages of other disorders such as Parkinson's disease. Among the growing population of persons older than 80, a significant cause for acute hospitalization, especially among institutionalized patients, is fever because of infection. In more than half of these patients, the infection has been traced to pneumonia.[17] Dementia may progressively attenuate a patient's ability to perform even the most basic aspects of daily function such as swallowing. Risk factors predisposing elderly demented patients to aspiration and subsequent bronchopulmonary disease, such as pneumonia, include central nervous system disorders affecting oropharyngeal function, esophageal and upper gastrointestinal motility disorders. Pneumonia rates may be further influenced by inactivity. When identifiable oropharyngeal, esophageal, or other deficits associated with dysphagia and aspiration are absent, factors such as mental status should be considered as contributing to aspiration risk. According to the Centers for Disease Control and Prevention, a primary risk factor predisposing institutionalized patients to prandial aspiration is a decreased level of consciousness.[18]

Unfortunately, the pathophysiology of these observed deficits remains unclear, because of the variety of etiologies for dementia. The day-to-day or even minute-to-minute variability of confusion, memory deficits, effects of medications used to control agitation and wandering, depression, and other factors related to management of the demented patient further complicate attempts to isolate causes for the apparent sensorimotor oropharyngeal deficits seen. Multiple biomechanical deficits have been described in groups with progressive dementia. The patient who has dementia may also display delayed initiation of oral transit, delayed onset of the pharyngeal response and its critical airway closure component, distractibility, and inability to initiate even the most simple responsive behaviors. The potential outcome of "swallowing" deficits and the failure to maintain adequate oral nutrition and hydration produce medical complications that exacerbate declining cognitive and sensorimotor performance in this population.

Patients with stroke and brain injury are known to exhibit variable periods of recovery, some of which may be prolonged. Neurodegenerative diseases, on the other hand, produce accumulating disability. Conversely, the duration of most instrumental assessments of swallowing function, rarely more than a few minutes, is brief compared to the period of recovery or the duration of a meal. Hence, the diagnostic picture should be painted with data from many forms of assessment and observation.

VI. OTHER FORMS OF NEUROGENIC DYSPHAGIA

The cranial nerves, the final common motor pathways to the oropharyngeal complex, have been thoroughly discussed in Chapter 2. This framework allows the reader to match isolated peripheral lower motor neuron lesions with specific sensorimotor deficits in the mouth, face, pharynx, larynx, and upper esophagus with their functional correlates in patients with oropharyngeal dysphagia. Isolated lower motor neuron damage can occur following numerous forms of injury to the skull base or peripheral structures within the swallowing system or because of treatment for other disease such as head and neck cancer.

The motor effectors of the cranial nerves related to oropharyngeal swallowing are summarized in Table 15-2. Sensory functions of the cranial nerves are summarized in Table 15-3. These may be used as guides to sensorimotor assessment in a patient with dysphagia.

Catastrophic disease affecting the peripheral nervous system can produce dramatic and rapid functional decline. Dysphagia among patients with motor neuron disease, multiple sclerosis (MS) and other neuromuscular disorders is commonly encountered by the acute care clinician and is discussed briefly. The conditions within this section are referred to as "peripheral disorders," although it is doubtful that there are any conditions that can be said to be strictly or inevitably peripheral. In reality, the clinician will rarely see patients presenting with these disorders in isolation.

Table 15-2. *Motor Functions of Cranial Nerves Related to Swallowing*

1. **Trigeminal (V)**
   Special visceral motor: muscles of mastication, tensor veli palatini, anterior digastric.

2. **Facial (VII)**
   a. General visceral motor: submandibular and sublingual salivary glands.
   b. Special visceral motor: muscles of facial expression and tension, stylohyoid, posterior digastric muscles.

3. **Glossopharyngeal (IX)**
   a. Special visceral motor: stylopharyngeus muscle.
   b. General visceral motor: parotid gland.

4. **Vagus (X)**
   Special visceral motor: palatoglossus, palatopharyngeus and levator veli palatini* (faucial arch) musculature.

5. **Hypoglossal (XII)**
   All intrinsic and extrinsic lingual musculature.

*Some texts implicate trigeminal in this muscle's function

Table 15-3. *Sensory Functions of Cranial Nerves Related to Swallowing*

1. Trigeminal (V)
General somatic sensory: face, oral, lingual, and hard palate mucosa: proprioception from temporomandibular joint and muscles of mastication.

2. Facial (VII)
a. Special visceral sensory: taste from anterior 2/3 of tongue.
b. General visceral sensory: input from soft palate and adjacent pharyngeal wall.
c. General somatic sensory: proprioception from facial musculature, stylohyoid, posterior digastric muscles.

3. Glossopharyngeal (IX)
a. General visceral sensory: mucosa of posterior 1/3 of tongue, tonsil and tonsillar fossa, upper pharynx, afferent limb of gag reflex.
b. Special visc
c. General somatic sensory: proprioception from stylopharyngeus (presumed).

4. Vagus (X)
a. General visceral sensory: pharyngeal, laryngeal, esophageal and tracheal mucosa.
b. Special visceral sensory: taste from epiglottis.
c. General somatic sensory: proprioception from soft palate (presumed).

5. Hypoglossal (XII)
General somatic sensory: proprioception from tongue and floor of mouth musculature.

A. Motor Neuron Disease (Amyotrophic Lateral Sclerosis (ALS))

There are many forms of motor neuron disease; some affect sensory and motor neurons, others specifically target motor neurons. Understanding the pathophysiology of the disease is fundamental to sorting through predicted and observed signs and symptoms such as dysphagia. Some, such as Charcot-Marie-Tooth syndrome, affect sensory and motor peripheral neurons; others, such as spinal muscular atrophy, attack lower motor neurons. ALS is a rapidly progressive neuron disease without sensory involvement that targets upper and lower motor neurons within and projecting from the brain, brainstem, and spinal cord. It may present as either a nonbulbar or bulbar type. In the latter, dramatic progressive loss of swallowing function is observed and may progress with surprising swiftness. Lower motor neuron signs result from damage to the motor nuclei in the spinal cord (anterior horn cells) and brainstem motor nuclei; upper motor neuron effects are because of damage to the corticospinal and corticobulbar tracts. The effects of coexistent central and peripheral motor denervation include signs of mixed upper and lower motor neuron damage as previously discussed. Atrophy with or without fasciculations may be observed in the tongue and face. Spasticity or

flaccidity may also be detected throughout affected regions. Patients with bulbar involvement tend to exhibit early signs of lingual and labial weakness, with progression to the muscles of mastication and airway protection (floor of mouth and intrinsic/extrinsic laryngeal muscles). The progressive loss of muscle function in patients with bulbar involvement produces difficulty controlling oral contents, including secretions, food, and liquids, which may be observed as drooling (anterior loss), loss of controlled transfer to the pharynx (posterior), or "pocketing" of residue in the buccal (lateral) cavities. Interestingly, many such patients exhibit awareness and respond to aspiration when eating or drinking, suggesting a degree of preserved sensory functions. The patient may be observed frequently clearing his or her throat. The use of supplemental respiratory muscles is often affected, disabling the effectiveness of the reflexive cough response to aspiration, and may render voluntary airway clearance maneuvers ineffective. The ultimate result of the disease is loss of the ability to sustain either nutrition or hydration because of profound fatigue, requiring enteral nutritional support of the patient's limited oral intake. Pulmonary complications typically ensue as the disease progresses.

B. Multiple Sclerosis (MS)

Multiple sclerosis often produces a mixed and fluctuating clinical picture, because of the frequent presence of damage to white matter in the brain, brainstem, and spinal cord. The result is spastic motor impairment, with severe sensory and cognitive involvement. It is characterized by progressive demyelination of neurons and neuron tracts within the central nervous system. Magnetic resonance imaging (MRI) has become essential in the detection of lesions within the subcortical white matter in patients with MS. Two types of the disease have been described: a chronic-progressive type and another characterized by cyclic periods of exacerbation and remission. In the former, patients may exhibit progressive sensorimotor deficits that stabilize briefly or for periods of months to years. The latter is characterized by a rapid onset of marked decompensation of sensorimotor performance from the pre-exacerbation baseline followed by a period of remission, during which some degree of functional return occurs. Such remission typically progresses to a level below that of the pre-exacerbation baseline, until the next exacerbation-remission cycle occurs.

Swallowing is affected by a combination of sensory and motor impairment affecting not only the oropharyngeal mechanism, but also by involvement of ventilatory and postural musculature, pain, and disturbances in cognitive performance. Initial exacerbation is typically devastating as patients often tend to have exhibited no documented warning of the disease and may become totally dependent on caregivers within hours to days of onset.

With both types of MS, loss of control of the oral bolus or secretions, disturbances in salivary flow, reduced range and speed of movement of oropharyngeal structures, and aspiration are commonly observed in the acute stages, although patients with remission tend to regain substantial function toward, but always short of, baseline. Aspiration occurs from a variety of interacting factors and is often unaccompanied by clinical evidence, such as coughing. The cognitive involvement reported among many patients with the disease tends to produce a form of denial of deficits and, in some, euphoria is observed. Both may produce a tendency for the patient to disregard findings of swallowing dianostic assessment and subsequent illness such as recurrent aspiration pneumonia, which have pointed out the serious health risks associated with aspiration while eating or drinking.

Enteral replacement of oral intake is often necessary, particularly during exacerbation periods, as many patients are seriously incapacitated. Despite remissions to the point of restored safety of oral intake, patients are often advised to retain an enteral route, such as a gastrostomy or button, for immediate resumption of a safe route for nutrition, hydration, and administration of medications during future exacerbations.

C. Myasthenia Gravis; Other Myopathies

A variety of neuromuscular diseases have been shown to contain a component of dysphagia within their respective syndromes. Groher has presented a summary of dysphagia among patients with a variety of neurologic diseases.[19] Many of these are more often classified as myopathies, because of their specific effects on muscle function resulting from biochemical or anatomic disorders affecting the neuromuscular junction. These include myasthenia gravis and some of the myotonic dystrophies. Despite the etiology, the diagnosis and management of dysphagia in these diseases follows the logical assessment of oropharyngeal and esophageal function with special consideration for each disease, itself.

In general, myopathies can be distinguished from neuropathies by electromyographic evidence of intramuscular rather than neural dysfunction, and the absence of signs of lost neuromuscular integrity, such as the lower motor neuron denervation signs described. Often, the motor deficits are symmetric. In progressive muscular dystrophy, atrophy may be undetected in the presence of weakness, because of replacement of muscle tissue by fat or connective tissue. Myasthenia gravis, a disorder of the neuromuscular junction, which reduces the supply of the available muscle-activating neurotransmitter, presents with global findings of rapid fatigability of muscles throughout the body. A patient's history provides the clinician with important information about types and patterns of symptoms. The myasthenic patient complains of loss of swallowing functions over the course of a meal that began with fairly intact function. This muscular fatigue pattern is similar with other activities. In assessment of the myasthenic patient with symptoms of dysphagia, the clinician should not only understand the disease, but also challenge oropharyngeal function under the conditions that induce fatigue (eg, perform a modified barium swallow study after the patient has eaten a full meal or at the end of the day) to enable observation of reported swallowing deficits present during eating of meals.

VIII. DIAGNOSIS OF NEUROGENIC DYSPHAGIA

Assessment of a patient with central or peripheral neurologic disease should include four main components. First, the clinician must collect a history of the development and path of the patient's disease or disorder preceding the swallowing consult. This involves careful review of the medical record and patient and, possibly, caregiver interview. The clinician must understand the patient's concomitant symptoms and his or her interaction with oropharyngeal and esophageal function related to swallowing. Second, a careful and comprehensive inventory of the patient's cognitive status and oropharyngeal plus related facial sensorimotor functions must be obtained. The patient's candidacy for instrumental assessment and oral intake is made at this time (see Chapters 11 and 12). Third, a modified barium swallow (MBS) must be performed when safe, not only to identify biomechanical deficits, but to provide information for expediting a plan of remediation whenever possible. The clinician must be proactively prepared to employ trials of potentially effective interventions during such instrumental assessment, rather than simply identifying the nature of the oropharyngeal deficits. Such assessment, when performed merely to identify the presence or absence of aspiration, is nothing more than an expensive screening tool. Finally, the clinician must possess a sound understanding of the disorder/disease process and its pathophysiology. Without these components, optimal outcomes in patient health cannot be attained.

IX. TREATMENT

The rehabilitation of dysphagia is a transdisciplinary art that unites the skills of many professionals. Careful analysis of the swallowing dysfunction often directly points to methods of rehabilitation of and compensation for deficits. The most important consideration in the management of neurogenic dysphagia is the notion that, with the exception of degenerative disease, progress and spontaneous recovery are likely. To ignore this results in allowing recovering patients to remain dependent on suboptimal oral intake conditions, often with devastating consequences for the quality of life. The importance of assessment and monitoring of changes in function cannot be understated in the management of the patient striving to recover from neurologic damage.

A. Rehabilitative Efforts

Improvement of function, the aim of rehabilitative efforts, may occur spontaneously or as the result of carefully planned treatment strategies. Important treatment considerations for neurologic populations include careful and realistic assessment of a patient's ability and motivation to perform the proposed rehabilitative regimen. The other critical ingredient is the clinician's expertise as an *oropharyngeal biomechanical engineer*. For example, gross strengthening exercises performed weekly or twice per week in the presence of a clinician are essentially useless. Theories of muscle re-education and strengthening in the exercise physiology literature clearly point to significant change in muscle strength, bulk, and flexibility resulting from more frequent performance of exercises (ie, repetitions several times per day) that logically target specific muscle groups in performance of a specific task. And even intensive strengthening will not improve the swallow of a patient whose dysphagia does not result from weakness. Knowing what and how much to do to improve function is the essence of good biomechanical rehabilitation.

B. Compensatory Efforts

Training a patient to compensate for deficits acquired as the result of neurological damage is dependent on the intactness of his or her trainability and motivation to accept and use trained techniques. The traditional methods of compensatory training involve posture modification, alteration of food consistencies, and other voluntary maneuvers designed to circumvent the health consequences of the oropharyngeal deficit (see Chapters 34 and 35). Training a patient to redirect a bolus or to protect the airway while swallowing are worthwhile endeavors only if it is reasonable to assume that the patient will be able to employ the techniques. Likewise, diet texture modification, if objectively proven to eliminate aspiration or improve a patient's swallowing effectiveness, should not be selected without a realistic prediction of whether the patient will indeed use the

intervention, despite the apparent "success" of the intervention observed during MBS testing. Failure to consider the real possibility of compliance during treatment selection can predictably result in counterproductive outcomes, such as reduced oral intake or aspiration. Furthermore, compensatory maneuvers and use of texture modified liquids and foods have not been systematically shown to produce improved swallowing or health outcomes or reduced illness in any dysphagic population, although careful assessment can document their effectiveness with selected individuals.

C. Prosthetic Augmentation of Anatomy

Prosthodontic augmentation may improve oropharyngeal swallowing function in some patients with persistent velopharyngeal incompetence, unilateral lingual paralysis, or combined structural and neurologic dysphagia, as is commonly seen in trauma cases (Chapter 36). In these cases, the speech pathologist can collaborate with a prosthodontist to design a special appliance that may improve oral preparatory and transit components of the swallow in some neurogenic patients. A palatal lift prosthesis, which may be added to the posterior aspect of an upper denture plate, may reduce nasal regurgitation and diminish escape of important intrabolus pressure, resulting in decreased postswallow aspiration risks because of oropharyngeal residue. Other appliances, such as augmented upper dentures to compensate for absent unilateral lingual movement, may be fabricated by the prosthodontist. These types of prostheses enable linguapalatal contact on the paralyzed side of the oral cavity, improving bolus containment and, again, permitting more efficient transfer of lingual driving forces to the bolus, reducing oral residue and its consequences. The clinician must possess a solid understanding of oral structure and function to make clear and appropriate recommendations for prosthetic augmentation of such deficits to the prosthodontist.

D. Surgical Intervention

Surgery to improve swallowing function and safety is discussed in Section VI, Chapters 38-49. Within the neurogenic populations, such options are infrequently considered, unless protracted deficits with resultant health consequences such as recurrent pneumonia or other pulmonary sequelae are present. A dramatic example of this scenario, in contrast to Case 15-1, is presented as Case 15-2. Radical surgical interventions should be considered only after recovery is stable and all less invasive interventions have been eliminated systematically and unsuccessfully.

CASE 15-2. Brainstem Cerebrovascular Accident

RD is a 53-year-old man who suffered a large infarction of the lateral and medial medulla and lateral/inferior mid-pons, resulting from embolic occlusion of one vertebral artery. Vascular imaging documented aberrant distribution of the posterior vessels resulting in the unusual territory affected. Initial fluorographic assessment demonstrated impaired but functional swallowing, which deteriorated over 6 to 8 months, during which further embolic events were presumed. Inability to manage oral secretions led to continuous coughing, rendering MRI impossible. He received antibiotics continuously for several months because of chronic lung infiltrates and exhibited profuse drooling. Reassessment revealed profound impairment with major aspiration before (Fig 15-2) and during (Fig 15-3) the swallow. Upper esophageal segment opening was observed; however, laryngeal closure was absent. Despite intact cognitive function, he exhibited motoric inability to compensate with trained maneuvers. Tracheostomy was performed, but did not eliminate the patient's distress or chronic respiratory disease, which nearly progressed to fibrosis. Laryngotracheal separation was proposed and performed. RD was immediately and thereafter free of respiratory illness, gained weight, and returned to part-time employment. Imaging was subsequently possible and documented the presumed and enlarged brainstem lesions. He communicated great satisfaction with his outcome.

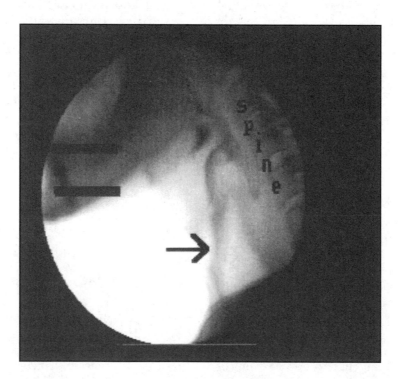

Fig 15-2. Aspiration before the swallow due to delayed pharyngeal response and absent laryngeal closure.

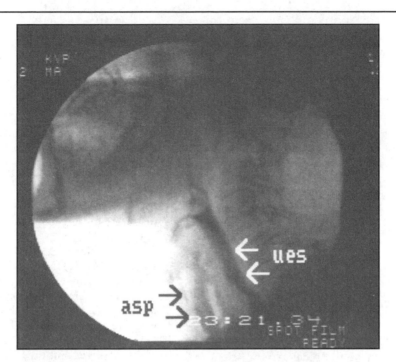

FIG 15-3. Aspiration during the swallow due to delayed and incomplete laryngeal closure. Nearly 50% of the bolus is consistently aspirated. Patient eventually underwent laryngotracheal diversion and successfully resumed safe oral intake.

Cricopharyngeal myotomy can be an effective surgical procedure in the management of the noncompliant upper esophageal sphincter (UES), as is common in brainstem stroke (see Chapter 42). However all efforts to adjudicate the deficit with less invasive interventions must be exhausted prior to making recommendations for surgical management. Likewise, the clinician must possess data to support the notion that such augmentation is expected to succeed. Impaired opening of the cricopharyngeal sphincter is a poor predictor of successful postmyotomy outcome; however it is the most readily available radiographic finding in the patient considered for myotomy or dilatation.[20] Ali et al have shown that fluorographically confirmed impairment of cricopharyngeal sphincter opening, together with manometrically documented high hypopharyngeal intrabolus pressures are more reliable predictors of improved postmyotomy cricopharyngeal compliance.[20]

Failure of the upper esophageal sphincter (UES) to distend may be the product of interruption of one or more normally occurring components of the swallow. The clinician must consider failure or interruption of (a) the normal preopening inhibition of UES tone, (b) the normal activity of suprahyoid muscles producing hyolaryngeal excursion that displaces the anterior wall of the UES and enables sphincter distension, and (c) the tissue elasticity or compliance properties of the normal

UES that allow the sphincter to be "pulled open." Such neuromotor, or physical, failures may eliminate several forces fundamental to bolus clearance through the UES, leaving the lingual driving forces alone to "push" each bolus into and through the sphincter. Cricopharyngeal myotomy is doomed to fail, if adequate lingual performance is not first documented to be adequate to serve as the remaining propulsive impetus.

The clinician should always exercise caution in decision making. Brain damage in particular carries with it a host of deficits that may critically affect clinical test interpretation and management decisions. The clinician must clearly understand and integrate the complex maze of cognitive, medical, and psychological issues carried by patients discussed in this chapter. Treatment of neurogenic dysphagia based on isolated biomechanical analysis will indeed fail without careful individualization of the plan to account for each patient's unique cluster of signs and symptoms.

X. CONCLUSION

In summary, carefully planned management of neurogenic swallowing disorders can effectively improve deglutitive function, when methods are systematically and objectively evaluated in the context of a patient's known neuromotor deficits and compliance/performance abilities. More radical and irreversible methods, such as surgery, should not be proposed until less invasive interventions fail to produce the desired outcomes.

This chapter describes the pathophysiology of neurogenic dysphagia. One may question whether or not certain stroke patients with dominant hemisphere damage and dysphagia have difficulty swallowing because of an apraxia. Does neglect explain the swallowing deficit in patients with nondominant hemisphere lesions? Can disease or site of lesion be predicted from the pattern of dysphagia? Must behavioral treatments always precede surgical ones? Must rehabilitative efforts always precede compensatory ones? Does etiology of the dysphagia influence the selection of specific behavioral treatment approaches? These questions are offered to stimulate discussion and research in the neuropathology of swallowing. Until these questions are prospectively answered, clinicians and clinical scientists are left to use the best diagnostic and treatment methods in their clinical art and science repertoire as the basis for management of dysphagia in patients with neurogenic disorders.

Frequently Asked Questions

1. Atrophy and fasciculations are the result of damage at which level of neuromotor organization?
   A. Lower motor neuron (nuclear, subnuclear, peripheral) damage produces this **flaccid paralysis.**

2. Why are soft palate and upper facial paresis not always clinically evident after unilateral cortical stroke?
   A. There are bilateral origins of motor outflow from the cortex to these sites. Also, unilateral UMN damage to tracts supplying these structures produces **spasticity**, hence appearance of these structures at rest may be undetectably asymmetric.

3. True or False: integrity of the gag reflex is a reliable predictor of oropharyngeal swallowing intactness.
   A. False. Individuals may possess various thresholds for a gag in response to noxious stimuli. Its presence or absence may merely reflect integrity of cranial nerve IX (afferent limb of gag reflex) or fibers from X (velar elevators, pharyngeal constrictors). The gag reflex is protective of the digestive system.

4. What are some general muscle activation disorders observed after upper motor neuron injury?
   A. Reduced strength due to disruption of higher level input including but not limited to cortical activation, reduced range and speed of motion due to spasticity, hyperreflexia, and hypertonicity due to reduced or absent inhibitory influences of higher subcortical center.

References

1. Buchholz D. Dysphagia associated with neurological disorders. *Acta Otorhinolaryngol Belg.* 1994;48:143-155.
2. Buchholz D. Neurogenic dysphagia: what is the cause when the cause is not obvious? *Dysphagia.* 1994;9:245-255.
3. Martin B, Corlew M. The incidence of communication disorders in dysphagic patients. *J Speech Hear Disord.* 1990;55:28-32.
4. Adams R, Victor M. (1989). *Principles of Neurology.* 4th ed. New York, NY: McGraw-Hill Book Company.
5. Cook I. Normal and disordered swallowing: new insights. *Bailliere's Clin Gastroenterol.* 1991;5:245-267.
6. Miller A. The search for the central swallowing pathway: the quest for clarity. *Dysphagia.* 1993;8:185-194.
7. Levine R, Robbins J, Maser A. Periventricular white matter changes and oropharyngeal swallowing in normal individuals. *Dysphagia.* 1992;7:142-147.
8. Martin R, Sessle B. The role of the cerebral cortex in swallowing. *Dysphagia.* 1993;8:195-202.
9. Robbins J, Levine R. Swallowing after unilateral stroke of the cerebral cortex: preliminary experience. *Dysphagia.* 1988;3:11-17.
10. Perlman A, Booth B, Grayhack J. Videofluoroscopic predictors of aspiration in patients with oropharyngeal dysphagia. *Dysphagia.* 1994;9:90-95.
11. Cherney L, Halper A. Swallowing problems in adults with traumatic brain injury. *Semin Neurol.* 1996;16:349-353.
12. Lieberman A, Horowitz L, Redmond P, Pachter L, Lieberman I, Leibowitz M. Dysphagia in Parkinson's disease. *Am J Gastroenterol.* 1980;74:157-160.
13. Ali G, Wallace K, Schwartz R, DeCarle D, Zagami A, Cook I. Mechanisms of oral-pharyngeal dysphagia in patients with Parkinson's disease. *Gastroenterology.* 1996;110:383-392.
14. Robbins J, Logemann J, Kirshner H. Swallowing and speech production in Parkinson's disease. *Ann Neurol.* 1986;19:283-287.
15. Leopold N, Kagel M. Pharyngo-esophageal dysphagia in Parkinson's disease. *Dysphagia.* 1997;12:11-18.
16. Winograd C, Jarvik L. Physician management of the demented patient. *J Am Geriatr Soc.* 1986;34:295-308.
17. Zarian D, Peter S, Lee S, Kleinfeld M. The causes and frequency of acute hospitalization of patients with dementia in a long-term care facility. *Natl Med Assoc.* 1989;81:373-377.
18. Centers for Disease Control and Prevention. Guidelines for prevention of nosocomial pneumonia. *Morbidity and Mortality Weekly Report.* 1997;46:3-11.
19. Groher M. Dysphagic patients with progressive neurologic disease. *Semin Neurol.* 1996;16:355-363.
20. Ali G, Wallace K, Laundl T, Hunt D, DeCarle D, Cook I. Predictors of outcome following cricopharyngeal disruption for pharyngeal dysphagia. *Dysphagia.* 1997;12:133-139.

CHAPTER 16

■ ■ ■

Neuromuscular Disorders

Susan M. Baser, M.D.

I. INTRODUCTION

Patients with neurogenic dysphagia can be effectively evaluated and managed, particularly if the dysphagia is recognized before development of medical complications such as aspiration pneumonia. Management is most cost effective and efficient when the assessment not only defines symptoms, but also when their underlying anatomic or physiologic cause and treatment is designed to eradicate the abnormalities in structure or function. The specific nature of the oropharyngeal dysphagia may also point to the nature of the underlying neurologic damage or disease process. Involvement of a speech-language pathologist early in the neurogenic patient's dysphagia care can speed recovery and reduce cost of treatment.

Causes of neurogenic dysphagia include stroke, head trauma, Parkinson's disease, motor neuron disease, and myopathy. Evaluation of the cause of unexplained neurogenic dysphagia should include a careful history, neurologic examination, magnetic resonance imaging (MRI) of the brain, blood tests (routine studies plus muscle enzyme studies, thyroid screening, vitamin B12 check, and antiacetylcholine receptor antibodies), electromyography (EMG) nerve conduction studies and, in certain cases, muscle biopsy or cerebrospinal fluid examination.

Many neurogenic disorders lead to dysphagia. One of the most common etiologies for unexplained neurogenic dysphagia may be cerebrovascular disease in the form of either confluent periventricular infarcts or small, discrete brainstem strokes, which may be invisible in MRI. The diagnosis of occult stroke causing pharyngeal dysphagia should not be overlooked, because this diagnosis carries important treatment implications.

Motor neuron disease producing bulbar palsy, pseudobulbar palsy, or a combination of the two can present with gradually progressive dysphagia and dysarthria with little, if any, limb involvement. Myopathies, especially polymyositis, and myasthenia gravis are potentially treatable disorders that must be considered. A variety of medications may cause or exacerbate neurogenic dysphagia. Psychiatric disorders can masquerade as swallowing apraxia. Once diagnosed, treatment for dysphagia should be directed toward the etiology of the symptom. Dysphagia secondary to myasthenia gravis and Parkinson's disease may improve when the underlying disease is treated.

II. AMYOTROPHIC LATERAL SCLEROSIS (ALS)

ALS has an incidence of around 2 per 100 000, with onset around age 60, although it may present earlier. Men are affected slightly more frequently than women, usually presenting with progressive, painless weakness. Neurological examination often shows upper motor neuron signs, increased tendon reflexes, and positive Babinski sign. The diagnosis of ALS requires the presence of lower motor neuron signs, upper motor neuron signs, and progression of the disorder. Upper limb muscles are affected more frequently than lower limb muscles, and bulbar muscles may be involved, with prominent dysarthria and dysphagia.

Patients with ALS survive for an average of 3 years after diagnosis, but patients with bulbar involvement frequently have shorter survival. Because of the progressive loss of function in bulbar and respiratory muscles, dysphagia may be an early and prominent problem or may occur only in the terminal phases of the disease. At least 73% of ALS patients have dysphagia before they require ventilatory support, and even a higher percentage have swallowing difficulty subsequently.[1]

Characteristically, patients have more problems with liquids and large pieces of food and find pureed or soft foods much easier to swallow. Secondary complications, such as nutritional deficiency and dehydration, compound the deteriorating effects of the disease and require careful monitoring.[2]

The patient with ALS can be managed as an outpatient by a team consisting of a nurse, physiotherapist, occupational therapist, speech-pathologist, nutritionist, respiratory therapist, and certain other consultants from time to time. The team's goal is to maintain physical function and extend the useful life of a patient through the skills that the team members are trained to provide.

For the patient with bulbar ALS and dysphagia, the accumulation of oral secretions may compound swallowing problems. Difficulty handling saliva can be an early and very disturbing symptom of bulbar ALS, often leading to aspiration and social isolation. Many therapeutic approaches have been suggested over the years to reduce salivary production, including the tricyclic amitriptyline. Some ALS patients benefit from treatment with beta antagonists to help to control thick secretions.[3]

Dysarthria may complicate the evaluation of dysphagia in an ALS patient. Communication is essential in the treatment of ALS patients, who may benefit from devices such as voice synthesizers and computer-assisted communication devices. In patients with prominent bulbar weakness, a palatal lift is sometimes useful. Spasticity may complicate the bulbar contribution to dysarthria and dysphagia in an ALS patient. In occasional patients, baclofen can be effective in relieving some of the upper motor neuron (UMN) impairment. Diazepam can occasionally be useful, but sedation and increased weakness can be a limiting adverse effect.

Pulmonary insufficiency, primarily a result of damage to motoneurons at the cervical level that innervate the diaphragm, is the proximate cause of death from ALS. Pulmonary function tests, especially spirometry, should be conducted at regular intervals and a modified barium swallow (MBS) or fiberoptic endoscopic evaluation of swallowing should also be done at least once. With careful monitoring, it is possible to anticipate and even correct a number of hazards, such as upper airway obstruction and aspiration. Some patients are candidates for gastrostomy and tympanic and chorda tympani neurectomy, but full knowledge of these patients' pulmonary function is essential before undertaking any surgical procedure.[4]

Early pulmonary impairment is a very poor prognostic sign. Bulbar involvement in ALS is often associated with a worse prognosis, because of the higher risk of pulmonary aspiration and malnutrition due to dysphagia. When dysphagia begins, it is important to monitor the patient's weight carefully and to begin discussions of percutaneous endoscopic gastrostomy (PEG) to increase caloric intake. Almost all patients with significant dysphagia have a caloric intake below that recommended by nutritional guidelines.[5] Thus, PEG can improve survival in elderly and young ALS patients with bulbar involvement. Adequate nutrition is maintained, medication is easier to administer, with complications of tube placement and care being negligible.[6]

III. INFLAMMATORY MYOPATHIES

The inflammatory myopathies include dermatomyositis, polymyositis, and inclusion body myositis. Although all of these diseases result in muscle weakness and dysphagia, each is unique in its clinical presentation. Inflammatory myopathies are a group of muscle diseases exhibiting inflammation and degeneration of skeletal muscle tissues. Thought to be autoimmune disorders, inflammatory cells surround, invade, and destroy normal muscle fibers, eventually resulting in muscle weakness.[7] The muscle weakness is usually symmetrical and develops slowly. Early signs of inflammatory myopathies include difficulty rising from a chair, climbing stairs, or lifting the arms. A patient may become exceedingly fatigued after prolonged standing or walking. In some cases, early signs include difficulty in swallowing or breathing.

A. Dermatomyositis

Dermatomyositis is one of the acquired inflammatory myopathies, affecting both children and adults, females more often than males. Dermatomyositis is characterized by a rash accompanying or, more often, preceding muscle weakness. The rash is described as patchy, bluish-purple discolorations on the face, neck, shoulders, upper chest, elbows, knees, knuckles, and back. Occasionally, muscle pain and tenderness occur and may be associated with fatigue, weight loss, and fever. Some patients may develop calcium deposits under the skin. The most common symptom, however, is proximal muscle weakness, producing difficulty rising from a sitting position, climbing stairs, lifting objects, or reaching overhead. Dysphagia occurs in at least one third of dermatomyositis patients.[8] Other problems complicating swallowing in the dermatomyositis include dryness of the mouth and prolonged posterior swallowing time.[9]

High dose prednisone is an effective treatment for many patients. Other nonsteroidal immunosuppressants, such as azathioprine and methotrexate, are often used.[8] Unfortunately, these drugs have adverse effects, especially after prolonged use. For patients who do not respond well to prednisone, intravenous administration of immunoglobulins (IVIg) has also proven effective.[11] Most cases of dermatomyositis respond to medical therapy. Dermatomyositis, however, is usually more severe and resistant to therapy in patients with cardiac or pulmonary problems.

B. Polymyositis

Polymyositis (PM) does not have the characteristic rash of dermatomyositis. More women than men are affected with polymyositis, which rarely affects people under the age of 20, although cases of childhood and infant polymyositis have been reported. As many as one third of polymyositis patients have muscle pain, but it is rarely the chief complaint. Onset of muscle weakness usually progresses slower than in dermatomyositis. Proximal limb and neck muscles are weakened; involvement of distal muscles varies. Dysphagia is common in polymyositis. As in dermatomyositis, dryness of the mouth and prolonged pharyngeal swallowing (ie, transit) complicate the dysphagia. Inability to breathe because of muscle failure is uncommon, but occurs more often in polymyositis than in dermatomyositis or inclusion body myositis.[8] Treatment is similar to dermatomyositis and includes prednisone, azathioprine, methotrexate, and IVIg.[10,11]

C. Inclusion Body Myositis

Inclusion body myositis is an inflammatory muscle disease characterized by slow and relentlessly progressive muscle weakness and atrophy. The disorder is very similar to polymyositis and is often the correct diagnosis in cases of polymyositis that are unresponsive to therapy. Onset of muscle weakness in inclusion body myositis is usually very gradual, taking place over months or years. It is different from polymyositis in that both proximal and distal muscles are affected and it occurs more frequently in men than women. Symptoms of the disease usually begin after the age of 50, although the disease can occur in any age group. About 1 in 10 cases of inclusion body myositis may be hereditary.[12]

Typical findings include weakness of the wrist flexors and finger flexors. Atrophy of the forearms is characteristic, and in the legs, atrophy of the quadriceps muscle is common, with varying degrees of weakness in other muscles. Falling is often the first noticeable symptom, and facial muscle weakness is present in a small number of patients.[12]

Unfortunately, there is as yet no known treatment for inclusion body myositis.[13] The disease is unresponsive

to corticosteroids and other immunosuppressive drugs. IVIg has shown some preliminary evidence for a slight beneficial effect in a small number of cases.[14] Physical therapy may be helpful in maintaining mobility. Other therapy is symptomatic and supportive. Inclusion body myositis is generally resistant to all therapies, and its rate of progression also appears to be unaffected by the present treatments.

IV. MUSCULAR DYSTROPHIES

The myriad of clinical presentations of all of the various muscular dystrophies is too much to detail in this chapter, so only brief descriptions of the most common disorders are included. Dysphagia occurs frequently in patients with the various forms of muscular dystrophies. Feeding difficulty and symptoms consistent with oropharyngeal, esophageal, and gastric dysfunction are frequent in patients with a variety of muscular dystrophies. Dysphagia is reported in 38% with limb-girdle syndrome, in 33% of those with myotonic muscular dystrophy, in 32% with spinal muscular atrophy, in 20% with Duchenne muscular dystrophy, and in 6% of those with facioscapulohumeral dystrophy.[9] Coordinated speech, swallowing, and nutritional support is essential in the diagnosis and treatment of neurogenic dysphagia associated with the muscular dystrophies.

A. Duchenne Muscular Dystrophy (DMD)

Duchenne muscular dystrophy (DMD) is the most common childhood form of muscular dystrophy, with usual age of onset at 2 to 6 years. Inheritance is X-linked and males are affected. Muscles first affected include the pelvic girdle, upper arms, and upper legs. It is usually slowly progressive. Early signs of DMD include frequent falling, difficulty getting up from a sitting or lying position, and a waddling gait. Another hallmark is the apparent enlargement of the calf and sometimes other muscles, which is due to an accumulation of fat and connective tissue in the muscle. Mild mental retardation has been noted in some affected individuals. Blood levels of creatine kinase are elevated. Breathing becomes affected during the later stages of DMD, leading to respiratory infections, and cardiac problems occur in the final stages, usually in the teens or early 20s. A defect in the gene that codes for the muscle protein, dystrophin, is the cause of the disease.

In addition to skeletal muscle involvement, visceral smooth muscle is affected in DMD, including gastric dilatation and intestinal pseudo-obstruction.[15] In 1990, Jaffe et al demonstrated dysphagia in virtually all Duchenne muscular dystrophy patients by 12 years of age; severe dysphagia and aspiration were common by age 18.[16] For individuals with DMD, prepharyngeal mechanisms contribute to dysphagia, including increased mandibular angle and weakness of masticatory muscles.[17]

For some individuals with muscular dystrophy, difficulties may be initially limited to abnormalities with macroglossia, mastication, temporomandibular joint (TMJ) motion, dental malocclusion, and prognathism.[9] Pharyngeal impairment in DMD is associated with the appearance of macroglossia and weakness of the pterygoid and superior constrictor muscles. Weakness of lip and cheek muscles and tongue elevators may become more pronounced as the disease progresses. Reduction in flexion and rotation of the cervical spine with scoliosis can also hamper swallowing. In DMD, neck hyperextension stretches the muscles that close the jaw, causing upper lip retraction with reduction in the ability to flex and rotate the neck.[16] Pharyngeal swallowing reflexes are eventually delayed because of impaired elevation and retraction of the tongue.[18] Sitting and balance difficulties can also hamper deglutition, which is also often affected by the presence of scoliosis and cervical and lumbar hyperlordosis.

Aspiration of food and saliva, weight loss, and pulmonary complications ultimately occur as dysphagia progresses. In DMD, ventilatory insufficiency with tachypnea decreases oral phase swallowing time and respiratory fatigue further hampers swallowing efforts. In DMD patients, weight loss correlates with increasing breathing impairment. The mean weight of DMD patients who are at the point of requiring ventilatory support is only 70 lb.[19] Weight will stabilize without resorting to parenteral means of delivering nutrition once adequate ventilatory assistance is provided.

B. Spinal Muscular Atrophies (SMA)

The SMAs constitute a group of neuromuscular disorders defined pathologically by degeneration of the anterior horn cells in the spinal cord, with the genetic defect in some localized to chromosome 5q11-q13.[20]

Many classification schemes have been proposed for SMA.[21] Briefly, three major subtypes of SMA are autosomal recessive and have onset in childhood. A smaller number show autosomal dominant or X-linked inheritance and onset begins later in life.

In spinal muscular atrophy type I (Werdnig-Hoffman), clinical features include onset in utero or before the age of 3 months, with hypotonia and weakness. Often the child is in a frog posture, with prominent respiratory problems, diphragmatic breathing, costal recession, and absent tendon reflexes. Affected children are intellectually typical. This disorder has a poor prognosis, with most patients dying within the first year.[22]

Patients with spinal muscular atrophy type 2 (intermediate) have onset of symptoms usually between 6 and 12 months, with symmetric weakness or proximal weakness, more in the legs than arms. Patients never learn to walk, muscle tendon reflexes are absent, scoliosis develops, and facial muscles are clinically spared. Patients have typical intellect.[23]

In spinal muscular atrophy type 3 (Kugelberg-Welander), symptoms begin between 1-20 years of age. Patients learn to walk but later loose this ability, often presenting with difficulties with walking, running, climbing, or jumping. Clinical features include slow progression, Gower's sign, proximal weakness with legs weaker than arms, and hypermobility of joints.[24]

Swallowing difficulties occur in over one third of patients with spinal muscular atrophy.[9] Bulbar and respiratory involvement is a prominent feature only in early onset, more severely affected SMA patients, with insufficient respiration, difficulty sucking and swallowing, accumulation of secretions, and a weak cry. The intercostal and accessory respiratory muscles are weakened, but the diaphragm is relatively spared, so a characteristic paradoxical breathing pattern and flaring of the lower portion of the rib cage are produced. Tongue fasciculations are commonly seen in type I SMA, and a limitation in the ability to open the mouth is also noted in SMA, further complicating dysphagia.[25,26]

Patients with severe SMA requiring intubation and tracheostomy have an extremely poor prognosis. However, each situation must be managed individually with careful attention to bioethical issues. Gastrostomy is needed less commonly than one might expect, but, when appropriate, should be carried out. Understandably, the therapeutic goals and management of patients with types II and III are quite different, because they have a much better prognosis.[23]

C. Myotonic Dystrophy

Myotonic dystrophy is an autosomal dominant disorder that results in skeletal muscle weakness and wasting, myotonia, and numerous nonmuscular manifestations including frontal balding, cataracts, gonadal dysfunction, cardiac conduction abnormalities, respiratory insufficiency, and hypersomnolence.[27] Age of onset ranges from early childhood to adulthood, with newborn onset in the congenital form of myotonic dystrophy. Muscle weakness is slowly progressive, with a wide variation in degree of weakness, even among members of a single family.

The gene defect in myotonic dystrophy has been mapped to chromosome 19, but the exact metabolic abnormalities responsible for this disorder are unknown.[28] Laboratory studies, including EMG, electrocardiography (ECG), and muscle biopsy, are helpful in evaluating patients for this disorder, but the clinical aspects and a careful family history are important in the diagnosis of myotonic dystrophy.

Gastrointestinal symptoms are found in a large proportion of patients suffering from this disease and may herald the onset of muscular disorders; in rare cases they are even the predominant feature of the disorder.[29] Involvement of the pharyngeal and gastrointestinal smooth and striated muscles results in velopharyngeal insufficiency, resulting in swallowing difficulties, gastrointestinal motility disorders, and anal incontinence.[30]

Radiologic features of dysphagia in myotonic dystrophy include a marked reduction in resting tone of both the upper and lower esophageal sphincters and a reduction in contraction pressure in the pharynx and throughout the esophagus. Radiology showed hypotonic pharynx with stasis and a hypo-, or amotile, often dilated, esophagus, and gastroesophageal reflux disease (GERD) in these patients.[31] Recurrent intestinal pseudo-obstruction has also been described.[32] The agent cisapride has been shown to be useful in the treatment of both gastroparesis and intestinal pseudo-osbstruction in these patients.[31,33] Cricopharyngeal myotomy is an effective treatment in some myotonic dystrophy patients where cricopharyngeal dysfunction is a predominant problem, but it is contraindicated when pharynx propulsion is severely impaired.[34]

D. Oculopharyngeal Muscular Dystrophy

Oculopharyngeal muscular dystrophy (OPMD) is a progressive neurological disorder characterized by gradual onset of dysphagia, ptosis, and facial weakness. The later stages of this slowly progressive disease may include weakness in the pelvic and shoulder muscles. OPMD is an autosomal dominant disorder that affects both males and females, with onset of symptoms in the 4th or 5th decade. Dysphagia is slowly progressive and may be a presenting symptom before a diagnosis is made.[35] Linkage of OPMD to 14q11.2-q13 has been reported in a series of French Canadian and American families.[36]

Dysphagia with weight loss and aspiration commonly occurs in oculopharyngeal muscular dystrophy. Both striated skeletal and smooth muscle are affected in oculopharyngeal muscular dystrophy, including very low striatal muscle mediated pharyngeal pressures, cricopharyngeal bar, and low lower esophageal sphincter pressure.[37] In oculopharyngeal dystrophy patients, cricopharyngeal myotomy is an effective treatment of dysphagia secondary to cricopharyngeal bar. However, a cricopharyngeal myotomy does not modify the final prognosis and is contraindicated in cases with pharyngeal aperistalsis.[38] Long-term follow up shows a recurrence of the swallowing and tracheobronchial symptoms in many cases of OPMD after cricopharyngeal myotomy.[39]

Upper esophageal sphincter (UES) dilatation with a Maloney bougie or an achalasia dilator may also be effective in some patients with moderate to severe dysphagia associated with with oculopharyngeal muscular dystrophy.[40]

E. Limb-Girdle Muscular Dystrophy

Limb-girdle muscular dystrophy is a slowly progressive form of muscular dystrophy with both autosomal recessive and dominant forms. Both males and females are affected, with the usual onset in adolescence or early adulthood. In the most common forms, the disease causes progressive weakness that starts in the hips and moves to the shoulders. The pectoralis, iliopsoas and gluteal muscles, hip adductors, and hamstrings were the most affected muscles. Distal muscle involvement occurs late in the course of the disease. Facial weakness is rare.[41]

A reclassification of the limb-girdle types of autosomal recessive muscular dystrophy based on genetic information has been made possible by major advances in the past several years. At least six different forms of limb-girdle type of autosomal recessive muscular dystrophy can be defined by their genetic basis, with at least two pathogenic mechanisms involved and that an autosomal dominant form can result from gene defects on chromosome 5.[42]

Limb girdle muscular dystrophy is not a common cause of dysphagia, but swallowing abnormalities are demonstrated in up to 30%, with demonstrated dysfunction of the pharyngeal striated muscle.[43] Some patients with a cricopharyngeal bar have had successful treatment of dysphagia by cricopharyngeal myotomy.[44]

F. Facioscapulohumeral Muscular Dystrophy

Facioscapulohumeral muscular dystrophy (FSHD) is a slowly progressive, autosomal dominant neuromuscular disorder, with onset in the teens or early adulthood. The disease affects specific muscles of the face, shoulder-girdle, and upper arm. The weakness spreads to the muscles of the abdomen, feet, upper arms, pelvic area, and lower arms, with severity from very mild to considerably disabling, with impairment of walking, chewing, swallowing, and speaking. The biochemical defect underlying FSHD is unknown and there are no specific tests that are diagnostic of FSHD. Genetic linkage studies have mapped the FSHD gene to chromosome 4q35.[45]

Difficulties in the pre-oral phase of swallowing occur in many of the muscular dystrophies, including FSHD.[9] Facial weakness and deformity may contribute to swallowing difficulty in FSHD. Individuals with facioscapulohumeral syndrome have a low incidence of dysphagia (less than 10%). But for persons with swallowing problems, evaluation and treatment are important.[46] Thirty-five percent of the patients with FSHD have spine deformity, which may contribute to dysphagia; however, most have had hyperlordosis.[47]

V. MYASTHENIA GRAVIS

Adult-onset myasthenia gravis is an acquired autoimmune disorder of neuromuscular transmission in which acetylcholine receptor antibodies attack the postsynaptic membrane of the neuromuscular junction. Most patients have ptosis, diplopia, dysarthria, and dysphagia. Weakness due to myasthenia gravis characteristically fluctuates, worsening throughout a day or with prolonged physical activity. The incidence of myasthenia has two peaks, the first occuring in the 2nd and 3rd decade with female predominance and the other in the 6th and 7th decade affecting mostly men.[48]

The onset is generally insidious with progression over weeks to months. However, a variety of conditions such as infections, emotional stress, or pregnancy may rapidly aggravate symptoms of myasthenia gravis. A number of medications with inhibitory effects on neuromuscular transmission, cholinergic blocking agents, and muscle relaxants can exacerbate myasthenia gravis. Penicillamine may even induce myasthenia gravis. Weakness in systemic musculature can be diffuse, but is usually more prominent in proximal areas such as the neck, shoulder, and hip girdle muscles.

Swallowing problems may be an early sign of myasthenia gravis and occur in approximately one third of those diagnosed. Dysphagia is the presenting sign of myasthenia gravis in neonates and in 6% to 15% of adult patients.[49] The bulbar and facial muscles are frequently affected, causing dysphagia, dysarthria, nasal speech, or weakness of mastication. Examination may show masseter weakness, bifacial weakness, poor gag reflex and palate elevation, dysarthria, or dysphonia. A weak tongue is very common when the bulbar musculature is involved. Dysphagia caused by bulbar weakness may result in aspiration pneumonia. Posterior tongue swallowing transit time is especially affected in myasthenia gravis.

Swallowing severity can fluctuate and it is therefore important that swallow is assessed and closely monitored by a speech-language pathologist. In its mild form, patients may experience a mild sensation of food sticking in the throat while eating semisolids. Liquids may be easier than solids and patients may fatique with chewing because of masseter weakness. Patients typically do well at the beginning of a meal, but tire at the end. Some patients may deteriorate to a point where there is total loss of ability to chew and swallow, causing aspiration.

Practical guidelines include eating slowly and resting between bites, as necessary, and, if fatigue is a problem late in the day, have the main meal earlier in the day. Patients should take meals when muscle strength is best, possibly 1 hour after medication such as Mestinon.

VI. ACQUIRED AND DEGENERATIVE CEREBRAL DISORDERS

A. Stroke

Stroke is detailed in greater description in Chapter 15, so only the most common neurologic presentations of dysphagia with stroke are described here. Briefly, dysphagia and aspiration are two devastating sequelae of stroke, accounting for nearly 40 000 deaths from aspiration pneumonia each year in the United States. Patients with an abnormal swallow on bedside assessment have a higher risk of chest infection and a poor nutritional state. The presence of dysphagia is associated with an increased risk of death, disability, length of hospital stay, and need for institutional care.[50]

Significant dysphagia and aspiration can occur in patients with a variety of stroke presentations, including unilateral hemispheric, bilateral hemisheric, and brainstem strokes. Motor and sensory deficits in the larynx and pharynx may play a significant role in the occurrence of dysphagia and aspiration in some stroke patients.[51] Aggressive identification, evaluation, and treatment of dysphagia in the stroke patient can diminish the risk of pneumonia, dehydration, calorie-nitrogen deficit, recurrent upper airway obstruction, and even death following stroke.

1. Localization

Patients who have experienced stroke should be individually evaluated for swallowing dysfunction, regardless of stroke location or size. Aspiration is a common problem following stroke in both large vessel and small vessel stroke, resulting in feeding difficulties and aspiration pneumonia. In an MRI study of patients with acute stroke who underwent a swallowing evaluation, aspiration was present in over one half. Patients with only small vessel infarcts had a significantly lower occurrence of aspiration compared to those with both large- and small-vessel infarcts.[52] Oropharyngeal dysphagia occurs in up to a third of patients presenting with a unilateral hemiplegic stroke, yet its neurophysiological basis remains unknown. Neurophysiological studies suggest that dysphagia after unilateral hemispheric stroke is related to the magnitude of pharyngeal motor representation in the unaffected hemisphere.[53]

In patients with ischemic middle cerebral artery (MCA) stroke, different patterns of MCA involvement is shown to be associated with certain deficits in swallowing. Patients with right hemisphere stroke show longer pharyngeal transit and higher incidences of laryngeal penetration and aspiration of liquid, as compared to patients with left sided strokes.[54]

In one large series, 30% of patients with single-hemisphere strokes had difficulty swallowing a mouthful of water, but in most of those who survived, the deficit resolved by the end of the first week. Strong correlations occur between dysphagia and speech impairment (comprehension and expression) in single-hemispheric stroke and facial weakness.[55]

In patients with bilateral strokes, up to 50% aspirate. Patients with aspiration are more likely to have posterior circulation strokes, abnormal cough, abnormal gag, and dysphonia. However, patients likely to aspirate can be best identified by the presence of an abnormal voluntary cough, an abnormal gag reflex, or both. The prediction of which patients are at-risk for aspiration was not improved by additional clinical information (ie, presence of dysphonia or bilateral neurologic signs).[56]

Wallenberg's syndrome (lateral medullary syndrome [LMS]) is due to thrombosis of the posteroinferior cerebellar artery, which results in ischemia of the lateral medullary region of the brainstem. In addition to vertigo, nystagmus, nausea, vomiting, Horner's syndrome, dysphonia, ataxia, falling to the side of the lesion, and loss of pain and temperature sensation to the ipsilateral head and contralateral body, this syndrome also leads to dysphagia with ipsilateral palatal paralysis. It differs from many other types of dysphagia in that tongue driving force and oropharyngeal propulsion pump force are greatly increased, in part due to the failure of pharyngoesophageal sphincter to open during swallowing.[57]

2. Evaluation of Swallowing

Aspiration pneumonias are frequent complications of swallowing disorders following cerebrovascular accidents. A simple bedside test is based on observation of some components of the oral and pharyngeal stages of the swallowing process and on a drinking test of 50 cc of clear liquids. The administration of this swallowing evaluation is associated with a marked reduction of frequency of aspiration pneumonia.[58] The Burke Dysphagia Screening Test (BDST) is highly sensitive in identifying stroke patients at-risk for developing pneumonia and recurrent upper airway obstruction.[59] Videofluoroscopic modified-barium swallow is also useful in documenting aspiration in stroke patients.[60]

3. Swallowing Therapy

Early screening and management of dysphagia in patients with acute stroke has been shown to reduce the risk of aspiration pneumonia, is cost effective, and assures quality care with optimal outcome.[61] Because of swallowing deficits, changes in the consistency of foods and other modifications for safe nutrition should be considered during the first month of recovery, even for unilateral stroke patients.[62] Direct therapy programs for chronic neurogenic dysphagia resulting from brainstem stroke show that functional benefits are long lasting without related health complications.[63]

B. Parkinson's Disease and Progressive Supranuclear Palsy

Aspiration related to swallowing is a major cause of morbidity and mortality in Parkinson's disease. Parkinson's disease is a progressive degenerative disorder characterized by loss of striatal dopamine. Peak age of onset is in the late 50s to early 60s, but Parkinson's disease can affect younger age groups. Progressive rigidity, bradykinesia, and tremor are hallmarks of this disease. Patients typically respond well initially to a variety of dopaminergic agents, but as the disease progresses, pharmacologic treatments are less effective. Prominent speech and swallowing disorders complicate the course in many Parkinson's disease patients, particularly in those with long-standing disease.

Oral and pharyngeal dysphagia in Parkinson's disease is multifactorial. Many prepharyngeal abnormalities of ingestion, including cognitive, drooling, jaw rigidity, impaired head and neck posture during meals, upper extremity dysmotility, impulsive feeding behavior, and impaired amount regulation and lingual transfer movements are common in more advanced patients. The motor disturbances of ingestion in Parkinson's disease reflect problems caused by akinesia, bradykinesia, tremor, and rigidity.[64] Some of the motor disturbances improve with treatment of the underlying neurological disease, but as symptoms progress, dysphagia becomes progressively disabling in these patients.

Pharyngeoesophageal motor abnormalities also play a role in dysphagia in Parkinson's patients. These abnormalities include low pharyngeal contraction, abnormal pharyngeal wall motion, impaired pharyngeal bolus transport, and manometric abnormalities, with incomplete upper esophageal sphincter relaxation.[65] Typical aberrations of lower esophageal sphincter (LES) function include an open or delayed opening of the LES and gastroesophageal reflux (GER). Other esophageal abnormalities include delayed transport, stasis, bolus redirection, and tertiary contractions.[66]

Cricopharyngeal function should be carefully evaluated in Parkinson's disease. The presence of a Zenker's diverticulum causing cricopharyngeal dysfunction should not be overlooked in Parkinson's patients. Cricopharyngeal myotomy has produced excellent and sustained improvement in swallowing in Parkinson patients with coexisting Zenker's diverticulum,[67] but is not recommended to treat other causes of dysphagia in Parkinson patients.

Progressive supranuclear palsy (PSP) is a progressive degenerative extrapyramidal disease that often masquerades as Parkinson's disease. Patients usually have onset at or over age 40, and experience rigidity with axial predominance, postural instability, frequent falls, and bradykinesia. PSP patients have a characteristic ophthalmologic feature of bilateral supranuclear ophthalmoplegia, typically with loss of down gaze, up gaze, then horizontal gaze. Other clinical manifestations of PSP include poor or absent response to levodopa, cervical dystonia with neck hyperextension, dysarthria and dysphagia, apraxias of eyelid opening, echolalia, and palilalia.

Similar to Parkinson's disease, dysphagia frequently complicates the course of PSP, with almost all PSP patients showing multiple abnormalities in swallowing. These defects include uncoordinated lingual movements, absent velar retraction or elevation, impaired posterior lingual displacement, and copious pharyngeal secretions. Tongue-assisted mastication, noncohesive lingual transfer, excessive spillage of the oral bolus into the pharynx prior to active transfer, vallecular bolus retention, abnormal epiglottic positioning, and hiatal hernias are also noted in about one half of PSP patients.[68] Unfortunately, PSP patients are not as responsive to dopaminergic pharmacologic treatment as Parkinson's patients and their dysphagia is more life-threatening and resistant to treatment. Early and aggressive swallowing evaluation and treatment is mandatory in PSP patients.

C. HEAD INJURY

The etiology of dysphagia and its treatment in patients with brain injury are multifactorial. There is a high correlation between swallowing dysfunction and prolonged hospitalization after head injury. The most common swallowing problems demonstrated by videofluorography barium swallow are prolonged oral transit and delayed swallowing reflex. Serial videofluoroscopy can also be used to document improved swallowing function and indicate when it is safe to stop of nasogastric tube feedings.[69]

Despite a large percentage of oral motor problems in severe head injury, most patients will become successful oral feeders after participating in organized dysphagia programs implemented by a head injury rehabilitation team. First, the resolution of cognitive problems and primitive oral motor reflexes improves outcome in neurogenic dysphagia after severe head injury. In nonoral feeders, the average time from injury to successful completion of their first oral meal is about 3 months.[70] Attention to details such as simple changes in the position of the patient during feeding can alter the incidence of aspiration in head injury patients.[71] Newer techniques in oral dysphagia rehabilitation range from specific oromotor exercises to audiovisual biofeedback.[72]

Frequently Asked Questions

1. How common is dysphagia in myasthenia gravis?
   A. Dysphagia may be a prominent feature of myasthenia gravis (MG) and may occur early in the course of the disease. Swallowing difficulties occur in about one-third of the MG patients.
2. How does ventilatory impairment influence dysphagia in muscular dystrophy patients?
   A. Aspiration and weight loss occur as the disease progresses. Ventilatory insufficiency and respiratory fatigue make swallowing more difficult. Control of ventilatory impairment will improve swallowing ability.
3. How important is evaluation of dysphagia in amyotrophic lateral sclerosis (ALS) patients?
   A. Patients with bulbar involvement have prominent dysphagia early. Dysphagia should be monitored closely with close attention to weight loss. PEG placement can prolong both survival and quality of life in these patients.

References

1. Mayberry JF, Atkinson M. Swallowing problems in patients with motor neuron disease. *J Clin Gastroenterol.* 1986;8:233-234.
2. Strand EA, Miller RM, Yorkston KM, Hillel AD. Management of oral-pharyngeal dysphagia symptoms in amyotrophic lateral sclerosis. *Dysphagia.* 1996;11:129-139.
3. Newall AR, Orser R, Hunt M. The control of oral secretions in bulbar ALS/MND. *J Neurol Sci.* 1996;139(suppl):43-44.
4. Hudson AJ Jr. Outpatient management of amyotrophic lateral sclerosis. *Semin Neurol.* 1987;7:344-351.
5. Kasarskis EJ, Berryman S, Vanderleest JG, Schneider AR, McClain CJ. Nutritional status of patients with amyotrophic lateral sclerosis: relation to the proximity of death. *Am J Clin Nutr.* 1996;63:130-137.
6. Mazzini L, Corrà T, Zaccala M, Mora G, Del Piano M, Galante M. Percutaneous endoscopic gastrostomy and enteral nutrition in amyotrophic lateral sclerosis. *J Neurol.* 1995;242:695-698.
7. Dalakas M. Immunopathogenesis of inflammatory myopathies. *Ann Neurol.* 1995;37:574-586.
8. Dalakas M. Polymyositis, dermatomyositis, and inclusion-body myositis. *N Eng J Med.* 1991;325:1487-1498.
9. Willig TN, Paulus J, Lacau Saint Guily J, Béon C, Navarro J. Swallowing problems in neuromuscular disorders. *Arch Phys Med Rehabil.* 1994;75:1175-1181.
10. Dalakas M. Current treatment of inflammatory myopathies. *Cur Opini Rheumatol.* 1994;6:595-607.
11. Dalakas M, Illa I, Dombrosia JM, et al. A Controlled Trial of high-dose intravenous immune globulin infusions as treatment for dermatomyositis. *N Eng J Med.* 329:27;1993-2000.
12. Sekul E, Dalakas M. Inclusion body myositis: New concepts. *Semin Neurol.* 1993;13:256-263.
13. Barohn R. The therapeutic dilemma of inclusion body myositis. *Neurology.* 1997;48:567-568.
14. Dalakas M, Sonies B, Dambrodia J, et al. Treatment of inclusion-body myositis with IVIg: a double-blind, placebo-controlled study. *Neurology.* 1997;48:712-716.

15. Bensen ES, Jaffe KM, Tarr PI. Acute gastric dilatation in Duchenne muscular dystrophy. *Arch Phys Med Rehabil.* 1996;77:512-514.
16. Jaffe KM, McDonald CM, Ingman E, Haas J. Symptoms of upper gastrointestinal dysfunction in Duchenne muscular dystrophy: case-control study. *Arch Phys Med Rehabil.* 1990;71:742-744.
17. Ashby DW. Bone dystrophy in association with muscular dystrophy. *Br Med J.* 1951;1486-1488.
18. Gilardeau C. Dystrophie a evolution rapide (stade non ambulatoire) et troubles de la deglutition-mastication. *Entretiens de Montpellier.* Paris: Edition Masson, 1991.
19. Bach JR, Tippett DC, McCrary MM. Bulbar dysfunction and associated cardiopulmonary considerations in polio and neuromuscular disease. *J Neurol Rehabil.* 1992;6:1212-1218.
20. Brzustowicz LM, Lehner T, Castilla LH, et al. Genetic mapping of childhood-onset spinal muscular atrophy to chromosome 5q11.2-13.3. *Nature.* 1990;344:540-541.
21. Dubowitz V. Chaos in classification of the spinal muscular atrophies of childhood. *Neuromusc Disord.* 1991;1:77-80.
22. Brandt S. Course and symptoms of progressive infantile muscular atrophy. *Arch Neurol Psychiatry.* 1950;63:218-228.
23. Fried K, Emery AEH. Spinal muscular atrophy type II. A separate genetic and clinical entity from type I (Werdnig-Hoffmann disease) and type ll (Kugelberg-Welander disease). *Clin Genet.* 1971;2:203-209.
24. Kugelberg E, Welander L. Heredofamilial juvenile muscular atrophy simulating muscular dystrophy. *Arch Neurol Psychiatry.* 1956;75:500-509.
25. Moosa A, Dubowitz V. Spinal muscular atrophy in childhood: two clues to clinical diagnosis. *Arch Dis Child.* 1973; 48:386-388.
26. Pearn JH, Hudgson P, Walton JN. A clinical and genetic study of spinal muscular atrophy of adult onset. *Brain.* 1978;101:591-606.
27. Jozefowicz RF, Griggs RC. Myotonic dystrophy. *Neurol Clin.* 1988;6:455-72.
28. Alberts MJ, Roses AD. Myotonic muscular dystrophy. *Neurol Clin.* 1989,7:1-8.
29. Rönnblom A, Forsberg H, Danielsson A. Gastrointestinal symptoms in myotonic dystrophy. *Scand J Gastroenterol.* 1996;31:654-657.
30. Sartoretti C, Sartoretti S, DeLorenzi D, Buchmann P. Intestinal non-rotation and pseudoobstruction in myotonic dystrophy: case report and review of the literature. *Int J Colorectal Dis.* 1996;11:10-14.
31. Costantini M, Zaninotto G, Anselmino M, et al. Esophageal motor function in patients with myotonic dystrophy. *Dig Dis Sci.* 1996;41:2032-2038.
32. Brunner HG, Hamel BC, Rieu P, Höweler CJ, Peters FT. Intestinal pseudo-obstruction in myotonic dystrophy. *J Med Genet.* 1992;29:791-793.
33. Champion MC. Management of idiopathic, diabetic and miscellaneous gastroparesis with cisapride. *Scand J Gastroenterol.* 1989;165(Suppl):44-53.
34. St Guily JL, Périé S, Willig TN, Chaussade S, Eymard B; Angelard B. Swallowing disorders in muscular diseases: functional assessment and indications of cricopharyngeal myotomy. *Ear Nose Throat J.* 1994;73:34-40.
35. Young EC, Durant Jones L. Gradual onset of dysphagia: a study of patients with oculopharyngeal muscular dystrophy. *Dysphagia.* 1997;12:196-201.
36. Stajich JM, Gilchrist JM, Lennon F, et al. Confirmation of linkage of oculopharyngeal muscular dystrophy to chromosome 14q11.2-q13. *Ann Neurol.* 1996;40:801-804.
37. Tiomny E, Khilkevic O, Korczyn AD, et al. Esophageal smooth muscle dysfunction in oculopharyngeal muscular dystrophy. *Dig Dis Sci.* 1996;41:1350-1354.
38. Périé S, Eymard B, Laccourreye L, et al. Dysphagia in oculopharyngeal muscular dystrophy: a series of 22 French cases. *Neuromuscl Disord.* 1997;7(suppl 1):S96-S99.
39. Fradet G, Pouliot D, Robichaud R, St Pierre S, Bouchard JP. Upper esophageal sphincter myotomy in oculopharyngeal muscular dystrophy: long-term clinical results. *Neuromuscl Disord.* 1997; 7(suppl 1):S90-S95.
40. Mathieu J, Lapointe G, Brassard A, et al. A pilot study on upper esophageal sphincter dilatation for the treatment of dysphagia in patients with oculopharyngeal muscular dystrophy. *Neuromuscl Disord.* 1997;7(suppl 1):S100-4.
41. van der Kooi AJ, Barth PG, Busch HF, et al. The clinical spectrum of limb girdle muscular dystrophy. A survey in The Netherlands. *Brain.* 1996;119:1471-1480.
42. Beckmann JS, Bushby KM. Advances in the molecular genetics of the limb-girdle type of autosomal recessive progressive muscular dystrophy. *Curr Opin Neurol.* 1996; 9:389-393.
43. Stübgen JP. Limb girdle muscular dystrophy: a radiologic and manometric study of the pharynx and esophagus. *Dysphagia.* 1996;11:25-29.
44. Johnson ER, McKenzie SW. Kinematic pharyngeal transit times in myopathy: evaluation for dysphagia. *Dysphagia.* 1993;8:35-40.
45. Wijmenga C, Frants RR, Hewitt JE, et al. Molecular genetics of facioscapulohumeral muscular dystrophy. *Neuromuscl Disord.* 1993;3:487-491.
46. Goldberg MH, McNeish L, Clarizzio LO. Correction of facial skeletal deformities in two patients with facioscapulo-humeral dystrophy. *J Oral Maxillofac Surg.* 1989; 47:996-999.
47. Kilmer DD, Abresch RT, McCrory MA, et. al. Profiles of neuromuscular diseases. Facioscapulohumeral muscular dystrophy. *Am J Phys Med Rehabil.* 1995;74:5 (suppl):S131-S139.
48. Pourmand R. Myasthenia gravis. *Dis Mon.* 1997;43:65-109.
49. Grob D. Myasthenia gravis. *Arch Intern Med.* 1961:108:615-638
50. Smithard DG, ONeill PA, Parks C, Morris J. Complications and outcome after acute stroke. Does dysphagia matter? *Stroke.* 1996;27:1200-1204.
51. Aviv JE, Martin JH, Sacco RL, et al. Supraglottic and pharyngeal sensory abnormalities in stroke patients with dysphagia. *Ann Otol Rhinol Laryngol.* 1996;105:92-97.
52. Alberts MJ, Horner J, Gray L, Brazer SR. Aspiration after stroke: lesion analysis by brain MRI. *Dysphagia.* 1992;7: 170-173.
53. Hamdy S, Aziz Q, Rothwell JC, et al. Explaining oropharyngeal dysphagia after unilateral hemispheric stroke. *Lancet.* 1997;350:686-692.
54. Robbins J, Levine RL, Maser A, Rosenbek JC, Kempster GB. Swallowing after unilateral stroke of the cerebral cortex. *Arch Phys Med Rehabil.* 1993;74:1295-1300.
55. Barer DH. The natural history and functional consequences of dysphagia after hemispheric stroke. *J Neurol Neurosurg Psychiatry.* 1989;52:236-241.

56. Horner J, Massey EW, Brazer SR . Aspiration in bilateral stroke patients. *Neurology.* 1990;40:1686-1688.

57. McConnel FMS, Cerenko D, Mendelsohn MS. Manofluorographic analysis of swallowing. *Otolaryngol Clin North Am.* 1988;21:625-636.

58. Gottlieb D, Kipnis M, Sister E; Vardi Y, Brill S. Validation of the 50 ml3 drinking test for evaluation of post-stroke dysphagia. *Disabil Rehabil.* 1996;18:529-532.

59. DePippo KL, Holas MA, Reding MJ. The Burke Dysphagia Screening Test: validation of its use in patients with stroke. *Arch Phys Med Rehabil.* 1994;75:1284-1286.

60. Teasell RW, Bach D, McRae. Prevlence and recovery of aspiration poststroke: a retrospective analysis. *Dysphagia.* 1994;9:35-39.

61. Odderson IR, Keaton JC, McKenna BS. Swallow management in patients on an acute stroke pathway: quality is cost effective. *Arch Phys Med Rehabil.* 1995;76:1130-1133.

62. Barer DH. The natural history and functional consequences of dysphagia after hemispheric stroke. *J Neurol Neurosurg Psychiatry.* 1989;52:236-241.

63. Crary MA. A direct intervention program for chronic neurogenic dysphagia secondary to brainstem stroke. *Dysphagia.* 1995;10:6-18.

64. Leopold NA, Kagel MC. Prepharyngeal dysphagia in Parkinson's disease. *Dysphagia.* 1996;11:14-22.

65. Ali GN, Wallace KL, Schwartz R, et al. Mechanisms of oral-pharyngeal dysphagia in patients with Parkinson's disease. *Gastroenterology.* 1996; 110:383-392.

66. Leopold NA, Kagel MC. Pharyngo-esophageal dysphagia in Parkinson's disease. *Dysphagia.* 1997;12:11-18,19-20.

67. Born LJ, Harned RH, Rikkers LF, et al. Cricopharyngeal dysfunction in Parkinson's disease: role in dysphagia and response to myotomy. *Mov Disord.* 1996;11:53-58.

68. Leopold NA, Kagel MC. Dysphagia in progressive supranuclear palsy: radiologic features. *Dysphagia.* 1997; 12:140-143.

69. Field LH, Weiss CJ. Dysphagia with head injury. *Brain Inj.* 1989;3:19-26.

70. Winstein CJ. Neurogenic dysphagia: frequency, progression, and outcome in adults following head injury. *Phys Ther.* 1983;63:1992-1997.

71. Drake W, ODonoghue S, Bartram C, Lindsay J, Greenwood R. Eating in side-lying facilitates rehabilitation in neurogenic dysphagia. *Brain Inj.* 1997;11:137-142.

72. Sukthankar SM, Reddy NP, Canilang EP, Stephenson L, Thomas R. Design and development of portable biofeedback systems for use in oral dysphagia rehabilitation. *Med Eng Phys.*1994;16:430-435.

CHAPTER 17

■ ■ ■

Iatrogenic Swallowing Disorders: Medications

Aijaz Alvi, M.D.

I. INTRODUCTION

Numerous medications have primary and secondary effects that affect swallowing. The effects of these medications are influenced by sex, age, body size, metabolic status, individual biological response, and concurrent use of other medications. The clinician must recognize the potential primary and side effects and optimize the desired effect of the medication versus its undesirable effect.

II. PATHOPHYSIOLOGY

In general, the effects of medications on swallowing can be divided into those that affect lubrication of the upper aerodigestive tract, those that affect motor function or coordination through influences on the central nervous system, and those that produce mucosal toxicity. Toxicity of the oral, pharyngeal, and esophageal tracts can be caused by direct effects or by allergic or idiosyncratic reactions (Table 17-1). Some medications will also have effects over the lower digestive tract that will indirectly affect swallowing. The following is a discussion of the most commonly prescribed medications with direct or indirect adverse effects on the aerodigestive tract.

A. Antibiotics

Antibiotics can indirectly cause difficulty in swallowing. Adverse effects, such as glossitis, stomatitis, and esophagitis, have been described for penicillin, erythromycin, chloramphenicol, and the tetracyclines. These effects are usually a result of an overdose or an allergic-type reaction. Sulfa can cause a Stevens-Johnson type reaction, resulting in extensive mucosal ulceration and glossitis. Aminoglycosides can increase Parkinsonian symptoms of weakness. Stomatitis and glossitis have been reported with trimethoprim and sulfonamide antibacterial agents.

Antituberculous medications such as isoniazid, rifampin, ethambutol, and cycloserine can cause confusion, disorientation, and dysarthria. Ethionate can cause stomatitis and a metallic taste. Antiviral agents such as acyclovir, amantadine, gancyclovir, and vidarabine can indirectly cause dysphagia with confusion, asthenia, and lingual facial dyskinesia. Amantadine can cause severe xerostomia and xerophonia in selected patients.[1] Alternatively, treatment of odynophagia secondary to a herpes infection with antiviral medications can often palliate these patients. Zidovudine (AZT) causes dysphagia in approximately 5%-10% of patients and tongue edema in 5% of patients. Chloroquine (Plaquenil) can cause stomatitis. Epigastric pain has been reported with primaquine and quinine.

B. Antineoplastic Agents

Antineoplastic agents can inhibit or prevent the development of neoplasms. These agents can affect swallowing mainly through inflammation, sloughing, and occasional superinfection of the aerodigestive tract mucosa.

Table 17-1. *Medications—Primary Effects on Swallowing*

Drug	Lubrication	Motor	Mucosal Toxicity	Allergic/Idiosyncratic	Other
Antibacterials				+	
Antituberculous		+			
Antivirals		+		+	
Antineoplastics			+		
Antihistamines	+				Sedation
Antitussives	+				Sedation/Constipation
Antimuscarinics/ Anticholinergic	+	+			
H2-Antagonists	+		+		Diarrhea
Vitamins			+		
Salicylates					
Anxiolytics		+			Sedation/Incoordination
Anticonvulsants	+	+			
Antipsychotics	+	+			
Antiparkinsonian	+	+			
Botulinum Toxin A		+			
Corticosteroids		±			
Immunosuppressants			+		
Antihypertensives					

(See Chapter 18.) This effect results in mucositis, stomatitis, pharyngitis, esophagitis, and esophageal ulceration (Fig 17-1). Patients feel burning pain, have loss of appetite, and weight loss. This effect is dose-dependent and is magnified when multiple agents are used concomitantly. Commonly used agents include 5-fluorouracil, cyclophosphamide, doxorubicin, methotrexate, and vinblastine. There are currently no effective drugs to prevent the onset of mucosal problems due to chemotherapy. Palliative topical preparations containing diphenhydramine hydrochloride, kaolin and pectin, antacids, sucralfate, steroids, and lidocaine hydrochloride have been used with varying degrees of success.

C. Antihistamines

Antihistamines (H1-receptor antagonists) are commonly used to treat allergies. However, because of their anticholinergic adverse side effects, medications in this class commonly exert a drying effect on the aerodigestive tract mucosa, causing difficulty in gastrointestinal motility during the swallowing process. Mucosal secretions can thicken and lubrication is reduced, making food "stick" as it goes down to the stomach. The degree of dryness varies with type of antihistamine, dosage, and concomitant medication use.

Commonly encountered antihistamines are those belonging to the alkylamine or chlorpheniramine family. Because they have been deregulated by the FDA (ie, are available as over-the-counter medications), these agents are being used with increasing frequency. Swallowing is not only affected by their drying effect but also by other adverse effects, such as sedation, disturbed coordination, and gastric distress. Central nervous system effects include ataxia, incoordination, convulsions, dystonia, and bruxism, which can lead to poor oral intake. Diphenhydramine is also present in some sleep aids. Promethazine is contained in several antitussive mixtures and can dry secretions. Some of

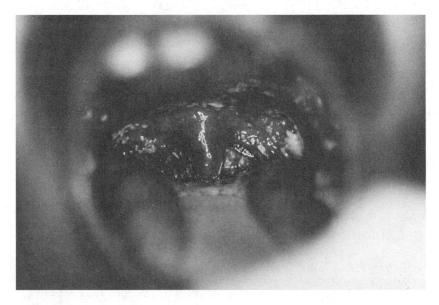

Fig. 17-1. Patient with oral mucositis and thrush after chemotherapy.

these name brand antihistamines are Actifed, Comtrex, Rynatan, and Benadryl. Newer antihistamines such as loratadine (Claritin) and terfenadine (Seldane) cause less dryness and are less sedating.

D. Mucolytic Agents/Salivary Stimulants and Substitutes

Lubrication is essential for optimal swallowing function. Dehydration can be caused by medications, medical conditions, or therapies. No medications, including mucolytic agents, substitute for adequate hydration and, indeed, these medications are dependent on adequate water intake. Patients should always be advised to drink ample amounts of water daily. However, mucolytics can be used to counter the effects of drying agents such as antihistamines. Guaifenesin is an expectorant that thins and increases secretions. Humibid and Robitussin are brand name drugs containing guaifenesin. It can be combined with decongestants such as phenylephrine hydrochloride/phenylpropanolamine (Entex) and pseudoephedrine hydrochloride (Deconsal), which reduce the viscosity of secretions and improve mucociliary flow. This type of drug is relatively safe, but should be prescribed by a physician.

Pilocarpine (eg, Salagen) is a cholinergic parasympathomimetic agent. It stimulates secretion of exocrine glands; therefore, the sweat, salivary, lacrimal, and intestinal glands are stimulated. It is indicated for xerostomia from salivary gland hypofunction caused by radiotherapy to the head and neck and may be useful in patients with Sjögren's disease. It seems to be more effective when given before beginning radiotherapy, as it only minimally affects glands that have been severely damaged from radiotherapy. It does have adverse effects such as cardiovascular instability, arrhythmia, and pulmonary edema.

Salivart is an artificial form of saliva that can also palliate patients with xerostomia. Its active ingredients are sodium carboxymethyl cellulose and sorbitol. It lubricates the oral cavity when sprayed into the mouth.

Antitussives containing codeine have a drying effect on the aerodigestive tract. Symptoms include dryness of the mouth, nose, and throat. Additionally, because codeine depresses the medullary center and is readily absorbed by the gut, sedation and constipation can result. Benzonatate (Tessalon perles) is a nonnarcotic oral antitussive agent. This drug is chemically related to the anesthetic, tetracaine. If perles are chewed or dissolved in the mouth, oropharyngeal anesthesia will rapidly develop. Although it is less sedating than codeine, it can cause mild sedation and constipation.

E. Antimuscarinics, Anticholinergics, and Antispasmodics

Antimuscarinics and antispasmodics are used for a variety of reasons, such as bradycardia, excessive oral secretions, motion sickness, and diarrhea. They inhibit the action of acetylcholine during transmission of neural impulses within the parasympathetic system. These medications vary in their site of action and adverse effects are often dose dependent. Salivary secretion is particularly sensitive to inhibition by antimuscarinic agents, which can completely abolish the copious water secretions induced by the parasympathetic system. The mouth becomes dry with swallowing and talking becomes difficult. The belladonna alkaloids have marked effects on gastrointestinal motility, as the parasympathetic system almost exclusively provides motor control of the gut. They aggravate gastroesophageal reflux (GER) by decreasing lower esophageal sphincter tone. Medications in this class include scopolamine, atropine, glycopyrrolate, atropine, and benzotropine mesylate (Cogentin).

Glucagon decreases lower esophageal sphincter pressure (increases GER) and has been use commonly to relieve esophageal impaction. The contraindications to its use include situations that can predispose to esophageal perforation (eg, presence of a sharp foreign body, esophageal diverticulum, or long-term impaction).[2]

F. Gastroenterologic Medications

Many of these medications treat acid reflux, esophagitis, and gut motility problems. Treatment of gastroesophageal reflux includes neutralization of gastric acid (antacids); inhibition of acid secretion with an H2 receptor antagonist such as cimetidine (Tagamet), ranitidine (Zantac), or famotidine (Pepcid); and blockage of the gastric proton pump (omeprazole, lansoprazole). In some patients antacids can cause constipation, diarrhea, bloating, and, occasionally, mucosal dryness. Drying effects associated with H2 blockers are more common within the gut as well as the eye. Gastric proton pump inhibitors are very effective in abolishing acid secretion in the gastric mucosa. Although the incidence of side effects is low, they can include diarrhea, abdominal pain, and nausea.

Prokinetic agents improve gut motility and speed gastric emptying. The two major drugs in this category are metoclopramide (Reglan) and cisapride (Propulsid). Because of the neurologic and extrapyramidal problems associated with metoclopramide, cisapride is becoming more popular. However, diarrhea, constipation, and pharyngitis have been reported with cisapride.

G. Vitamins

Vitamins are not innocuous medications. Vitamin A is often contained in multivitamin tablets. Overdosage of Vitamin A causes hypervitaminosis syndrome, which includes dermatologic, gastric, skeletal, and cerebral and optic nerve edema. Fissures of the lips, dry mouth, and abdominal discomfort can result. A similar stomatitis can result with vitamin E overdosage. Water soluble vitamins, such as vitamins B and C, are not significantly stored by the body and are easily excreted. Excess of these vitamins can have a diuretic effect.

H. Analgesics

Salicylates (aspirin) and nonsteroidal anti-inflammatory agents can alleviate symptoms of odynophagia and minor throat irritation. However these agents can cause ulceration of the mouth, throat burning, mucosal hemorrhage, glossitis, and dry mouth. Acetaminophen is the best substitute. The use of such analgesics should be carefully monitored and persistent pain should be investigated.

Morphine decreases the duration and magnitude of lower esophageal sphincter relaxation. This effect occurs through opioid receptors and is consistent with an action at the level of the inhibitory neural pathways.[3]

I. Neurologic Medications

1. Anxiolytics

Benzodiazepines are anxiolytic, sedative, and hypnotic drugs commonly prescribed to patients with symptoms of anxiety. Commonly prescribed benzodiazepines are alprazolam (Xanax), chlordiazepoxide (Librium), diazepam (Valium), and lorazepam (Ativan). The main adverse effects are drowsiness, confusion, and impaired motor coordination. These drugs have a high addictive potential, which is exhibited by symptoms of withdrawal, including potential seizures, if the drug is abruptly stopped.[1] Significant dysphagia can result from chronic use of benzodiazepines. Reported effects include hypopharyngeal retention, cricopharyngeal incoordination, aspiration, and drooling. It has been suggested that benzodiazepines can inhibit discharges from interneurons in the nucleus of the tractus solitarius or nucleus ambiguus, both of which are critical to the pharyngeal phase of swallowing. This action is reversible with cessation of the benzodiazepine.[4]

Clozapine (Clozaril) has effects at adrenergic and muscarinic acetylcholine receptors. Such differential effects could alter the tight control and coordination of peristalsis.[5] This effect is reversible with dosage reduction, but clozapine should be used with caution in patients with preexisting esophageal dysfunction. Midazolam seems to have a depressive effect on the swallowing reflex that persists even after the recovery of normal consciousness. Propofol by itself, however, does not seem to have such an effect.[6]

2. Anticonvulsants

Phenobarbital is a sedative and anticonvulsant that is becoming less popular in use. Its adverse effects are similar to the tricyclic antidepressants: dry mouth, sweating, hypotension, and tremor. Phenytoin (Dilantin) is chemically related to phenobarbital and is primarily used to treat epilepsy. The most common adverse effects include central nervous system signs such as ataxia, slurred speech, incoordination, and dystonia. Gingival hyperplasia, pseudolymphoma, Stevens-Johnson syndrome, and constipation are also reported adverse effects. There is no antidote and supportive care is necessary in cases of overdosage. This is a class IV drug and is habit forming.

Carbamazepine (Tegretol) is an anticonvulsant used primarily for seizures. The most severe adverse reactions have been observed in the hematopoietic system (aplastic anemia) and skin (Stevens-Johnson syndrome). Digestive symptoms can also be serious, such as glossitis, stomatitis, and dryness of the mouth.

3. Antipsychotics

Antipsychotic medications primarily work by dopamine antagonism. Commonly used drugs in this class include haloperidol (Haldol), chlorpromazine (Thorazine), thioridazine (Mellaril), and prochlorperazine (Compazine). These medications can have anticholinergic effects, such as dry mouth, nasal congestion, and hypotension. Approximately 14% of patients receiving long-term antipsychotic medications develop tardive dyskinesia ranging from tongue restlessness to disfiguring choreiform and/or athetoid movements leading to significant swallowing and feeding problems. Unfortunately, there is no cure for this condition once it develops.[1]

Life-threatening dysphagia can occur after prolonged neuroleptic therapy. Neuroleptic drugs can induce extrapyramidal symptoms such as dystonia, akathisia, and tardive dyskinesia. Gastrointestinal complications can cause weight loss and aerophagia. Contrast radiography have revealed poor contractions in the upper esophagus, a hypertonic esophageal sphincter, and hypokinesia of the pharyngeal muscles.[7]

4. Anti-Parkinson's Agents

Levodopa, dopamine receptor agonists, amantadine hydrochloride, and MAO inhibitors can have significant peripheral and central adverse effects. Anticholinergic adverse effects include dryness, impaired vision and urination, confusion, and headache. Levodopa may improve swallowing in Parkinson's patients mainly by improving oral and pharyngeal stages of swallowing.[8] However, it can cause gastrointestinal discomfort, dyskinesia, and oral dryness.

5. Botulinum Toxin A

Botulinum Toxin A (BOTOX) seems to benefit patients with swallowing problems after total laryngectomy. Injection of this medication is performed transcutaneously under videofluoroscopic guidance. Multiple injections are needed to achieve the desired effect.[9] However, botulinum toxin A can cause dysphagia when used during treatment for spasmodic dysphonia.

This is presumably due to the imbalances in muscle activity that slows swallowing and disrupts the usual laryngeal muscle pattern for swallowing. Patients with reports of dysphagia prior to botulinum toxin A use may be more predisposed to significant dysphagia after treatment with botulinum toxin A.[10]

J. Corticosteroids

Corticosteroids are potent anti-inflammatory agents. Although they are effective in managing acute laryngitis, their role in dysphagia is unclear. Physicians should be familiar with the dose relationships of the various steroids and should be aware of their contraindications. Adverse effects include gastric irritation, blurred vision, mood changes, and uncontrolled infection. Corticosteroids may have an alleviating effect on dysphagia in patients with systemic diseases, such as sarcoidosis and autoimmune diseases, that affect the swallowing mechanism.[11] It is not clear if the steroids improve the swallowing mechanism directly or indirectly by controlling the systemic disease.

K. Immunosuppressants

Azathioprine (Imuran) is an immunosuppressive antimetabolite primarily used for the prevention of rejection in renal homotransplantation. It has also been used in the treatment of severe rheumatoid arthritis. The principal adverse effects are hematologic and gastrointestinal. The effects are dose and duration dependent. Nausea and vomiting can occur within the first few months of therapy. These symptoms can be accompanied by fever, malaise, and myalgia.

Cyclosporin (Sandimmune) is a potent immunosuppressive agent used in the prevention of rejection of organ transplantation. It is used in conjunction with corticosteroids. The principal adverse reactions include renal dysfunction, hypertension, hirsutism, and gum hyperplasia. Gastritis, hiccups, dysphagia, gastrointestinal bleeding, and peptic ulcer occurs in less than 2% of patients. These symptoms can be worsened by the concomitant use of corticosteroids.

L. Antihypertensives

Almost all of the antihypertensive agents have some degree of parasympathomimetic effect and, thus, dry the mucous membranes. They are commonly used in combination with diuretic agents that also promote dehydration. Verapamil (Calan) is known to decrease gastrointestinal transit time and can cause gastric distress, diarrhea, and dryness. These symptoms are uncommon if the drug is titrated upward within the recommended dosage.

Captopril (Capoten) is a competitive inhibitor of angiotensin I converting enzyme. Because angiotensin I converting enzyme inhibitors affect the metabolism of eicosanoids and bradykinin, anaphylactoid and allergic reactions can result. The most serious side effect is angioedema, which occurs in about 1 in 1000 patients. This results in swelling of the oral cavity and larynx, which can lead to airway obstruction. This reaction can result many months after the initiation of therapy. Dysgeusia occurs in about 2% to 4% of patients and is reversible. Cough has been reported in approximately 0.5%-2% of patients.[1]

III. CONCLUSION

Numerous medications can have positive and negative influences on the swallowing mechanism, through either primary or secondary side effects. The degree of swallowing dysfunction depends on a variety of factors, including type and dosage of medication, patient's medical condition, age, sex, and other medication interaction with other medications.

It is essential that all physicians who take care of patients with swallowing complaints be familiar with the potential effects of their patients' medications on swallowing. This chapter has reviewed some of the major classes of medications that can affect swallowing; however, these classes are not inclusive and any ingested substance should be suspect as a cause of swallowing dysfunction.

Frequently Asked Questions

1. What is angioedema commonly associated with?
   A. Antihypertensive agents
2. What is Stevens-Johnson syndrome, associated with oral ulcers and blisters, most commonly caused by?
   A. Sulfa

3. What can antihistamines lead to?
   A. Oral dryness

References

1. Sataloff RT, Hawkshaw M, Rosen DC. Medications: effects and side effects in professional voice users. In: Sataloff RT, ed. *Professional Voice—The Science and Art of Clinical Care.* San Diego, Calif: Singular Publishing Group; 1997:457-469.
2. Maglinte DD. Pharmacoradiologic disimpaction of lower esophageal foreign bodies—should we abandon it? *Dysphagia.* 1995;10:128-130.
3. Penagini R, Picone A, Bianchi PA. Effect of morphine and naloxone on motor response of the human esophagus to swallowing and distention. *Am J Physiol.* 1996;271:675-680.
4. Dantas RO, Nobre-Souza MA. Dysphagia induced by chronic ingestion of benzodiazepine. *Am J Gastroenterol.* 1997;92:1194-1196.
5. McCarthy RH, Terkelsen KG. Esophageal dysfunction in two patients after clozapine treatment. *J Clin Psychopharmacol.* 1994;14:281-283.
6. D'Honneur G, Rimaniol JM, el Sayed A, Lambert Y, Duvaldestin P. Midazolam/propofol but not propofol alone reversibly depress the swallowing reflex. *Acta Anaesthesiol Scand.* 1994;38:244-247.
7. Hayashi T, Nishikawa T, Koga I, Uchida Y, Yamawaki S. Life-threatening dysphagia following prolonged neuroleptic therapy. *Clin Neuropharmacol.* 1997;20:77-81.
8. Tison F, Wiart L, Guatterie M, et al. Effects of central dopaminergic stimulation by apomorphine on swallowing disorders in Parkinson's disease. *Movement Dis.* 1996;11:729-732.
9. Crary MA, Glowasky AL. Using botulinum toxin A to improve speech and swallowing function following total laryngectomy. *Arch Otolaryngol Head Neck Surg.* 1996;122:760-763.
10. Holzer SE, Ludlow CL. The swallowing side effects of botulinum toxin A injection in spasmodic dysphonia. *Laryngoscope.* 1996;106:86-92.
11. Geissinger BW, Sharkey MF, Criss DG, Wu WC. Reversible esophageal motility disorder in a patient with sarcoidosis. *Am J Gastroenterol.* 1996;91:1423-1426.

CHAPTER 18

■ ■ ■

Iatrogenic Swallowing Disorders: Chemotherapy

Sanjiv S. Agarwala, M.D.
Ibraham Sbeitan, M.D.

I. INTRODUCTION

Chemotherapy, either by itself or in combination with radiation, is now an accepted modality for the treatment of head and neck cancer. Not only is it a logical choice for the patient with unresectable disease, but it is also an option for patients with advanced, surgically resectable disease as an approach to organ preservation and as an alternative to surgery that could severely compromise a patient's functional ability or social standing. Chemotherapy is also being tested in the adjuvant setting in combination with radiation therapy for patients with features suggestive of a high risk for recurrence.

The mucosal lining of the oral and pharyngeal areas has a rapid epithelial turnover rate that renders it vulnerable to the effects of cytotoxic chemotherapy, particularly in combination with radiation. Mucositis results from the shedding of cells of the outer epithelium at a rate that exceeds their replacement. Oral mucositis is a commonly observed adverse effect of chemotherapy for head and neck cancer and its management follows a multi-disciplinary approach by the medical oncologist, radiation oncologist, head and neck surgeon, and the nursing staff caring for the patient. The incidence of oral mucositis due to cancer chemotherapy has been estimated at 30%-35% overall, but with concurrent radiation/chemotherapy for head and neck cancer, this number may be closer to 100%.

II. CHEMOTHERAPEUTIC AGENTS IMPLICATED IN ORAL MUCOSITIS

The chemotherapeutic agents most commonly implicated in oral mucositis are the antimetabolites. These include 5-fluorouracil (5-FU), methotrexate, and the purine antagonists. Other offending agents are doxorubicin and other antitumor antibiotics, procarbazine, and hydroxyurea. Among these, the most commonly used for head and neck cancer are 5-FU and methotrexate. Mucositis is a much less frequent problem with the taxanes (paclitaxel and docetaxel) and platinum analogues (cisplatin and carboplatin), drugs that are also used with some frequency, particularly in combination regimens for locally advanced and metastatic disease. However, almost any chemotherapeutic agent can worsen the mucositis from radiation therapy, when given concurrently.

The severity of mucositis induced by 5-FU is schedule dependent. Oral mucositis is dose limiting for 5-FU when given by a bolus 5-day intensive course, whereas diarrhea is more frequent with the continuous infusion. Mucositis induced by 5-FU is exacerbated by leucovorin. As would be expected, combinations of drugs are more likely to cause mucositis than single agents.

III. DIAGNOSIS

Symptoms of mucositis include pain, xerostomia (dryness of the oral mucosa), and pain on mastication and swallowing (odynophagia). A burning sensation in the mouth is often followed by sensitivity to hot, cold, spicy, and salty food. With current chemotherapy and chemoradiation regimens, mucositis generally begins within 7-10 days of initiating chemotherapy and may persist for up to 6 weeks after regimen completion. When severe oral intake may be compromised with consequent effects on nutrition and hydration, it is important that all members of the health care team use a standardized assessment for the severity of mucositis. The Common Toxicity Scale is a useful way to grade the degree of mucositis in patients undergoing chemotherapy or radiation therapy (Table 18-1). Swallowing difficulty is often aggravated by the xerostomia caused by radiation.

The first sign on physical examination is usually erythema of the soft palate, the ventral surface of the tongue, or the buccal mucosa (Table 18-2). Desquamation of the mucous membranes indicates a more advanced process. Edema of the lateral tongue borders may also be observed. Ulceration of the mucosal membranes can occur, weakening the mucosal barrier and allowing secondary infection. Candidiasis is the most common oral infection in patients undergoing radiation therapy and may present as whitish plaques on the mucous membranes.[1]

Table 18-1. *Common Toxicity Criteria (CTC) Grading System for Mucositis*

Grade	
0	None
1	Painless ulcers, erythema, or mild soreness
2	Painful erythema, edema, or ulcers, but can eat
3	Painful erythema, edema or ulcers, and cannot eat
4	Requires parenteral or enteral support

Table 18-2. *Clinical Presentation and Sequelae of Mucositis*

Symptoms
• Pain
• Dysphagia
• Odynophagia
• Heartburn, nausea, and vomiting
• Bleeding (with thrombocytopenia)

Signs
• Erythema
• Swelling
• Ulcers
• Pseudomembranes
• Superinfection, eg, Candida, viruses

Sequelae
• Intolerable pain requiring hospitalization and parenteral narcotic analgesia
• Decreased intake dehydration
• Mucosal breakdown and secondary infection that could become systemic

IV. PREVENTION

Perhaps, the old adage, "Prevention is better than cure" is nowhere more applicable than in the management of a patient undergoing chemotherapy or chemoradiation at risk for oral mucositis (Table 18-3).

A. General Measures

Most of these have never been proven to be effective in randomized trials, but make logical sense.

1. General Oral Hygiene

Maintenance of good oral hygiene by means of regular, gentle tooth brushing with a soft brush is important, as is adequate hydration. Both these measures would serve to reduce the chance for secondary bacterial and fungal infections, factors known to aggravate direct effects of chemotherapy on the mucosa.

2. Mouthwashes

Accumulated dental plaque contributes significantly to the development of oral inflammation. Various mouthwashes are available and no conclusions can be drawn as to the superiority of one over the other. Any mouthwash is capable of promoting moisture, removing solid debris, and reducing plaque formation. Suggested agents include tap water, saline, sodium bicarbonate, and hydrogen peroxide. The alcohol content in most over-the-counter mouthwashes ranges from 6-27%. Alcohol produces a burning sensation, may aggravate inflammation, and cause dryness of the mucous membrane.[2] Prophylactic chlorhexidine mouthwashes may have the best antibacterial effect and have been shown in one study to significantly reduce the incidence of oral mucositis in chemotherapy patients.[3,4] These preparations are bacteriostatic at low concentrations and bactericidal at high concentrations against both gram posi-

Table 18-3. *Management of Mucositis*

Prevention:
Oral Hygiene maintenance
Soft bland diet
Avoid irritants:
  Tobacco
  Alcohol
  Spices
Maintenance of nutrition, moisture, and hydration
Cryotherapy: Ice chips, best described with 5-FU chemotherapy
Pharmacologic
  Sucralfate
  Pilocarpine
  Allopurinol mouth washes

tive and negative bacteria. Some studies have formally evaluated the role of "mucositis prevention protocols," including the described measures, with inconclusive results.[5,6] Antifungal mouthwashes such as Nystatin, clotrimazole, and fluconazole, have recently gained in popularity, but lack convincing evidence of efficacy.

3. Other

The Ora-Swab, a grooved applicator, has been shown to be as effective as a toothbrush in maintaining general oral hygiene and is useful for patients with established mucositis when brushing becomes painful.[7] Other potentially useful devices include, the Suction Ora-Swab (Sage Inc, Crystal Lake, IL) and oral irrigators. Moisturizing agents such as Moistir Moisturizer (Kingswood Laboratories Inc, Carmel, IN) and Mouth Moisturizer (Sage Inc, Crystal Lake, IL) and synthetic saliva are other adjuncts to the specific measures described in the next section.

B. Specific Measures

1. Cryotherapy

The short half life of 5-FU (5-20 minutes) led to the evaluation of oral cryotherapy in prevention of 5-FU induced mucositis. The hypothesis that temporary oral vasoconstriction would decrease 5-FU exposure to the oral mucosa was tested in a randomized, controlled, cross-over clinical trial. Patients receiving their first dose of 5-FU were randomized to receive oral cryotherapy with ice chips 5 minutes prior to drug administration and continuing for 30 minutes, or to a control group of 5-FU alone. A marked reduction in stomatitis was noted in the treatment group.[8] A subsequent trial in 179 patients testing two different durations of cryotherapy (30 and 60 minutes), compared with observation, also showed a benefit for both the treatment groups.[9] This technique is not applicable for 5-FU continuous infusion, which is the usual method that 5-FU is administered in combination with cisplatin in patients with head and neck cancer.

2. Sucralfate

Sucralfate is a poorly absorbed aluminum salt of sucrose octasulfate that is used in peptic ulcer disease treatment. Its ability to form a mechanical pastelike barrier and bind to ulcerated tissue has led to its evaluation in several trials.[10,11] One small, randomized, double-blind trial did show a small benefit in patients treated with cisplatin/5-FU chemotherapy.[12]

3. Pilocarpine

A healthy adult produces approximately 1.5 L of saliva in 24 hours. This complex secretion of the salivary glands acts to maintain oral moisture and serves as a deterrent to colonization of bacterial and fungal species. The degree of xerostomia caused by radiation therapy may be enhanced by radiation-sensitizing chemotherapy drugs. Furthermore, a single dose of radiation therapy has been shown to reduce salivary flow from major glands.[13] Two randomized trials showed that pilocarpine is effective for the treatment of postradiation-induced xerostomia.[14,15] Pilocarpine has recently been approved by the Food and Drug Administration for this indication. There is accumulating evidence that pilocarpine may be more effective when introduced early in the treatment course. By preventing xerostomia, pilocarpine may be useful in addition to other measures aimed at mucositis prevention in patients undergoing chemoradiation.

4. Other

Allopurinol is another agent that has been evaluated for the treatment of radiation-induced xerostomia. Positive data from early pilot studies did not successfully withstand the scrutiny of a placebo-controlled, double-blind randomized trial.[16] Prophylactic acyclovir also failed to show benefit in a randomized, controlled study.[17] Topical application of Vitamin E was tested against placebo in a small study of 18 patients treated with chemotherapy.[18] Six of 9 patients randomized to vitamin E had resolution of their oral lesions within 4 days of starting therapy. However, the small numbers preclude any firm conclusions being made from this study.

V. TREATMENT

The treatment for mucositis can be evaluated according to severity.

A. Mild-Moderate Mucositis

Local anesthetics are effective in providing symptomatic relief. These are available as sprays, rinses, or gels. Most agents are effective within 5 minutes and have a short duration of action of an hour or less. The potential for systemic absorption with viscous lidocaine or diphenhydramine, with attendant adverse effects needs to be kept in mind. A solution of salt and baking soda in water is often soothing to the oral mucosa and can be effective as an adjunct. Compounds that act as physical barriers, such as benzocaine in a hydroxypropylcellulose base, and sucralfate can relieve symptoms of pain and burning and may help prevent further damage to the oral mucosa. Zilactin (Zila Pharmaceuticals, Phoenix, AZ) is a gel containing tannic acid that acts as a local anesthetic and can relieve pain for up to 6 hours. Another "barrier agent" is Orahesive (Convatec Squibb Co., Princeton, NJ), a thin dressing that can be applied to painful areas and provide pain relief for up to 30 hours.

B. Severe Mucositis

It is sometimes not appreciated that the pain of mucositis can be disabling and often requires narcotic analgesics for adequate control. Analgesics such as acetaminophen and codeine may be effective in the early stages. Narcotics such as morphine should preferably be administered round the clock instead of on demand as this will provide better pain control. Severe pain may necessitate hospitalization for continuous morphine infusions or patient-controlled analgesia. Nutritional status needs to be considered, and patients not having a feeding tube for nutritional support may require inpatient or home parenteral administration of fluid and nutritional support.

VI. FUTURE DIRECTIONS

Innovative therapies that may add to the therapeutic armamentarium for the prevention and treatment of mucositis are currently undergoing evaluation. Keratinocyte growth factor (KGF) was first described in 1989.[19] It is a growth factor produced by mesenchymal cells whose effects are restricted to tissue that expresses the receptor KGFR, and has a stimulatory effect on epithelial cells from a wide variety of tissues, but no direct effects on other tumor types. Increased production of KGF is a normal response to epithelial cell injury and may represent an attempt by the surrounding stroma to repair tissue damage.[20] In preclinical studies, recombinant KGF (rHuKGF) has been shown to improve weight maintenance and survival in animals treated with 5-FU chemotherapy. This agent is undergoing phase I and II trials in the USA to evaluate its ability to reduce the severity of mucositis in patient with head and neck cancer undergoing chemotherapy and radiation.

VII. CONCLUSION

In summary, mucositis and its sequelae are common effects of chemotherapy and chemotherapy radiation combinations that require a multi-disciplinary approach to management. Both prevention and treatment are important. Appropriate and rapid intervention by a health care team is needed to ensure adequate patient compliance and maximize chances for a successful outcome of the planned therapy for the underlying disease.

Frequently Asked Questions

1. Which are the commonly implicated drugs in chemotherapy-induced mucositis and what is the usual time course?
   A. The antimetabolites class of chemotherapy agents are the most common offenders. These include 5-fluorouracil (5-FU), a common component of combination chemotherapy and chemotherapy-radiation regimens for HNC and another important drug, methotrexate. The taxanes, paclitaxel, and docetaxel, plus the platinum analogues, cisplatin and carboplatin, also cause mucositis, but to a lesser degree. Mucositis is caused by 5-FU when given by the bolus 5-day administration than by the continuous infusion method. Mucositis usually begins 7-10 days after chemotherapy is initiated and may persist for the duration.

2. What are the features useful in the diagnosis of mucositis?
   A. Early symptoms are often nonspecific and include pain, xerostomia, odynophagia, intolerance for spicy food, and anorexia. Compromised oral intake can lead to deleterious effects on nutrition and hydration. Examination of the oral mucosa shows features ranging from erythema to ulceration and secondary infection. The most useful grading system is the Common Toxicity Scale.

3. What is the optimal treatment of chemotherapy induced oral mucositis?
   A. General measures such as good oral hygiene and various mouthwashes are helpful. Specific measures include cryotherapy for 5-FU induced mucositis, analgesics, local anesthetics, and if necessary, parenteral fluid and nutritional support.

References

1. Jacob R. Management of xerostomia in the irradiated patient. *Clin Plast Surg.* 1993;20:507-516.
2. Madeya ML. Oral complications from cancer therapy: part 2--nursing implications for assessment and treatment. *Oncol Nurs Forum.* 1996;23:808-819.
3. Richards RME, McCague GJ. In vivo estimation of the antimicrobial activity of proprietary mouthwashes. *Pharm J.* 1988; 2:1226-1227.
4. Ferretti GA, Raybould TP, Brown AT, et al. Chlorhexidine prophylaxis for chemotherapy- and radiotherapy-induced stomatitis: a randomized double-blind trial. *Oral Surg Oral Med Oral Pathol.* 1990;69:331-338.
5. Beck S. Impact of a systemic oral care protocol on stomatitis after chemotherapy. *Can Nurs.* 1979;2:185-199.
6. Kenny SA. Effect of two oral care protocols on the incidence of stomatitis in hematology patients. *Can Nurs.* 1990; 13:345-353.

7. Beck S. Prevention and management of oral complications in the cancer patient. In: Hubbard SM, Greene PE, Knofb T, eds. *Current Issues in Cancer Nursing Practice.* St. Louis; Lippincott; 1991:1-12.

8. Mahood DJ, Dose AM, Loprinzi CL, et al. Inhibition of fluorouracil-induced stomatitis by oral cryotherapy. *J Clin Oncol.* 1991:9;499-452.

9. Rocke LK, Loprinzi CL, Lee JK, et al. A randomized clinical trial of two different durations of oral cryotherapy for prevention of 5-fluorouracil-related stomatitis. *Cancer.* 1993; 72:2234-2238.

10. Pfeiffer P, Hansen O, Madsen EL, May O. A prospective pilot study on the effect of sucralfate mouth-swishing in reducing stomatitis during radiotherapy of the oral cavity. *Acta Oncol.* 1990;29:471-473.

11. Solomon RA. Oral sucralfate suspension for mucositis. *N Engl J Med.* 1986;315:459-460.

12. Pfeiffer P, Madsen EL, Hansen O, May O. Effect of prophylactic sucralfate suspension on stomatitis induced by cancer chemotherapy. *Acta Oncol.* 1990;29:171-173.

13. Leslie MD, Dische S. The early changes in salivary gland function during and after radiotherapy given for head and neck cancer. *Radiother Oncol.* 1994;30:26-32.

14. Johnson JT, Ferretti GA, Netheny WJ, et al. Oral pilocarpine for post-irradiation xerostomia in patients with head and neck cancer. *N Engl J Med.* 1993;329:390-395.

15. LeVeque FG, Montgomery M, Potter D, et al. A multicenter, randomized, double-blind, placebo-controlled, dose-titration study of oral pilocarpine for treatment of radiation-induced xerostomia in head and neck cancer patients. *J Clin Oncol.* 1993;11:1124-113.

16. Loprinzi CL, Cianflone SG, Dose AM, et al. A controlled evaluation of an allopurinol mouthwash as prophylaxis against 5-fluorouracil-induced stomatitis. *Cancer.* 1990;65: 1879-1882.

17. Vander Vliet W, Erlichman C, Elhakim T. Allopurinol mouthwash for prevention of fluorouracil-induced stomatitis. *Clin Pharm.* 1989;8:655-658.

18. Wadleigh RG, Redman RS, Graham ML, Krasnow SH, Anderson A, Cohen MH. Vitamin E in the treatment of chemotherapy-induced mucositis. *Am J Med.* 1992;92:481-484.

19. Finch PW, Rubin JS, Miki T, Ron D, Aaronson SA. Human KGF is FGF-related with properties of a paracrine effector of epithelial cell growth. *Science.* 1989;245:752-755.

20. Werner S, Peters KG, Longaker MT, et al. Large induction of keratinocyte growth factor expression in the dermis during wound healing. *Proc Natl Acad Sci USA.* 1992;89: 6896-6900.

CHAPTER 19

■ ■ ■

Iatrogenic Swallowing Disorders: Radiotherapy

Sanjeev Bahri, M.D.
Elmer Cano, M.D.

I. INTRODUCTION

Dysphagia is a common adverse effect of radiation therapy for head and neck cancers. The etiology of dysphagia following radiation therapy is multi-factorial and can be divided into acute and late effects. Acute effects present during and immediately following a course of irradiation, and late effects manifest themselves from several months to years after completion of radiation therapy. The acute phase of dysphagia is primarily secondary to radiation effects on mucosa (erythema, pseudomembranous mucositis, ulceration), taste buds (decreased, altered, or loss of taste acuity), and salivary glands (thickened saliva secondary to decreased serous secretions).[1] It is further complicated by surgical procedures that may be done prior to radiation. Late effects include injury to salivary glands resulting in xerostomia and damage to connective tissue (fibrosis) resulting in trismus and poor pharyngeal motility. Rehabilitation specialists, physical therapists, nutritionists, and speech-language pathologists are part of the team to implement rehabilitation of swallowing during both the acute and late effects stages.

II. PATHOPHYSIOLOGY

The acute and late effects of radiation on normal tissues of the head and neck are dependent on time-dose factors such as dose per fraction, number of fractions, number of fractions per day, interfraction interval, total dose, and the duration over which dose is delivered. Experimental data and the linear quadratic biologic formulation suggest that acutely responding tissues are less severely affected than the late responding tissues by larger dose per fraction. Additionally, multiple daily fractions result in increased acute reactions without significant increase in late effects. The injury over both the acute and late responding tissues is directly proportional to the volume of the target organ. Furthermore, the incidence of late complications in normal tissues appears to be influenced by tumor-related factors, such as size of the primary tumor and local invasiveness/destruction of the normal structures. For example, a bulky base of tongue primary tumor may result in destruction of the taste buds as well as fibrosis disrupting the swallowing mechanism, neither reversing, despite a complete response of the tumor to irradiation. Taylor et al[4] reported on the impact of the time-dose factors on late complications in 784 patients with carcinoma of the pharynx and larynx. One interesting finding was the direct effect of primary tumor size on the incidence of late effects. Larger tumors were associated with higher complication rate.

III. MUCOUS MEMBRANES

Acute reactions involving the mucous membranes of the upper aerodigestive tract result in dysphagia due to pain and superimposed infections. Irradiation induces mitotic death of the basal cells of the mucosa, as this is a rapidly renewing system.[1] With a standard course of radiation therapy (180-200 cGy/fraction, 5 daily fractions per week), there is a 2-week delay from the start of therapy before the onset of mucositis. This is the time required for the basal cells to mature. Mucosal erythema is noted as early as 2 weeks into therapy with a dose of 2000-3000 cGy. This progresses to patchy mucositis (pseudomembranes) after a dose of 4000-5000 cGy, generally during the 4th or 5th week after initiation of therapy. With doses greater than 5000 cGy, patchy mucositis progresses to confluent mucositis and ulceration. Increases in dose per fraction results in an increase in the severity of mucositis and in a more acute onset. Following the completion of radiation therapy, healing and re-epithelialization occurs within 2 to 3 weeks, resulting in significant improvement in swallowing.

Late complications involving the mucosa of the upper aerodigestive are primarily related to atrophy, manifested by pallor and thinning, submucosal fibrosis, manifested as induration and diminished pliability, and occasionally chronic ulceration and necrosis with resultant exposure of the underlying bone/soft tissue.

Diagnosis of mucositis is made primarily by physical examination. A grading scale to score the severity of mucosal reaction helps clinicians to determine the intervention, prophylactic and therapeutic, required. Table 19-1 outlines the Radiation Therapy Oncology Group (RTOG) grading scale for acute and late complications of irradiation.

Acute reactions involving the mucous membranes usually require temporary intervention to manage odynophagia. Topical solutions usually containing a mixture of lidocaine, diphenhydramine, and liquid antacid (eg, Mylanta, Maalox) are very effective in relieving the symptoms during the early phases of radiotherapy. As the mucosal reaction worsens, most patients require additional systemic analgesics usually containing narcotics (eg, Roxicet, Lortab, Percocet).

Because of breakdown of the mucosal barrier, secondary *Candida* or microbial infections can result in further pain and delayed healing. Compliance with a thorough oral hygiene protocol can decrease the risk of superimposed infections. However, despite such efforts, antibiotics and antifungal agents are often required. Additionally, mucoprotective agents, such as sucralfate (Carafate), are effective in promoting mucosal healing. Recently, animal data have shown that thiol compounds like amifostine (WR-2721), oxygen free-radical scavengers, are effective in reducing the acute confluent mucositis by a factor of 1.7 and necrosis by 1.2 in dogs.[5] In the near future, similar agents will be available for clinical use.

IV. SALIVARY GLANDS

The irradiation fields used for the treatment of head and neck carcinomas frequently include one or more of the salivary glands (parotid, submandibular, and sublingual). In humans, the parotid glands are purely serous, the submandibular glands are made of serous and mucous acini, and the minor salivary glands are predominantly mucous secreting.[6] The normal human salivary glands produce approximately 1000-1500 cc of saliva per day. The parotid accounts for about 60%-65% of the salivary flow, the submandibular contributes 20%-30%, and sublingual glands 2%-5%.[7] Irradiation of the normal salivary glands results primarily in injury to the serous acini with no significant effect on the mucous acini.[8] Fajardo and Berthrong[9] reported histopathologic changes 10-12 weeks postinitiation of fractionated irradiation to 5000-7000 cGy. They described loss of serous acini, distortion or dilatation of acinar ducts, aggregation of plasma cells and lymphocytes, and mild fibrosis. Six months after radiation therapy, the gland

Table 19-1. *The Radiation Oncology Group (RTOG) Grading Scale for Acute and Late Complications of Irradiation*

RTOG Grade	Acute	Late
0	No change over baseline	None
1	Injection/may experience mild pain not requiring analgesics	Slight atrophy and dryness
2	Patchy mucositis that may produce an inflammatory serosanguinous discharge/may experience moderate pain requiring analgesics	Moderate fibrosis but asymptomatic; slight field contracture; <10% linear reduction
3	Confluent fibrinous mucositis / may include severe pain requiring narcotics	Severe induration and loss of subcutaneous tissue; field contracture >10% linear measurement
4	Ulceration, hemorrhage, or necrosis	Necrosis

parenchyma is replaced by fibrosis with heavy collagen deposits and no recognizable acini.

A decrease in the salivary flow can be detected 24-48 hours after initiation of standard fractionated irradiation and it continues to decline through the course of therapy. In addition to the decrease in flow, there is increase in viscosity, and decreased pH and IgA in saliva.[10] As the serous acini are primarily affected, the saliva becomes thick, sticky, and resulting in dry mouth and difficulty with mastication and swallowing. Most patients are unable to clear these thick secretions. These changes promote for increased yeast flora of the oral cavity. If greater than 50% of the major salivary glands are in the irradiation fields, patients develop xerostomia (chronic dry mouth) several months to years after irradiation. These patients may have partial or no recovery. They develop an impaired ability to chew, swallow, or talk. These patients are also at a high risk for developing dental caries due to change in the microflora and recurrent *Candida* infections.

Rubin and Casarett[3] reported that the TD 5/5 (dose at which 5% of patients will develop xerostomia at 5-year follow-up after irradiation) following partial or whole organ irradiation was 5000 cGy and the TD 50/5 (dose at which 50% of patients develop xerostomia at 5 years follow up after irradiation) was 7000 cGy.

Acute and late effects on salivary gland are primarily diagnosed on the basis of subjective patient complaints and findings on physical exam. Table 19-2 indicates the RTOG grading scale for the severity of irradiation injury.

Xerostomia results from permanent injury to the salivary glands. The most effective treatment for xerostomia is prevention. During the course of irradiation, maintenance of good oral hygiene is extremely important. One percent sodium fluoride gel and sodium bicarbonate oral rinses are recommended for prophylaxis of dental caries. Additionally, modifications of the treatment technique and field orientation to minimize the volume of major salivary glands that will be irradiated can help decrease the severity of dry mouth. Exclusion of more than 50% of both the parotid glands is adequate to prevent severe xerostomia.[11]

Once xerostomia develops, its treatment primarily consists of administering saliva substitute (water and glycerin mixture) and salivary gland stimulants such as pilocarpine hydrochloride, bromohexine, and anethole-trithione.[1] Of these agents, pilocarpine hydrochloride has shown some very promising results. Pilocarpine is a cholinergic agonist that simulates the smooth muscle and exocrine glands by its action the postganglionic cells. This results in increased excretion of saliva and sweat. Greenspan and Daniels conducted a double-blind study of xerostomia[12] with 12 patients that showed at least a temporary relief in symptoms of xerostomia. The benefit was noted in patients with residual salivary gland function. Subsequently, a multi-institutional randomized double-blind prospective study was conducted.[13] One hundred sixty-two patients irradiated for head and neck cancers receiving a minimum dose of 4000 cGy who had xerostomia were enrolled and randomized between pilocarpine and placebo. The researchers found a clinically significant benefit for symptomatic treatment of postirradiation xerostomia. The results were obtained with continuous treatment with pilocarpine, taking doses greater than 2.5 mg 3 times a day for 8-12 weeks. LeVeque et al[14] evaluated 16 patients irradiated for oral and oropharyngeal carcinomas treated with pilocarpine (5 mg qid) given during therapy and continued 30 days after irradiation. During the radiation treatments, ≥ 50% of the parotid glands were included in the radiation field receiving ≥ 5000 cGy. The authors reported that 30% of the flow was preserved, resulting in subjective improvement of the

Table 19-2. *The RTOG Grading Scale for Severity of Irradiation Injury*

RTOG Grade	Acute	Late
0	No change over baseline	None
1	Mild mouth dryness/slightly thickened saliva/may have slightly altered taste such as metallic taste/these changes do not result in alteration in feeding behavior, such as increased liquids with meals	Slight dryness of mouth; good response to stimulation
2	Moderate to complete dryness/ thick, sticky saliva/markedly altered taste	Moderate dryness of the mouth; poor response to stimulation
3	No classification	Complete dryness of mouth; no response to stimulation
4	Acute salivary gland necrosis	Fibrosis

dry mouth as compared to the postirradiation administration of pilocarpine. Additionally, objectively scored oral mucositis was 60% less than historical controls with associated decrease in subjective oral/oropharyngeal pain or dysphagia. These results have led to a placebo-controlled, double-blind, randomized trial currently underway.

In an effort to prevent permanent injury to the salivary glands, protective agents such as WR-2721 may be available in the future. Data from Takahashi and colleagues showed decrease in radiation-induced salivary gland injury as measured by the Gallium citrate salivary uptake 6 months or more following irradiation.[15] They documented an increase in salivary flow as compared to patients irradiated without WR-2721. However, difficulty in administration as well as some of the side effects have prevented the routine use of this drug.

V. CONCLUSION

Dysphagia is a symptom that results from irradiation effects primarily on the mucous membranes, taste buds, and salivary glands. The acute and late toxicity resulting from irradiation of these tissues can be complicated by various factors, such as prior surgery, concurrent chemotherapy, tumor extent, and preirradiation organ status. Aggressive approach to prevention and symptomatic treatment of both the acute and late effects is crucial to maintenance of good quality of life in patients irradiated for head and neck cancers. Team coordination of a nutritionist, physical therapist, and speech-language pathologist can provide management with food supplements, physical therapy to improve muscle flexibility, and treatment of dysphagia that may accompany radiation therapy.

Frequently Asked Questions

1. Does the use of pilocarpine concurrently with radiation therapy increase the risk of late injury to the salivary gland?
    A. There is no data to support increased risk of salivary gland injury with concurrent use of pilocarpine with radiation therapy. Pilocarpine does not stimulate the acinic cells to produce saliva, but rather stimulates the ducts to increase the secretion of saliva. There would be a theoretical increase in risk of injury if pilocarpine was inducing cell mitosis/reproduction.
2. What are the indications for the use of pilocarpine?

   A. Patients being irradiated to the head and neck region where ≥ 50% of both the parotid gland with or without the inclusion of submandibular glands. In addition, the salivary glands would receive ≥ 4000cGy to ≥ 50% of the gland volume.

References

1. Cooper JS, Fu K, Marks J, Silverman S. Late effects of radiation therapy in the head and neck region. *Int J Radiat Oncol Biol Phys.* 1995;3:1141-1164.
2. Fajardo LF. Salivary glands and pancreas. In: *Pathology of Radiation Injury.* New York: Masson Publishing; 1982:77-87.
3. Rubin P, Casarett GW. *Oral Cavity and Pharynx in Clinical Radiation Pathology.* Philadelphia: WB Saunders; 1968: 120-152.
4. Taylor JMG, Mandenhall WM, Lavey RS. Dose, time and fraction size issues for late effects in head and neck cancers. *Int J Radiat Oncol Biol Phys.* 1992;22:3-11.
5. Utley JF, King R, Giansanti JS. Radioprotection of oral cavity structures by WR-2721. *Int J Radiat Oncol Biol Phys.* 1978;4:643-647.
6. Reith EJ., Ross MH. *Atlas of Descriptive Histology.* New York, NY: Harper & Row; 1969:100-103.
7. Lavelle CLB. *Saliva. Applied Oral Physiology.* Boston: Wright; 1988.
8. Kashima HK, Kirkham WR, Andrews JR. Postirradiation sialoadenitis. *Am J Roentgen Radiat Ther Nucl Med.* 1965;94: 271-291.
9. Fajardo LF, Berthrong M. Radiation injury in surgical pathology. part III. *Am J Surg Pathol.* 1981;5:279-296.
10. Franzen L, Funegard U, Ericson T, Henriksson R. Parotid gland function during and following the radiotherapy of malignancies in the head and neck: a consecutive study of salivary flow and patient discomfort. *Eur J Cancer.* 1992;28: 457-462.
11. Mira JG, Wescott WB, Starcke EN, Shannon IL. Some factors influencing salivary function when treating with radiotherapy. *Int J Radiat Oncol Biol Phys.* 1981;7:535-541.
12. Greenspan D, Daniels TE. Effectiveness of pilocarpine in postradiation xerostomia. *Cancer.* 1987;59:1123-1125.
13. LeVeque FG, Montgomery F, Potter D, et al. A multicenter randomized, double-blind, placebo-controlled, dose-titration study of oral pilocarpine for treatment of radiation-induced xerostomia in head and neck cancer patients. *J Clin Oncol.* 1993;11:1124-1131.
14. LeVeque FG, Fontenesi J, Devi S, Aref A, Klein B, Leung Y. Salivary gland sheltering using concurrent pilocarpine (PC) in irradiated head and neck cancer patients. *J Clin Oncol.* 1996; Abstract 1665.
15. Takahashi I, Nagai T, Miyaishi K, Maehara Y, Miibe H. Clinical study of the radioprotective effect of amifostine (YM-08310, WR2721) on chronic radiation injury. *Int J Radiat Oncol Biol Phys.* 1986;12:935-938.

CHAPTER 20

■■■

Tracheotomy/Endotracheal Intubation

Roxann Diez Gross, M.A.
David E. Eibling, M.D.

I. INTRODUCTION

It is well recognized that dysphagia frequently accompanies airway interventions such as tracheotomy. Aspiration of salivary secretions around an indwelling oral or nasal endotracheal tube is well documented, but dysphagia in this setting is not a clinical problem as most of these patients are unable to eat by an oral route. However, following tracheotomy, aspiration that presents as tracheal drainage represents a problematic and common "complication." In actuality, dysphagia is really a *sequela*, as it is an expected effect of tracheotomy.

Unfortunately, experience with the management of dysphagia and aspiration occurring in patients with a tracheotomy is often limited or inconsistent. Physicians and nurses often fail to recognize that many of the clinical problems developing in tracheotomized patients are the result of dysphagia and aspiration. One of the most common errors is the assumption that copious tracheal secretions following a tracheotomy are due to "bronchorrhea," when the secretions are aspirated saliva. Primary physicians, nurses, therapists, and speech-language pathologists are often reluctant to manage these patients because of fear engendered by inadequate knowledge and experience. Patients may be either routinely fed an oral diet, resulting in occasional bouts of aspiration pneumonia; or, conversely, treatment policies may dictate that all patients with a tracheotomy be maintained on a nonoral diet, resulting in

inappropriate restriction for some patients. Physicians frequently assume that tracheal secretions and episodes of pneumonia are unavoidable and fail to pursue the clinical problem and seek remedies. Moreover, with customarily severe time constraints, they do not have the luxury of spending what may be hours of direct contact with this population, limiting their ability to identify and correct problems. The same constraints often limit the abilities of nursing personnel to participate in the rehabilitation of the swallowing disorders that occur in patients with tracheotomies. In most institutions, this role is assumed by the speech-language pathologist, usually working with a multidisciplinary *dysphagia team*.

This chapter describes the physiologic changes that impact swallowing function following tracheotomy. An understanding of changes associated with the a tracheotomy will lead to the employment of an orderly algorithm to enhance the rehabilitation of swallowing function. Chapter 37, which discusses evaluation and treatment of patients with a tracheotomy, suggests strategies that clinicians may use to safely evaluate and manage this population.

II. INDICATIONS FOR TRACHEOTOMY

Tracheotomy is performed for a wide variety of reasons, some of which are listed in Table 20-1. These indi-

Table 20-1. *Indications for Tracheotomy*

Airway obstruction

    Laryngeal stenosis or tumor

    Acute infectious processes such as epiglottitis, Ludwig's angina, and so on

    Congenital malformations of the upper airway, such as Pierre Robin sequence

    Bilateral vocal fold paralysis.

Respiratory failure

Pulmonary toilet

cations can essentially be subdivided into three major categories: airway obstruction, ventilatory support, and pulmonary toilet (see Chapter 37).

Patients may undergo tracheotomy for a combination of factors. For example, patients who are undergoing extirpative head and neck oncologic surgery often require a tracheotomy for all of the listed indications. An understanding of the indications for tracheotomy is very helpful when assessing the ability of a patient to tolerate oral feedings following the procedure.

III. PHYSIOLOGICAL EFFECTS OF TRACHEOTOMY

It has been recognized for many years that the presence of a tracheotomy is associated with aspiration. It is estimated that between 43% to 83% of patients with tracheotomy tubes will manifest signs of dysphagia, usually aspiration. Cameron and colleagues first identified aspiration in patients with tracheotomies by placing blue dye on the tongue and then examining tracheal secretions for the presence of the dye. They were able to detect dye in 63% of a randomly selected group of patients.[1] In an interesting study in which they quantified aspiration in tracheotomized patients by the use of scintigraphy, Muz and coworkers demonstrated that aspiration associated with the presence of a tracheotomy is reversible merely by occluding the tube.[2] Their findings suggest that it is the physiologic change associated with *opening the trachea to atmospheric pressure* that is responsible for the effect, not merely the presence of the tube in the neck.

The observation that tracheotomy promotes aspiration has been noted previously and for years has been taken into consideration when managing patients after head and neck surgery. Many head and neck oncologic centers routinely withhold oral feedings from patients who have undergone extirpative head and neck surgery as long as the tracheostomy is in place. The dysphagia that results from the surgical procedure is aggravated by the presence of the open airway. Some centers therefore employ postoperative management protocols that mandate oral feeding not be resumed until the patient has been decannulated and the stoma has closed. This technique is particularly valuable in those patients who have undergone resection of the base of the tongue, pharyngeal wall, or supraglottic larynx.

A number of factors associated with the presence of a tracheotomy may contribute to aspiration in these patients. Clinicians, however, must consider that these patients are also likely to have dysphagia and aspiration that is secondary to neurologic disease or other underlying factors, such as prior head and neck surgery. Physiologic changes that occur following tracheotomy include a wide range of effects, some obvious and some not so obvious (Table 20-2).

A. Airway Pressure Changes

A major factor contributing to aspiration is that tracheotomy results in a reduction in airway resistance, both inspiratory and expiratory. Inhalatory resistance is reduced, with normal nasal resistance of approximately 3 cm H_2O/liter/min resistance during inhalation. The resistance to inhalation in a patient with a tracheostomy may be considerably less, but is ultimately a factor of the diameter of the tube and if it is obstructed with secretions. Expiratory resistance during respiration is provided by the vocal folds, with a constant resistance of about 8 to 10 cm/H_2O/liter/min. This "braking" helps maintain lung inflation through physiologic prolongation of the expiratory phase. Pressure measurements during swallowing are similar with an occluded airway and are lost with an open airway.[3] This pressure is present in the trachea following glottic closure during swallowing, and peaks at about 8 to 10 cm/H_2O. Subglottic air pressure seems to be critical to swallow function, as its restoration reverses, at least in part, the disordered swallowing function that accompanies tracheotomy.

B. Expiratory Speaking Valves

It is well known that decannulation or even tube occlusion will enhance swallowing function in a patient with a tracheotomy. However, this is not feasible in all patients. An alternative strategy is to place an expiratory speaking valve (Passy-Muir valve or Montgomery valve) on the open tracheotomy tube, which restores subglottic air pressure during swallowing (Fig 20-1). Several clinical studies have demonstrated that aspiration is reduced or eliminated in many patients with the use of a speaking valve.[4-6] The beneficial effect of a valve strengthens the fact that subglottic air pressure is a critical factor in swallowing efficiency, probably through restoring proprioceptive cues.

Loss of subglottic pressure prevents an effective cough and glottic closure reflexes are altered or delayed in its absence. In addition, there is an "uncoupling" of the normal coordination between swallowing and respiration, suggesting that in the "normal" patient, there are proprioceptive cues accompanying glottic closure that assist with this timing. These effects are reversible with decannulation or, if that is not possible, valving of the tracheotomy tube.

C. Laryngeal Elevation

Laryngeal elevation is another key component of the swallowing mechanism. The vertical motion of the larynx is dependent on the function of the suprahyoid musculature, and results in shortening of the pharynx and simultaneous active opening of the cricopharyngeal sphincter. It is well recognized that laryngeal ele-

Table 20-2. *Physiologic Changes Following Tracheotomy*

1. Loss or change in airway resistance.
2. Inability to generate subglottic air pressure during the swallow.
3. Reduced ability to produce an effective cough.
4. Loss of sense of smell.
5. Loss of phonation.
6. Reduced mucosal sensitivity.
7. Reduced true vocal fold closure and coordination.
8. Disruption of the respiration/swallowing cycle.
9. Foreign body effect.
10. Reduced laryngeal elevation during deglutition.

vation is reduced following tracheotomy, and probably plays a significant role in the dysphagia associated with the procedure. Mechanical tethering may account for some of this reduction, but it is likely that disruption of protective (ie, sphincteric) reflexes may also play a role. With a fresh incision, the discomfort associated with laryngeal motion may lead to splinting, with resultant reduced elevation and possibly some of the profuse aspiration of saliva that is frequently encountered immediately following the procedure.

It has been postulated that the surgical technique utilized in the procedure may alter laryngeal elevation; therefore, some surgeons elect to use a vertical incision to theoretically reduce inhibition of laryngotracheal motion. The technique of suturing a flap of the tracheal wall to the skin may also potentially reduce laryngeal elevation. Most likely, the reduction in laryngeal motion is multi-factorial and is not due to any single factor.

D. Glottic Closure

Bolus transit (ie, swallowing) is a function of timing and distance. The pharynx is a common pathway for both deglutition and gas exchange, but air exchange must cease prior to deglutition and resume following completion of swallowing. Lung protection is provided by cessation of respiration and glottic closure. In the typical individual, swallowing is timed to occur during expiration. This relationship is lost in patients with severe respiratory disease, and is probably also lost in the presence of a tracheotomy.

Glottic closure during swallowing is an extremely basic reflex, mediated by the superior laryngeal nerve (uncrossed) requiring only 18 to 25 milliseconds. This rapid response demonstrates that the reflex arc is located in the lower brainstem and does not require input from higher centers. Sasaki and coworkers demonstrat-

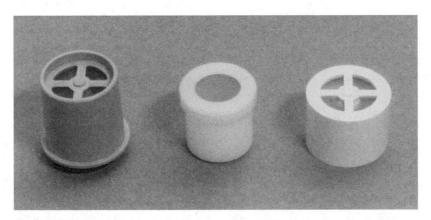

Fig 20-1. Three speaking valves. The Passy-Muir valve for ventilators, left; the Montgomery valve, middle; and the Passy-Muir valve, right.

ed in a cat model that the glottic closure reflex could be elicited by stimulation of any cranial nerve.[6] Reflexive glottic closure is triggered during swallowing by the presence of food and water on the supraglottic mucosa. The laryngeal surface of the epiglottis and the other supraglottic structures are richly endowed with receptors, including water receptors. Interruption of this sensory input by superior laryngeal nerve or high vagal nerve interruption will limit reflex glottic closure and contribute to aspiration. Aviv demonstrated that this reflex is dependent on the sensory threshold of the pharyngeal mucosa, which is affected by aging, stroke, and a variety of other disease processes.[7]

Disruption of the integrity of the subglottic airway by the presence of a tracheotomy will also blunt or eliminate this reflex. The reasons for this are probably multifactorial, but it seems clear that loss of subglottic air pressure may be one of the basic factors in the blunting of this reflex. Sasaki et al demonstrated in an animal model that the presence of a tracheotomy reversibly increased the reflex threshold as well as its latency.[8] This effect was also noted in humans, with reduction or loss of normal phasic glottic closure with tracheotomy. This effect was noted to be dependent on the time that the tracheotomy was in place and was reversible. They noted that glottic closure did not revert to normal immediately following decannulation or plugging of the tracheotomy tube. This finding supports the clinical observation that decannulation is safest when performed in a stepwise fashion, especially following prolonged intubation. Endoscopic laryngeal examination of a patient with a tracheotomy will often demonstrate this finding and it is especially evident in chronically ventilated patients.

E. Pharyngeal Transit

Safe deglutition requires that the bolus must traverse the pharynx during the period that the glottis is closed. Bolus transit from the tongue base to the esophagus requires less than a second in the typical individual. Prolongation of bolus transit time, as well as disruption of the glottic closure will result in food or liquid being in the pharynx while the glottis is open and, thus, places the individual at-risk for aspiration. Pharyngeal transit velocity is dependent on a number of factors, including the structural integrity of the pharynx, the tongue base driving force, extent of pharyngeal shortening and laryngeal elevation, constrictor muscle strength and coordination, and appropriate timing of cricopharyngeal opening. It has been demonstrated that this transit time can be prolonged in the presence of a tracheotomy and that this effect is reversible by restoration of subglottic air pressure with an expiratory speaking valve.[3] Restricted range of motion of pharyn-

geal structures such as may be associated with the tethering of the larynx by the presence of a tracheotomy tube is likely to also affect transit time. Previous radiation to the neck can result in decreased motion because of tissue edema and induration.

F. Neurologic Motor Dysfunction

Many illnesses that require tracheotomy are also associated with neurologic dysfunction and deconditioning. These disease processes affect the pharyngeal and laryngeal muscles just as they do such other body parts as extremities. When combined with the pharyngeal disuse and deconditioning associated with a tracheotomy, the effects of the disease process are compounded. The longer a patient is ventilator dependent, the more problematic will be the weaning process. In a similar vein, the longer a patient has a tracheostomy bypassing his or her upper airway, the more profound will be the effect on pharyngeal muscle tone. In contrast, patients without neurologic disease, deconditioning, or defects in the integrity of their oral cavity or pharynx often have no dysphagia associated with a tracheotomy. Common examples are individuals with isolated bilateral vocal fold paralysis or those who require tracheotomy for the management of severe sleep apnea.

G. Respiratory Failure

Tracheotomy is often performed to facilitate the management of patients with respiratory failure. This group of patients is particularly prone to develop complications of dysphagia and associated aspiration pneumonia. A variety of physiologic changes occur in respiratory failure, including rapid respiratory rates, drying of the oral and pharyngeal mucosa, thickening of mucus, loss of the physiologic timing of deglutition, and inability to cough and clear aspirated material. These patients have often lost considerable weight, and what muscle bulk they do have is concentrated in the muscles of respiration. These changes can be summarized by recognizing that the individual is concentrating his or her efforts on moving air and that other functions, such as deglutition, are secondary. Pneumonia is a frequent occurrence in these patients and it can be hypothesized that aspiration due to disordered deglutition is a common factor. Evidence supporting this hypothesis is that continuous suction of secretions from the subglottic airway above the tracheotomy tube cuff has been demonstrated to reduce the incidence of pneumonia. The combination of borderline pulmonary function, often with the requirement for assisted ventilation; inability to generate enough force to cough and clear secretions; and the generalized deconditioning associated with pulmonary failure combine to place this group at a high risk for developing complications of dysphagia following tracheotomy. The weaker and more inactive the patient, the greater the likelihood of aspiration pneumonia.

V. CONCLUSION

The performance of a tracheotomy disrupts the normal swallowing mechanism and contributes to aspiration. The severity of this effect varies from patient to patient, but is particularly problematic in patients with other disease processes that result in dysphagia, deconditioning, or pulmonary failure. The mechanism of the alteration is multi-factorial, but loss of subglottic air pressure is a major contributing factor. Therapy should be directed toward restoration of this intact, closed system by either decannulation, plugging, or valving of the tracheostomy tube. These therapeutic modalities are discussed in detail in Chapter 37.

Frequently Asked Questions

1. Why does tracheotomy result in a dramatic increase in tracheal secretions—"bronchorrhea"?
   A. The tracheal secretions seen following tracheotomy are due to aspiration of oral pharyngeal secretions into the trachea. The reasons for this aspiration are multi-factorial, but disruption of the normal closed subglottic air space is probably a major cause.
2. Why does swallowing improve following decannulation?
   A. Disruption of normal swallowing function by the presence of a tracheostomy is reversible following tracheostomy tube removal. In most instances improvement in swallowing function with decrease in aspiration can be seen immediately, whereas in other cases some time may be required for complete restoration of laryngeal and pharyngeal reflexes to normal.
3. How can swallowing function be enhanced in a patient for whom, decannulation is not feasible?

   A. If decannulation is not feasible, some patients will demonstrate improved swallowing function by use of a expiratory speaking valve which will restore subglottic air pressure while still permitting inspiration through the tube.
4. Why does aspiration occur even with a tracheostomy tube cuff inflated?
   A. The tracheostomy tube cuff occludes the airway when inflated, but this occlusion is not absolute. Moreover, the presence of the cuff prevents normal air flow through the subglottic airway and larynx. Pooling of aspiral secretions above the tracheostomy tube cuff is common, and leakage around the cuff into the distal airway eventually occurs. For many patients, the use of a cuffless tube with an expiratory speaking valve, or decannulation, will result in less aspiration than with an inflated tracheostomy tube cuff.

References

1. Cameron JL, Reynolds J, Zuidema GD. Aspiration in patients with tracheostomies. *Surg Gynecol Obstet.* 1973;136:68-70.
2. Muz J, Mathog, REH, Miller PR, Rosen R, Borrero G. Detection and quantification of laryngotracheopulmonary aspiration with scintigraphy. *Laryngoscope.* 1987;94:1185-1190.
3. Eibling DE, Gross RD. Subglottic air pressure: a key component of swallowing efficiency. *Annals of Otol Rhinol Laryngol.* 1996;105:253-258.
4. Dettelbach MA, Gross RD, Mahlmann J, Eibling DE. The effect of the Passy-Muir Valve on aspiration in patients with tracheostomy. *Head Neck.* 1995;17:297-302.
5. Stachler RJ, Hamlet SL, Choi J, Fleming S. Scintigraphic quantification of aspiration reduction with the Passy-Muir valve. *Laryngoscope.* 1996;106:231-234.
6. Sasaki CT, Suzuki M. Laryngeal reflexes in cat, dog, and man. *Arch Otolaryngol.* 1976;102:400-402.
7. Aviv JE. Sensory discrimination in the larynx and hypopharynx. *Otolaryngol Head Neck Surg.* 1997;116:331-334.
8. Sasaki CT, Suzuki M, Horiuchi M, Kirchner JA. The effect of tracheostomy on the laryngeal closure reflex. *Laryngoscope.* 1977;84:1428-1433.

CHAPTER 21

■ ■ ■

Surgery of the Oral Cavity, Oropharynx, and Hypopharynx

Lisa T. Galati, M.D.
Jonas T. Johnson, M.D.

I. INTRODUCTION

Swallowing is a common problem for patients presenting with tumors of the oral cavity, oropharynx, or hypopharynx. Swallowing dysfunction may result from tumor infiltration or obstruction and from surgical extirpation. Although a very frustrating and common problem, dysphagia in the head and neck cancer patient can be reduced through reconstructive efforts and postoperative swallowing rehabilitation. In this chapter the normal oral phase of swallowing is discussed to introduce the role of each component of oral cavity, oropharyngeal, and hypopharyngeal anatomy. The effects of surgical alteration, through resection and reconstruction, are also described, focusing on the resulting swallowing disorder, its pathophysiology and its treatment.

A brief review of the normal swallow is indicated because alteration of even an apparently minor component of the normal swallowing mechanism may result in dysphagia postoperatively (Table 12-1). Food placed into the oral cavity is prepared by the teeth and tongue for distal transit. While the bolus is being prepared, the lips keep it within the oral cavity. As the tongue elevates, it makes contact with the hard and soft palate in an anterior to posterior direction. This stripping action generates what is known as the tongue driving force

Table 21-1. *Normal Swallowing Mechanism*

Oral Cavity
1. Bolus preparation
   a. Teeth
   b. Tongue
2. Tongue driving force
3. Closure of oral cavity by lips

Oropharynx
1. Oropharyngeal propulsion pump
   a. Soft palate
   b. Lateral pharyngeal wall
   c. Tongue base
2. Velopharyngeal competency, soft palate

Hypopharynx
1. Muscular propulsion
   a. Constrictors
   b. Piriform sinuses
   c. Cricopharyngeal function

and the bolus is propelled back into the oropharynx.[1] At this stage, the oral phase is complete. As the food enters the oropharynx, the soft palate elevates, approaches the posterior pharyngeal wall, and closes the nasopharynx. Simultaneously, the tongue base elevates and the larynx elevates, closing the epiglottis over the introitus of the larynx and the true and false vocal folds adduct. In the oropharynx, the bolus is propelled inferiorly by the oropharyngeal propulsion pump, which is the positive pressure generated by the tongue base, the oropharyngeal walls, and the soft palate.[1] This positive pressure is necessary to propel the bolus into the hypopharynx. Once in the hypopharynx, the bolus is further advanced by the suction pump action (negative pressure) created by the hypopharyngeal walls on laryngeal elevation and by the contraction of the inferior and middle constrictor muscles. As the hypopharyngeal musculature contracts, the cricopharyngeus muscle relaxes, allowing the bolus to enter the cervical esophagus. This basic mechanical overview of the swallowing mechanism is, of course, orchestrated by complex voluntary and involuntary muscular coordination mediated by the sensory input from the entire upper aerodigestive tract, which is vital to proper swallowing. These important concepts are discussed as each anatomic site is reviewed.

II. PATHOPHYSIOLOGY

The basic principle of extirpative surgery for head and neck cancer is to completely excise tumor with a normal tissue margin. Efforts to save normal structures are important, but should not compromise the complete resection of the tumor. Tumor invasion or resection of healthy structures will alter the normal swallowing mechanism. Whether or not important structures are sacrificed, reconstruction is planned to maximize functional rehabilitation (Table 21-2).

The boundaries of the oral cavity are the lips anteriorly and the junction between the hard and soft palate posteriorly. If a perpendicular line is dropped from the hard palate, the tongue, floor of mouth, retromolar triangle, and mandibular and maxillary alveoli are within the boundaries of the oral cavity. Anatomical or functional alteration of any of these stuctures can interfere with the oral phase of swallowing (Table 21-3).

The lips serve as a sphincter to prevent drooling and spillage from the oral cavity. The orbicularis oris is crucial to the sphincteric function of the lips. This muscle is divided during lip splitting procedures and must be carefully reapproximated during closure to restore function. The loss of lower lip sensation secondary to mental nerve injury makes sphincteric control difficult if not impossible. One must consider this when planning mandibular osteotomies. The osteotomy should be placed anterior to the mental foramen so that the mentum and lips do not become insensate. Microstomia that results from lip resection may hinder swallow-

Table 21-2. *Reconstruction Options for Various Sites*

Secondary intention

Small tumors (1 cm) of the tongue, floor of mouth, soft palate, posterior pharyngeal wall

Primary closure

Small tumors (1-2 cm) of the tongue, floor of mouth, tonsillar fossa, alveolar ridge

Split thickness skin graft

Floor of mouth, posterior pharyngeal wall, tonsillar fossa

Regional myocutaneous flaps

Pectoralis major

Tonsillar fossa

Temporalis

Total palatectomy

Free flaps

Fasciocutaneous (radial forearm)

Floor of mouth, tonsillar fossa, posterior pharyngeal wall

Osteofascial (iliac crest, scapula, fibula)

Mandiblectomy, maxillectomy

Table 21-3. *Causes of Abnormal Oral Phase Swallowing*

Loss of oral sphincter

1. Resection of lip
2. Poor reapproximation of orbicularis oris
3. Marginal mandibular and lingual nerve section

Dental extractions

Floor of mouth resection

1. Loss of glossoalveolar sulcus
2. Tethering of anterior tongue

Tongue resection

1. Improper bolus preparation
2. Pumping force diminishment

Hard palate resection

1. Loss of oronasal separation
2. Nasal regurgitation

Mandibulectomy

1. Loss of dentition
2. Altered oral sphincter

ing by creating difficulty in getting food into the mouth. It also causes problems for denture wearers who will have difficulty inserting prostheses through a smaller orifice. Motor denervation of the lower lip secondary to sacrifice of the marginal mandibular nerve often manifests itself as loss of sphincteric control, resulting in drooling. A more common problem, however, is lip biting during chewing because of lack of control of the lower lip. Although these seem to be minor components of the entire swallowing mechanism, each of these added to other problems of the oral cavity, oropharynx, or hypopharynx can result in significant swallowing dysfunction.

The floor of mouth is considered a sulcus for saliva and food particles; however, when obliterated by surgery, the lack of this sulcus and the loss of mobility of the anterior tongue become a major impairment during the preparation of the food bolus. During resection of a tumor involving the floor of mouth, there are two major issues that should be considered to provide the patient with the best chance for normal swallowing postoperatively. First, during resection, all efforts should be made to protect the lingual nerve to preserve sensation to the tongue. The lingual nerve is quite vulnerable as it courses up from the submandibular triangle toward the tongue. The second consideration is the reconstruction. Small defects in the floor of mouth should be closed primarily if possible. Alternatively, very small defects can be allowed to heal by secondary intention. Larger defects require resurfacing of the floor of mouth and separation of the oral cavity from the deep tissues of the neck. Reconstruction of the floor of mouth using a split thickness skin graft preserves maximal tongue mobility. A thin split thickness skin graft measuring approximately 0.015 of an inch is sutured to the defect in the floor of the mouth and a bolster of xeroform gauze is secured over the graft with tie-over sutures.

Local muscle flaps, such as a tongue or platysma flap, may also be used to reconstruct the floor of mouth. Although tongue flaps are hardy and reliable, the loss of tongue mobility is a considerable hurdle for a patient to overcome during the postoperative swallowing rehabilitation. Platysma flaps, with or without a split thickness skin graft, are useful in reconstructing the floor of mouth, especially if there is concern about healing of a skin graft over exposed mandibular periosteum in a patient who has been irradiated. Most patients reconstructed with a split thickness skin graft require a tracheotomy during the early postoperative period to secure the airway and, more importantly, to provide a safe and effective means to evacuate tracheobronchial secretions that become difficult to cough up and swallow with the xeroform bolster in place.

Regional flaps, such as the pectoralis major myocutaneous flap, are often too bulky for this area. The most commonly used microvascular free flap for floor of mouth reconstruction is the radial forearm free flap, which is thin and pliable. Some reconstructive surgeons reinnervate the radial forearm flap so that the patient eventually will have a sensate reconstruction site. Regardless of the method of reconstruction, the concern is of scar contracture later in the patient's recovery. A freely mobile tongue in the immediate postoperative period may lose some mobility, if scarring results in tethering anteriorly or laterally to the floor of mouth. This problem seems to be less significant when the sulcus is reconstructed with a split thickness skin graft. However, the success of this technique requires the skin graft to be sutured in place, forming a deep pouch to account for wound and graft contraction.

The anterior tongue is extremely important to the oral phase of swallowing. Following partial glossectomy, near-normal swallowing and normal speech can be predicted, if the patient can protrude the tongue past the sublabial crease. Small defects of the mobile tongue are repaired primarily. Large defects often cause the loss of tongue driving force and inability to propel the bolus posteriorly, which disrupts the sequence of events during the oral phase. In the case of a large anterior tongue defect, the bolus is often improperly prepared and because of the lack of proper control it may be presented to the oropharynx prematurely. This does not allow for sufficient laryngeal protection and therefore may result in aspiration. Alterations of the anterior tongue also produce abnormal anterior propulsion of the bolus. Food and saliva will spill out of the oral cavity because of poor tongue mobility, a problem worsened if the oral sphincter has been altered.

Tumors of the hard palate that require partial or total maxillectomy affect both speech and swallowing. Resection results in loss of oronasal separation, which causes leakage of food into the nose and hypernasal speech with decreased intelligibility. Unilateral maxillectomy is usually best reconstructed with a dental prosthesis. (See Chapter 36.) This provides oronasal separation and replaces missing dentition. Total bilateral palatectomy requires flap reconstruction because there is no structure to anchor a prosthesis. The use of unilateral or bilateral temporalis muscle transposition flaps is a reliable way to achieve oronasal separation. However, a denture cannot be worn, because the ridge necessary to hold the plate in place is absent. Free microvascular flaps can be used to reconstruct large palatal defects and have the advantage of restoring a more normal facial contour as well as the capability for dental rehabilitation. Iliac crest, fibula, radial forearm, and scapula free flaps can be used to reconstruct large defects. Dental implants, placed into the vascularized bone graft, allow the use of a denture after a total palatectomy. Reconstruction using free tissue microvascular transfers, although requiring longer operating time, increased cost, and additional surgical training, provides a significant improvement in the rehabilitation of these patients.[2]

The remaining major components of the oral cavity are the mandible and teeth. Many patients undergoing resection of oral cavity tumors require full dental extraction. Lack of dentition hinders the ability to prepare the food bolus and limits the variety of food tolerable by the patient. Although the problems associated with segmental mandibular defects seem obvious (loss of teeth and muscles of mastication), one must consider the challenges posed by the marginal mandibulectomy.

If the marginal mandibulectomy is performed as part of the extirpation of a floor of mouth tumor, the ability to reconstruct an adequate sulcus may prohibit the patient from wearing a denture postoperatively.

Segmental defects in the midline of the mandible must be reconstructed to prevent inward rotation of the ascending rami and an "Andy Gump" deformity. Without reconstruction of the midline arch defects, a patient will lose proper chewing, oral sphincter control, laryngeal suspension and elevation, and the tongue driving force. Mandibular reconstruction plates may be used in combination with a myocutaneous flap to close the bone and soft tissue defects. Reconstruction of this area using microvascular free flaps yields better cosmetic and functional results than metal plates. The use of radial forearm flaps is limited by the the small bone volume. The radial forearm flap is considered less viable than the fibula free flap. The fibula free flap, because of its segmental blood supply, can be harvested in lengths up to 25 cm and is our prefered method of reconstruction. Alternatively, scapular free flaps may be used, but require repositioning of the patient and prolongs the operative time because simultaneous tumor resection and flap harvesting is impossible. The posts for dental implants can be placed during the initial reconstruction.

Resection of the lateral mandible also poses a complex problem in reconstruction and deglutition. Loss of soft tissue and the muscles of mastication (masseter and pterygoids) causes swallowing dysfunction by hindering a patient's ability to chew. Although the bulk of reconstuctive flaps can replace the loss of soft tissue, the restoration of the masticatory function of the masseter, temporalis muscle, and pterygoids is not possible. Often the bony defects are not reconstructed, leaving the patient without normal dentition or occlusion postoperatively. Edentulous patients or patients with medical problems that limit operative time are best managed by primary closure of the soft tissues and no bony reconstruction. Reconstruction plates may be inserted in combination with a myocutaneous flap, if the condyle remains. Free flap reconstruction of the lateral mandible is similar to the midline mandible reconstruction.

The oropharynx begins at the soft palate anteriorly and includes the tongue base, tonsillar pillars, tonsils, and posterior wall of the pharynx from the level of the soft palate to the level of the hyoid bone. Surgical defects of the oropharynx can cause significant dysphagia and pose challenging problems in reconstruction (Table 21-4).

Tumors of the soft palate are challenging to treat while maintaining normal postoperative function. Resection of even small tumors may result in velopharyngeal insufficiency and abnormal speech. After soft palate resection, patients often have nasal regurgitation. The reconstruction options are limited and defects

Table 21-4. *Dysphagia After Oropharyngeal Cancer Resection*

Soft palate
    1. Loss of oropharyngeal suction pump
    2. Velopharyngeal insufficiency
Tonsil
    1. Altered mobility of lateral pharyngeal wall
Tongue base
    1. Loss of laryngeal protection
        a. Loss of sensation
        b. Loss of laryngeal elevation

in the soft palate are best managed by dental prostheses with extensions to close the nasopharyngeal isthmus.

Although resection of small tonsil tumors usually poses no permanent problem with postoperative swallowing, wide-field tonsillectomy for squamous cell carcinoma may result in significant scar contracture of the lateral pharyngeal walls. This, in turn, leads to decreased lateral pharyngeal wall mobility which alters oropharyngeal propulsion. As stated earlier, this may seem to be a small component in the entire scheme of the normal swallowing mechanism, but when added to a second defect, this may cause significant difficulty in swallowing. Most of these defects are closed primarily or with a split thickness skin graft, but larger defects must warrant careful consideration in terms of reconstruction. Pectoralis myocutaneous flaps can be used for large defects, but as mentioned earlier, are often too bulky for tonsillar fossa defects. The radial forearm free flap is a better choice, because of its pliability and thinness.

The tongue base is extremely important in normal swallowing. The muscles of the base of tongue assist in elevation of the larynx and are essential for the oropharyngeal propulsion pump and for adequate oral cavity-pharyngeal separation. Although partial resection is well tolerated, large defects often cause dysphagia. Reconstruction of large defects of the base of the tongue requires a sensate flap. Insensate flaps in this area usually result in poor swallowing because of aspiration. Insensate, adynamic flaps should be avoided whenever the area of the defect has residual mobility and potential to function. Scarring at the tongue base can also limit anterior tongue mobility; therefore, not only is the oropharyngeal phase of swallowing affected by the resection of the tongue base but the oral phase can also be affected.

In the hypopharynx, piriform sinus tumors are the most common. The majority of these tumors are treated with total laryngectomy and swallowing disorders in this situation are discussed in Chapter 22. Resection of hypopharyngeal tumors arising on the posterior pharyngeal wall poses several problems for swallowing rehabilitation (Table 21-5). Small defects (less than 2 cm)

Table 21-5. *Dysphagia After Surgery of the Hypopharynx*

Piriform sinus

   1. Scarring of lateral pharyngeal wall

   2. Injury to superior laryngeal nerve and loss of sensation

Posterior pharyngeal wall

   1. Adynamic insensate flap reconstruction

   2. Scarring and aspiration

can be closed primarily or the edges can be stitched to the prevertebral fascia. Reconstruction with a split thickness skin graft or radial forearm free flap provides a satisfactory closure of larger defects. However, neither one restores motility and lack of contraction leads to significant postoperative aspiration. Also, the reconstruction in this area is almost always devoid of sensation, which further weakens laryngeal protection. Another very important yet seldomly mentioned problem unique to hypopharyngeal reconstruction is the scarring that occurs along the posterior pharyngeal wall. Patients lose the normal gliding action of the hypopharynx on the prevertebral fascia because of scarring of the posterior hypopharyngeal wall to the prevertebral fascia. Examination of patients who have undergone reconstruction using a radial forearm free flap or a split thickness skin graft may reveal scarring that has resulted in small, horizontal shelves along the posterior pharyngeal wall. These shelves hold and divert the food bolus anteriorly into the larynx and may retain secretions and ingested food. When enough food or saliva accumulates, the material is dumped anteriorly into the introitus of the larynx and can result in significant aspiration. In this situation, scar revision is an attractive option; however, the shelves often reform and more aggressive measures of airway protection must be taken.

One last point regarding the hypopharynx is the important anatomic relationships found during surgery. The lateral pharyngotomy incision is either through the piriform sinus or the lateral pharyngeal wall at a level between the superior laryngeal and hypoglossal nerves. Patients with small tumors reconstructed by primary closure with seemingly normal postoperative anatomy can suffer significant aspiration, if the superior laryngeal nerve (SLN) is damaged during the extirpative phase. Sensation of the ipsilateral hemilarynx and hypopharynx, provided by the superior laryngeal nerve, is extremely important and great care must be taken to preserve this structure during resection of hypopharyngeal tumors through the lateral pharyngotomy approach. Total pharyngectomy is performed in combination with a total laryngectomy and is discussed in Chapter 22.

Although the above mentioned techniques and their pitfalls should always be kept in mind, oncologic resection often requires sacrifice of many structures that are important for swallowing; therefore, the management of dysphagia is an integral part of treatment of the head and neck cancer patient. In the early post-op period, nutrition and airway protection are prime considerations. Enteral feedings through a nasogastric or gastrostomy tube are implemented as soon as normal bowel activity resumes. Nursing care of enteral tubes and tracheotomy must be diligent to maximize nutrition and pulmonary toilet.

III. DIAGNOSIS

Patients with dysphagia that persists despite intensive swallowing therapy need to be evaluated in order to pinpoint the area causing the dysphagia. The most commonly used method to assess the oropharyngeal and hypopharyngeal phases of swallowing is the modified barium swallow (MSBS). Functional fiberoptic endoscopic evaluation of swallowing (FEES) has gained popularity because of the lack of radiation exposure, the ability to be performed at bedside, and ease in which it is performed. The patient is examined with a flexible endoscope while eating food stained with food coloring. One major drawback is that the oral phase cannot be evaluated by this technique; therefore, for a patient with an oral cavity defect, the best method to evaluate postoperative dysphagia is with the MBS.

IV. TREATMENT

Once the cause of dysphagia is identified, the options for treatment range from simple measures such as changes in food texture to more aggressive maneuvers. (See Chapters 34-37.) Texture changes in food are important to enhance sensation. The most challenging texture for patients with dysphagia is thin liquids because of the rapid transit time and the lack of sensory cues given by the thin liquid. Products such as Thick-It[R] thicken liquids and other thin foods so that sensation is improved and the transit time is increased, allowing for laryngeal protection. Some patients with aspiration may be managed by complete withdrawal of thin liquids, with only pureed or soft foods offered. In carefully selected patients, liquids may be allowed if they are carbonated, because the bubbles in these beverages supply more sensory cues than noncarbonated beverages.

The next step in swallowing therapy involves muscular training. Speech-language pathologists can teach a patient exercises to strengthen the tongue and palatal muscles, so that improved strength and coordination in this area will provide a more normal swallow. The Mendelsohn maneuver has been shown to greatly improve swallowing function in patients with oral cavity or oropharyngeal defects.[3] Patients are first shown how the larynx is elevated during swallowing. They are then instructed to maintain this elevation during the entire swallow or for 2 to 3 seconds, if possible. This maneuver keeps the arytenoids close to the tongue base and the tongue base close to the posterior pharyngeal wall, both important in prevention of aspiration. The most drastic measure in swallowing therapy is total avoidance of swallowing. Nasogastric tube feeding is normally considered a temporary measure while a patient is learning to swallow after surgery. Percutaneous endoscopic gastrostomies or open gastrostomy tubes provide an excellent route for feeding that can be temporary or permanent. Surgical separation of the airway from the pharyngoesophageal tract is reserved for patients with intractable aspiration. (See Chapter 44.)

Frequently Asked Questions

1. How is reconstruction of floor of the mouth best achieved?
   A. With a thin split thick skin graft that restores its contour and function. A split thickness skin graft is ideal for flood of mouth reconstruction because it is thin and pliable, unlike myocutaneous flaps which are too bulky for this area. The contour of the sulcus can be recreated and tongue mobility is improved because the skin graft limits tethering from scarring.
2. Reconstruction of lateral mandibular defects is used for which patients?
   A. Reconstruction of the lateral mandible should be considered for patients with teeth to maintain normal occlusion. Fibula free flaps are currently favored because of the length of bone available.
3. Which factors contribute to dysphagia after resection of hypopharyngeal tumors?
   A. Loss of sensation, altered constrictor function, and horizontal scar bands. Loss of bulk does not play a role in swallowing after hypopharyngeal resection. Injury or resection of the superior laryngeal nerve (SLN) results in loss of sensation to the hypopharynx and supraglottic larynx, which increases the likelihood of aspiration. Scarring of the constrictor muscles can lead to incoordinated contractions that will also adversely affect swallowing and horizontal scar bands or "shelves" can retain food, which is then dumped anteriorly into the introitus of the larynx.

References

1. McConnel FM. Dysphagia. In *Current Therapy in Otolaryngology Head and Neck Surgery*, St. Louis, Mo: Mosby; 1994: 491-498.
2. Anthony JP, Foster RD, Sharma AB, Kearns GJ, Hoffman WY, Pogrel MA. Reconstruction of a complex midfacial defect with the folded fibular free flap and osseointegrated implants. *Ann Plat Surg.* 1996;37:204-210.
3. Lazarus C, Logemann JA, Gibbons P. Effects of maneuvers on swallowing function in a dysphagic oral cancer patient. *Head Neck.* 1993;15:419-424.

CHAPTER 22

■■■

Pathophysiology of Swallowing Disorders After Laryngectomy

Lisa T. Galati, M.D.
Eugene N. Myers, M.D.

I. INTRODUCTION

Dysphagia after laryngectomy is quite common and can result from a myriad of causes. In this chapter we discuss our approach to limiting the effects of swallowing dysfunction, including careful preoperative planning and flawless operative technique.

Preoperative assessment includes the consideration of a patient's general medical condition, extent of disease, and form of reconstruction. Patients undergoing partial laryngectomy may have a modified barium swallow (MBS) examination preoperatively, if there is a history of swallowing difficulty or aspiration. The patient's expectations must be carefully discussed, because cooperation after surgery is crucial for relearning of the act of swallowing. Postoperatively, cricopharyngeal spasm, stricture, reflux, and recurrent tumor are just some of the etiologies that must be included in the differential diagnosis when treating the laryngectomy patient with dysphagia. A systematic approach to diagnosing and treating postoperative dysphagia is included.

II. TOTAL LARYNGECTOMY

A. Pathophysiology

After total laryngectomy, the trachea and esophagus are permanently separated. Technical aspects of the recon-struction of the pharynx (ie, surgical closure procedures), as well as healing may affect swallowing. The neopharynx created after total laryngectomy is formed by a 2-layer closure of the mucosa and musculature of the piriform sinus and tongue base. Closure of the mucosa is reinforced by closure of a second layer that includes the inferior constrictor muscles and tongue muscles. The cricopharyngeus, which is divided when the larynx is removed, is not used in the reinforcing layer, as this leads to narrowing and tightness in the neopharynx.

The geometric pattern of the closure is a source of controversy. Vertical, horizontal, or T-shaped closures are most commonly used, but innovative techniques, such as the tobacco pouch closure (Figs 22-1 and 22-2), are attempts to simplify this part of the procedure, which is often considered the most tedious and worrisome. The immediate goal of pharyngeal reconstruction is a widely patent conduit to facilitate swallowing and a strong closure line to avoid pharyngo-cutaneous fistulization. The most reliable method is the vertical closure, using a running inverting stitch of 3-0 vicryl or 3-0 chromic. Horizontal and T-shaped closures should be used when required by defect to have the least tension on the suture line.

Total laryngectomy extended to include either the base of tongue or a piriform sinus makes primary closure difficult. Large defects in the base of tongue result

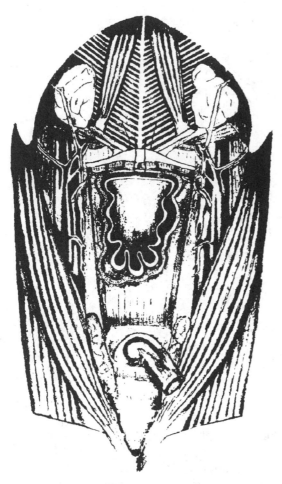

FIG 22-1. Circumferential suture for tobacco pouch closure. (From "Pharyngeal Closure Following Total Laryngectomy: The 'Tobacco Pouch' Technique," by C. Gavilan, M. Cerdeira, and J. Gavilan, 1993, p. 300. *Operative Techniques in Otolaryngology, 4.* Reprinted with permission.)

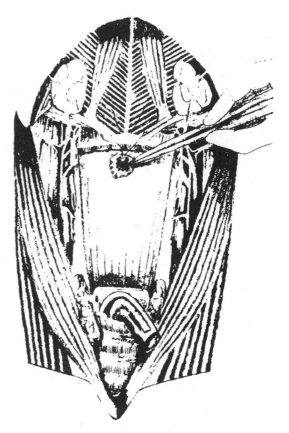

FIG 22-2. Cinching of tobacco pouch closure. (From "Pharyngeal Closure Following Total Laryngectomy: The 'Tobacco Pouch' Technique," by C. Gavilan, M. Cerdeira, and J. Gavilan, 1993, p. 301. *Operative Techniques in Otolaryngology, 4.* Reprinted with permission.)

in wide gaps superiorly that can be closed vertically, but in some cases the resultant tension on the suture line is excessive. Advancement flaps from the tongue base can provide more surface area for closure and reduce tension on the suture line. A flap, 2 cm in width and 3-4 cm in length is based on the lateral aspect of the base of tongue on the side of the defect. The flap is undermined and sewn into the defect to recreate the anterior wall of the neopharynx (Figs 22-3 and 22-4).

Resection of the piriform sinus often hinders an optimal closure because the hypopharyngeal mucosal remnant is small. If the width of the remaining mucosa is less than 4 cm, the probability of postoperative dysphagia is high. Small strips of pharyngeal mucosa (1.5-2 cm) can be successfully closed over a nasogastric tube, but even with healing without fistula formation, the postoperative function will be compromised.[1] This situation is worse in patients who will receive radiation therapy. In that situation, normal swallowing is not at-

tainable using this technique and patients usually are limited to a liquid diet. Tracheoesophageal puncture (TEP) speech is also difficult, if not impossible, because the tight neopharynx provides little surface capable of vibration.

There are several options for closure of pharyngeal remnants that are less than 2 cm wide. Pectoralis myofascial flaps may be used for patients undergoing total laryngectomy with partial pharyngectomy. During this technique the mucosal edges are sutured to the fascia of the pectoralis muscle after the pharynx has been stented with a Montgomery salivary bypass tube. The pectoralis myofascial flap may also be tubed to reconstruct a circumferential defect but, because of its bulk and the superior results with free flaps, it is not frequently used for this purpose.

State-of-the-art reconstruction in such cases is a jejunal free flap. This technique involves the sacrifice of the remaining posterior wall pharyngeal mucosa after which a segment of small bowel is anastomosed to the BOT and esophagus (Fig 22-5). The jejunal segment maintains peristaltic movement and patients are able to achieve good TEP speech. Total laryngectomy for sub-

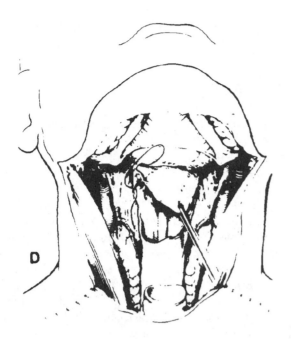

FIG 22-3. Advancement of tongue base flap. (From "Tongue Flap Repair of Postlaryngectomy Hypopharyngeal Stenosis," by T. Calcaterra, 1986, p. 618. *Laryngoscope, 96.* Reprinted with permission.)

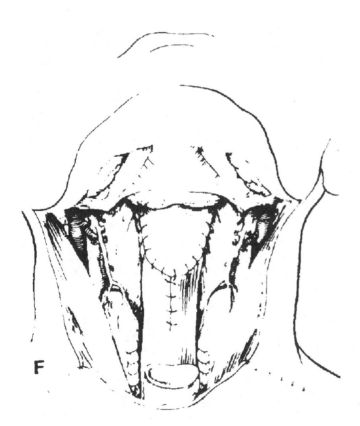

FIG 22-4. Closure of neopharynx. (From "Tongue Flap Repair of Postlaryngectomy Hypopharyngeal Stenosis," by T. Calcaterra, 1986, p. 619. *Laryngoscope, 96.* Reprinted with permission.)

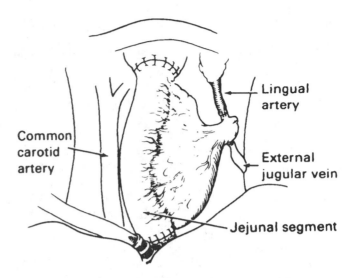

FIG 22-5. Jejunal free flap reconstruction of pharynx. (From "Reconstruction of the Hypopharynx Following Extensive Loss of Mucosa," by G. Sambataro, C. Oldini, and R. F. Mazzola, 1984, p. 692. *Laryngoscope, 94.* Reprinted with permission.)

glottic primaries may require gastric pull up, if total esophagectomy is necessary. Jejunum free flap is not an option in these patients, because the distal anastomosis is difficult and unsafe to perform in the mediastinum. Tubed radial forearm free flaps are also a good option for reconstruction of the pharynx, especially for patients who have had abdominal surgery and jejunum is not available.

Postoperatively, patients receive nasogastric feedings when they feel hungry or have shown signs of normal bowel function, usually on postoperative day 2. Early vomiting secondary to feedings that were started too early may be disastrous to the newly reconstructed pharynx. Fistulization occurs in up to 75% of these patients.[2] Enteral feedings in patients undergoing free flap reconstruction is either through a gastrostomy or a jejunostomy tube, placed during the harvest of the viscus. The best way to gauge readiness for oral intake is the patient's ability to swallow saliva. When the patient relies on bedside suction for less than 50% of saliva clearance, oral intake may be started. In most patients without prior irradiation this occurs on postoperative day 5 to 7. Patients with prior irradiation are started on oral feedings on postoperative day 10, if their ability to swallow saliva is restored. Patients who have had a free-flap or gastric pull up need to undergo a barium swallow to assess the integrity of the anastomosis. For the first 2 weeks of oral intake, all patients are instructed to eat a soft or soft mechanical diet (soups, puddings, liquids, soft-cooked eggs).

B. Diagnosis

Swallowing disorders may be as simple as dysphagia secondary to radiation xerostomia or as frustrating as a slowly healing pharyngocutaneous fistula (Table 22-1). Patients with xerostomia show a completely dry mouth or small amounts of thick white strands of saliva. Some patients may have slight hypertrophy of the submandibular glands. In each case, a careful examination is necessary to avoid overlooking a recurrent or new tumor.

Dysphagia may result from a tightly closed neopharynx—scarring narrows the already compromised pharynx and patients are unable to eat solids. Pooling of secretions in the hypopharynx is the most usual finding and mandates further evaluation with a barium swallow esophagogram to assess the degree of narrowing and the presence of tumor. Esophagoscopy with biopsy is performed to rule out recurrence.

Pharyngocutaneous fistula formation is one of the most dreaded complications of total laryngectomy, as it prolongs recovery time and delays the ability to eat by mouth. Early signs of fistula formation are erythema and edema (*peau d'orange*) of the skin, which is followed by suture line dehiscence and finally by drainage of saliva and food from the neck.

Formation of an anterior neopharyngeal pouch may lead to dysphagia after total laryngectomy, if the pouch is large and retains food and debris. As many as 35%-100% of postlaryngectomy patients have been noted to have an anterior neopharyngeal pouch, the posterior wall of which is formed by a fibrous band referred to as the neoepiglottis. The pouch is believed to be secondary to a healed fistula, incoordinated contraction of the constrictor muscles, radiation therapy, vertical closure, or a combination of these. A neopharyngeal pouch leads to dysphagia in 10%-40% of laryngectomy patients.[3,4]

Occasionally, patients will complain of leakage around or though the TEP. If the TEP prosthesis does not fit properly or is worn out, secretions can leak through the tract from the esophagus into the trachea. The tract must be carefully examined to rule out recurrent tumor. Biopsy is necessary if there is suspicious tissue at the TEP site. Leakage may also occur around the

Table 22-1. *Dysphagia After Total Laryngectomy*

1. Stricture
   a. Small hypopharyngeal mucosal remnant
   b. Tight reapproximation of constrictors/cricopharyngeus
   c. Radiation therapy
   d. Fistula healing by secondary intention
2. Tumor
3. TEP
4. Xerostomia
5. BOT resection
6. Total laryngopharyngectomy
   a. Stenosis of jejunal free flap
   b. Gastric pull-up complication

prosthesis. This is treated by inserting a larger diameter prosthesis.

C. Treatment

Once the etiology of the swallowing disorder has been identified and recurrent tumor has been ruled out, treatment is fairly straightforward. Patients complaining of xerostomia can be treated with cholinergic agents and increased fluid intake.

Stenosis of the neopharynx can be ameliorated by bougienage in the less severe cases, but some may require augmentation of the pharyngeal lumen with a pectoralis myofascial flap or jejunal microvascular flap. Dysphagia in a patient after reconstruction with a microvascular jejunum flap is most often due to stricture of the distal anastomosis. Dilatation is used to improve transit of solid food, but occasionally surgical revision of the anastomosis is necessary.

Patients who undergo a gastric pull up may suffer dumping (cramping and diarrhea immediately after eating) and abnormal motility, which cause diarrhea, regurgitation, and early satiety. Small frequent meals and upright positioning are often sufficient to manage these sequelae.

Patients who have a fistula are kept NPO during healing, and nutrition must be maintained by nasogastric tube or central intravenous hyperalimentation. Antibiotics are given to aid in healing. The wound is packed with gauze to create a controlled fistula. This directs the salivary flow away from the carotid and tracheostoma to protect the artery and prevent aspiration of secretions. In select cases, esophagostomy is an option to establish a controlled fistula. Primary esophagostomy, at one time a relatively common procedure resulting in "three stomas," is rarely indicated with current reconstruction options. Patients undergoing total laryngopharyngectomy in whom operating time must be limited because of medical reasons or because of inability to reconstruct the defect during the time of resection can be closed in conjunction with formation of a esophagostomy. The superior, oropharyngeal mucosa is sewn to the skin, creating the first of the three stomas. The upper cervical esophagus, sewn to an opening in the skin, is the second fistula, through which a feeding tube is inserted for post-op feeding. The skin flap closure and tracheostoma are then completed and the patient is allowed to recover until ready for the second procedure (Fig 22-6).

Treatment of neopharyngeal pouches aims to eliminate retention of food in the pouch and consists of dilatation of the pharynx for smaller pouches and endoscopic laser resection of larger pouches. The strategy with laser endoscopy is similar to the approach for endoscopic treatment of Zenker's diverticulum. A portion

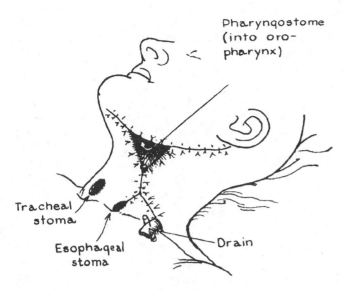

FIG 22-6. Three stomas after total laryngopharyngectomy. (From *Surgery of the Head and Neck*, by H. Martin, 1957, p. 359. Philadelphia: Lippincott-Raven.

of the neoepiglottis is excised to prevent the pouch from retaining food and debris.[4] Open techniques, in which the pouch mucosa is excised and the neopharyngeal edges are reapproximated, have been replaced by endoscopic procedures, because of patient preference and ease of performance.

Management of a leaking TEP requires a change of the prosthesis, which is usually sufficient to alleviate this problem. More severe cases of aspiration caused by an enlarged TEP may require closure of the tract. Prostheses that are too large can cause dysphagia by creating a foreign body sensation and partial obstruction of the esophageal lumen.

III. PARTIAL LARYNGECTOMY

A. Introduction

The discussion of dysphagia after partial laryngectomy is more complex for the simple reason that there is no separation of the trachea and esophagus. Aspiration is the most common manifestation of dysphagia in the patient undergoing certain types of conservation surgery. Altered sensation, movement, and anatomy cause all patients to have dysphagia during the immediate postoperative period, if not longer.

The typical vertical hemilaryngectomy specimen includes the true vocal fold, a portion of the false vocal fold, and nearly one half of the thyroid cartilage. The classic method of reconstruction is reapproximation of thyroid perichondrium and a second layer closure of the strap muscles. Even though one true vocal fold is missing, these patients tend to compensate well be-

cause both arytenoids and the supraglottis, with its rich sensory innervation, are intact. Thus, aspiration is usually a problem of the early postoperative period. Sacrifice of the superior laryngeal nerve (SLN) or one arytenoid can severely hinder post-operative swallowing. Normally, the traditional hemilaryngectomy patient can swallow on postoperative day 9 or 10.

Patients with extended hemilaryngectomy, in which the arytenoid, cricoid, or SLN are removed, often require months of post-op swallowing therapy. Employing compensatory techniques such as head turning (toward the operated side) and breath holding, most patients will improve and be able to eat a normal diet.

The standard supraglottic laryngectomy includes removal of the epiglottis, false vocal folds, and the superior half of the thyroid cartilage. Reconstruction consists of reapproximation of the tongue base to the thyroid perichondrium and closure of the lateral portion of the hypopharynx. One of the most important aspects of the reconstruction is the closure of the tongue base to the perichondrium. It must be made by approximating the perichondrium to the anterior portion of the cut edge of the tongue, ie, tongue musculature, and not the posterior mucosal margin (Fig 22-7). This creates a ledge that diverts the bolus posterior to the glottis. Closure of the perichondrium to the mucosa of the tongue base creates a direct path for the food from the oropharynx to the laryngeal inlet. Preservation of the SLN, when possible, is also important, because normal endolaryngeal sensation will aid in regaining normal swallowing function.

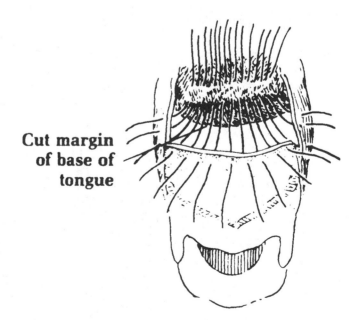

Cut margin of base of tongue

FIG 22-7. Anastomosis of tongue base muscle to perichondrium. (From *Atlas of Laryngeal Surgery*, by C. W. Cummings, C. W. Sessions, E. A. Weymukker, and P. Wood, 1984, p. 291. St. Louis, Mo: Mosby Co. Reprinted with permission.)

Swallowing after supraglottic laryngectomy requires intensive therapy, which in many cases takes months. Dysphagia after supraglottic laryngectomy occurs because many normal sensory cues are altered and some of the food bolus is presented directly to the vocal folds after passing through the oropharynx. Preservation of the SLN provides for sensation at the glottic level. However, the laryngeal surface of the epiglottis contains the richest sensory innervation in the larynx, and patients need time to adjust to this loss. With training, the patient should be able to coordinate swallowing and airway protection.

Supracricoid laryngectomy is a conservation procedure indicated for the removal of the entire glottis and paraglottic and pre-epiglottic spaces. The cricoid, hyoid, and at least one arytenoid are preserved. The key step to assure safe swallowing postoperatively is to suture the arytenoid to the anterior cricoid cartilage, which allows the arytenoid to make contact with the base of tongue during swallowing and prevent aspiration. Preservation of the recurrent and superior laryngeal nerves is imperative to provide a safe airway and swallowing mechanism, and some consider sacrifice of either of these nerves a contraindication to completion of the supracricoid laryngectomy. After decannulation, swallowing therapy usually begins on postoperative day 7. Most patients accommodate quickly and aspiration is not a common problem. Soft foods and liquids are given for the first 2 weeks to avoid stress on the healing anastomosis and a normal diet is then resumed.

B. Pathophysiology

In conservation laryngeal surgery, there are several factors that contribute to postoperative dysphagia. The tracheotomy causes dysphagia for several reasons. First, the tracheostomy tube limits the upward mobility of the trachea and larynx, which is an imperative aspect for normal swallowing. Loss of normal subglottic pressure causes loss both of true vocal fold proprioception and effective cough. True vocal fold adduction is inefficient without normal proprioception (afferent-efferent reflex) and can result in aspiration. Decannulation is attempted in all patients, but unfortunately is impossible in some cases. The previously mentioned problems can be partially circumvented with the use of a Passy-Muir valve, which allows ingress of air but closes on expiration. This causes a build-up of subglottic pressure, which enables the patient to cough effectively.

The timing of decannulation is determined by the patient's performance. In a patient with a vertical hemilaryngectomy, deflation of the cuff is attempted 9-10 days after surgery. At that point, patients should be able to tolerate their secretions. After 1 day with the cuff down, the tracheotomy tube is downsized to a #4 cuffless tube,

which is then capped. If the capped tube is tolerated for 24 hours, the patient is decannulated. Oral feedings are not begun until the stoma is almost completely closed, usually 2 to 3 days after decannulation. The method of decannulation is the same for patients with supraglottic laryngectomy, but is not initiated until postoperative week 2 or 3. The first attempt at cuff deflation should not be made before postoperative day 14, because aspiration will occur. However, if the patient has slackening need for bedside suction for saliva clearance, deflation of the cuff can be attempted. The same steps as detailed previously are followed to decannulate these patients, but requires a much longer time (sometimes 2-3 weeks) to achieve.

Gastroesophageal reflux (GER) is an important consideration in the management of patients who underwent a partial laryngectomy. Gastric secretions bathing the arytenoids can cause edema significant enough to cause retention of secretions, aspiration, and dysphagia. All patients undergoing conservation surgery should receive GER prophylaxis. Some believe that cricopharyngeal myotomy leads to reflux and do not routinely use it. In supracricoid laryngectomy, the myotomy is not recommended because the arytenoids are the major component of the reconstruction and even small amounts of reflux can compromise laryngeal function and airway protection.

Extended resections beyond standard conservation procedures may also cause prolonged dysphagia. Excision of an arytenoid, the base of tongue, or piriform sinus will often double or triple the rehabilitation time. The normal contours of the base of the tongue and piriform sinuses are very important to guide food and saliva around the larynx and into the esophagus. Therefore, alteration of these structures by resection and scarring may lead to rerouting of food and saliva from the oropharynx directly into the laryngeal inlet. Loss of the arytenoid, which results in a fixed hemilarynx and compromised airway protection, is poorly tolerated. Compensatory maneuvers and diet modification can lessen the severity of these problems. Gastrostomy can be useful in cases of prolonged dysphagia for several reasons: (1) The discomfort of a long-standing nasogastric tube is eliminated; (2) the rehabilitation can progress without the pressure to get the patient back to "normal" as soon as possible; and (3) there is elimination of friction, and therefore no edema or ulceration caused by the nasogastric tube resting on the arytenoids. Also, it is important to consider that patients with a nasogastric tube rarely go out in public because the tube attracts too much attention. A feeding gastrostomy therefore provides patients with more confidence to resume social activities.

Dysphagia that develops progressively after the initial recovery period should raise the suspicion of recurrent tumor. Although scarring may cause swallowing problems months after surgery, recurrent cancer must be ruled out. Accompanying symptoms of pain, weight loss, and bleeding should heighten the suspicion of malignancy, with esophagoscopy necessary to make the diagnosis.

C. Diagnosis

Dysphagia after partial laryngectomy requires a physical examination that is focused on vocal fold mobility and sensation (Table 22-2). Gentle palpation of the supraglottic structures and the remaining vocal cord with the tip of the flexible laryngoscope will elicit laryngeal closure if normal innervation exists. If examination of the patient with persistent dysphagia is normal, a modified barium swallow (MBS) may provide useful information. Findings may include cricopharyngeal achalasia, requiring myotomy; abnormal phases of swallowing, such as aspiration due to incoordinated pharyngeal contraction; or improper laryngeal elevation.

D. Treatment

Patients undergoing partial laryngectomy require postoperative swallowing therapy. There are several maneuvers that improve swallowing and decrease the incidence of aspiration. (See Chapters 34 and 35.) After vertical hemilaryngectomy, turning the head toward the operated side dircts the food toward the remaining hemilarynx and improves swallowing efficiency and safety. Approximately 2 weeks after supraglottic laryngectomy, if healing is normal, patients can be taught the supraglottic swallow. (See Chapter 35.) In cases of refractory aspiration, the arytenoid or cricoid cartilage is reconstructed using a muscle transposition flap or autogenous cartilage. Some patients may require a completion laryngectomy to restore a safe airway and normal swallowing.

Table 22-2. *Dysphagia After Conservation Laryngeal Surgery*

1. Aspiration
   a. Loss of sensation (superior laryngeal nerve)
   b. Resection of tongue base or arytenoid
2. Cricopharyngeal achalasia
3. Poor pulmonary function
4. Tracheostomy

E. Controversy

Cricopharyngeal myotomy has traditionally been recommended after supraglottic laryngectomy. Division of the muscular fibers creates a more accommodating esophageal inlet. The narrowing created by the muscle can be easily palpated in preparation for the myotomy. Anatomically, the muscle is found posterior to the cricoid cartilage and rotation of the larynx allows easy localization of the cricopharyngeus. As a nasogastric tube is inserted into the esophagus and two Babcock clamps are placed at either end of the muscle, the nasogastric tube is grabbed. The muscle is divided until the radio-opaque stripe on the tube is visible through the remaining mucosal layer (Fig 22-8). A small strip of the cricopharyngeal muscle is then excised to prevent reapproximation of the cut edges through scarring. Recently, however, the use of cricopharyngeal myotomy has been questioned. A study carried out by the World Health Organization showed that cricopharyngeal myotomy conferred no benefit in swallowing function. Many believe that myotomy not only does not improve swallowing, but promotes incoordinated pharyngeal contractions and GER.

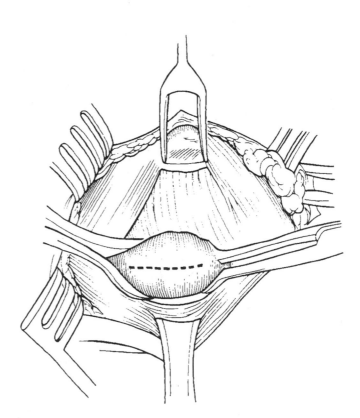

FIG 22-8. Cricopharyngeal myotomy over Babcock clamp. (From *Operative Otolaryngology—Head and Neck Surgery*, E. N. Myers, ed., 1997, p. 470. Philadelphia, Pa: W. B. Saunders. Reprinted with permission.)

VI. CONCLUSION

A standard, stepwise approach to dysphagia is important in the laryngectomee to identify the cause and rule out recurrent cancer. Careful preoperative evaluation of the extent of the disease and a clear strategy for reconstruction are the first steps taken toward minimizing complications that cause swallowing dysfunction. A multi-disciplinary approach, with the help of a nutritionist, speech-language pathologist, oncologist, and reconstruction surgeons offers the optimal management for the patient undergoing laryngectomy.

Frequently Asked Questions

1. Aspiration is more likely in patients who have
   A. A vertical hemilaryngectomy with one arytenoid resected. Extended conservation procedures increase recovery time of normal swallowing by 2 to 3 times. Excision of one arytenoid greatly increases the incidence of aspiration.
2. Long-term dysphagia after total laryngectomy
   A. Results in pooling of secretions and poor TEP speech. Dysphagia after laryngectomy is common and is manifested as pooled secretions in the hypopharynx, difficulty swallowing solids, and inability to phonate. Scarring and narrowing of the neopharynx cause dysphagia and poor TEP speech.
3. Decannulation
   A. Is based on a patient's ability to tolerate secretions and plugging of tracheotomy tube. The best measure to assure successful decannulation after par-

tial laryngectomy is the patient's ability to swallow secretions and breathe around a plugged tracheotomy tube. Of all of the conservation procedures, supraglottic laryngectomy usually requires the longest time to decannulation.
4. Closure of the neopharynx
   A. May result in neopharyngeal pouch formation if there is a breakdown. Formation of a neopharyngeal pouch is usually the result of breakdown of the neopharyngeal suture line. Food and debris may collect and form a small pouch that persists after healing. Most neopharyngeal closures are done vertically. However, the most important decision in closure is creation of a suture line with the least amount of tension, which can be achieved with a T-closure.

References

1. Hui Y, Wei WI, Yuen PW, Lam LK, Ho WK. Primary closure of pharyngeal remnant after total laryngectomy and partial pharyngectomy: how much residual mucosa is sufficient? *Laryngoscope.* 1996;106:490-494.
2. Tomkinson A, Shone GR, Dingle A, Roblin DG, Quine S. Pharyngocutaneous fistula following total laryngectomy and post-operative vomiting. *Clin Otolaryngol.* 1996;21: 369-370.
3. Kirchner JA, Scatliff JH. Disabilities resulting from healed salivary fistula. *Arch Otolaryngol.* 1962;75:60-68.
4. Davis RV, Vincent ME, Shapshay SM, Strong MS. The anatomy and complication of "T" versus vertical closure of the hypopharynx after laryngectomy. *Laryngoscope.* 1982; 93:16-22.

CHAPTER 23

■ ■ ■

Skull Base Surgery

Anna M. Pou, M.D.
Ricardo L. Carrau, M.D.

I. INTRODUCTION

Patients undergoing skull base surgery are at risk for injury to the lower cranial nerves, brainstem, brain parenchyma, and soft tissues of the upper aerodigestive tract, depending on tumor location. Injury to these vital structures can lead to dysfunction of speech, swallowing, and airway protection. In addition to the mentioned deficits, patients undergoing skull base surgery frequently need reconstruction with insensate soft tissue flaps, which may compound a deficit because of large anesthetic areas and bulk. These patients frequently need enteral tubes, prolonged intubation and ventilation, and tracheotomies that further compound the swallowing deficits (see Chapter 20).

II. PATHOPHYSIOLOGY

Injuries to the brain or brainstem include a variety of mechanisms, such as ischemic or hemorrhagic vascular events, encephalomalacia due to retraction, or even resection of tissue as part of an oncologic resection. Any of these mechanisms will produce lesions similar to those produced by strokes affecting the specific affected area, including cognitive, motor, and sensory deficits (see Chapters 15 and 16). Similarly, the muscles and mucosa of the upper aerodigestive tract may be injured, if it is traversed as part of the surgical approach to the tumor or resected as part of the extirpative surgery. These lesions produce deficits similar to those produced

by other types of head and neck oncologic surgery (see Chapter 22) and compound other neurological deficits.

The cranial nerves most commonly injured are the trigeminal (cranial nerve V), facial (cranial nerve VII), glossopharyngeal (cranial nerve IX), vagus (cranial nerve X), and hypoglossal (cranial nerve XII). All of these nerves provide sensory and/or motor innervation to the mouth, pharynx, and larynx that help initiate and control swallowing.[1,2] Deficits in these cranial nerves affect the oral and pharyngeal phases of swallowing and often lead to aspiration. Thus, injury to multiple cranial nerves increases patient morbidity, functional deficits, and length of rehabilitation.

In skull base surgery, injury to the vagus nerve is usually proximal to the nodose ganglion and thus involves both the recurrent and superior laryngeal nerves (high vagal lesion). A high vagal injury leads to ipsilateral laryngeal anesthesia and vocal fold paralysis. In addition, it also produces paralysis of the ipsilateral soft palate, loss of vagus-mediated relaxation of the cricopharyngeus muscle, and discoordination of the pharyngeal musculature by elimination of the vagal contribution to the pharyngeal plexus. Therefore, a high vagal lesion, in addition to other cranial nerve or neurological deficits, produces marked postoperative deglutition and airway morbidity.

Normal swallowing consists of an orderly sequence of events resulting in the neuromuscular coordination of oral, pharyngeal, and esopharyngeal muscular contractions, each with varying degrees of dependence on central control. Swallowing is evoked by motor neurons in the lateral precentral gyrus and, more importantly, the brainstem.[2] The key to this coordinated sequence is intact sensory input that can trigger the swallowing center in the medulla, which will then act as a central pattern generator producing sequential muscle contraction. Sensory feedback may also modify the motor output of selected muscles.[3,4] (See Chapters 2 and 3.)

The act of swallowing is divided into four phases: oral preparatory, oral, pharyngeal, and esophageal.[5] The oral and oral preparatory phases are the voluntary phases of swallowing during which the bolus is prepared by mastication (cranial nerve V) and mixed with saliva. The action of the tongue (cranial nerve XII) is crucial during this time. The oral aperture (lips) and the buccal musculature are controlled by the facial nerve and are important for the prevention of drooling, retention of food in the gingivobuccal gutter, and delay in the oral phase. At the end of the oral phase, the tongue positions the bolus against the hard palate. Afferent receptors in the anterior tonsillar pillars, posterior tongue, soft palate, and oropharynx are the probable initiators of the pharyngeal phase.[2] These impulses are carried via cranial nerves IX and X. Therefore, alterations during these phases of swallowing secondary to direct cranial nerve (cranial nerves V, VII, IX, X, XII) or brainstem/brain injury may result in premature spillage of the bolus into the hypopharynx or delay the triggering of the pharyngeal phase. This, in turn, will result in failure to trigger the glottic closure reflex, and the bolus will spill into an open glottis.[5]

The next phase of swallowing is the pharyngeal phase, which is involuntary. During this phase of swallowing, velopharyngeal closure and laryngeal elevation occurs. There is also sequential contraction of the constrictor muscles, which creates a peristaltic wave that sweeps the bolus down. These events are timed with spontaneous laryngeal closure that begins at the level of the true vocal folds and proceeds in an inferior-to-superior direction. As the peristaltic wave reaches the cricopharyngeal level, there is reflex relaxation of the muscle, mediated by cranial nerve X, which facilitates the entrance of the bolus into the esophagus.[2,6] Cranial nerves IX and X are the mediators of the afferent and efferent impulses of this phase of swallowing. Injury to cranial nerve X will not only cause impaired pharyngeal peristalsis via the pharyngeal plexus, but will also impair glottic closure. Cricopharyngeal dysfunction can also lead to aspiration by interfering with smooth transition of the bolus from the hypopharynx into the esophagus. Furthermore, velopharyngeal insufficiency will cause nasal regurgitation and partial loss of the intraluminal pressure generated by the base of tongue and constrictor muscles.

The esophageal phase is the final phase of swallowing. After the bolus enters the esophagus, it is carried to the stomach by spontaneous peristalsis. Transport of the bolus is also aided by gravity and negative pressure created by diaphragmatic activity.

III. DIAGNOSIS

Following skull base surgery, the surgeon is usually aware of the areas of injury, as it reflects the area corresponding to the surgical field. Nevertheless, a complete history and physical examination should be performed to elucidate the degree of dysfunction and its impact on the patient's lifestyle. (See Chapter 4.) The patient should be questioned about repeated throat clearing, chronic cough, slurred speech, tongue biting, paresthesia, nasal regurgitation, weight loss, history of pneumonia, and changes in quality and strength of voice. The physical examination should consist of a neurological evaluation of all cranial nerves, particularly V, VII, IX, X, and XII. An examination of the oropharynx and hypopharynx, in addition to indirect and flexible laryngoscopy or videolaryngoscopy, are performed to ascertain the presence of gross motor or sensory deficits. Gross sensory deficits of the oropharynx may be ascertained with the use of tongue blade or swabs. The swabs may be dipped into liquids at different temperatures to grossly test thermal sensitivity.[4]

Pooling of secretions, the presence of frank aspiration, and the ability to clear secretions with a cough should be noted. Indirect laryngoscopy should determine vocal fold position, movement, and tone. Sensation of the larynx and pharynx is assessed using the tip of the flexible laryngoscope.

The maximal phonation time (MPT) is also determined, as it gives information about the severity of the glottic gap. It is defined as the greatest length of time over which phonation can be sustained steadily for the /a/ sound.[7]

Radiologic studies provide additional information regarding the severity of a patient's dysphagia and his or her ability to swallow different test substances. The modified barium swallow (MBS) is considered to be the "gold standard" for the evaluation and rehabilitation of swallowing disorders and is recommended for all patients who are able to undergo this test. This test is performed by a speech-language pathologist and a radiologist. It examines the function of the oral cavity, pharynx, and esophagus during swallowing. It can also be used to assess the effects of various head positioning maneuvers on swallowing function. Therefore, it has significant treatment implications, in addition to its diagnostic usefulness.

The fiberoptic endoscopic evaluation of swallowing (FEES) also provides information regarding the structural and functional deficits of swallowing. A great advantage of this test is that it can be performed at the bedside; this diminishes cost and it benefits those who cannot travel to a radiology suite. The FEES, however, is unable to assess esophageal disease or to identify aspiration during the pharyngeal phase of swallowing.[8,9]

IV. TREATMENT

A. Nonsurgical

Nonsurgical options for treating the swallowing problem include diet modification, swallowing retraining, and postural compensation techniques (Table 23-1).[10] (See Chapters 34-37.) Consultation with a speech-language pathologist is critical during the patient assessment and training process; the speech-language pathologist tailors compensatory maneuvers to each patient's needs. Nonsurgical interventions, alone, may eliminate aspiration or may be used in conjunction with surgical intervention to treat aspiration.

B. Surgical Treatment

Many surgical treatments for aspiration have been described[10] (Table 23-2).

Recently, laryngeal framework surgery (thyroplasty and arytenoid adduction) for the management of aspiration due to high vagal lesions has proven to be a very reliable method.[4,11] Advantages of medialization thyroplasty over other medialization procedures, include intraoperative monitoring of the vocal folds (position, closure, etc) under physiologic conditions, minimal al-

Table 23-1. *Nonsurgical Treatment of Aspiration*

Diet modification:
NPO
Change in bolus size
Change in food consistencies
Changes in temperature and taste
Thermal sensitization

Swallowing retraining:
Supraglottic swallow
Mendelson maneuver
Multiple swallows
Frequent throat clearing

Postural compensation techniques:
Sitting upright
Lying on side

Head position maneuvers:
Chin tuck
Head lift
Rotating head to side of lesion

Oral motor exercises:
Lip seal
Tongue retraction and elevation
Tongue strengthening

Table 23-2. *Surgical Treatment of Aspiration*

Tracheotomy
Gastrostomy tube
Vocal fold medialization:
Injection
Implantation
Arytenoid adduction

Cricopharyngeal myotomy
Laryngeal closure:
Laryngeal stenting
Glottic closure
Supraglottic closure

Laryngotracheal separation
Laryngectomy

teration of the vocal fold vibratory characteristics, local anesthesia, adjustability of prosthesis, and potential reversibility. Arytenoid adduction, however, should be considered permanent; it requires partial dissection of the posterior cricoarytenoid and interarytenoid muscles of the larynx, with possible injury to the terminal end of the recurrent laryngeal nerve (RLN) that innervates these muscles.[12]

By improving the sphincteric function of the glottis with laryngeal framework surgery, the incidence of aspiration is decreased through vocal fold medialization and improvement in glottic closing pressure, which is essential to normal swallowing.[13-15]

Cricopharyngeal myotomy, in addition to laryngeal framework surgery, also decreases the incidence and amount of aspiration following skull base surgery.[16] Laryngeal framework surgery and cricopharyngeal myotomy have successfully helped in avoiding tracheotomy, promoting early swallowing, and shortening hospital stays[4,11] in the rehabilitation of patients undergoing skull base surgery who have multiple cranial nerve deficits.

V. CONTROVERSIES

There is controversy about the timing of vocal fold medialization, cricopharyngeal myotomy, and gastrostomy tube placement. If the vagus nerve has been sacrificed during skull base surgery, one can predict that the patient will have dysphonia and dysphagia. The degree of dysphagia/aspiration will also be affected by the presence of additional neurologic deficits. In this cohort of patients, it is common for multiple neurologic deficits to be present.[4] Netterville et al[11] advocate the use of thyroplasty at the time of initial surgical resection. This practice achieves immediate glottic competency, leading to the avoidance of tracheotomy, early swallowing, and decrease in number of hospital days. Cricopharyngeal myotomy is also recommended for patients presenting with clinical (ie, pooling of secretions in pyriform sinus) and/or radiologic evidence (ie, pooling of barium, achalasia) of cricopharyngeal muscle dysfunction.[4] Montgomery et al[16] compared the efficiency of thyroplasty and cricopharyngeal myotomy in treating dysphonia, aspiration, and dysphagia secondary to different etiologies. These two procedures were performed simultaneously in one group of patients and sequentially in a second group of patients. It was concluded that, with both cranial nerves IX and X paralysis, it is best to perform these procedures simultaneously and as soon as possible, even when there is a possibility of nerve function return. A gastrostomy tube should be placed in anyone who is unable to maintain adequate oral intake secondary to severe dysphagia/aspiration. The most efficient time to place a gastrostomy tube is unknown. However, placement should occur early in treatment to avoid the increase in postcricoid/interarytenoid edema, and gastroesophageal reflux, which is associated with nasal feeding tubes; these changes can influence the degree of dysphagia.

Frequently Asked Questions

1. Which patients should undergo a modified barium swallow postoperatively?
   A. A modified-barium swallow should be ordered for any patient who complains of, or shows signs/symptoms of dysphagia/aspiration, and patients with known sacrifice of cranial nerves, particularly cranial nerves IX, X, and XII.

2. When should a speech-language pathologist be consulted?
   A. A speech-language pathologist should be consulted when a patient presents with dysphonia/dysphagia. Evaluation and subsequent compensatory maneuvers can be taught using the modified-barium swallow.

3. If vocal fold medialization is not performed primarily—that is, at the time of surgical resection—when should it be performed?
   A. As soon as the patient is able to undergo the medialization procedure ± CPM.

4. Will all primary thyroplasties need to be revised?
   A. Some primary thyroplasties will need to be revised because of progressive vocal fold atrophy and decrease in vocal fold tension. This is dependent on the level and severity of the neural lesion, which will dictate the level of reinnervation. Even with subclinical reinnervation, the vocal fold will maintain tone and bulk. In addition, only 20% to 30% will need revision because of initial malposition or undermedialization.

5. When is an arytenoid adduction performed?
   A. An arytenoid adduction is performed when the vocal fold paralysis is permanent and there is a large posterior glottic chink ± vocal folds at different levels.

References

1. Larson C. Neurophysiology of speech and swallowing. *Semin Speech Language.* 1985;6:275-291.
2. Miller AJ. Neurophysiological basis of swallowing. *Dysphagia.* 1986;1:91-100.
3. Miller AJ. The search for the central swallowing pathway: the quest for clarity. *Dysphagia.* 1993;8:185-194.
4. Pou AM, Carrau RL, Eibling DE, Murry T. Laryngeal framework surgery for the management of aspiration in high vagal lesions. *Am J Otolaryngol.* 1998;19:1-7.
5. Logemann J. *Evaluation and Treatment of Swallowing Disorders.* San Diego, Ca: College-Hill Press; 1983.
6. Miller A. Deglutition. *Physiol Rev.* 1983;62:129-184.
7. Kent RD, Kent JF, Rosenbek, JC. Maximum performance tests of speech production. *J Speech Hear Disord.* 1987;52:367-387.
8. Langmore SE, Schatz K, Olsen N. Fiberoptic endoscopic examination of swallowing safety: a new procedure. *Dysphagia.* 1988;2:216-219.
9. Bastian RW. Videoendoscopic evaluation of patients with dysphagia: an adjunct to the modified barium swallow. *Otolaryngol Head Neck Surg.* 1991;104:339-350.
10. Pou A, Carrau RL, Eibling DE, Murry T, Ferguson BJ. Laryngeal framework surgery for the treatment of aspiration. In: Friedman M, ed. *Laryngeal and Tracheal Reconstruction.* Philadelphia, Pa: WB Saunders Co; in press.
11. Netterville JL, Stine RE, Luken ES, Civantos FJ, Ossoff RH. Silastic medialization and arytenoid adduction: the Vanderbilt experience. A review of 116 phonosurgical procedures. *Ann Otol.* 1993;102:413-424.
12. Isshiki N, Tanabe M, Sawada M. Arytenoid adduction for unilateral vocal cord paralysis. *Arch Otolaryngol.* 1978;104:555-558.
13. Iwanaga Y, Maeyama T, Umezaki T, Shin T. Intracordal injection increases glottic closing force in recurrent laryngeal nerve paralysis. *Otolaryngol Head Neck Surgery.* 1992;107:451-456.
14. Eibling DE, Gross RD. Subglottic air pressure: a key component of swallowing efficiency. *Ann Otol Rhinol Laryngol.* 1996;105:253-258.
15. Slavit DH, Maragos NE. Physiologic assessment of arytenoid adduction. *Ann Otol Rhinol Laryngol.* 1992;101:321-327.
16. Montgomery WW, Hillman RE, Varvares MA. Combined thyroplasty type I and inferior constrictor myotomy. *Ann Otol Rhinol Laryngol.* 1994;103:858-862.

CHAPTER 24

■ ■ ■

Thyroid Surgery

Lisa T. Galati, M.D.

I. INTRODUCTION

Understanding the pathophysiology and management of swallowing disorders after thyroidectomy is important, because these patients often complain of a swallowing problem at some point in their postoperative course. The etiologies range from self-limited dysphagia caused by pain or swelling to more serious and sometimes permanent causes such as vocal fold paralysis (Table 24-1). In this chapter the different causes and management of postthyroidectomy dysphagia are discussed so that clinicians can formulate a systematic approach to diagnosing and treating this particular type of swallowing disorder.

II. PHYSIOLOGY

The normal swallowing sequence was described in Chapter 3. Several key anatomic sites may be affected by thyroidectomy and can cause dysphagia. The normal pharyngeal phase of swallowing entails the coordinated functions of sensation and contraction. The hypopharynx and larynx receive sensory innervation from the superior laryngeal nerve. The area innervated by this branch of the vagus nerve extends from the tip of the epiglottis to the subglottis. Sensory cues received from this area trigger laryngeal protection maneuvers and relaxation of the cricopharyngeus muscle.

Laryngeal protection during swallowing begins as the larynx is elevated. As the larynx is elevated, the arytenoids approximate the epiglottis and true vocal fold closure begins. As the true folds approximate each other, the false folds begin to adduct. After the false vocal folds reach the midline, the epiglottis tips posteriorly toward the arytenoids and the aryepiglottic folds contract. All of these functions depend on a normal recurrent laryngeal nerve (RLN).

III. PATHOPHYSIOLOGY

One of the most common complaints after thyroid surgery is odynophagia with dysphagia. Although patients

Table 24-1. *Etiology of Dysphagia After Thyroid Surgery*

Pain
Aspiration secondary to vocal fold paralysis and/or hypopharyngeal anesthesia
Cricopharyngeal achalasia
Esophageal injury
Scarring of skin to trachea

with this complaint do not have a mechanical or functional alteration of swallowing, they are unable to tolerate solids and liquids because of pain. As the larynx is elevated during swallowing, the upper trachea traverses the thyroid bed (surgical site) and causes pain, usually lasting 2 to 5 days. A large hematoma or seroma may compress the trachea posteriorly causing partial obstruction of the esophageal lumen. Many patients experience a tightening sensation that begins approximately 2 weeks after surgery. This is due to scarring and contraction of the deep tissues in the wound and may persist for 4 to 6 weeks.

During the ligation of the superior thyroid vessels, injury to the superior laryngeal nerve (SLN) can be avoided by clamping the vessels as close as possible to the thyroid gland (Fig 24-1). Patients in whom the SLN nerve is injured often suffer from aspiration because of loss of sensation and the additional loss of motor innervation to the cricothyroideus muscles, which increase true vocal fold tension and aid in adduction. However, aspiration occurs more often with bilateral nerve injury.

Injury to the distal RLN may cause aspiration because of uncompensated vocal fold paralysis. Patients most often complain of choking when drinking liquids, but this usually improves as the compensatory mechanisms improve the glottic closure. Identification of the RLN during thyroid surgery is the most prudent way to avoid injuring the nerve. There are several landmarks that are reliable during surgery. The RLN runs in the

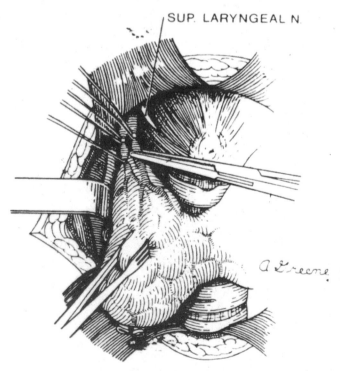

FIG 24-1. Ligation of superior thyroid vessels and avoidance of superior laryngeal nerve. (From Cady B and Ross R. *Surgery of the Thyroid and Parathyroid Glands.* 3rd ed. Philadelphia: WB Saunders; 1991:197. Reprinted with permission.)

tracheoesophageal groove, which is easily palpable during thyroid surgery and serves as a consistent landmark. The RLN can also be identified in the triangle formed by the lower pole of the thyroid lobe, the common carotid artery, and the trachea. Alternatively, the nerve can be identified at the cricothyroid joint where it enters the larynx.

During thyroid surgery, the motor innervation of the pharyngeal musculature may be injured, causing dysphagia. The cricopharyngeus muscle serves as a sphincter and is in tonic contraction in its normal resting state (Fig 24-2). Parasympathetic innervation causes the relaxation of the cricopharyngeus that is necessary to allow a food bolus to pass and initiate the esophageal phase of swallowing.

Parasympathetic fibers reach the cricopharyngeus via the recurrent laryngeal nerve. Sympathetic fibers reach the constrictors as the pharyngeal plexus, which travels along the posterior aspect of the pharynx (Fig 24-3) and maintain cricopharyngeal contraction. If the RLN or vagus nerve is injured, the parasympathetic fibers will be disrupted and the cricopharyngeus cannot relax.

Esophageal injury is a rare complication of thyroid surgery. It may occur during dissection in the tracheoesophageal groove in attempts to identify the RLN or, more commonly, it may be the result of resection of an infiltrative thyroid carcinoma. Vertical fibers of the cervical esophageal muscles are in danger of injury when the thyroid and trachea are rotated medially (Fig 24-4).

Failure to close the strap muscles at the end of the procedure results in scarring of the skin flap to the underlying trachea. If the scarring is severe, this may tether the laryngotracheal complex, preventing its ascent during swallowing and leading to dysphagia.

IV. DIAGNOSIS

Diagnosis of the etiology of dysphagia in the thyroidectomy patient should begin with a clinical evaluation and consideration of the differential diagnosis (see Table 24-1). The wound is examined for proper healing and, if the trachea and larynx are noted to glide normally on swallowing, complications related to scarring can be excluded. Flexible laryngoscopy or mirror examination of the larynx is focused on vocal fold mobility, laryngeal sensation, and clearance of secretions. If one vocal fold is paralyzed, the extent of compensation (size of glottic chink) should be noted. Sensation is tested by gently touching the flexible endoscope to the epiglottis to elicit the cough reflex, which is mediated by the superior laryngeal nerve. The external branch of the superior laryngeal nerve is examined by observing rotation of the larynx on phonation. As the frequency of the pitch increases, the anterior commissure will rotate toward the side of the injured superior laryngeal nerve. Pooling of saliva in the esophageal inlet may indicate cricopha-

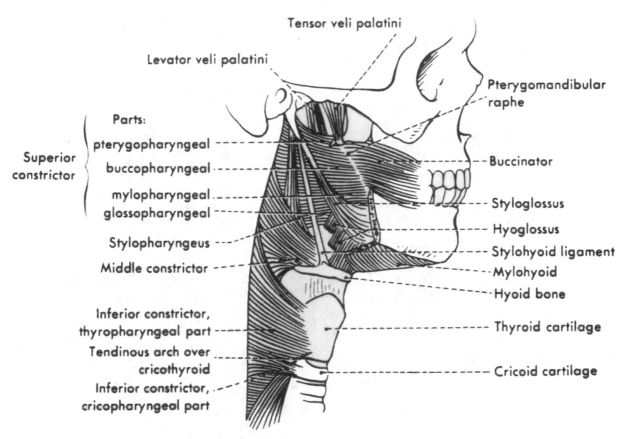

FIG 24-2. Cricopharyngeal and thyropharyngeal portions of the inferior constrictor. (From Hollinshead WH. *Anatomy for Surgeons: The Head and Neck.* 3rd ed. Philadelphia: Harper and Row; 1982:399. Reprinted with permission.)

ryngeal achalasia and this finding should be studied further with modified barium swallow (MBS). Cricopharyngeal achalasia is readily identified on modified barium swallow as an anterior bulge of the muscle on lateral view. (See Chapter 11.) Modified barium swallow may also demonstrate the rare case of esophageal injury or stricture.

V. TREATMENT

Patients with dysphagia caused by wound pain and splinting of the strap muscles are best managed with the application of ice, analgesics, and a soft diet. Aspiration secondary to superior laryngeal nerve injury usually occurs when both nerves are injured. Management of RLN paralysis includes initial avoidance of thin liquids, compensatory maneuvers and adduction exercises to improve swallowing, and vocal fold medialization, if aspiration or poor voice quality persists. (See Chapters 34 and 35.)

Treatment of cricopharyngeal achalasia includes cricopharyngeal myotomy or botulinum toxin injection of the muscle. Esophageal lacerations should be repaired with absorbable stitches that invert the mucosa. Strictures may result at the site of repair and may cause dys-

phagia. Management of esophageal stricture is dictated by the degree of narrowing. Mild narrowing may be treated with bougienage. Severe stenosis of the esophagus may require resection and reconstruction with free microvascular grafts or a gastric pull up. Finally, the problem of skin flaps that have healed directly to the trachea can be corrected by re-elevating the skin flaps and approximating the medial borders of the strap muscles.

Frequently Asked Questions

1. Which of the following structures is *not* at-risk for injury during thyroid surgery: phrenic nerve, recurrent laryngeal nerve, esophagus, trachea?
   A. Phrenic nerve. The phrenic nerve travels in an inferomedial direction across the anterior scalene muscle, lateral to the carotid artery, which is the lateral limit of dissection during thyroid surgery.
2. A patient is recovering from a total thyroidectomy. While in the recovery room, he becomes stridorous. What is the appropriate management?
   A. Check vitals, examine the neck for hematoma, employ flexible laryngoscopy at bedside, and

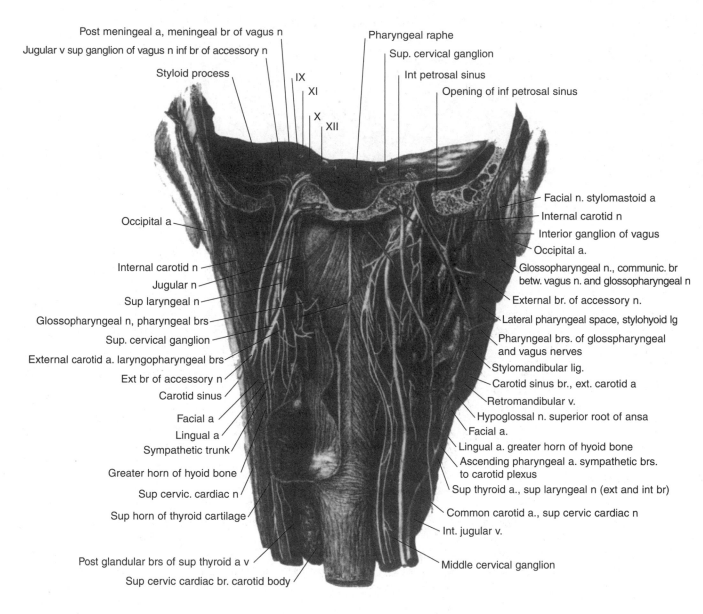

Post meningeal a, meningeal br of vagus n
Jugular v sup ganglion of vagus n inf br of accessory n
Styloid process
IX
XI
X
XII
Pharyngeal raphe
Sup. cervical ganglion
Int petrosal sinus
Opening of inf petrosal sinus

Occipital a
Internal carotid n
Jugular n
Sup laryngeal n
Glossopharyngeal n, pharyngeal brs
Sup. cervical ganglion
External carotid a. laryngopharyngeal brs
Ext br of accessory n
Carotid sinus
Facial a
Lingual a
Sympathetic trunk
Greater horn of hyoid bone
Sup cervic. cardiac n
Sup horn of thyroid cartilage
Post glandular brs of sup thyroid a v
Sup cervic cardiac br. carotid body

Facial n. stylomastoid a
Internal carotid n
Interior ganglion of vagus
Occipital a.
Glossopharyngeal n., communic. br betw. vagus n. and glossopharyngeal n
External br. of accessory n.
Lateral pharyngeal space, stylohyoid lg
Pharyngeal brs. of glosspharyngeal and vagus nerves
Stylomandibular lig.
Carotid sinus br., ext. carotid a
Retromandibular v.
Hypoglossal n. superior root of ansa
Facial a.
Lingual a. greater horn of hyoid bone
Ascending pharyngeal a. sympathetic brs. to carotid plexus
Sup thyroid a., sup laryngeal n (ext and int br)
Common carotid a., sup cervic cardiac n
Int. jugular v.
Middle cervical ganglion

Fig 24-3. Sympathetic and parasympathetic innervation of the pharynx. (From Pernkopf E. *Atlas der topigraphischen und angewandten Anatomie des Menchen.* 3rd ed. Baltimore, Md: Urban and Schwarzenberg; 1987: 336. Reprinted with permission.)

secure the airway. If the postthyroidectomy patient is hemodynamically stable, but having difficulty breathing, the first step in the assessment should include examination of the neck, followed by either evacuation of the hematoma at the bedside or flexible laryngoscopy if there is no evidence of hematoma. Stridor may be the result of laryngospasm, bilateral vocal fold paralysis, or hypocalcemia (which normally occurs 8-24 hours after surgery, but occasionally occurs in the immediate postoperative period). Management must include immediate stabilization of the airway via intubation, cricothyroidotomy, or tracheotomy. Unilateral vocal fold paralysis does not cause stridor.

3. What is the best management of unilateral vocal fold paralysis?
   A. Speech-language therapy is needed, along with either temporary or permanent vocal fold medialization if speech and swallowing do not improve.

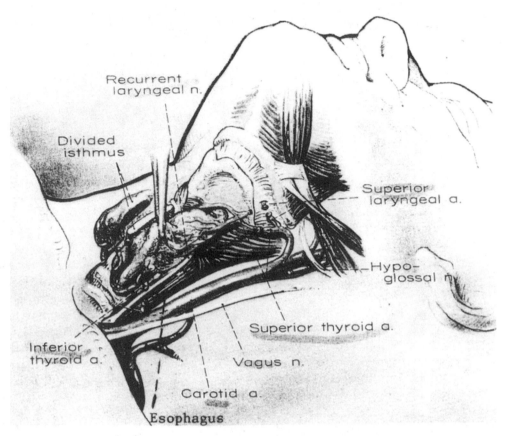

FIG 24-4. Esophagus in relation to thyroidectomy surgical site. (From Hollinshead WH. *Anatomy for Surgeons: The Head and Neck.* 3rd ed. Philadelphia: Harper and Row; 1982:413. Reprinted with permission.)

References

1. Cady B, Rossi R. *Surgery of the Thyroid and Parathyroid Glands.* 3rd ed. Philadelphia, Pa: WB Saunders; 1991:197.

2. Hollinshead WH. *Anatomy for Surgeons: The Head and Neck.* 3rd ed. Philadelphia, Pa: Harper and Row; 1982:399, 413.

3. Pernkopf E. *Atlas der topigraphis chen und angewandten Anatomie des Menchen.* 3rd ed. Baltimore, Md: Urban and Schwarzenberg; 1987:336.

CHAPTER 25

■ ■ ■

Swallowing Disorders After Cervical Spine Surgery

Kristin Drennen, M.D.
William Welch, M.D., F.A.C.S.
Ricardo L. Carrau, M.D.

I. INTRODUCTION

Dysphagia following anterior cervical spine surgery is a commonly encountered complication. Although the literature reports that dysphagia in the immediate postoperative period ranges from 35% to 80%[1-3] our experience is that all patients exhibit some degree of dysphagia. The difference among the various reports lies in how dysphagia is defined and how inquisitive clinicians are during the postoperative period. Postoperative dysphagia is expected because the surgical approach to anterior cervical spine requires dissection around the strap muscles, the ansa cervicalis, the pharyngeal nerve plexus, the pharyngoesophagus, the larynx, the recurrent laryngeal nerve (RLN), the superior laryngeal nerve (SLN), and sometimes the hypoglossal nerve, all of which are part of the swallowing mechanism. Fusion of the cervical spine may require bulky plates placed between the spine and the pharyngoesophagus, which may cause some mechanical obstruction, diversion of the bolus, or tethering of the pharyngeal musculature. In addition, many patients have preoperative dysphagia caused by osteophytes and/or motor dysfunction of the pharynx and esophagus. These factors, combined with postoperative edema and scarring, all contribute to dysphagia. Postoperative dysphagia is usually of short duration and requires mini-mal rehabilitation. However, prolonged postoperative dysphagia has been noted in 5% to 12% of patients.[1,2]

II. SURGICAL PROCEDURE

The anterior approach to cervical spine surgery was first described by Chipault, a French anatomist, in 1895,[4] but was not popularized until the late 1950s by Robinson and Smith, Dereymaeker and Mulier, and Cloward.[5-7] At a Cervical Research Society Meeting Cloward was introduced by John Collis as "a pioneer in surgery" (a pioneer being the one with arrows in his back) for his work in this approach.[8] Indeed, it was not a popular approach initially. An example of the negative criticism directed toward the surgeon who used the anterior approach may be found in the editorial comments of B.M. Cameroy, *American Journal of Orthopedics*, 1966.[9] He described "The Brave Anterior Cervical Approach" in which the surgeon traversed "a haunted, enchanted, anatomical forest," wove his way through numerous vital structures, escaped the carotid and vertebral arteries, the vagus nerve, the internal jugular vein and phrenic nerves, the mesh of the brachial plexus, but "tripped rather heavily on the recurrent laryngeal nerve." Dr. Cameroy continues, "I would never be able to muster the courage for this dangerous, anterior approach unless there were no posterior avenues available or unless there were some reasons why a simple, safe, successful, posterior fusion could not be performed." He concludes that he and most of his colleagues, "remain the conservative cowards: afraid for my patients and their structures."[9(p29)]

The anterior approach can be time-consuming, tedious, and difficult in certain situations and may be associated with significant morbidity. A summary of the complications of anterior cervical spine surgery (early dysphagia; prolonged dysphagia; hematoma; recurrent laryngeal nerve injury; superior laryngeal nerve injury; and/or esophargeal perforation) by literature review is listed in Table 25-1.[1-3, 10-16] Spine surgeons, however, have become extremely familiar with the anterior cervical approach as cervical pathology often causes ventral compression of the spinal cord and nerve roots. The ventral approach to the cervical spinal cord and nerve roots is often the most direct method to correct lesions such as disc rupture, spondylitic changes, tumors, infections, and other pathologic changes.

A brief description of the surgical approach is provided to illustrate the surgical trauma. The standard anterior cervical approach begins with a skin incision directed along the antero-medial border of the sternocleidomastoid muscle or transversely in a skin fold.[17] The incision can be placed on the right or left side of the neck, depending on the surgeon's preference and the patient's pathology. Subplatysmal flaps are dissected and the strap muscles are identified. Blunt or sharp dissection of the areolar tissue between the sternocleidomastoid muscle and the strap muscles expose the carotid sheath. The carotid sheath and its contents are retracted laterally while applying simultaneous medial retraction of the esophagus and trachea. The recurrent laryngeal nerve has a variable course, but generally travels in the tracheoesophageal groove and, thus, is covered by the thyroid gland. Identification and/or dissection of the recurrent laryngeal nerve are not necessary. The fascia overlying the longus coli muscles is

cut. The muscles are dissected free from the vertebral bodies using electrocautery and blunt subperiosteal dissection. Toothed retractor blades are placed under the lateral longus coli muscles for lateral retraction. Blunt retractor blades are used for superior-inferior retraction and along the medial longus coli muscles. It is important to avoid compression of the tracheoesophageal groove and the cricothyroid joint with the retractor blades, as compression may result in RLN injury.

The anterior longitudinal ligament, spinal osteophytes, and spinal column are directly exposed after the esophagus is identified, retracted, and protected. Further surgery is directed at the underlying pathology. For example, discectomy is performed by identifying the correct interspace and incising and removing the anterior longitudinal ligament. Mechanical distractors are then placed in the interspace, and the disc material is removed with forceps and curettes. Osteophytes can be removed from the vertebral end plates as necessary.

Interspace fusion is performed by inserting allograft or autograft bone into the interspace under compression. Corpectomy is effected by removing the intervertebral discs above and below the vertebral segment and inserting graft bone under compression. Instrumentation is performed by securing a plate across the vertebral segments to be fused. The plate is secured with cancellous screws and most instrumentation systems have a mechanism by which the screws are affixed to the plate. This creates a constrained system, increases the biomechanical stability, and prevents the screws from coming loose.

III. PATHOPHYSIOLOGY

Postoperative swallowing disorders after cervical spine surgery can be categorized by etiology: (1) surgical disruption of anatomical structures and (2) postoperative sequelae. Surgical disruption of anatomical structures are discussed first. As stated previously, the approach to the anterior cervical spine often requires division of the omohyoid muscle and the ansa cervicalis, which will cause paralysis of the infrahyoid strap muscles and may impair the laryngeal motion associated with swallowing. In addition, the innervation of the pharyngoesophagus is often divided or injured by retraction (compression or stretching). The innervation to the cricopharyngeus muscle and upper esophageal region is through the parasympathetic vagal input, which arises in the dorsal motor nucleus and the nucleus ambiguus, and through sympathetic input from the superior cervical sympathetic ganglion. The latter joins the pharyngeal plexus, composed of the branches of the glossopharyngeal and vagus nerves. This plexus travels in the retropharyngeal space, adjacent to the con-

Table 25-1. *Complications of Anterior Cervical Approach*

Early dysphagia	100%[1-3]
Prolonged dysphagia	5-11%[1,10,19]
Hematoma	1-3%[1,10-13]
RLN injury	1-16%[11]
SLN injury	1%[14,15]
Esophageal Perforation	0.2-0.9%[14]

RLN = recurrent laryngeal nerve

SLN = superior laryngeal nerve

strictor muscles that they supply and is at-risk for injury by retraction or dissection.

Injury to the SLN, the RLN, or the hypoglossal nerve can be secondary to accidental disruption of the nerve or by traction injury. Injury to the SLN will cause anesthesia of the ipsilateral supraglottic area and may predispose the patient to aspiration. Injury to the RLN may lead to aspiration by impairing the sphincteric function of the glottis, which is the most important of the three major tiers of airway protection. Dissection around the hypoglossal nerve is necessary for fusion of spinal levels C2 and C3, and injury to this nerve will cause impairment of the oral and pharyngeal phases of swallowing. Traction or compression of the SLN, RLN, or vagus nerve is a more common and often overlooked mechanism of injury than is accidental transection. Numerous studies have demonstrated the potential for significant neural damage with nerve stretch greater than 12%.[18] Netterville et al reported that the risk of traction injury to the right RLN is greater than the risk to the left nerve, because the right nerve has a shorter course around the subclavian than does the left around the aortic arch.[19] This is discussed further in section VI of this chapter.

Postoperative edema develops to varying degrees from blunt and/or sharp trauma to the lateral pharyngeal and esophageal walls. Edema is usually mild and may cause minor symptoms. Occasionally, major transmural edema can completely obstruct the pharyngoesophageal lumen, leading to total dysphagia, aspiration, or even airway compromise. An improperly drained wound, flawed technique, or a coagulopathy may contribute to a postoperative hematoma in the retropharyngeal space and, similarly, can compress the pharyngoesophagus or cause airway obstruction.[20] Scarring and adhesion formation between the pharyngoesophagus, prevertebral muscles, and the fused cervical spine can also cause dysphagia, as described by Elies.[21] These adhesions tether the pharyngoesophagus to the cervical spine, preventing the normal sliding motion that occurs with every swallow.

Transoral approaches to the anterior cervical spine are associated with an even higher incidence of postoperative difficulty. These approaches include the transoral-transpharyngeal, transoral-transpalatal-transpharyngeal, LeFort I osteotomies-transpharyngeal, and midline mandibulotomy-transpalatal-transpharyngeal approach (Trotter approach). In our experience, the latter two approaches are rarely necessary for the treatment of cervical spine disorders, as the first two approaches provide the required exposure and are associated with less morbidity.[22] Both the transoral-transpharyngeal, with or without a soft palate split (ie, transpalatal), involve the exposure of the high cervical spine via a midline incision of the posterior pharyngeal wall and lateral retraction of the anterior paraspinal musculature. The decision of whether to split the soft palate or not depends on the site of lesion, dentition, and anatomical idiosyncracies of each patient. Edentulous patients with a short and pliable soft palate can be approached sparing the soft palate incision, as their nasopharynx can be easily exposed with retraction of the velum. Transoral approaches require the use of special retractors that often cause compression injury of the pharyngeal and tongue musculature. Edema, contusion, or even ischemic injury to the neuromuscular unit or sensory innervation are not uncommon. In addition, these approaches often require securing the airway with a tracheotomy, which by itself will cause swallowing difficulties. (See Chapters 20, 37, and 38.) Thus, the transoral-transpharyngeal approaches, although not associated with damage to the laryngopharynx innervation, are associated with direct muscle injury to the oral, oropharyngeal, and hypopharyngeal areas.

Another unique problem associated with the transpalatal approach is postoperative velopharyngeal insufficiency (VPI). Splinting of the palatal muscles because of pain and inflammation, palatal shortening due to the midline incision/scar, and surgical division of Passavant's ridge all combine to cause VPI. Breakdown of the palatal split repair also contributes to VPI. Postoperatively, the patient may suffer from hypernasal speech, nasal regurgitation, and lack of adequate oropharyngeal separation (the base of tongue does not approximate the soft palate) with early spillage of the oral bolus into the pharynx. The loss of a velopharyngeal seal also affects the base of tongue pump, as some of the positive pressure generated by this mechanism escapes into the nasal cavity.

IV. DIAGNOSIS

Evaluation of postoperative dysphagia begins at the bedside with a complete clinical evaluation. Significant points in the patient's history are symptoms of dysphagia of solids or liquids, symptoms of aspiration or gastroesophageal reflux, and a prior history of aspiration pneumonia. It is important to identify the onset and progression of these symptoms and if they preceded the surgery. Ideally, a patient presenting with preoperative dysphagia should undergo a preoperative swallowing evaluation.

Examination of a patient should include evaluation of the neck wound for signs of possible hematoma, infection, salivary fistula, quality of voice, adequacy of the airway, and ability to swallow. A muffled voice or stridor suggest edema or hematoma of the pharynx or larynx. A weak, breathy, or hoarse voice suggests a vocal fold motion impairment. Similarly, inability to alter pitch of the voice may be secondary to edema, denervated strap muscles, or a superior laryngeal nerve injury (loss of motor innervation to the cricothyroid muscle). Bedside observation of attempts to swallow thick or thin liquids provides information regarding the severity of the dysphagia and of possible aspiration. However, it is important to note that aspiration may be silent. The quality of a patient's voice after a swallow may suggest aspiration or retention of secretions/food, manifested as a wet or gurgly voice and the need to frequently clear the throat. It is also important to know that a young robust patient may be able to compensate well for an RLN injury and have a normal voice without aspiration until years later, when the ability to compensate declines. Therefore, a normal bedside examination that does not include laryngeal visualization does not rule out postoperative complication. Monitoring the weight of a patient with prolonged postoperative dysphagia also allows assessment of the severity of the dysphagia.

Flexible fiberoptic laryngoscopy allows for the assessment of the laryngeal and pharyngeal anatomy and range of motion. Edema, hematoma, vocal fold and arytenoid mobility, adequacy of glottic closure, laryngeal sensation, pooling of secretions at the vallecula or hypopharynx and aspiration should be noted. Ideally, a preoperative flexible laryngoscopy should be performed on all patients. A preoperative assessment is most important, however, if dysphagia, hoarseness, or signs of aspiration are present (Fig 25-1A and 25-1B). Similarly, if significant dysphagia, hoarseness, or aspiration persist until postoperative day 3, fiberoptic laryngoscopy should be used to evaluate the degree of edema and to evaluate for possible complications such as impairment of vocal fold motion.

A swallow evaluation can be performed by a speech pathologist at bedside. (See Chapter 5.) Fiberoptic endoscopic evaluation of swallowing (FEES) (see Chapter 12) and modified barium swallow (MBS) (see Chapter 11) are used to assess prolonged dysphagia and postoperative aspiration. The MBS allows for better evaluation of all phases of swallowing and is more sensitive for oral problems and pharyngeal tethering than FEES. FEES, however, may be done at the bedside. The MBS is useful in identifying which phase of swallowing is affected, the severity of the swallowing problem, and the degree of aspiration. In addition, the speech pathologist can train the patient on proper use of compensatory maneuvers, such as body posture and neck position. This evaluation is an important first step in rehabilitation, as discussed in the next section.

Postoperative dysphagia may be secondary to mechanical obstruction, tethering, or flow disruption due to large bulky plates used for fusion of the spine, or by a dislodged plate, screw, or graft (Tables 25-2 and 25-3). A lateral X ray of the neck, barium swallow, or esophagogram help to evaluate this problem (Fig 25-2).

A postoperative wound hematoma that compresses the pharynx or esophagus is generally not subtle. If necessary, however, a CT of the neck with contrast can help to differentiate a hematoma from edema in some cases to identify which patients will benefit from surgical drainage.

V. TREATMENT

Certain surgical techniques may help to reduce the occurrence of postoperative dysphagia. Johnston and Crockard recommend that the prevertebral space be entered in the lower cervical region with blunt dissection performed from an inferior to superior direction.[23] They further recommend avoiding high dissection along the carotid artery to avoid injury to the pharyngeal branches of the vagus nerve. Other techniques to potentially reduce the incidence of postoperative dysphagia include reducing or avoiding prolonged esophageal retraction, confirming that the retractor blades are under the longus coli muscles and do not injure the esophagus directly, removal of large osteophytes, and, finally, one should ascertain that the fixation screws are flush with the plate and appropriately restrained.

The first step in treating postoperative dysphagia is identifying the cause (Table 25-4). Generally, mild dysphagia in the first 1 to 2 days postoperatively is from edema and division of the omohyoid and ansa cervicalis. As the edema resolves and the patient compensates for the alteration in the strap musculature, this mild postoperative dysphagia resolves and no treatment or further evaluation is necessary. At times, pain alone can prevent normal swallowing function and this can be treated with narcotic analgesia. If severe dysphagia, stridor, or signs of airway compromise are present or if dysphagia, hoarseness, or alteration in pitch persist beyond postoperative day 3, evaluation with flexible laryngoscopy, MBS, and/or FEES is indicated.

It is also important to identify which phase of swallowing is impaired. A thorough assessment of this by a speech pathologist, followed by instructions for swallowing exercises and compensatory mechanisms, will speed the recovery of swallowing dysfunction and also will help to decrease the patient's anxiety and frustration associated with the postoperative deficit.

Patients with severe dysphagia or aspiration should receive tube feeds via nasogastric tube until swallowing function improves. Occasionally, when prolonged dysphagia is present, a gastrostomy tube is necessary. These patients should receive prophylactic medications against gastroesophageal reflux (GER), including H_2 blockers and a prokinetic agent. GER can compound and prolong a swallowing difficulty.

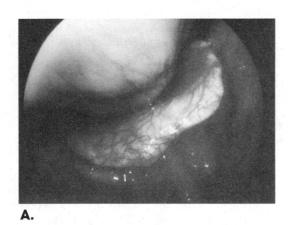

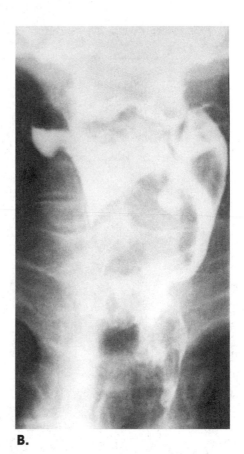

A.

B.

Fig 25-1. A. Fiberoptic endoscopy view of large osteophyte opposing the epiglottis. **B.** Anteroposterior view of a barium esophagogram showing diversion of the barium flow by the osteophyte.

Table 25-2. *Etiological Factors for Postoperative Dysphagia After Anterior Cervical Spine Surgery*

Pain	Muscles, pharynx/larynx, (post ET)
Edema	Pharynx, larynx, neck
Hematoma	Retropharyngeal space
Infection/abscess	Retropharyngeal space
Interruption of motor innervation	Ansa cervercalis RLN Pharyngeal plexus
Injury to sensory innervation	SLN Pharyngeal plexus
Mechanical factors	Perforation Bulky reconstruction plate Adhesions

ET = endotracheal tube

RLN = recurrent laryngeal nerve

SLN = superior laryngeal nerve

Table 25-3. *Etiological Factors for Postoperative Dysphagia After Transoral Spine Surgery*

Tracheotomy	Tethering, pain, loss of supraglottic pressure
Pain	Tongue, pharynx
Edema	Pharynx, tongue
Interruption of neuromuscular function	Anterior tongue Base of tongue
Mechanical factors	Bulky plate/graft Posterior pharyngeal wall adhesions
VPI	Palatal shortening Wound breakdown

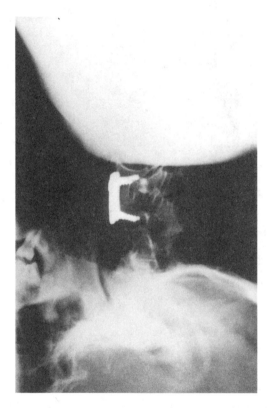

FIG 25-2. Lateral soft tissue radiogram of the neck illustrating a reconstruction plate over the anterior spine.

An impairment of the vocal fold motion that is associated with aspiration or significant hoarseness may be treated initially with a Gelfoam injection and later with a medialization laryngoplasty (see Chapters 39-41) if fold function does not return or if the RLN is known to be divided.

Perforations of the esophagus have been well described as a complication of the anterior cervical spinal approach. These perforations can be noted during the surgery, in the immediate postoperative period, or later.[24,25] Transmural perforations are the most serious type because they allow the esophageal bacteria to invade an otherwise sterile field. Injuries to the serosa are fairly common and generally of little consequence, other than contributing to postoperative dysphagia. Muscular injuries are potentially more serious.

During the surgery, the spine surgeon may be concerned that a direct, transmural esophageal injury has occurred. If the surgeon is confident that a significant injury has occurred, an otolaryngologist should immediately be consulted for assistance and confirmation. A tear may be repaired primarily and the patient placed NPO for a few days to a week. Should the spine surgeon be concerned that an injury has occurred, he or she may ask the anesthesiologist to irrigate a diluted mixture of methylene blue into the nasogastric tube while slowly removing the tube. Should the mixture leak into the surgical wound, a transmural injury has been identified and appropriate therapy needs to be instituted.

If esophageal perforation is suspected postoperatively, this should be evaluated by a barium swallow (Fig 25-3). Treatment should include intravenous antibiotics with coverage for oral flora and anaerobes. The indications and timing for surgical repair are controversial and depend on the mechanism of injury (retractor or drill), extent of the injury, experience of the surgeon, presence of a free bone graft, unstable bone or hardware, and so on. Small postoperative leaks caused by retractor injury can be observed with a large defect in a patient who required decompression and bone grafting needing repair as soon as possible. Large defects often require the use of muscle flaps (eg, sternohyoid muscle) to "cover" the defect.

Occasionally, the bone graft or plates need to be revised to treat dysphagia caused by their bulk. However, any revision surgery is associated with increased risk to the recurrent and superior laryngeal nerves and pharyngoesophagus because of scarring and should be performed 6-8 weeks postoperatively, when the spine is stable.

In cases where postoperative edema is contributing to dysphagia, systemic steroids are often beneficial and allow a more rapid recovery of swallowing dysfunction.

Table 25-4. *Problem-Oriented Treatment*

Hematoma	Drainage, correct etiology
Pain	R/O infection, extrusion of plate
	Narcotics
Edema	R/O infection, perforation
	Steroids
Tracheotomy	Decanulation protocol
Perforation	Antibiotics
	Observation versus repair
VPI	Observation
	Palatal lift prosthesis versus surgical lengthening
Bulky plate or graft	Revise after spine is stable (6-8 weeks postoperatively)

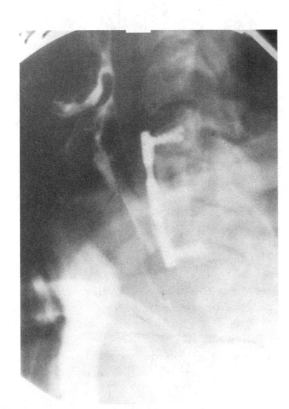

FIG 25-3. Esophagogram demonstrating an esophageal leak from "drill trauma" during a cervical spine decompression.

All hematomas should be evacuated and the wound properly drained. The best treatment for a hematoma is proper drainage of the wound and careful perioperative management of coagulation disorders.

VI. CONTROVERSIES

Many spine surgeons prefer to approach the cervical spine from the right side of the neck because this approach is easier for the right-handed surgeon. Howev-

er, as described by Netterville et al, the right RLN is at greater risk for traction injury than the left, because the right nerve has a shorter course around the subclavian artery and less redundancy in its course[19] (Figs 25-4, 25-5, 25-6).

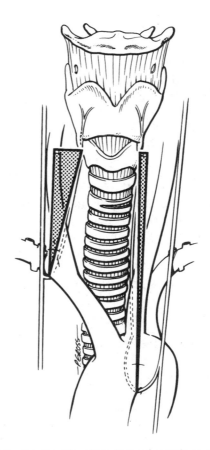

FIG 25-4. Anatomic drawing of each recurrent laryngeal nerve (RLN). Superimposed right triangles resolve course of each RLN into vertical and horizontal components. Right RLN has shorter, more oblique course than left RLN.[19(Fig 1)] From Netterville et al. Reprinted with permission from Annals Publishing Company.

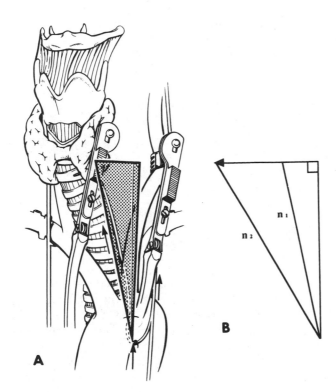

FIG 25-5. A. Anatomy and **B.** Geometry of left RLN during anterior cervical exposure. Because of longer, more vertical course of left RLN, horizontal displacement of larynx to right by Cloward retractor stretches left RLN only slightly.[19(Fig 2A, 2B)] Reprinted with permission from Annals Publishing Company.

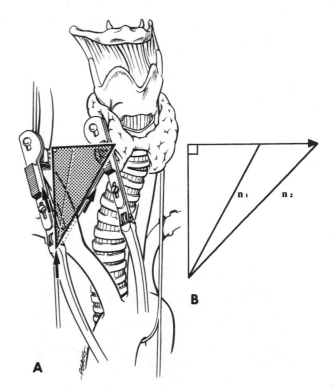

FIG 25-6. A. Anatomy and **B.** Geometry of right RLN during anterior cervical exposure. Because of shorter, more oblique course of right RLN, horizontal displacement of larynx to left by Cloward retractor stretches right RLN significantly.[19(Fig 3A, 3B)] Reprinted with permission from Annals Publishing Company.

When the larynx is retracted laterally to allow access to the anterior cervical spine, the strain is greater on the right nerve than it is on the left. (See Figs 25-1, 25-2, and 25-3.) In Netterville et al's study with neck dissections on 10 cadavers, the right-sided approach to C7 resulted in an average in situ stretch on the ipsilateral RLN of 12%-24% with 3 cm and 4 cm of Cloward retraction, respectively.[19] Many studies have demonstrated the potential for significant neural damage with nerve stretch greater than 12%.[18]

Frequently Asked Questions

1. What is the innervation of the cricopharyngeus muscle and upper esophagus?
   A. Parasympathetic vagal input from the dorsal motor nucleus and nucleus ambiguous and sympathetic input from the superior cervical ganglion.
2. What is a modified barium swallow sensitive for?
   A. A barium swallow evaluates the integrity of the esophagus from the level of the cricopharyngeus to the lower esophageal sphincter and may reveal aspiration. A modified barium swallow evaluates the phases of swallowing, as well as penetration, and is more sensitive for aspiration than is a fiberoptic endoscopic evaluation of swallowing.
3. Why does the left-sided approach to anterior cervical spine surgery place the recurrent laryngeal nerve at less risk for injury?
   A. The left recurrent laryngeal nerve has a longer course and more redundancy and is therefore at less risk for traction injury.

References

1. Bertalanffy H, Eggert HR. Complications of anterior cervical discectomy without fusion in 450 consecutive patients. *Acta Neurochir (Wien)*. 1989;99:41-50.
2. Stewart M, Johnston RA, Stewart I, Wilson JA. Swallowing performance following anterior cervical spine surgery. *Brit J Neurosurg*. 1995;9:605-609.
3. Cloward RB. Complications of anterior cervical disc operation and their treatment. *Surgery*. 1971;69:175-182.

4. Chipault A. *Chirurgie Operatoire du Systeme Nerveux: Tome I. Chirurgie Cranio-cérébrale. Tome II. Chirurgie de la Moelle et des Nerfs.* Paris: Rueff et Cie; 1894-1895.

5. Robinson RA, Smith GW. Anterolateral cervical disc removal and interbody fusion for cervical disc syndrome. *Bull Johns Hopkins Hosp.* 1955;96:223-224. Abstract.

6. Dereymaeker A, Mulier J. Nouvelle cure chirurgicale des discopathies cervicales. La méniscectomie par voie centrale suivie d'arthrodèse par greffe intercorporéale. *Neuro-Chirurgie;* 1956;2:233-234.

7. Cloward RB. The anterior approach for removal of ruptured cervical disks. *J Neurosurg.* 1958;15:602-617.

8. Cloward RB. The anterior surgical approach to the cervical spine: the Cloward procedure: past, present, and future. The presidential guest lecture, Cervical Spine Research Society. *Spine.* 1988;13:823-827.

9. Cameroy BM. The brave anterior approach. *Am J Orthop.* 1966;8:29.

10. Watters WC III, Levinthal R. Anterior cervical discectomy with and without fusion. results, complications, and long-term follow-up. *Spine.* 1987;19:2343-2347.

11. Lunsford LD, Bissonette DJ, Zorub DS. Anterior surgery for cervical disc disease. Part 2. Treatment of cervical spondylotic myelopathy in 32 cases. *J Neurosurg.* 1980;53:12-19.

12. Bulger RF, Rejowski JE, Beatty RA. Vocal cord paralysis associated with anterior cervical fusion: considerations for prevention and treatment. *J Neurosurg.* 1985;62:657-661.

13. Husag L, Probst C. Microsurgical anterior approach to cervical discs: review of 60 consecutive cases of discectomy without fusion. *Acta Neurochir Wien.* 1984;73:229-242.

14. Cuatico W. Anterior cervical discectomy without interbody fusion: an analysis of 81 cases. *Acta Neurochir Wien.* 1981;57:269-274.

15. Tew JM Jr, Mayfield FH. Complications of surgery of the anterior cervical spine. *Clin Neurosurg.* 1976;23:424-434.

16. Capen DA, Garland DE, Waters RL. Surgical stabilization of the cervical spine: a comparative analysis of anterior and posterior spine fusions. *Clin Orthop.* 1985;196:229-237.

17. Carrau RL, Cintron FR, Astor F. Transcervical approaches to the prevertebral space. *Arch Otolaryngol Head Neck Surg.* 1990;116:1070-1073.

18. Weisberg NK, Spengler DM, Netterville JL. Stretch-induced nerve injury as a cause of paralysis secondary to the anterior cervical approach. *Otolaryngol Head Neck Surg.* 1997;116:317-326.

19. Netterville JL, Koriwchak MJ, Winkle M, Courey MS, Ossoff RH. Vocal fold paralysis following the anterior approach to the cervical spine. *Ann Otol Rhinol Laryngol.* 1996;105:85-91.

20. Welsh LW, Welsh JJ, Chinnici JC. Dysphagia due to cervical spine surgery. *Ann Otol Rhinol Laryngol.* 1987;96: 112-115.

21. Elies W. Esophageal complications following ventral cervical disc surgery. *HNO.* 1979;27:380-381.

22. Welch WC, Ragoowansi A, Carrau RL. Transoral resection of the odontoid. *Op Tech Orthopaed.* 1998;8:8-13.

23. Johnston FG, Crockard HA. One-stage internal fixation and anterior fusion in complex cervical spinal disorders. *J Neurosurg.* 1995;82:234-238.

24. Kelly MF, Spiegel J, Rizzo KA, Zwillenberg D. Delayed pharyngoesophageal perforation: a complication of anterior spine surgery. *Ann Otol Rhinol Laryngol.* 1991;100: 201-205.

25. English GM, Hsu SF, Edgar R, Gibson-Eccles M. Oesophageal trauma in patients with spinal cord injury. *Paraplegia.* 1992;30:903-912.

CHAPTER 26

■ ■ ■

Pathophysiology of Swallowing and Gastroesophageal Reflux

Brendan Levy, M.D.
Michele A. Young, M.D.

I. ANATOMY AND PHYSIOLOGY OF THE SWALLOWING MECHANISM

A. Anatomy

Structurally, the physical properties of the swallowing mechanism consist of the oral cavity and its component parts, the pharynx, upper esophageal sphincter (UES), esophageal body, and the lower esophageal sphincter (LES) (Fig 26-1). The UES is a tonically contracted group of skeletal muscles separating the pharynx from the esophagus. The major component of the sphincter is the cricopharyngeus muscle. Other contributors to this 2-3 cm sphincter include portions of the inferior constrictor muscle and the muscles of the cervical or proximal esophagus. The posterior border of the cricoid also contributes a passive component to the sphincter. The esophageal body is a muscular tube extending 20-25 cm in length from its origin just caudal to the cricopharyngeus muscle to its termination at the gastric cardia. The longitudinal muscle layer and the circular muscle layer constitute the outermost and innermost layers spanning the length of the esophageal body. At the top of the esophageal body, both muscle layers consist of skeletal muscle fibers. Approximately 5 cm distal to the UES, nonstriated smooth muscle fibers begin to intermingle with the striated muscle. Generally, there are fibers of both skeletal and smooth muscle for approximately 10 cm distal to the cricopharyngeus muscle. The smooth muscle increases proportionately with distance from the UES. Thus, the caudal half of the esophageal body, including the lower esophageal sphincter, is composed entirely of smooth muscle fibers. Gross and histologic examinations of the LES have failed to identify a specific sphincteric structure. Endoscopically, the squamous mucosa lining the esophagus appears pale and glossy and is distinguishable from the reddish, velvety columnar lining of the stomach. The junction between the squamous and columnar mucosa forms a circumferential line, often called the Z-line. In the absence of disease, the mucosal squamocolumnar junction may correspond to the anatomic gastroesophageal junction.

B. Physiology

The events associated with the normal swallow in the striated region, specifically the oral cavity and the pharynx, occur very rapidly and in a precisely timed manner. The beginning of the involuntary elements of the swallow, the apposition of the soft palate to the pharyngeal wall is a contraction that lasts over 0.9 seconds and generates a pressure greater than 180 mm Hg. It is the beginning of a moving contraction front, pharyn-

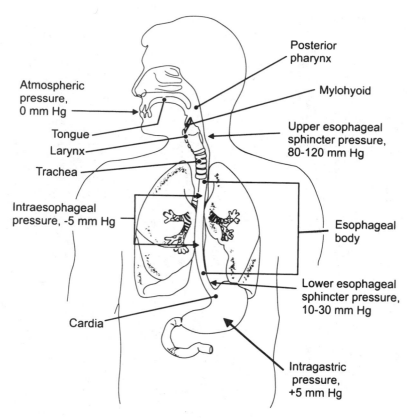

FIG 26-1. The relationship of the major structures and sphincters constituting the swallowing mechanism. The normal pressure relationships of the upper esophageal sphincter, esophageal body, lower esophageal sphincter, and the stomach are also shown. Using atmospheric pressure at zero as reference derived the pressures shown.

geal peristalsis, that transverses the oropharynx and hypopharynx at about 15 cm/sec to reach the UES in about 0.7 seconds. The tonically contracted UES relaxes during the pharyngeal peristaltic sequence. The relaxation begins after the onset of swallowing and lasts 0.5-1.0 seconds, after which the sphincter contracts with an increase in force such that the pressure may exceed twice the pressure of the resting tone for approximately a second prior to returning to baseline.[1] The UES also relaxes with belching and emesis to allow retrograde movement of material from the esophagus to the pharynx. Resting sphincter pressure minimizes entrance of air into the gastrointestinal tract from respiration. Equally important is its function to prevent refluxed material from the esophagus into the pharynx.

Although the primary function of the esophageal body is passage of ingested material from the pharynx to the stomach, recent studies indicate that the esophagus is not merely a hollow conduit for food passage, but rather has several active functions for acid control and mucosal protection. The esophageal body may secrete bicarbonate, possess a cellular mechanism to transport hydrogen ions actively out of the epithelial

cells, and secrete mucin and epidermal growth factor in response to acid and pepsin. The esophagus shortens by 10% on swallowing through longitudinal muscle contraction.[2] Contraction of the circular muscle causes a squeezing motion required for peristalsis and sphincter control. A caudally progressing front of contraction of the circular muscle layer begins at the top of the esophageal body following UES relaxation. This contraction is preceded by a brief fall in intraesophageal pressure that is a result of entry of the swallowed bolus into the esophagus. The peristaltic contraction occurs and proceeds throughout the length of the esophageal body, with the velocity varying at different levels within the esophagus.[3] The contraction requires 5-6 seconds to traverse the esophageal body. The force of the peristaltic contraction also varies among the different points of the esophageal body and is expressed as generated intraluminal pressure. The force of the contraction front is dependent on the age of the patient, bolus, volume, temperature and intraabdominal pressure.

The LES is a specialized segment of smooth muscle in the distal esophagus that relaxes with swallowing, permitting entrance of the bolus into the gastric cavity and preventing gastroesophageal reflux (GER) in its resting state. Although the LES is difficult to define by gross observation, several physiologic characteristics distinguish it from adjacent, nonsphincteric muscles. Serially cut and stretched muscle strips from the esophageal body, LES, and stomach reveal that tension generated by similar increments in length produce substantially greater force in sphincteric than in nonsphincteric muscle. Because drugs that antagonize neural function do not affect this process, this increased force is likely myogenic.[4] Further, this increased force can be abolished using agents that inhibit muscle contraction. The sphincter muscle also possesses an increased sensitivity to many excitatory agents compared to that of the adjacent tissues, suggesting a greater influence on sphincter tone by nerves and hormones. LES relaxation begins approximately 2-3 seconds after initiation of the swallow—thus starting well after the peristaltic contraction began in the proximal esophageal body. The relaxation lasts 5-10 seconds and is followed by a transient contraction, which may be twice the pressure of the resting tone. The muscle tone returns to basal level following the hypercontraction.[2] Normal swallowing also involves the fundic portion of the stomach, which relaxes almost simultaneously with the onset of LES relaxation. Intragastric pressure falls just prior to the arrival of a swallowed bolus, because of a reactive relaxation of the smooth muscle cells of the stomach. After passage of the bolus, the pressure in the stomach returns to basal levels. A reflex pathway involving afferent and efferent neurons mediates this process, termed "receptive relaxation." Because relaxation occurs with each swallow, large volumes can be accommodated with minimal rise in intragastric pressure.

1. Innervation

Deglutition, or swallowing, may be initiated voluntarily or reflexively. Once initiated, it proceeds as a coordinated involuntary reflex. Coordination occurs in the central nervous system (CNS) within the reticular formation of the brainstem. This area has been termed the swallowing center and it is located within the medulla of the brainstem. Cranial nerves V (trigeminal), IX (glossopharyneal), and X (vagus) carry afferent impulses from the sensory receptors surrounding the oropharynx to their corresponding nuclei in the brainstem. Efferent impulses from the nucleus ambiguus housed within the swallowing center are carried to the pharyngeal musculature via the motor portions of cranial nerves V (trigeminal), VII (facial), IX (glossopharyngeal), X (vagus), and XII (hypoglossal) (Fig 26-2). The swallowing center also interacts with other areas of the brainstem and cortex involved with respiration and speech.

The LES has an increased sensitivity to many excitatory agents compared to that of the adjacent muscle tissue. For example, norepinepherine produces LES contraction and esophageal body relaxation. Agents that mimic acetylcholine (ACh) increase basal sphincter tone. LES tone is decreased by agents such as isoproternol and by the gastrointestinal (GI) hormone motlin. Vasoactive intestinal peptide (VIP) and Nitric oxide (NO) function as inhibitory neurotransmitters that relax the LES. Numerous pharmocologic agents and food products influence LES pressure. The vagus nerve carries preganglionic fibers, whose cell bodies are housed in the dorsal root ganglion, which release ACh. One of the effector neurons releases ACh and excites the smooth muscle fibers, whereas the other postganglionic neuron inhibits smooth muscle by releasing noncholingeric, nonadrenergic inhibitory neurons. Recently, LES relaxation was produced in the human LES when muscle strips were treated with sodium nitroprusside, or a NO donor. NO and, to a lesser degree, VIP are the primary inhibitory neurotransmitters functioning in this mechanism.

2. Process of Swallowing

The process of swallowing can be divided into four consecutive phases: preparatory, oral, pharyngeal, and esophageal. In the preparatory phase, the bolus is processed through mastication into a bolus suitable for transport throughout the GI tract. This phase includes a breakdown of the bolus into an appropriate size, shape, and consistency to mix with saliva. During the oral phase, sequential squeezing of the tongue, which propels the bolus into the pharynx, generates a peristaltic wave. Contraction of the mylohyoid muscle lifts the back of the tongue, thrusting the bolus into the posterior pharynx. Elevation of the soft palate and posterior portion of the tongue prevents nasal and oral regurgitation, respectively. Interruption of respiration, closure of the laryngeal inlet and vocal folds, and elevation and anterior displacement of the larynx prevent pulmonary aspiration of the bolus. The oral phase of swallowing is under voluntary control and is dependent on cranial nerves V (trigeminal), VII (facial), and XII (hypoglossal).

The pharyngeal phase of swallowing is controlled reflexively and involves protection of the airway and further onward propulsion of the bolus. Pharyngeal peristalsis provides the force to propel the food through the UES and into the esophagus. During the pharyngeal phase of swallowing, approximation of the soft palate to the posterior nasopharyngeal wall accompanied by contraction of the superior constrictor muscles results in narrowing of the upper pharynx. Concurrently, the larynx is elevated and displaced forward causing relaxation of the UES. Closure of the vocal folds, following

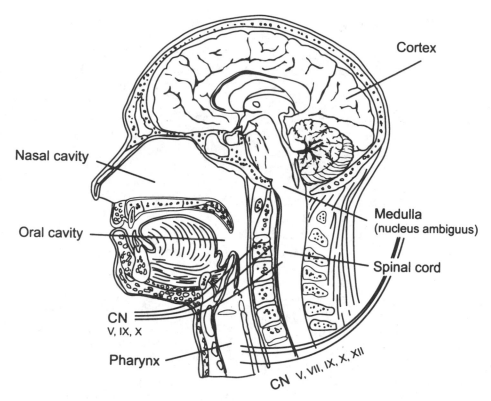

FIG 26-2. The neural control of the swallowing mechanism schematic. Both afferent and efferent limbs are shown. Included are the cranial nerves involved in the swallowing process.

UES relaxation, coupled with apposition of the base of the tongue to the posterior wall, increases the intrapharyngeal pressure, thereby assisting the propulsion of the bolus into the esophagus. Pharyngeal clearance is accomplished by the contraction of the pharyngeal constrictors, which creates a peristaltic wave down the esophagus. The pharyngeal phase is completed by downward displacement of the larynx.

Active peristalsis or sequential contraction of the esophagus and relaxation of the LES characterizes the esophageal phase of swallowing. Esophageal distention by the bolus also acts as a stimulus for peristalsis. The bolus is propelled through the esophagus by a contraction above and relaxation below the bolus. This relaxation is referred to as descending inhibition.[3] Primary peristalsis occurs when a swallow induces peristaltic activity, with secondary peristalsis being the initiation of a propagated contraction wave in the absence of a swallow. Distention by a bolus, such as retained esophageal contents that was not completely cleared by the primary swallow or refluxed gastric contents, provides adequate stimulation for the initiation of secondary peristalsis. Initiation of secondary peristaltic contractions is involuntary and normally is not sensed. The primary esophageal peristaltic wave is a continuation of the peristaltic wave that originated in the pharynx shortly following the initiation of a swallow. This wave passes from the pharynx to the striated muscle portion of the esophagus through the smooth muscle portion of the distal esophagus. Once the peristaltic wave reaches the distal esophagus, the LES is relaxed to allow the bolus to enter the stomach.

II. Gastroesophageal Reflux Disease

Gastroesophageal reflux (GER), defined as the retrograde movement of gastric contents from the stomach through the lower esophageal sphincter (LES) and into the esophagus, may or may not be symptomatic. When symptomatic signs of tissue injury are produced the patient is said to have gastroesophageal reflux disease (GER) disease. The prevalence of GER disease is difficult to estimate, because of symptom variability and limitations inherent in the diagnostic studies used in the evaluation of GER disease. A study that surveyed presumably typical hospital staff and employees found that 7% of the people interviewed have daily heartburn.[5] The prevalence of monthly heartburn was estimated to be 36%-44%.[6,7] A randomized study of 2000 subjects demonstrated a prevalence of 58.1% of white patients with symptoms of heartburn and/or acid regurgitation. The prevalence of weekly or more frequent episodes of heartburn or acid regurgitation was 19.4%.[8]

The classic symptoms of heartburn, water brash, and

regurgitation are well recognized. Advances in diagnostic technology have shown that the frequency of GER disease is much greater than can be appreciated by evaluating patients only for the classic symptoms. The availability of prolonged ambulatory esophageal pH recording has revealed that many other symptoms can be attributed to acid reflux disease. Persons with GER disease frequently complain of noncardiac chest pain, regurgitation of gastric contents, water brash (stimulated salivary secretion by esophageal acid), dysphagia, and sometimes odynophagia (pain on swallowing).

GER disease has also been associated with numerous extraesophageal symptoms, including pharyngitis, laryngitis, hoarseness, chronic cough, asthma, and pulmonary aspiration.[9,10] Acid reflux-induced symptoms referable to the oropharyngeal, laryngeal, and respiratory tracts are termed "atypical reflux" symptoms. Table 26–1 contrasts the typical, or esophageal, symptoms of GER disease with the atypical or extraesophageal, symptoms. Interestingly, these extraesophageal manifestations of GER disease may be the primary presentation in a large subset of patients. In fact, erosive, ulcerative esophagitis has been reported to occur in up to 40% of patients presenting with symptoms of pharyngitis, laryngitis, and asthma. Similarly a study performed at a Veteran's Administration hospital demonstrated that patients with erosive esophagitis and esophageal stricture were shown to have a 1.5-2-fold increase in the prevalence of sinusitis, pharyngitis, aphonia, laryngitis, and laryngeal stenosis compared to the general veteran population.[9] Barrett's metaplasia, a compensatory change in the esophageal mucosa from squamous to specialized intestinal epithelium, occurs in up to 10%-15% of patients with atypical presentations of GER disease.[11] Although these oropharyngeal symptoms are important causes of illness and health care utilization, patients who suffer from these conditions often do not have typical symptoms of esophageal reflux. Therefore, it is imperative for physicians managing the upper aerodigestive tract, chiefly otolaryngologists, to fully understand the pathology and varied symptom spectrum of gastroesophageal reflux (GER).

III. PATHOGENESIS OF GASTROESOPHAGEAL REFLUX

The pathogenesis of GER disease is multi-factorial, resulting in an imbalance between the protective or defensive factors and the aggressive factors (Table 26-2). Protective or defensive mechanisms include the competency of the antireflux barrier, esophageal acid clearance, and esophageal epithelial tissue resistance.[12] The aggressive factors include the constituents of the refluxate. Acid, pepsin, and bile acids are the toxic components of the refluxate contributing to GER disease.[13] The degree of injury that can be attributed to each of these agents varies with the pH and the tissue examined. Microscopic and macroscopic abnormalities have been induced in dogs by brief reported exposure of their subglottic regions to acid. Experimental studies indicate that acid and pepsin are capable of creating significant mucosal injury when applied to the upper airway. Pretreatment with histamine receptor 2 antagonists has been shown to reduce the degree of subglottic mucosal injury in these experimental animals. Furthermore, treatment with H2RAs resulted in shorter time to re-epithelization of the tissue following induction of subglottic stenosis in animals.[14]

A. Competence of antireflux barrier

Lower esophageal sphincter (LES) competence is the most important barrier to GER. The LES is a localized region of tonically contracted smooth muscle at the gastroesophageal junction, which is best described as a 2-4-cm zone of increased pressure in the distal esophagus. LES pressure is measured in mm Hg with a minimum pressure of 6-10 mm Hg greater than intragastric pressure needed to prevent GER disease. Gut hormones that are innervated by excitatory and inhibitory neurons of the vagus nerve alter the amplitude of this zone. Food, alcohol, smoking, drugs, and hormones affect the sphincter (Table 26-3). Normally, the LES relaxes after

Table 26-1. *Symptoms of Gastroesophageal Reflux*

Esophageal	Extraesophageal
Heartburn	Pharyngitis
Acid regurgitation	Laryngitis
Waterbrash	Hoarseness
Dysphagia	Globus hystericus
Odynophagia	Chronic cough
	Asthma
	Pulmonary aspiration

Table 26-2. *Determinants of Reflux Injury*

Protective	Injurious
Competency of antireflux barrier	Reflux constituents
Esophageal acid clearance	• Acid
Epithelial tissue resistance	• Pepsin
	• Bile

Lower Esophageal Sphincter Dysfunction

Inappropriate or transient LES relaxation (TLESRs)

Increased intra-abdominal pressure or stress induced reflux

Incompetent or reduced LES pressure or spontaneous free reflux swallowing to allow the food bolus to pass unobstructed into the stomach. Following passage of the bolus, the LES returns to its resting pressure, which is normally 10-25 mm Hg above intragastric pressure. This gastroesophageal gradient helps prevent reflux of gastric contents. Dysfunction of this sphincter may lead to GER disease through three mechanisms: (1) inappropriate, or transient LES relaxation (TLESR); (2) increased abdominal pressure, or stress-induced reflux; or (3) incompetent, or reduced, LES pressures or spontaneous free reflux.

It has been demonstrated that most episodes of reflux in normal people are related to TLESR.[15] LES pressures frequently fall to levels that are incompetent for all or part of a day because of physiologic temporary relaxation and cyclic variations in pressure. These TLESRs represent a decrease in LES that is not associated with swallowing or primary or secondary peristalsis. These relaxations allow for passage of acid into the esophagus, this, however, does not occur with every LES relaxation. TLESRs are the most important cause of GER, both in healthy individuals and in patients with esophagitis. TLESRs provide a measure for reflux in patients with normal sphincter pressures.

Stress reflux results when intra-abdominal pressure exceeds LES pressure during coughing, Valsalva's maneuver, straining, or wearing tight abdominal garments. Reflux episodes associated with increased intra-abdominal pressure are usually noted when LES pressures are relatively low and intra-abdominal pressure overcomes the LES pressure. Patients with chroni-

cally low basal LES pressures, usually with LES pressures of less than 10 mm Hg are particularly vulnerable to reflux during times of increased intra-abdominal pressure.[15] High intra-abdominal pressures tend to force open the hypotensive LES more readily and allow for reflux of gastric contents. The specific mechanism responsible for sphincter hypotension is not clear, but there are various factors that have been shown to alter LES tone. As illustrated in Table 26-3, ingestion of fat, alcohol, chocolate, mint, and some medications (calcium channel blockers, theophylline, beta agonists, alpha antagonists, and birth control pills) can produce a decrease in the resting LES pressure. Spontaneous free reflux occurs readily during periods of very low LES pressures. This form of reflux is most common in patients with a hypotensive sphincter, usually with LES pressures of less than 6 mm Hg. Because of smooth muscle atrophy and fibrosis, patients with progressive systemic sclerosis and very low sphincter pressures frequently suffer from spontaneous free reflux.

The LES is only one component to the antireflux barrier. The diaphragm crura work in conjunction with the LES to prevent reflux. The esophagus normally penetrates the diaphragm in the same location as the LES. In the presence of a hiatal hernia, the LES is located or intermittently slides above the diaphragmatic crura. This leads to an anatomic disruption of the diaphragmatic sphincter. Wright and Hurwitz demonstrated in 1979 that there is a significant relationship between the presence of a hiatal hernia and reflux esophagitis.[16] It has also been demonstrated that regardless of the LES pres-

Table 26-3. *Substances Influencing Lower Esophageal Sphincter Pressure*

	Increase LES Pressure	Decrease LES Pressure
Hormones	Gastrin	Secretin
	Norepinephrine	Cholecystokinin
	Acetylcholine	Glucagon
	Motilin	Nitric Oxide
		Pancreatic Polypeptide
		Substance P
Pharmacologic agents	Metoclopramide	
	Cisapride	Cholinergic Agonists
	Domperidone	Alpha Adrenergic Agonists
	Prostaglandin F2	Beta Adrenergic Antagonists
		Anatacids
	Protein	Diazepam
		Calcium Channel Blockers
		Theophylline
		Morphine
		Dopamine
		Prostaglandin E2 , I2
Diet		Fat
		Chocolate
		Caffeine
		Mint
		Ethanol

sure, patients with hiatal hernias were more prone to stress reflux than were patients without a hernia.[17] These reflux episodes probably occur because the diaphragmatic crus do not contract completely following intra-abdominal pressure events—thus permitting transmitted intragastric pressure to overcome the LES easily. Once GER disease occurs, esophageal peristalsis serves to clear the esophageal contents into the hiatal hernia, which then acts as a reservoir of gastric contents awaiting further intra-abdominal pressure events, transient LES relaxations, or free reflux events leading to repetition of the reflux cycle.

B. Esophageal Acid Clearance

Esophageal clearance mechanisms are probably the second most important factor in the control of GER. Esophageal acid clearance is normally considered a two-step process consisting of esophageal peristalsis, which clears the majority of the refluxate, while the swallowed alkaline saliva neutralizes the residual acid. Thus, both abnormal esophageal peristalsis and decreased salivary production may contribute to the pathogenesis of GER disease. However, no specific defect in esophageal clearance has been identified as the cause of reflux esophagitis. Although failed peristaltic sequences are ineffective in clearing acid from the esophagus thereby prolonging esophageal acid exposure, it has been demonstrated that peristaltic dysfunction occurs in a minority of patients with symptomatic reflux disease.[8] It has been suggested that peristaltic dysfunction may result from the acid reflux, itself, and may not be the cause of the reflux. Thus, it is unclear whether the peristaltic abnormalities found in patients with GER disease are primary abnormalities or a secondary result from repeated acid injury. Acid neutralization by swallowed saliva is a well recognized mechanism of clearing residual esophageal acid. Significant differences between resting saliva or stimulated parotid secretion in patients with reflux esophagitis and in healthy controls have not been demonstrated.[19] Saliva production may be impaired by medication or disease, and this can subsequently affect acid neutralization. During sleep, the amount of saliva produced and the frequency of swallows are reduced, thus diminishing the availability of saliva to neutralize refluxed gastric contents.

Gravity also affects esophageal clearance, returning refluxed materials to the stomach in the absence of peristalsis when the patient is in the upright position. Esophageal damage resulting from presumed inactivity of protective clearance mechanisms has generated significant concern. Studies have shown prolonged acid clearance during sleep or nocturnal reflux induces arousal from sleep, which then facilitates swallowing and subsequent acid clearance.[20] In contrast, some investigations have demonstrated that normal acid clearance times could be preserved during sleep, with only a minimal degree of wakening required to allow for swallowing.[21] Delays in arousal induced by CNS depressants (alcohol, sedatives, and hypnotics) can contribute to the development of GER disease. The duration of acid exposure correlates better with the severity of esophagitis than the frequency of reflex events, as it reflects the ability of the esophagus to clear acid. Generally, the duration of acid exposure reflects the ability of the esophagus to clear acid. The constant emptying of gastric contents ensures that gastric stasis and subsequent increases in gastric pressure, with resulting GER, does not occur.[15]

C. Tissue Epithelial Resistance

Nonkeratinized squamous epithelium provides the initial defense of the esophagus against refluxed acid. This specialized epithelium acts to retard hydrogen ion penetration and injury. Esophagitis develops when hydrogen ions leak into the mucosa, causing acidification and cell necrosis. There are tight junctions within the epithelium that retard the diffusion of noxious substances.[22] Following damage to the superficial cell layer, the esophageal mucosa becomes increasingly vulnerable to injury. There are mechanisms for the protection of the esophageal basal cells from the injurious effects of acid reflux. Two mechanisms for exchange of hydrogen ions operate within the esophageal mucosa to regulate the pH of the basal cells lining the esophagus.[23] The $Na+/H+$ exchanger and $Na+$-dependent $Cl/HCO3$ exchanger function to return the luminal pH to nonacidic levels following intracellular acidification, which occurs after acid reflux. The blood supply to the esophagus also plays an important protective role. It provides nutrients and delivers $HCO3$ to the intracellular space. The blood supply to the esophageal mucosa increases in response to the stress of luminal acid.[24]

D. Mediators of Tissue Injury

As previously mentioned, hydrogen ions are potentially damaging to the esophageal mucosa. Other known noxious stimuli are pepsin and bile salts. The degree of mucosal damage by hydrogen seems to be potentiated by adding pepsin to the reflux material.[25] Pepsin, which becomes activated at low pH, is a proteolytic enzyme secreted by the stomach and participates in acid-induced esophageal injury. Bile acids have also been implicated in the development of esophagitis.[26] This is especially important following gastric surgery, which tends to predispose the reflux of duodenal contents into the stomach. A study by Hirschowitz, comparing patients with esophagitis to those without, showed that neither the amount nor the composition of gastric secretions determined the presence or absence of esophagitis.[27] He postulated that the amount of time that the refluxed material was in contact with the esophageal mucosa might be a determining factor in the formation of esophagitis. This confirmed the importance of transient LES relaxations and abnormal acid clearance mechanisms in the pathogenesis of GER disease.

IV. PATHOPHYSIOLOGY OF EXTRAESOPHAGEAL-RELATED GER DISEASE

It has been estimated that 25% of patients with GER disease have symptoms isolated to the upper aerodigestive tract.[28] Disorders of the aerodigestive tract known or suspected of being related to GER include: laryngitis, chronic cough, globus, granuloma, subglottic stenosis, laryngeal cancer, asthma, and several disorders in infants such as apnea and recurrent bronchopulmonary infections. The relationship of these symptoms to specific reflux episodes or provocative situations is less obvious than typical esophageal complaints. Nevertheless, these symptoms are frequently associated with GER disease and may commonly be the sole manifestation of GER. Furthermore, medical and surgical antireflux therapies have been used to treat hoarseness, chronic cough, globus, and subglottic stenosis with promising results. Many of the symptoms and findings occur secondary to reflux as a consequence of the direct effect of gastric contents on the underlying tissue or through neural stimulation. The cricopharyngeus, or UES, serves a purpose similar to the LES, protecting the pharynx and larynx from the harmful effects of refluxed gastric acid. Although there is a paucity of literature concerning the UES and reflux, investigators have speculated that UES dysfunction may contribute to the extra-esophageal disorders of GER. The cricopharyngeus muscle has been implicated in the development of Zenker's diverticulum. It is thought that incoordination and spasm of this muscle leads to the development of a diverticulum. Zenker's diverticulum is formed by the protrusion of the posterior hypopharyngeal mucosa between fibers of the inferior constrictor and cricopharyngeus muscles (Fig 26-3). There is agreement in the literature that there is a significant relationship between GER disease and cricopharyngeal muscle spasm, which is believed to be an important component in the development of the diverticulum.[29]

Several lines of evidence suggest that acid may cause hyperactive airway disease. Although exact mechanisms by which GER triggers bronchospasm or laryngospasm is unclear, several possible mechanisms have been proposed. As shown in Fig 26-4, they include:

macroaspiration of gastric contents, microaspiration of gastric contents, and vagally mediated reflux bronchoconstriction. Aspiration of refluxed gastric contents into the tracheobronchial tree or laryngeal inlet has been offered as an explanation for the association of GER disease and bronchospasm and reflux laryngitis. Scintigraphic studies have demonstrated the aspiration of gastric contents after eating a ^{99}Tc radiolabeled meal. Lung scans performed in patients with a ^{99}Tc meal were found to be positive in 75% of patients with both pulmonary symptoms and GER disease.[30] Subsequent studies with either pulmonary or laryngeal symptoms have not confirmed these original observations. Microaspiration of minute amounts of gastric contents at low pH into the tracheal bronchial tree may also cause bronchosconstriction and reflux laryngitis. Animal studies have demonstrated that stimulation of tracheal receptors located in the upper airway epithelium is associated with vagally mediated reflex bronchoconstriction.[31] Tracheal acidification has been shown to produce marked increases in airway resistance, with these effects abolished following a surgically induced bilateral vagotomy. The reflux of gastric contents may induce bronchoconstriction by stimulating esophageal mucosal receptors, which subsequently initiates a vagal nerve mediated reflex bronchial constriction. Intraesophageal HCL challenges infused into dogs caused a significant fall in the ratio of total respiratory resistance/functional residual capacity. In human studies, significant increases in total respiratory resistance and reduced flow rates at 25% of vital capacity were seen shortly following intraesophageal acid infusions, but not after infusion of normal saline or infusions of neutralized gastric contents.[32] These findings can be negated by anesthetizing the esophageal receptors, by blocking the vagus nerve surgically or chemically, and by neutralization of the gastric acidity.

A. Subglottic Stenosis

Subglottic stenosis is most commonly associated with traumatic events such as endotracheal intubation. A relationship between subglottic stenosis and GER disease has been substantiated in both human and animal studies. Synthetically prepared gastric juice at pH 1.4 or 4.0 applied to the larynx and trachea of rabbits for periods of 1-4 hours demonstrated gross and microscopic changes of local submucosal hemorrhage, edema, inflammation, and ulceration.[14] The changes progressively worsened as the pH was lowered and the duration of contact was increased. Case reports using antireflux therapies in the treatment of subglottic stenosis have been promising. Treatment with reflux precautions, antacids, and H2 receptor antagonists have been shown to provide symptomatic improvement

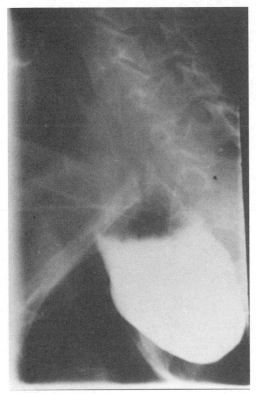

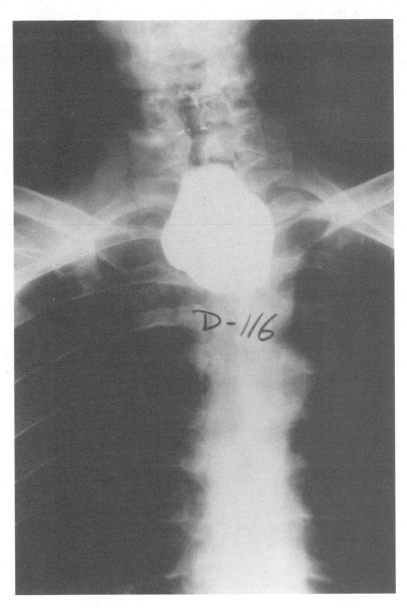

FIG 26-3. A barium swallow depicting a Zenker's diverticulum. Two views are shown: a lateral (**A**) and an anterior posterior view (**B**).

and increases in airway diameter in patients with recalcitrant subglottic stenosis. Further, abnormal acid reflux was found in over 40% of intubated patients who subsequently developed laryngeal or tracheal stenosis. Therefore, a strong association between GER disease and the development of laryngeal or tracheal stenoses has been suggested.

B. Chronic Laryngitis and Hoarseness

GER has also been implicated in the pathogenesis of chronic laryngitis and hoarseness.[33,34] Fifty-five percent of patients with idiopathic hoarseness are estimated to have GER disease.[34] Nonspecific chronic laryngitis is a term applied to persistent complaints of voice change, hoarseness, and throat irritation and discomfort for which no etiology can be found. Delahunty and Ardan

advocated that such symptoms be renamed acid laryngitis and postulated that these signs and symptoms are caused by gastric contents bathing the pharynx and posterior larynx. Most often the laryngoscopic examination is normal.[35] However, when severe, the arytenoids and posterior third of the true vocal folds may be edematous and erythematous. Pachyderma laryngis, a thickening of the mucosa of the posterior glottis is a common finding in these patients and is clinically indistinguishable from acid laryngitis. Pathologic changes may not correlate well with clinical complaints of hoarseness, globus sensation, burning pharyngeal discomfort, or nocturnal coughing. Chronic acid exposure, however, may lead to contact granulomas, ulcers, plaques, or nodularity in the interarytenoid region and posterior larynx. Gastric juices applied for a few minutes daily to the vocal folds of dogs for 6 weeks resulted in the formation of a granuloma. These changes did

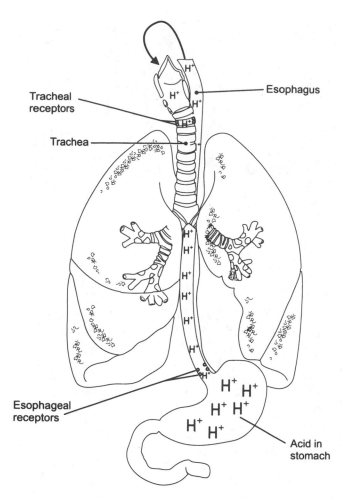

FIG 26-4. The proposed pathophysiology of atypical reflux-induced symptoms. Three mechanisms have been implicated in the pathogenesis of this type of reflux-induced injury. They include macroaspiration, micoraspiration, and vagally mediated reflex bronchoconstriction.

not occur with the application of saliva to the vocal folds of the experimental dogs. A clinical correlation between granulomas, contact ulcers, and GER has been substantiated with the use of ambulatory 24-hour pH monitoring.

Globus hystericus, the sensation of a lump in the throat, or a choking sensation, in the absence of a swallow is a disorder for which there is currently no definite etiology. However, some researchers feel that GER disease may be an underlying in the etiology of this disorder.[35,36] GER disease was reported in 64% of patients reporting globus who were studied by ambulatory pH monitoring, endoscopic gastroesophageal junction biopsies, esophageal manometry, and Bernstein acid perfusion tests. These findings have been supported by other studies using 24-hour ambulatory dual pH monitoring. Treatment with medical antireflux therapies including, antacids, H2 receptor antagonists, and/or pro-

kinetic agents resulted in improvement in 70% of the patients. Proposed mechanisms by which GER disease could induce a globus sensation include direct tissue irritation, esophageal dysmotility, referred discomfort from esophagitis mediated by the vagal afferents, or cricopharyngeal hypertension.

C. Oropharyngeal Dysphagia

GER disease has also been implicated in the etiology of oropharyngeal dysphagia, difficulty in passing a food bolus from the oropharynx into the upper esophagus. It has been reported that 50% of patients with GER disease experience cervical dysphagia at some time.[28] It is, however, important to distinguish oropharyngeal dysphagia from globus, which, in contrast, is often relieved by swallowing. The pathophysiology of acid-induced dysphagia is not understood. Relaxation of the UES to a bolus initiates esophageal peristalsis and the esophageal phase of swallowing. Response of the sphincter to acid reflux is relatively variable and inconsistent. Both elevated and reduced UES tone has been reported in patients with intraesophageal acidification. Episodic premature cricopharyngeal sphincter contractions have also been suggested as a mechanism for dysphagia. Although acid reflux appears to have an important etiologic role in oropharyngeal dysphagia further research is needed to elucidate the mechanism responsible for this association.

D. Chronic Cough

Cough represents a very common complaint among patients and the prevalence of GER disease-associated cough ranges from 10% to 40%.[37] There are two proposed mechanisms of GER disease-associated cough: (1) acid in the distal esophagus stimulating an esophageal-tracheobroncial cough reflex and (2) microaspiration or macroaspiration of esophageal contents in to the larynx and tracheobronchial tree.[38] The cough reflex appears to be vagally mediated with distal esophageal acid exposure, rather than proximal esophageal acid exposure triggering this reflex arc. The relationship between pulmonary symptoms (aspiration, wheezing or asthma, and nocturnal cough) and pH evidence of GER was evaluated in a large series of patients. The results of this investigation demonstrated that typical reflux symptoms of heartburn and regurgitation were not reliable indicators of GER. Clearance of acid from the esophagus in the upright position in these patients was not significantly different from patients with a primary respiratory disorder. Conversely, patients with reflux and asthma or cough showed significantly delayed esophageal acid clearance when supine.

E. Summary

Further advances in our diagnostic abilities, specifically an increased use of ambulatory pH monitoring, have improved our ability to diagnose extraesophageal manifestations of GER disease. Many of these symptoms may be the sole presentations of GER in these patients. It is important that the clinician is aware of these atypical presentations of GER disease. Furthermore, improved diagnostic measures and the use of clinical therapeutic trials will help us better understand the pathophysiology of these atypical symptoms.

Frequently Asked Questions

1. What is the most important mechanism responsible for GER?
   A. TSLERs is considered to be the most important mechanism responsible for GER in both normal individuals as well as in patients with GER disease. LES pressure is also one of the prime factors contributing to the presence or absence of GER. The next most important mechanism responsible for GER is esophageal peristalsis.
2. How do you treat patients with atypical GER symptoms?
   A. Because only a small amount of GER is needed for patients to experience atypical presentations of GER such as, hoarseness, cough, and asthma, a greater degree of acid suppression therapy will likely be required in the treatment. High doses of a proton pump inhibitor can be used as both a clinical trial in the diagnosis of atypical GER and for the treatment.
3. Can GER be an etiologic factor for patients with hoarseness, cough, or asthma in the absence of typical symptoms of GER?
   A. Absolutely, approximately half of patients with atypical presentations of GER do not experience the typical GER symptoms of heartburn and acid regurgitation.

References

1. Goyal RK, Cobb BW. Motility of the pharynx, esophagus and esophageal sphincters. In: Johnson LR, ed. *Physiology of the Gastrointestinal Tract.* New York, NY: Raven Press; 1981:359-391.
2. Christensen J. Motor functions of the pharynx and esophagus. In: Johnson LR, ed. *Physiology of the Gastrointestinal Tract.* New York, NY: Raven Press; 1987:595-612.
3. Humphries TJ, Castell DO. Pressure profile of esophageal peristalsis in normal humans as measured by direct intraesophgeal transducers. *Am J Dig Dis.* 1997;22:641-645.
4. Knauer CM, Castell JA, Dalton CB, Nowak L, Castell DO. Pharyngeal/upper esophgeal sphincter pressure dynamics in humans: effects of pharmocological agents and thermal stimulation. *Dig Dis Sci.* 1990;35:774-780.
5. Barret NR. Chronic peptic ulcer of the oesophagus and "oesophagitis." *Br J Surg.* 1950;38:175-181.
6. The Gallup Organization. *A Gallup Organization National Survey: Heartburn Across America.* Princeton, NJ: The Gallup Organization; 1988.
7. Nebel OT, Forne MF, Castell DO. Symptom as gastroesophageal reflux: incidence and precipitating factors. *Am J Dig Dis.* 1976;21:953-956.
8. Locke GR, Talley NJ, Fett SL, Zinmeister AR. The prevalence and impact of gastroesophageal reflux disease in the United States: population based study. [Abstract]. *Gastroenterology.* 1994;106:A15.
9. El-Serag HB, Sonnenberg A. Comorbid occurrence of laryngeal and pulmonary disease with esohpagitis in United States military veterans. *Gastroenterology.* 1997;113: 755-760.
10. Waring JP, Lacayo L, Hunter J, Katz E, Suwak B. Chronic cough and hoarseness in patients with severe gastroesophageal reflux disease. *Dig Dis Sci.* 1995;40:1093-1097.
11. Deschner WK, Benjamin SB. Extraesophageal manifestations of gastroesophageal reflux disease. *Am J Gastroenterol.* 1989;84:1-5.
12. Helm JF, Dodds WJ, Pelc LR, Palmer DW, Hogan WJ, Teeter BC. Effect of esophageal emptying and saliva on clearance of acid from the esophagus. *N Engl J Med.* 1984; 310:284-288.
13. Orlando RC. Esophageal epithelial resistance. *J Clin Gastroenterol.* 1986;8(Suppl):12-16.
14. Little FB, Koufman JA, Kohut RI, Marshall RB. Effect of gastric acid on the pathogenesis of subglottic stenosis. *Ann Otol Rhinol Laryngol.* 1985;94: 516-519.
15. Dodds WJ, Dent J, Hogan WJ, Helm JF, Hauser R, Patel GK, Egide MS. Mechanisms of gastroesophageal reflux in patients with reflux esophagitis. *N Engl J Med.* 1982;307: 1547-1552.
16. Wright RA, Hurwitz AL. Relationship of hiatal hernia to endoscopically proven reflux esophagitis. *Dig Dis Sci.* 1979; 24:311-313.
17. Sloan S, Kahrilas PJ. Hiatal hernia with or without a hypotensive LES predispose to stress reflux. [Abstract]. *Gastroenterology.* 1991;100:A164.
18. Kahrilas PJ, Dodds WJ, Hogan WJ, Kern M, Arndorfer RC, Reece A. Esophageal peristaltic dysfunction in peptic esophagitis. *Gastroenterology.* 1986;91:897-904.
19. Sonnenberg A, Steinkamp U, Weise A, Berges W, Weinbeck M, Rohner HG, Peter P. Salivary secretion in reflux esophagitis. *Gastroenterology.* 1982;83:889-895.
20. Orr WC, Robinson MG, Johnson LF. Acid clearance during sleep in the pathogenesis of reflux esophatitis. *Dig Dis Sci.* 1984;26:423-427.
21. Orr WC, Johnson LF, Robinson MG. Effect of sleep on swallowing, esophageal peristalsis, and acid clearance. *Gastroenterology.* 1984;86:814-819.
22. Yassin TM, Toner PG. Fine structure of squamous epithelium and submucosal glands of human esophagus. *J Anat.* 1977;23:705-721.
23. Tobey NA, Reddy SP, Khalbuss WE, Silvers SM, Cragoe ES, Orlando RC. Na+-dependent and -independent Cl-/HCO3- exchangers in cultured rabbit esophageal epithelial cells. *Gastroenterology.* 1993;104:185-195.

24. Hollworth ME, Smith M, Kvietys PR, Granger DN. Esophageal blood flow in the cat: normal distribution and effects of acid perfusion. *Gastroenterology*. 1986;90:622-627.

25. Goldberg HI, Dodds WJ, Gee S, Montgomery C, Zboralske FF. Role of acid and pepsin in acute experimental esophagitis. *Gastroenterology*. 1969;56:223-230.

26. Vaezi MF, Singh S, Richter JE. Role of acid and duodenogastric reflux in esophageal mucosal injury: review of animal and human studies. *Gastroenterology*. 1995;108:1897-1907.

27. Hirschowitz BI. A critical analysis, with appropriate controls, of gastric acid and pepsin secretion in clinical esophagitis. *Gastroenterology*. 1991;101:1149-1158.

28. Henderson RD, Woolf C, Marryatt G. Pharyngoesophageal dysphagia and gastroesophageal reflux. *Laryngoscope*. 1976;86:1531-1549.

29. Gaynor EB. Otolaryngologic manifestations of gastroesophageal reflux. *Am J Gastroenterol*. 1991;86:801-808.

30. Shay SS, Abreu SH, Tsuchida A. Scintigraphy in gastroesophageal reflux disease: a comparison to endoscopy, LESp, and 24-hr pH score, as well as to simultaneous pH monitoring. *Am J Gastroenterol*. 1992;87:1094-1101.

31. Exahros ND, Logan WD, Abbott OA, Hatcher CR. The importance of pH and volume in tracheobronchial aspiration. *Dis of Chest*. 1965;47:167-169.

32. Mansfield LE, Hameister HH, Spaulding HS, Smith NJ, Glab N. The role of the vagus nerve in airway narrowing caused by intraesophgeal hydrocholic acid provocation and esophageal distention. *Ann Allergy*. 1981;47:431-434.

33. Ward PH, Zwitman D, Hanson D, Berci G. Contact ulcers and granulomas of the larynx: New insights into their etiology as a basis for more rational treatment. *Otolaryngol Head Neck Surg*. 1980;88:262-272.

34. McNally PR, Maydonovitch CL, Prosek RA, Collette RP, Wong RKH. Evaluation of gastroesophageal reflux as a cause of idiopathic hoarseness. *Dig Dis Sci*. 1989;34:1900-1904.

35. Delahunty JE, Ardran GM. Globus hystericus—a manifestation of reflux esophagitis? *J Laryngol Otol*. 1970;84:1049-1054.

36. Cherry J, Siegel CI, Margulies SI, Donner M. Pharyngeal localization of symtoms of gastroesophageal reflux. *Ann Otol Rhinol Laryngol*. 1970;79:912-914.

37. Ing AJ, Ngu MC, Breslin AB. Pathogenesis of chronic persistent cough associated with gastroesophageal reflux. *Am J. Respir Crit Care Med*. 1994;149:160-1607.

38. Harding SM, Richter JE. The role of gastroesophageal reflux in chronic cough and asthma. *Chest*. 1997;111:1389-1402.

CHAPTER 27

■ ■ ■

Disorders of Esophageal Motility

Sukhdeep Padda, M.D.
Michele A. Young, M.D.

I. INTRODUCTION

Advances in manometric, scintigraphic, and radiographic techniques have brought a better understanding of motility disorders of the esophagus. These disorders, which may be primary or secondary, have a varied etiology with direct effects over the mucosal lining, muscle, or neural plexus.

II. ESOPHAGEAL MOTILITY DISORDERS

A. Achalasia

Achalasia is the most recognized and understood motor disorder of the esophagus. It is uncommon, with an annual incidence in the United States and Europe estimated at 1.1 per 100,000 population. It initially presents in individuals between 20 and 60 years of age. Men and women are affected equally. Classically, patients present with long-standing, slowly progressive dysphagia for both solids and liquids.[1] Regurgitation is common and unprovoked, occurring during or shortly after a meal. Weight loss is common. Chest pain clinically mimicking cardiac angina is frequently reported. Heartburn from gastroesophageal reflux (GER) is very uncommon. Patients do, however, complain of bitter or sour regurgitant material. This is a result of retained food in the esophagus fermenting and causing a lactic acidosis. Although the etiology of achalasia is unknown,

it is characterized by the degeneration of neural elements in the wall of the esophagus, particularly at the LES. The pathogenesis is due primarily to a reduction in the number of ganglion cells in the myenteric plexus and secondarily to damage to the vagus nerve, most notably myelin degeneration. The degree of ganglion cell loss appears to be related to the duration of the disease.[2] Ganglion cells are nearly absent in patients reporting symptoms for a minimum of 10 years.

Achalasia means "failure to relax" and describes a cardinal feature of this disorder: absent or incomplete LES relaxation. Also required for the diagnosis of achalasia is esophageal aperistalsis, which is most easily identified with esophageal manometry. Radiographic imaging has a clear role in the identification and diagnosis of achalasia. An air-fluid level within a dilated esophagus may be seen on a standard chest X ray. The normally present gastric air bubble is frequently absent on posterior-anterior and lateral chest views in patients with achalasia. Barium esophagography is an appropriate screening test for this disorder. In a recumbent patient with achalasia, the contrast material either sits in an atonic dilated esophagus or moves to and fro without propulsion because of lack of peristalsis. On barium swallow, the distal esophagus is typically dilated and the barium column tapers at the contracted LES. The distal segment of the esophagus tapers giving the appearance of a "bird's beak" (Fig 27-1). The endoscopic appearance of the esophagus in achalasia varies with the stage of the disease. Early in the disease process, the

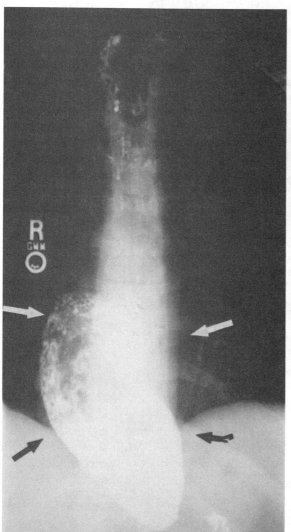

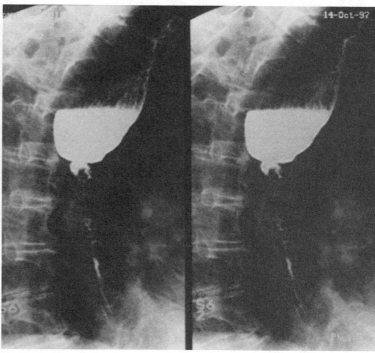

Fig 27-1. This barium esophagogram allows easy delineation of the dilated esophagus as marked by the arrows. The distal segment narrows at the lower esophageal sphincter with the appearance of a "bird's beak." An anterior posterior (**A**) and a lateral view (**B**) are shown.

esophageal mucosa may appear normal. With disease progression, there is progressive dilation and tortuosity of the esophagus, giving the appearance of a sigmoid colon. Poor esophageal clearance frequently results in mucosal plaques, erosions, and ulcerations. During endoscopy, increased pressure is usually required to pass the endoscope through the tonically contracted LES. The diagnosis of achalasia, however, is confirmed manometrically with esophageal manometry studies.

B. Diffuse Esophageal Spasm (DES)

Intermittent dysphagia, chest pain, and repetitive contractions of the esophagus characterize diffuse esophageal spasm (DES). The onset of the disorders may occur at any age, with the mean age of presentation occurring at approximately 40 years. A greater prevalence is seen in women. Angina-like chest pain is the most frequently reported symptom, occurring in 80%-90% of patients with manometrically confirmed DES.[3] The pain may be relat-

ed to swallowing, but it also may occur independent of eating. Dysphagia is present in 30%-60% of patients with DES. Clinically, dysphagia is intermittent, with daily severity varying from mild to severe. Food impaction and weight loss occur very rarely. The etiology of DES is not known and there is a paucity of literature regarding the pathophysiology. Diffuse muscular thickening in the distal esophagus has been reported in some patients with severe disease. Changes in vagal fibers have been found inconsistently by electron microscopy.[4]

Although esophageal manometry is required for the diagnosis, a barium study of the esophagus with fluoroscopy can reveal the abnormality. However, barium radiographic studies of the esophagus are most often normal in DES. Transit of barium through the esophagus may be markedly reduced, resulting in nonpropulsive contractions that often trap the barium between contracted segments, thereby indenting the barium-filled smooth muscle portion of the esophagus (Fig 27-2). The radiographic findings may be variable, as contractions are intermittent. These abnormal contractions

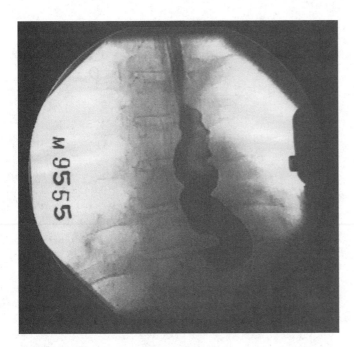

FIG 27-2. This barium esophagogram shows the indentations caused by the tertiary contractions typically seen in diffuse esophageal spasm.

are often elicited by giving a bolus of food or fluid. The distorted radiographic appearance of the esophagus is that of a "corkscrew" or of a "rosary bead." Nonperistaltic waves within the esophagus may result in barium being retained within a transient outpouching of the esophagus, giving the radiographic appearance of a diverticulum. Thickening of the esophageal wall may be demonstrated with high film resolution. There are no characteristic endoscopic findings in DES. Manometric findings are limited to the smooth muscle segment of the esophagus. Nonperistaltic or simultaneous contractions following a majority of the swallows is the most reliable criteria in the definition of DES. Less consistent but also observed are abnormalities of the contraction wave, such as increased amplitude or duration and intermittent episodes of repetitive contractions associated with increased baseline esophageal pressure. The diagnosis of DES is generally reserved for patients demonstrating nonperistaltic sequences in at least 30% of wet swallows. A hallmark characteristic of DES is the presence of unpropagated contractions intermixed with normal peristalsis.

C. Nonspecific Esophageal Motility Disorder (NEMD)

Certain motility abnormalities may be found during esophageal manometry studies in patients with dysphagia who have no evidence of other systemic diseases. These are collectively called nonspecific esopha-

geal motility disorders (NEMD). A clear distinction between the nonspecific esophageal motility disorder and classic primary esophageal motility disorders such as achalasia and DES is often not possible. The radiographic and endoscopic findings in these disorders are also nonspecific and most often normal; therefore, the diagnosis needs to be confirmed manometrically. Patients with NEMD constitute approximately 25%-50% of the abnormal motility studies performed in the diagnosis of chest pain and dysphagia.[5]

The etiology of this group of disorders is unknown. In some cases, the motor abnormalities may be induced by the irritation of refluxed gastric juice. However, this is not always true, as it can also be a primary event unrelated to the presence of reflux. With manometry, one can find manometric abnormalities that suggest the diagnosis of nonspecific esophageal motility disorder. Manometric findings included in this group are: high amplitude peristaltic contractions, reduced amplitude of peristaltic contractions, a change in the morphology of the waveform, such as an increased number of multi-peaked or repetitive contractions, prolonged duration of contractions, and abnormal LES function with normal peristalsis, such as a hypertensive LES with normal relaxation or normal pressure LES with incomplete relaxation.

Table 27-1 summarizes the most common manometric findings seen with esophageal motility disorders.

D. Upper Esophageal Sphincter Dysfunction and Motility Disorders of the Pharynx

Pharyngeal dysphagia is frequently a result of (1) a failure of the driving force or propulsion, (2) obstruction to flow, or (3) a combination of the first two causes. Failure of propulsive forces resulting in pharyngeal dysphagia is generally due to defects in the brainstem, cranial nerves, myoneural junction, or muscles. Amyotrophic lateral sclerosis (ALS), postpolio syndromes, and myasthenia gravis can lead to motor abnormalities in the pharynx. Patients may present with what appears to be a delayed swallow. There may be diminished laryngeal elevation and epiglottic tilting, which can lead to poor pharyngeal and cervical peristalsis. Pharyngeal dysphagia resulting from an obstruction to flow is almost always due to a mass lesion or incomplete UES relaxation. Poor compliance of the UES can cause incomplete relaxation during swallowing, leading to a rise in hypopharyngeal pressure. As a result, a pharyngoesophageal, or Zenker's, diverticulum may develop. Impairment of relaxation or opening of the sphincter may affect the smooth coordination of swallowing. Impairment of cricopharyngeal relaxation results in a prominent bar across the cricopharyngeal region, and paralysis of the suprahyoid pharyngeal muscles may

Table 27-1. *Common Manometric Abnormalities in Esophageal Motility Disorders*

Achalasia

Incomplete or absent LES relaxation
Esophageal aperistalsis
Increased intraesophageal pressure
High LES pressure

Diffuse Esophageal Spasm

Nonperistalsis intermixed with normal peristalsis
Abnormalities in the contraction wave
Simultaneous contractions

Nonspecific Motility Disorders

Hypertensive LES
Isolated incomplete LES relaxation
High amplitude peristalsis
Reduced amplitude peristalsis

---

cause paralytic achalasia of the UES.[6] A diagnosis of cricopharyngeal achalasia is frequently suggested when impaired transfer of barium from the pharynx to the upper esophagus is seen radiographically (Fig 27-3A and 27-3B). Primary abnormal UES relaxation has been described only in rare cases of central nervous system lymphoma or oculopharyngeal muscular dystrophy.[7] A secondary cause in adults is previous neck surgery, including pharyngectomy, laryngectomy, or tracheostomy placement.[8] Most cases of cricopharyngeal achalasia represent the inadequate transfer of barium through a poorly opening sphincter resulting from weak pharyngeal forces, poor elevation of the hyoid, or decreased elasticity of the cricopharyngeal muscle despite adequate UES muscle relaxation.

E. Secondary Motility Disorders

Systemic diseases such as diabetes mellitus, amyloidosis, and most notably progressive systemic sclerosis (PSS) can produce esophageal dysmotility and dysphagia. An estimated 50%-90% of patients with PSS have esophageal involvement.[9] Esophageal motility studies reveal the characteristic findings of PSS to include reduced LES pressure and reduced amplitude of peristalsis in the distal two thirds of the esophagus or esophageal aperistalsis. Peristalsis is frequently maintained in the striated, or proximal, portion of the esophagus and upper esophageal sphincter pressure and relaxation are generally unimpaired. The esophageal dysmotility found in these patients specifically, very low LES pressures combined with poor or absent esophageal peristalsis, may result in clinically significant GER, peptic strictures, and Barrett's esophagus.[9] Thus, progressive dysphagia for solids and liquids may

be a major complaint, but acid reflux is likely the pathophysiological mechanism of their complaint.

F. The Curling Phenomenon

Curling is an alteration in esophageal motility frequently seen in elderly individuals. It represents tertiary contractions, that are nonpropulsive. During the fluoroscopic portion of the barium swallow examination, tertiary contractions appear as ring-like contractions that occur and disappear, recurring at short intervals until a peristaltic wave appears. Tertiary contractions appear on the radiograph as a "beaded esophagus" or "corkscrew esophagus." Patients with more severe and rigorous curling frequently have dysphagia. Diverticula may also develop in the mid or distal esophagus as a result of esophageal dysmotility. Esophageal diverticula are outpouchings of one or more layers of the esophageal wall. These diverticula occur primarily in three locations within the esophagus. They are: (1) immediately above the UES (Zenker's diverticululum), (2) near the mid point of the esophagus (traction diverticulum), and (3) immediately above the LES (epiphrenic diverticulum). With the exception of a Zenker's diverticulum, these are often temporary and may disappear with the passage of the contractile activity. Barium esophagography readily demonstrates the presence of these diverticula and curling.[10]

G. Presbyesophagus

Presbyesophagus is a term used to describe esophageal dysmotility associated with the typical aging process. Although most patients are asymptomatic, moderate dysphagia may be noted specifically with solid foods. The primary peristaltic contractions are diminished and an increased degree of curling is seen on the barium swallow. Generally the distal half of the esophagus is more involved than the proximal segment.[11] Furthermore, relaxation of the lower esophageal sphincter may be impaired with resultant dilatation of the lower esophagus.

III. MECHANICAL OBSTRUCTION

Mechanical obstruction of the esophagus can occur from varied causes ranging from benign webs and rings to malignant lesions. The primary cause of solid food dysphagia is an anatomical defect in the esophagus most commonly resulting from peptic strictures and carcinoma. Benign peptic strictures are radiographically smooth, vary in length, and usually involve the mid to distal esophagus. Peptic strictures are a compli-

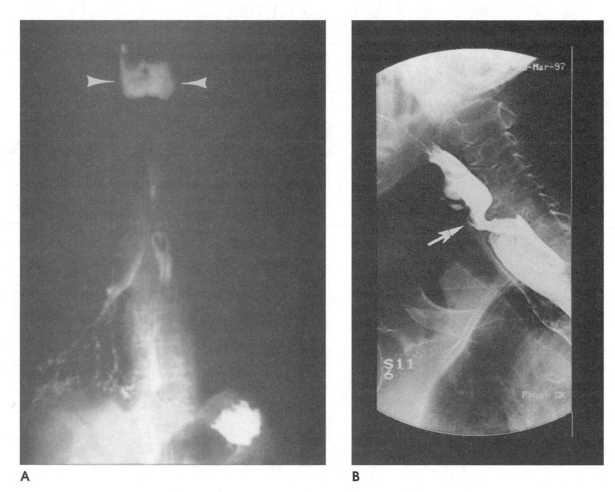

FIG 27-3. This barium esophagogram is an example of cricopharyngeal achalasia. In the anterior posterior view (**A**), the barium is pooling in the pharynx because of a poorly compliant UES. In the lateral view (**B**), a thickened cricopharyngeal muscle, the arrow shows a cricopharyngeal bar.

cation of long-standing GER that has not been adequately treated. Therefore, patients with peptic strictures have a long history of heartburn and frequent use of over-the-counter antisecretory medications. Generally patients with esophageal cancer are older and have rapidly progressive dysphagia and weight loss. An early carcinoma causes an eccentric luminal filling defect. Alternatively, some lesions may form flat plaque-like lesions that may remain asymptomatic until the advanced stages of the disease. Rarely the lesion may be ulcerative with a rim of neoplasm around the ulcer similar to an ulcerative carcinoma of the stomach. The findings on barium esophogram in advanced esophageal carcinoma can de divided into three major categories: polypoid, infiltrative, and ulcerative, with some overlap between the categories.[12] The most common presentation of an advanced esophageal carcinoma is that of a polypoid intraluminal mass. An exophytic cancer may produce either a localized or extensive polypoid defect. The mass may have the characteristic appearance of an "apple-core," lesion with circumferential involvement by the cancer leaving only a narrowed, irregular lumen.

In the early stages, esophageal carcinoma may be totally asymptomatic or be manifested only by mild, nonspecific symptoms for which the patient may not seek medical attention. As the disease progresses and the tumor grows, symptoms of advanced esophageal carcinoma appear. Progressive dysphagia is the most common presenting complaint, occurring in over 90% of patients. Dysphagia usually signifies that more than 50% of the esophageal lumen is occluded. It typically begins with solids and can progress to the point at which liquids or even saliva cannot be swallowed. Anorexia and weight loss occurs in approximately 75% of patients with advanced esophageal carcinoma. Bleeding from esophageal carcinoma is most frequently occult and can lead to iron deficiency anemia. Cough may result from aspiration pneumonia or tracheoesophageal fistula. Sinus tracts often form in the late stages of carcinoma of the esophagus and these are seen as irregular extensions into adjacent mediastinal structures.

Local invasion of the cancer can produce pleural effusions and empyema. Hoarseness suggests involvement of the recurrent laryngeal nerve (RLN). Histologically, there are two primary tumor types in the esophagus. Squamous cell carcinoma of the esophagus is the most common neoplasm worldwide. In the United States, African Americans have a four- to five-fold increased risk compared to the white population. It has been estimated that at least 90% of the risk for squamous cell cancer of the esophagus in North America and Europe can be attributed to alcohol and tobacco. The overall incidence of this cancer type in the United States is decreasing. On the contrary, the incidence of adenocarcinoma of the esophagus is increasing markedly, especially in white males. The reason for this increase is not clear.

Adenocarcinoma almost exclusively results from Barrett's esophagus, which is a result of long-term exposure of the esophagus to gastric acid. With the advent of very strong antisecretory agents, such as, the proton-pump inhibitors, perhaps this form of cancer will begin to decline. Flexible fiberoptic endoscopy with direct vision biopsy and cytology represents the single most important test in the diagnosis of carcinoma and in the differentiation of the cell types. The accuracy of endoscopic brush cytology in upper gastrointestinal malignancies is most commonly reported as 70%-90%.[13] By combining cytology with multiple endoscopic biopsies, accuracies of 90%-100% can be attained.[13] Rarely, both biopsy and cytology fail to diagnose a cancer in cases with endoscopic or radiographic evidence of carcinoma. Finally, endoscopic ultrasound is being used to identify the depth of tumor invasion. This is especially important in determining treatment options.

Patients with intermittent dysphagia for solids have esophageal webs or rings. A Schatzki's ring is a lower esophageal mucosal ring, which is located at the level of the squamocolumnar junction (Fig 27-4). The rings consist of mucosa and submucosa and are covered by squamous epithelium on the proximal side and either columnar epithelium or several millimeters of squamous epithelium on the distal or gastric side. The actual or true ring is circumferential and less than 3 mm in thickness. The incidence of these rings is estimated at 13% of the population however, only those with luminal narrowing of <13 mm are symptomatic. Esophageal webs are reported in 7% of the patients presenting with dysphagia.

Although esophageal mucosal injury is most often secondary to GER disease, injury can also result from infectious agents and pill ingestion. The clinical presentation may be identical to GER disease, including chest pain, heartburn, and dysphagia. Herpes simplex, cytomegalovirus, and candida may invade or colonize the esophageal mucosa and cause inflammation of the mucosa. Clinically significant esophagitis is most commonly seen in immunocompromised patients. Although not a common cause of esophagitis, mucosal injury as a result of ingested pills should be considered in the differential diagnosis of dysphagia. Delayed esophageal transit resulting from esophageal dysmotility increases

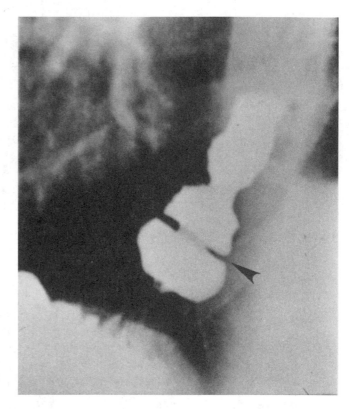

FIG 27-4. This barium esophagogram shows a typical Schatzki's ring in the distal esophagus as indicated by the arrow.

the amount of mucosal contact with the pill, thus increasing the likelihood of injury.

III. SUMMARY

The process, of swallowing involves sequential, complex movements. Dysfunction in this process is common and can result from multiple etiologies. Because of the complexity of this process, several different disciplines are involved in the diagnostic and management of patients presenting with dysphagia. The gastroenterologists will likely devote their portion of the evaluation to the esophagus, utilizing endoscopy, esophageal manometry, and 24-hour ambulatory pH monitoring. The best utilization of health care dollars are multi-disciplinary centers devoted to the diagnosis and treatment of swallowing disorders. These centers typically include a speech-language pathologist, neurologist, otolaryngologist, radiologist, and gastroenterologist.

Frequently Asked Questions

1. What are the manometric requirements for the diagnosis of achalasia?
   A. To diagnose achalasia the patient must have two manometric abnormalities:

1. esophageal aperistalsis
2. incomplete or absent LES relaxation
2. Do patients with achalasia have heartburn?
   A. Patients with achalasia rarely have heartburn from GER. They may complain of heartburn-like symptoms; however, these symptoms are most frequently secondary to lactic acid from the fermenting food usually found in the esophagus of patients with achalasia.
3. What are the manometric requirements for the diagnosis of DES?
   A. There are many manometric features associated with DES; however, the intermixing of simultaneous contractions with normal peristalsis must be present for the diagnosis of DES to be made.

References

1. Reynolds JC, Parkman HP. Achalasia. *Gastroenterol Clin North Am.* 1989;18:223-255.
2. Cassela RR, Brown AL, Sayre GP Ellis HF Jr. Achalasia of the esophagus: pathologic and etiologic considerations. *Ann Surg.* 1964;160:474-487.
3. Richter JE, Castell DO. Diffuse esophageal spasm: a reappraisal. *Ann Intern Med.* 1984;100:242-246.
4. Gillies M, Nicks R, Skyring A. Clinical, manometric, and pathological studies in diffuse esophageal spasm. *Br Med J.* 1967;2:527-531.
5. Hsu JJ, O'Connor MK, Kang YM, Kim CH. Nonspecific motor disorder of the esophagus: a real disorder or a manometric curiosity. *Gastroenterology.* 1993;104:1281-1284.
6. Goyal RK, Patterson WG. Esophageal motility In: Woods JD, ed. *Handbook of Physiology—The Gastrointestinal System, II.* Bethesda, Md: American Physiological Society; 1989:865.
7. Castell JA, Castell DO, Duranceau A, Topart P. Manometric characteristics of the pharynx, upper esophageal sphincter, esophagus, and lower esophageal sphincter in patients with oculopharyngeal muscular dystrophy. *Dysphagia.* 1995;10:22-26.
8. Bonanno PC. Swallowing dysfunction after tracheostomy. *Ann Surg.* 1971;174:29-33.
9. Garrett JM, Dubose TD, Jackson JE, Norman JR Esophageal and pulmonary disturbances in myotonia dystrophica. *Arch Intern Med.* 1969;123:26-32.
10. Russell CO, Hill LD, Holmes ER 3d, Hull DA, Gannon R, Pope CE 2d. Radionuclide transit: a sensitive screening test for esophageal dysfunction. *Gastroenterology.* 1981;80 (5 pt 1):887-892.
11. Hollis JB, Castell DO. Esophageal function in elderly man. A new look at "presbyesophagus." *Ann Intern Med.* 1974; 80:371-374.
12. Wiot JW, Felson B. Cancer of the gastrointestinal tract. Radiographic differential diagnosis. *JAMA.* 1973;226:1548-1553.
13. Winawer, SJ, Sherlock P, Belladonna JA, Melamed M, Beattle EJ Jr. Endoscopic brush cytology in esophageal cancer. *JAMA.* 1975;232,1358-1363.

CHAPTER 28

■ ■ ■

Pathophysiology of Zenker's Diverticulum

Andrew N. Goldberg, M.D.
David E. Eibling, M.D.

I. INTRODUCTION

A diverticulum in the hypopharynx may be discovered in the evaluation of a patient with dysphagia. This pouch, termed "Zenker's diverticulum," was first described by Abraham Ludlow in 1764 as a "preternatural bag" in the pharynx.[1] However, it was the seminal work by Friedrich Albert von Zenker in 1877 that defined not only the anatomic relationships of the diverticulum, but the pathophysiology that results in its formation, particularly the relationship to the cricopharyngeus muscle.[2] This chapter discusses the pathophysiology of Zenker's diverticulum, as well as the diagnosis and treatment options for this disorder.

II. PATHOPHYSIOLOGY

Many possible etiologies of Zenker's diverticulum had been proposed prior to Zenker's description. Cherry stones, hard bread, bird bones, and lead shot had all been found within a diverticulum, leading to the proposal that they played an etiologic role. Trauma from a blow to the neck and pharyngeal burns had also been described in conjunction with the discovery of a pouch and, thus, a traumatic etiology had been entertained.[3] The role of muscular discoordination in conjunction with a muscular defect was first put forward by Bell, who combined his expertise as an anatomist, neurologist, and surgeon.[4] He felt that a food bolus would en-ter the pharynx and be propelled into the hypopharynx only to meet a cricopharyngeus that had not yet opened. Over time, the pressure generated by this discoordinated movement was thought to create a pulsion diverticulum.

Zenker's diverticulum appears to be found almost exclusively in humans. Lower animals have a continuous outer longitudinal and a continuous inner circular layer of musculature. In humans, the larynx is located in a more caudal position, giving the circular fibers of the esophagus a more oblique course.[3] An area of relative weakness is thereby created, vulnerable to forces within the lumen of the espohagus and subsequent herniation. In 1908, Killian defined the most common area of weakness through which the diverticulum forms, Killian's triangle,[5] although two other nearby areas of muscular weakness can also become a site for herniation[3] (Fig 28-1). Killian's triangle is located between the lower pharyngeal constrictor and the most superior fibers of the cricopharyngeus; Killian-Jamieson's area is between the oblique and transverse fibers of the cricopharyngeus; Laimer's triangle is formed between the cricopharyngeus and the most superior circular fibers of the esophagus.

Virtually all investigators recognize high intrabolus pressures in the hypopharynx as the etiologic mechanism of the pulsion diverticulum described as Zenker's diverticulum.[6] However, the mechanism by which a high intrabolus force comes about is less well agreed on. Theories include congenital weakness,[7] high pres-

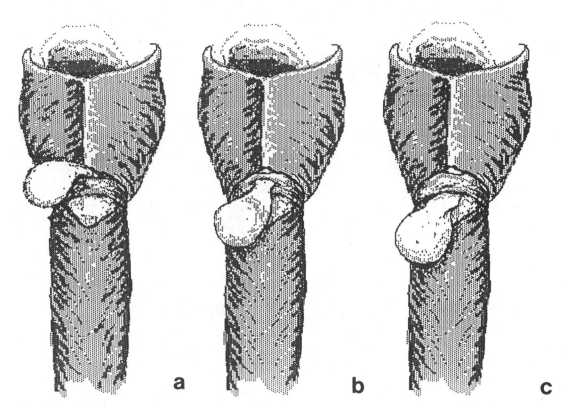

FIG 28-1. Sites of herniation of Zenker's diverticulum viewed from the posterior larynx/hypopharynx: (a) Killian's triangle, (b) Killian-Jamieson's area, (c) Laimer's triangle. Illustrations by Urban Knutsson, MD. (Reprinted with permission from Scandinavian University Press for Westrin KM, Ergun S, Carlsoo B, Zenker's diverticulum—a historical review and trends in therapy. *Acta Otolaryngologica (Stockh)*. 1996;116:351-360.)

sures in the cricopharyngeal segment related to gastroesophageal reflux,[8] discoordination of the pharyngoesophageal segment,[9] and incomplete opening or other disorders of the cricopharyngeus.[6,10]

A congenital etiology is supported by the higher incidence of Zenker's diverticulum in racial groups with an elongated neck, such as Northern Europeans. A low incidence in the Asian population, an increased incidence in certain families, and the finding of a large-sized Killian's triangle in afflicted patients contributes to this assertion.[7]

Although an association of gastroesophageal reflux (GER), hiatal hernia, and Zenker's diverticulum has been shown in epidemiologic studies, causality has not been proven. Although many point to increased cricopharyngeal pressure in patients with hiatal hernia, reflux, and Zenker's diverticulum, clinical experience does not demonstrate a strong association. The clinician should nevertheless evaluate the patient for reflux by history and upper endoscopy, treating significant reflux as warranted.[11]

Technical considerations are of paramount importance when evaluating the literature on manometric and dynamic changes during swallowing. Some of the first manometric studies that demonstrated early upper

esophageal sphincter relaxation, premature closure, and incoordination may have suffered from methodologic flaws that occurred with movement of the pressure sensor with sphincter movement.[12] More recent studies done with simultaneous manography and videoradiography point to disorders of the cricopharyngeus. There is still controversy, however, over what method of pressure monitoring should be used.

Using simultaneous videoradiography, and a perfused side hole manometry catheter, Cook and colleagues determined that there was no pharyngo-sphincteric incoordination and sphincter relaxation was adequate, but there was inadequate opening of the cricopharyngeus muscle. With a larger bolus size, the intrabolus pressure increased, creating the force behind the pulsion etiology for the diverticulum. Measurements of hyoid bone excursion failed to show any difference between controls and patients, reducing the possibility that inadequate laryngeal elevation caused inadequate opening of the sphincter. Timing of upper esophageal relaxation, opening, and closure as well as the duration of opening did not differ between patients and controls. Timing of hyoid movement was also equal in patients and controls.[6] These findings, along with the discovery of fibro-adipose tissue replacement of muscle fibers and fiber degeneration in the cricopharyngeus, contribute to the conclusion that increased hypopharyngeal pressure is a consequence of inadequate opening of the cricopharyngeus secondary to muscle fibrosis.[13,14]

McConnel et al dispute those findings, because of technical limitations of the measuring device.[10] Using a solid state manometry catheter rather than a perfused side hole sleeve manometry catheter, premature contracture, spasm, and acalasia of the cricopharyngeus muscle were all seen. Other abnormal dynamics of swallowing were also seen which contributed to increased hypopharyngeal pressures and pulsion diverticulum formation.[10]

The general pathophysiology in the formation of Zenker's diverticulum appears to be well agreed upon and differs little from the original descriptions of Bell and Zenker. High intrabolus forces in the hypopharynx caused by incomplete opening[6] or other cricopharyngeal dysfunction[10] causes the formation of a pulsion diverticulum in a natural area of muscular weakness, Killian's triangle. The precise pathophysiology that leads to the high intrabolus forces remains a subject of controversy.

III. DIAGNOSIS

Multiple symptoms can be associated with this pouch, such as dysphagia, aspiration, and postswallowing cough, as it may serve as a stagnant reservoir for material[15] (Table 22-1). The typical patient is elderly, above age 60, with a 2:1 male preponderance and commonly recalls a history of complaints for many years. Those with a classic constellation of symptoms are sent immediately for contrast videofluoroscopy where a diagnosis can be easily established. Contrast readily pools in the pouch, demonstrating the size of the pouch and filling defects caused by debris in the pouch. Patients with less

Table 28-1. *Symptoms of Zenker's Diverticulum**

Symptom	Patients (%)
Dysphagia	48 (100)
Aspiration	20 (42)
Postdeglutitive cough	17 (35)
Regurgitation	14 (29)
Noisy swallowing	13 (27)
Weight loss (>10 lbs)	13 (27)
Recumbent cough	10 (21)
Sore throat	8 (17)
Unable to swallow	8 (17)
Halitosis	2 (4)

*Adapted from Schmidt PJ, Zuckerbraun L. Treatment of Zenker's diverticula by cricopharyngeal myotomy under local anesthesia. *Am Surg.* 1992;58:710-716.

distinctive symptoms are sometimes treated for reflux or other conditions initially, with the true diagnosis becoming apparent later. Persistence of dysphagia, whether typical for Zenker's diverticulum or not, warrants further investigation with contrast videofluoroscopy. Diverticula are commonly observed in the left neck, as the cervical esophagus normally curves slightly to the left. Staging of Zenker's diverticulum by symptomatology and contrast videofluoroscopy divides patients into three stages[16] (Table 28-2) which can aid in formulating a treatment plan.

Endoscopy is not necessary to make the diagnosis, but is recommended prior to definitive therapy to eliminate other pathology in the esophagus. Care should be taken when diagnostic endoscopy is performed, as the endoscope may not pass easily into the esophagus, but into the pouch, putting the patient at-risk for perforation.

Physical findings may be present in some cases, but are commonly subtle. Halitosis may be detected by the examiner from stagnant undigested food present in the pouch. An external mass in the neck, most commonly on the left, may be palpated, or gurgling may be heard or felt with a hand placed on the patient's neck during a swallow. Office laryngoscopy may reveal erythema of the larynx or hypopharynx from regurgitation or pooling of secretions in the hypopharynx.

Cancer has rarely been detected in a Zenker's pouch, with an overall incidence of 0.3%-0.25%. Because of this low risk, the rationale for surgery is treatment of dysphagia and not the risk of cancer.[17]

IV. TREATMENT

Treatment for Zenker's diverticulum is surgical. With the possible exception of initiating a low-residue diet, no nonsurgical treatment is known to be effective in relieving symptoms or eliminating the diverticulum.

The three stages described lend themselves to different treatment strategies[16] (see Table 28-2). Stage I diverticula can be observed if symptoms are tolerated by the patient. Follow-up of the patient is recommended, although no specific guidelines for re-evaluation have been recommended. Yearly follow-up appears to be a logical interval.

Symptomatic patients who desire surgical removal and can tolerate anesthesia are candidates for excision. Local anesthesia has occasionally been used, but general anesthesia is usually recommended. A complete discussion of surgical options for treatment of Zenker's diverticulum is described in Chapter 48.

V. CONTROVERSIES

The etiology of Zenker's diverticulum is a subject of considerable debate as outlined in the section on pathophysiology. The common pathway of each theory, how-

Table 28-2. *Staging of Zenker's Diverticulum**

Stage I	Small herniation of mucosa, with minimal symptoms
Stage II	Larger herniation, with regurgitation of food during and between meals, nocturnal cough, halitosis, dysphagia, bronchitis, dysphonia, gurgling sound, local pain
Stage III	Diverticulum reaches into mediastinal cavity with nutritional difficulties and possibly cachexia and dehydration

*Adapted from Lahey FH, Warren KW. Esophageal diverticula. Surg Gynecol Obstet. 1954;98:1-28.

ever, appears to be increased pressure in the hypopharynx with herniation through an area of natural weakness in the muscular wall.

Surgical treatment options are many and include a range of options from open cricopharyngeal myotomy for small diverticula to myotomy with excision of the sack. Endoscopic options vary in the means used to incise the wall between the diverticulum and the esophagus. An electrocautery, laser, and endoscopic stapler are among the methods used to safely divide the wall and the cricopharyngeus that lies within. The reader is referred to Chapter 47 on surgical management of Zenker's diverticulum for further explanation.

Frequently Asked Questions

1. Are there nonsurgical treatments that show future promise for the treatment of Zenker's diverticulum?
   A. As the etiology of Zenker's diverticulum is felt to be a cricopharyngeus dysfunction, injection of Botulinum toxin may be a nonsurgical method for treatment. The role may be limited to small diverticula. This method has been used successfully in patients with cricopharyngeal acalasia.
2. What percentage of Zenker's diverticulum protrude into the right neck?
   A. Approximately 10% of diverticula protrude into the right neck. All others are found on the left side.
3. If the primary disorder is cricopharyngeal dysfunction, can a myotomy alone be performed without diverticulectomy or diverticulopexy?
   A. In isolated cases of patients with very small, symptomatic diverticula, a myotomy alone can be performed, or the diverticulum can be imbricated into the esophagus.

References

1. Ludlow A. A case of obstructed deglutition, from a preternatural dilation of, and bag formed in, the pharynx. *Med Observ Inq.* 1769;3:85-101.

2. Zenker FA, von Zeimssen H. Krankheiten des Oesophagus. In: Zeimssen H, ed. *Handbuch der speziellen Pathologie und Therapie.* vol 7 (suppl). Leipzig: FC Vogel; 1877:187.

3. Westrin KM, Ergun S, Carlsoo B, Zenker's diverticulum—a historical review and trends in therapy. *Acta Otolaryngol (Stockh).* 1996;116:351-360.

4. Bell C. *Surgical Observations.* London: Longmans, Greene, and Co; 1816:64-70.

5. Killian G. Ueber den Mund der Speiserohre. *Z Ohrenh.* 1908;55:1.

6. Cook IJ, Gabb M, Panagopoulos, V. Pharyngeal (Zenker's) diverticulum is a disorder of upper esophageal sphincter opening. *Gastroenterology.* 1992;103:1229-1235.

7. van Overbeek JJM. Meditation on the pathogenesis of hypopharyngeal (Zenker's) diverticulum and a report of endoscopic treatment in 545 patients. *Ann Otol Rhinol Laryngol.* 1994;103:178-185.

8. Hunt PS, Connell, AM, Smiley TB. The cricopharyngeal sphincter in gastric reflux. *Gut.* 1970;11:303-306.

9. Barthelen W, Feussner H, Haning, C, Holscher AH, Siewert JR. Surgical therapy of Zenker's diverticulum: low risk and high efficiency. *Dysphagia.* 1990;5:13-19.

10. McConnel FM, Hood D, Jackson K, O'Connor A. Analysis of intrabolus forces in patients with Zenker's diverticulum. *Laryngoscope.* 1994;104:571-581.

11. Feussner H, Siewert JR. Zenker's diverticulum and reflux. *Hepatogastroenterology.* 1992;39:100-104.

12. Chiao GZ, Kahrilas PJ. Zenker's diverticulum: new pieces to the pathogenesis puzzle. *Am Gastroenterol.* 1993;88: 1796-1797.

13. Cook IJ, Blumbergs P, Cash K, Jamieson GG, Shearman DJ. Structural abnormalities of the cricopharyngeus muscle in patients with pharyngeal (Zenker's) diverticulum. *J Gastroenterol Hepatol.* 1992;7:556-562.

14. Zaninotto G, Costantini M, Boccu C, et al. Functional and morphological study of the cricopharyngeal muscle in patients with Zenker's diverticulum. *Br J Surg.* 1996;83:1263-1267.

15. Schmidt PJ, Zuckerbraun L. Treatment of Zenker's diverticula by cricopharyngeal myotomy under local anesthesia. *Am Surg.* 1992;58:710-716.

16. Lahey FH, Warren KW. Esophageal diverticula. *Surg Gynecol Obstet.* 1954;98:1-28.

17. Giuli R, Lerut T, Aelvoet C, Leclef Y, Gruwez, JA. Rosetti M. Diverticula. In: Giuli R, McCallum RW, eds. *Benign Lesions of the Esophagus and Cancer.* Berlin: Springer Verlag; 1989:11-16.

CHAPTER 29

■ ■ ■

Autoimmune Disorders

Ahmed M.S. Soliman, M.D.
Farrel J. Buchinsky, M.D.

I.   INTRODUCTION

The immune system is a complex, multi-layered, system that functions to protect the body from foreign substances. The immune system consists of both specific and nonspecific limbs. Specific immunity differentiates self from nonself and includes cellular and humoral components. The cellular immune system is composed of a variety of cells produced in the lymph nodes and bone marrow and includes T cells, B cells, null cells, eosinophils, neutrophils, basophils, and mast cells. The humoral immune system is made up of highly specific antibodies produced by B cells. The immune response is carried out by direct or indirect effects of the antibodies, through phagocytosis or by cellular toxicity.[1]

Autoimmune diseases are characterized by production of either antibodies that react with host tissue or immune effector T cells that are autoreactive to endogenous self-peptides. In some cases, autoantibodies may arise from normal T and B cell responses to foreign organisms or substances that contains antigens that cross-react with similar antigens in body tissues; this phenomenon is known as molecular mimicry.

The first description of the autoimmune phenomenon was in the early 1900s by Ehrlich who coined the term "horror autotoxicus." Since then, many of these diseases have been reclassified as collagen-vascular diseases, rheumatic diseases, neuromuscular diseases, or immunologic diseases of connective tissue. A realistic

classification system is described in Table 29-1 in which putative autoimmune disorders are classified as highly probable, probable, or possible based on the currently available data. Autoimmune disorders may also be categorized as organ-specific or organ-nonspecific. Organ specific diseases include Hashimoto's thyroiditis, epidermolysis bullosa, and myasthenia gravis; organ-nonspecific diseases include rheumatoid arthritis, scleroderma, Sjögren's syndrome, and sarcoidosis.

Autoimmune disorders may affect swallowing by several different mechanisms, which present with both systemic and organ-specific effects, producing intrinsic obstruction as well as external compression, abnormal motility, or inadequate lubrication.

II. AUTOIMMUNE DISORDERS

A. Sjögren's Syndrome

Sjögren's syndrome is the combination of keratoconjunctivitis sicca and xerostomia due to infiltration of the lacrimal and salivary glands with lymphocytes. This is due to a systemic autoimmune process that may also affect other organs, including the airway, gastrointestinal tract, kidneys, vagina, and central and peripheral nervous system. Primary Sjögren's syndrome is not associated with other diseases. Secondary Sjögren's is defined as the association of the listed symptoms

Table 29-1. *Disorders in Which Autoimmunity is Thought to Play a Role**

	Disorder	Mechanism of Evidence†
Highly probable	Hashimoto's thyroiditis	Cell-mediated and humoral thyroid cytotoxicity
	Systemic lupus erythematosus	Circulating and locally generating immune complexes
	Goodpasture's syndrome	Anti-basement membrane Ab
	Pemphigus	Epidermal acantholytic Ab
	Receptor autoimmunity	
	Grave's disease	TSH receptor Ab (stimulatory)
	Myasthenia gravis	Acetylcholine receptor Ab
	Insulin resistance	Insulin receptor Ab
	Autoimmune hemolytic anemia	Phagocytosis of Ab-sensitized RBCs
	Autoimmune thrombocytopenic purpura	Phagocytosis of Ab-sensitized platelets
Probable	Rheumatoid arthritis	Immune complexes in joints
	Scleroderma with anti-collagen Abs	Nucleolar and other nuclear Abs
	Mixed connective tissue disease	Ab to extractable nuclear Ag (ribonucleoprotein)
	Polymyositis	Nonhistone ANA
	Pernicious anemia	Antiparietal cell, microsomes, and intrinsic factor ABs
	Adiopathic Addison's disease	Humoral and (?) cell-mediated adrenal cytotoxicity
	Infertility (some cases)	Antispermatozoal Abs
	Glomerulonephritis	Glomerular basement membrane Ab, or immune complexes
	Bullous pemphigoid	IgG and complement in basement membrane
	Sjögren's syndrome	Multiple tissue Abs, a special nonhistone ANA (SS-B)
	Diabetes mellitus (some)	Cell-mediated and humoral islet cell Abs
	Adrenergic drug resistance (some with asthma or cystic fibrosis)	*beta*-Adrenergic receptor Ab
Possible	Chronic active hepatitis	Smooth muscle Ab
	Primary biliary cirrhosis	Mitochondrial Ab
	Other endocrine gland failure	Specific tissue Abs in some cases
	Vitiligo	Melanocyte Ab
	Vasculitis	Some cases: Ig and complement in vessel walls, low serum complement
	Post-MI, cardiotomy syndrome	Myocardial Ab
	Urticaria, atopic dermatitis, asthma (some cases)	IgG and IgM Abs to IgE
	Many other inflammatory, granulomatous, degenerative, and atrophic disorders	No reasonable alternative explanation

*From *The Merck Manual of Diagnosis and Therapy*, Edition 16, p. 340, edited by Robert Berkow. Copyright 1992 by Merck & Co, Inc, Rahway, NJ. Used with permission.

†ANA = antinuclear antibody; Ab = antibody; Ag = antigen; Ig = immunoglobulin; TSH = thyroid-stimulating hormone.

with particular autoimmune diseases, such as rheumatoid arthritis, systemic lupus erythematosus, scleroderma, and dermatomyositis.

Johan van Mikulicz Radecki first described a patient with enlargement of the lacrimal and salivary glands in 1888. In 1933, Henrik Sjögren described the association of keratoconjunctivitis sicca with xerostomia, and rheumatoid arthritis.

The exact prevalence of primary Sjögren's syndrome in the general population is an issue of debate, because of varying inclusion criteria. Using serologic antibody markers in random blood donors, frequency is approximated at 1 in 2500. Ninety percent of patients are women and there is a strong association with the histocompatibility antigens HLA-B8 and HLA-DR3. Etiologic factors considered include viral infection, genetic factors, and abnormalities of immune regulation.[1,2]

Clinical features of Sjögren's syndrome include dry, itchy, or painful eyes; if severe, it may lead to filamentary keratitis in which there are epithelial filaments of varying sizes and length on the corneal surface. Oral symptoms include xerostomia that requires patients to drink water to swallow food and oral pain. Involvement of the exocrine glands of the upper respiratory tract leads to dryness of the nasal passages and tracheobronchial tree. Patients may complain of hoarseness, chronic cough, and dysphagia. Other features may include dry skin, hypothyroidism, and nephrocalcinosis.

On examination, the patients will have decreased tearing as measured by a Shirmer I test (<6 mm/5 min). Instillation of Rose Bengal dye in the lower conjunctival sac will give a "raccoon" appearance, as the dye is retained in areas of devitalized conjunctiva and corneal epithelium. Oral examination will show lack of normal salivary pooling sublingually. In addition, patients may have caries, erythema of the hard palate, and oral candidiasis, as well as angular cheilitis. Examination of the neck may reveal enlarged parotid glands and possible adenopathy.

Swallowing complaints in Sjögren's syndrome patients include food getting stuck in the oral cavity and oropharynx in contrast to the substernal level as reported by scleroderma patients. Heartburn and discomfort in the distal esophagus may also be reported. Saliva normally functions to lubricate the bolus. In Sjögren's syndrome patients, there is lack of unstimulated and stimulated salivary flow. A decrease of 33% in salivary flow was correlated with a subjective sensation of dysphagia.[3] The basic pH of saliva also functions to neutralize stomach acid. Its absence contributes to the heartburn sensation. Gastric biopsies in Sjögren's syndrome patients also show an increased incidence of chronic atrophic gastritis; they may also have elevated serum gastrin and decreased pepsinogen levels. This all results in a lower pH in the stomach. Abnormal esophageal motility has recently been demonstrated including defective peristalsis in more than 30% of Sjögren's syndrome patients.[3] It most closely correlates with severe dysphagia.

Laboratory findings may include leukopenia (WBC < 4000/mm^3) and increased levels of paraproteins and cryoglobulins. A polyclonal hypergammaglobulinemia is seen in 50% of patients. Antinuclear antibodies in a speckled or homogeneous pattern are present in 65% of patients. Rheumatoid factors are present in 90% of cases. Antibodies to the salivary gland duct antigens, SS-A and SS-B are also detected but are not specific to Sjögren's syndrome, as they are found in rheumatoid arthritis without Sjögren's syndrome and in systemic lupus erythematosus. Diagnosis of Sjögren's syndrome is made based upon demonstration of an elevated number of lymphocytic foci in parotid or minor salivary gland biopsy specimens.[2]

Swallowing complaints are addressed with symptomatic therapy. Avoidance of medications with anticholinergic effects is advised. The patient must drink frequently to lubricate food and prevent caries. Artificial saliva preparations and oral pilocarpine may also be of benefit. Antacids, H2 blockers, proton pump inhibitors, and prokinetic agents are helpful in treating the gastroesophageal reflux (GER) symptoms. The recent finding of defective peristalsis suggests that medications used for other esophageal motility disorders may be helpful in Sjögren's syndrome patients with severe dysphagia. Systemic corticosteroids and cytotoxic drugs are reserved for the life-threatening involvement of the lungs, kidneys, or central nervous system and are generally not used for dysphagia.

B. Rheumatoid Arthritis

Rheumatoid arthritis is a chronic relapsing inflammatory arthritis, usually affecting multiple diarthrodial joints with a varying degree of systemic involvement. The female to male ratio is 3:1. The peak prevalence is at 35 to 45 years of age. Polygenic inheritance appears to prevail, as does the association with HLA-DR4 major histocompatibility antigen.

Soranus made descriptions of RA as early as the second century AD, although it was not until more recently that it became known as a clear-cut entity. An estimated prevalence in 1994 was 5 million cases in the United States, slightly less than 1% of the population. The lifetime costs associated with rheumatoid arthritis exceeded $32000 per case in 1994 dollars.

Etiological factors in rheumatoid arthritis include genetics, hormones, and psychosomatic factors. The exact etiology is unknown. Theories include production of antibodies reactive to the Epstein-Barr virus and to joints, with the latter the primary area of involvement. The inflammatory response is believed to be due to immune complexes composed of altered IgG and anti-IgG rheumatoid factors in synovial fluid.

Clinical features consist of lymphadenopathy, weight loss, low-grade fever, morning stiffness, and fatigue. Presentation may be rapid or insidious; it may involve a single or multiple joints, including the cervical spine. Manifestations on physical examination include ulnar deviation of the fingers, "boutonniere" deformity, subcutaneous nodules, and nail fold thrombi. Other manifestations are pleurisy, pulmonary fibrosis, pericarditis, nerve entrapment syndromes, Sjögren's syndrome, and dysphagia. rheumatoid arthritis is the most common disease associated with secondary Sjögren's.

Laboratory abnormalities in rheumatoid arthritis include the presence of rheumatoid factors, antinuclear antibodies, C1q binding, and sometimes a depressed total hemolytic complement level. Diagnosis of rheumatoid arthritis is made according to the American Rheumatism Criteria (Table 29-2).[4] Seven criteria are required for classic rheumatoid arthritis, with 5 needed for the diagnosis of definite rheumatoid arthritis and 3 for probable rheumatoid arthritis. Symptoms and signs must be present for at least 6 weeks.

Juvenile rheumatoid arthritis is a variant that occurs in individuals younger than 16 years and can be classified based on modes of onset. Its immunologic and etiologic features are similar to rheumatoid arthritis. Seventy percent of patients with the juvenile form, however, have spontaneous and permanent remission by adulthood.

The dysphagia associated with rheumatoid arthritis is related to xerostomia, temporomandibular joint (TMJ) arthritis, a decrease in the amplitude of the peristaltic pressure complex in the proximal, striated part of the esophagus, as well as from cervical spine arthritic

Table 29-2. *American Rheumatism Criteria for Rheumatoid Arthritis*†*

1. Morning stiffness
2. Pain on motion or tenderness in at least 1 joint
3. Swelling of at least 1 joint
4. Swelling of at least 1 other joint
5. Symmetrical joint swelling of the same joint, right and left
6. Subcutaneous nodules
7. Roentgenographic changes typical of RA
8. A positive serum test for rheumatoid factors
9. Poor mucin clotting of synovial fluid
10. Characteristic histological changes in RA

*Seven criteria are required for classic rheumatoid arthritis, while five are needed for the diagnosis of definite rheumatoid arthritis and three for probable rheumatoid arthritis. Symptoms and signs must be present for at least 6 weeks.

†From Condemi JJ. The autoimmune diseases (review). *JAMA.* 1992;268: 2882-2892. Used with permission.

disease. Approximately 28% of patients with rheumatoid arthritis complain of dysphagia; 21% complain of xerostomia. Dysphagia correlates with disease severity.[5] Rheumatic laryngeal involvement such as cricoarytenoid joint fixation is also common in rheumatoid arthritis. Thirty-five percent of patients with laryngeal involvement have dysphagia.

Treatment of the dysphagia is focused on hydration and artificial saliva for the xerostomia. TMJ dysfunction (ie, trismus, mastication problems) is treated with nonsteroidal anti-inflammatory agents and mechanical exercises. Corticosteroids are reserved for severe disease. Local injections into the TMJ may be helpful in selected cases. Management of the systemic effects of rheumatoid arthritis that have persisted for greater than 3-6 months with sulfasalazine, antimalarials, and intramuscular gold injections may also help the dysphagia. Methotrexate, azathioprine, and penicillamine have also been used, but adverse effects are common. Cyclophosphamide is reserved for extreme cases.

C. Progressive Systemic Sclerosis

Systemic sclerosis (scleroderma) is a diffuse disorder characterized by progressive fibrosis and vascular changes. Most notably, there is a thickening of the skin, but there can also be variable involvement of the internal organs such as the gastrointestinal tract, the heart, lungs, and kidneys.

The estimated incidence is about 8 per million per year. Women are affected 4 times more commonly than men are and all racial groups are affected equally. The incidence is highest for those individuals between the ages of 30 and 50.

The underlying target and effector arms of this autoimmune disease have not been elucidated, although the presence of certain nuclear antibodies is associated with scleroderma. It appears as if T-cell hyperactivity may bring about both the vascular changes and the collagen overproduction.

Systemic sclerosis has several clinical patterns that range from mild and insidious skin thickening to severe and rapidly progressive internal organ fibrosis, which can be fatal. The CREST syndrome (calcinosis, Raynaud's phenomenon, esophageal dysmotility, sclerodactyly, telangiectasias) is just one clinical subtype of scleroderma with limited skin involvement.

The fact that hypomotility is so prevalent and demonstrable so early has made it a useful diagnostic feature. Barium swallow has purposefully not been mentioned, as it is considered insensitive and is not likely to detect esophageal stricture. The commonest and the earliest symptom in people with progressive systemic sclerosis is Raynaud's phenomenon.[10] Patients will complain of numb, cold, or tingling fingers secondary to cold exposure. Classically, a three-stage process evolves over a half-hour period. The attack commences with pallor and sweating of the fingers or hands and then moves to a phase of cyanosis and pain. Finally, the skin turns red and the patient experiences tingling, throbbing, and edema. Dysphagia is the second most common symptom of this disorder. Dysphagia is usually first noticed while swallowing solids or taking liquids while recumbent.

There are several proposed mechanisms by which these patients experience dysphagia.[6] The swallowing disorder is primarily due to poor motility through the inferior two thirds of the esophagus. The easiest mechanism to understand is the fibrotic sclerosing of the intramural smooth muscle. This is in keeping with the changes seen in the skin or any of the other organs affected by the systemic process. However, earlier in the course of the disease, when fibrosis is not so prevalent, many patients may demonstrate esophageal motility disorders. It is thought that the process may start as a neuropathic process affecting the intramural nerve (Auerbach's) plexus that coordinates the smooth muscle activity. Later, a myopathic process may develop. Lastly, in the late stages of the disease one may find lower esophageal stricture secondary to peptic ulceration. Lower esophageal sphincter incompetence is well known in this disease and years of gastroesophageal reflux (GER) may culminate in Barrett's esophagitis or stricture. Some have even speculated that very tight sclerodermatous skin around the neck or sclerodermatous involvement of the upper esophageal sphincter could result in transfer dysphagia and nasal regurgitation.[7]

Esophageal dysfunction can be shown by manometry (Figure 29-1), cineradiography, and radionuclide scintigraphy.[8] A cross-sectional study of 300 patients showed esophageal hypomotility in more than 80% of

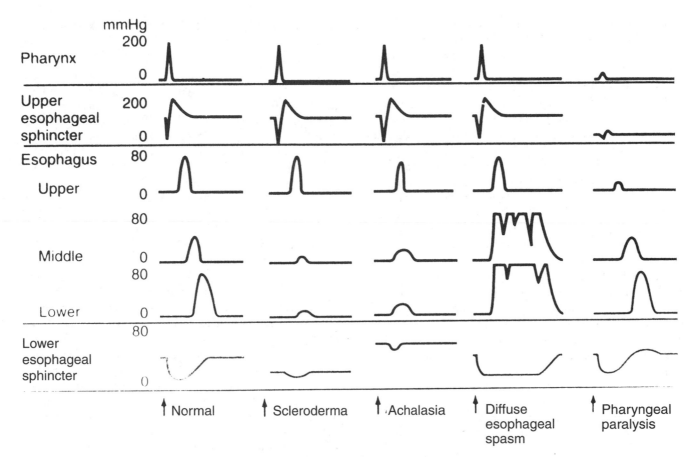

FIG 29-1. Motility patterns in selected esophageal and pharyngeal disorders. In normal subjects, the upper and lower esophageal sphincters appear as zones of high pressure. With a swallow, pressure in the sphincters falls and a contraction wave starts in the pharynx and progresses down the esophagus. In scleroderma, the lower part of the esophagus (smooth muscle) shows a reduced amplitude of contractions, which may be peristaltic or simultaneous in onset, and hypotension in the lower sphincter. In diffuse esophageal spasm, the lower part of the esophagus shows simultaneous-onset, large-amplitude, prolonged, repetitive contractions. (From Goyal RK. Diseases of the esophagus. In: Fauci AS, ed. *Harrison's Principles of Internal Medicine.* 14th ed. McGraw-Hill; 1998:1588-1596. Used with permission.)

the sample.[6,9] Although the severity of the dysphagia correlates with that of the hypomotility, it is important to note that the hypomotility precedes the symptoms of dysphagia. Roughly half of the patients with a demonstrable delay in esophageal transit will not have dysphagia.

The diagnosis can often be made on clinical grounds in a patient who has sclerotic skin above the wrist (90% specific) and at least one of the following features: esophageal dysmotility, Raynaud's phenomenon, restrictive lung disease, arthritis, contractures, pericarditis, and small or large bowel involvement. Various antinuclear antibody (ANA) tests are also useful.[4] Patient sera will often produce a speckled nuclear or a nucleolar staining pattern on fixed tissue substrates when detected by indirect immunofluorescence. This nonspecific finding is present in 90% of patients. The anticentromere antibody is relatively sensitive and specific for that subset of patients with the CREST syndrome and may be present from an early stage.

There is no proven treatment for scleroderma.[10] D-penicillamine has received some cautious optimism, but it is not well tolerated and its efficacy appears to be limited to early diffuse scleroderma with minimal internal organ involvement. The management of this disease is almost exclusively symptomatic and supportive. The dysphagia can be minimized by diligent chewing and by reducing the bolus size. Esophageal motility can be improved by metoclopramide or cisapride. For the uncommon occurrence of esophageal stricture, mechanical dilation can be tried. The reflux esophagitis can be treated by the standard lifestyle and dietary modifications, with or without the addition of antacids and/or various acid secretion inhibitors.

D. Systemic Lupus Erythematosus (SLE)

Systemic lupus erythematosus is a multi-system, inflammatory disorder that is associated with a variety of autoantibodies against many different tissue components. The incidence of newly diagnosed cases is 8 per 100 000 per year. Generally, the disease runs a chronic course yielding a prevalence of 1 per 2000. The prevalence is approximately 9 times higher in women than in men and affects African American women more than their white counterparts. The highest prevalence of 1 in 250 is found in African American women between the ages of 20 and 64.[4]

There is a myriad of clinical findings associated with the disorder. Common nonspecific manifestations include Raynaud's phenomenon, fever, fatigue, malaise, weight loss, splenomegaly, lymphadenopathy, and signs of vasculitis. On the other hand, there are less common symptoms and signs that are more specific to the disease. These include malar rash, discoid rash, photosensitivity, painless oral ulcers, nonerosive arthritis, serositis such as pleuritis or pericarditis, renal disorder, seizures, psychosis, hemolytic anemia, leukopenia, and thrombocytopenia. Almost all patients will have circulating antinuclear antibodies detected by indirect immunofluorescence. Antinuclear antibodies are relatively more specific for SLE if they are present in high concentration. One particular antibody, antidouble stranded DNA is highly specific to SLE. There are many more immunological associations with this disease that are not specific and are found in many other collagen-vascular disorders. They are interesting to note because they either elucidate pathophysiological phenomena or explain abnormal laboratory results. For instance, tissue deposition of circulating immune complexes with the subsequent activation of complement and resultant depressions of complement levels are important in the development of renal insufficiency and some of the dermatological manifestations of SLE.

Despite the multitude of nonspecific clinical manifestations of SLE, deglutition disorders are uncommon. The incidence of dysphagia in several groups of patients have ranged from 1.5% to 12%.[9] No studies have specifically addressed this issue, but, nevertheless, several case reports describe patients with dysphagia and/or chest pain attributed to esophageal dysmotility. Manometry has shown multi-peak, broad, high amplitude contractions associated with retrosternal pressure. These findings are typical of diffuse esophageal spasm (Fig 29-1).[8] Other reports have shown mild esophageal dilation, diminution of peristalsis and, on occasion, this has been associated with manometric characteristics typically seen in scleroderma: impaired or absent peristalsis in conjunction with lower esophageal sphincter pressure. To reiterate, the vast majority of SLE patients do not experience dysphagia and have normal esophageal transit studies.

Treatment of the underlying disorder ranges from nonsteroidal anti-inflammatory agents, through the antimalarials to prednisone. In severe unresponsive cases, high-dose steroid therapy and other immunomodulators such as cyclophosphamide have been administered.

E. Polymyositis and Dermatomyositis

This group of disorders is characterized by skeletal muscle inflammation. The muscle is damaged by an inflammatory infiltrate of lymphocytes and plasma cells that typically results in symmetrical weakness, with the proximal muscles being most affected. The diagnosis is usually confirmed by detecting an increased concentration of serum creatine phosphokinase and transaminase. Electromyography (EMG) will direct the physician to the optimal site for a muscle biopsy, the histopathology of which can be diagnostic. The etiology is considered to be autoimmune and is associated with a variety of antinuclear antibodies. Focal deposits of IgG, IgM and complement have been detected in the muscle and skin of patients with dermatomyositis. These disorders have also been associated with viral infections such as influenza, coxsackievirus, rubella, and HIV.

The incidence is less than scleroderma or systemic lupus erythematosus. The annual incidence was estimated at eight cases per million people in a recent Swedish study.[25] Females are affected twice as often as males. The commonest age of onset is from 40 to 60 years.

Although dysphagia does not feature prominently in descriptions of this disease, a couple of series have shown that about two thirds of these patients have demonstrable delayed esophageal transit.[11] These findings have prompted investigators to speculate that the esophageal smooth muscle may be involved in the inflammatory process. Another report described three patients with pharyngeal dysphagia who on subsequent biopsy of their cricopharyngeus and omohyoid muscles were seen to have an inflammatory myopathy.[12] The videofluoroscopic swallow study showed prominence of the cricopharyngeus muscle, decreased epiglottic tilt and moderate or severe residue in the pharyngeal recesses. Neither of these descriptions is intuitively typical. First, the inflammatory process usually attacks skeletal muscle as opposed to smooth muscle. Second, the inflammatory process predominantly affects limb girdle muscles as opposed to small muscles within the neck. Given that these muscles were affected, theoretically a myositic process could affect any muscle of importance to any stage of swallowing.

Polymyositis and dermatomyositis are treated with corticosteroids. Progress is gauged by muscle strength and by following creatine phosphokinase levels. Azathioprine is added if the response to steroids is inadequate. In about 10% of adult cases, the disease is associated with malignancy. In these cases, resection will lead to an improvement of the myositis. It is unclear how these therapies relate to the swallowing disorders described above.

F. Mixed Connective Tissue Disease

The diagnosis and classification of many of autoimmune collagen-vascular disease is frequently difficult and confusing. Many clinical features and laboratory studies can be found in several of the disorders and often there is an overlap of features from several disorders. It has become clear that some patients do indeed have an overlap syndrome of several disorders. Mixed connective tissue disease is characterized by features of progressive systemic sclerosis, systemic lupus erythematosus, and polymyositis/dermatomyositis. Just as in these 3 entities, one sees the presence of antinuclear antibodies and autoantibodies specifically to ribonucleoproteins, so too one sees these findings in mixed connective tissue disease. Similarly, the swallowing disorders described under each of the component disorders can occur in mixed connective tissue disease. Of the 3 component entities, scleroderma is the most closely associated with a swallowing disorder and, thus, it stands to reason that most of the deglutition disorders of mixed connective tissue disease closely resemble those of scleroderma. Usually the frequency of these phenomena and their intensity are reduced in mixed connective tissue disease compared to scleroderma.

In a recent study of 34 mixed connective tissue disease patients, heartburn and dysphagia were identified in a third to a half of the patients. Almost two thirds had no peristalsis or low-amplitude peristalsis. Ten patients were prospectively studied before corticosteroid therapy. It appeared that the dysmotility was responsive to this medical therapy.[26]

G. Giant Cell Arteritis

Giant cell arteritis, also known as temporal arteritis, is an inflammatory disorder of vessels that originate from the arch of the aorta, but that can also affect more peripheral arteries. Almost every patient is 50 years or older.[13] The disease is closely associated with the clinical syndrome of polymyalgia rheumatica in which there is aching and morning stiffness in the torso and proximal extremities. The annual incidence of temporal arteritis is about 20 per 100 000 population over the age of 50. Northern Europeans and their descendants have a higher incidence.

The clinical presentation varies widely but a severe piercing headache is the commonest symptom (70%-90%). Another well-known symptom is visual disturbance (blurred vision, diplopia, visual loss) occurring in 20% to 40% of individuals. The incidence of blindness is about 15%, but it is relatively rare if not developed before the commencement of steroid therapy, hence the need to expeditiously confirm the diagnosis and commence prednisone (50 mg daily) promptly. In an attempt to confirm the diagnosis, an erythrocyte sedimentation rate (greater than 50 mm/hr) should be sought before commencing therapy, and a superficial temporal artery biopsy should be obtained as soon as convenient, but certainly within 10 days of starting the prednisone.

For diagnosis, the superficial temporal artery is most frequently biopsied. Microscopic examination shows granulomatous inflammation of the intima and inner part of the media: lymphocytes, epithelioid cells, and giant cells predominate. The intima becomes thickened and in so doing narrows the vessels and can eventually occlude the vessel. Many of the symptoms of temporal arteritis are directly attributed to this process. Blindness may be the result of ophthalmic arteritis; temporal artery tenderness and headache can be due to vasculitis of the superficial temporal artery. None of the branches of the external carotid artery are immune from this process. When the ascending pharyngeal artery, the lingual artery, or the deep temporal and the masseteric artery are affected, dysphagia secondary to deglutition claudication, tongue claudication, or jaw claudication can ensue. Masticatory claudication is common and is experienced by roughly half to two thirds of those with temporal arteritis.[13,14] Lingual and/or deglutition claudication is not common and is experienced by slightly fewer than 10% of patients. Treatment of the temporal arteritis with prednisone will resolve the dysphagia within 1 to 2 weeks.[15] Rarely, marked narrowing of the vessel can lead to gangrene of the tongue.

H. Autoimmune Bullous Diseases

Autoimmune bullous disorders are a heterogeneous group of rare disorders that are caused by direct antibody, immune complex, or complement deposition. The clinical characteristics depend on the epidermal, subepidermal, or mucosal involvement. The latter is the main cause of swallowing dysfunction. Autoimmune bullous disorders include pemphigus, bullous pemphigoid, cicatricial pemphigoid, herpes gestationis, epidermolysis bullosa acquisita, bullous systemic lupus erythematosus, dermatitis herpetiformis, and linear immunoglobulin A bullous dermatosis. Of these, cicatricial pemphigoid, herpes gestationis, and dermatitis herpetiformis have minimal to no involvement of the mucosa. The following discussion thus focuses on the remaining group.

1. Pemphigus

Pemphigus vulgaris is a rare, chronic intraepidermal bullous disease. The worldwide incidence is 0.1-0.5 cases per 100 000 population. It is more common among Ashkenazi Jews. Pemphigus is caused by immunoglobulin G (IgG) directed against desmoglein 3 in skin and mucosal desmosomes. This results in splitting in the suprabasilar layer. Histologically, the hallmark is loss of cohesion among keratinocytes or epithelial mucosal cells with clumps of acantholytic cells floating in the blister fluid.

Oral lesions precede cutaneous disease in 70% of cases. The oral cavity is the only site of involvement in 50% of cases. Most commonly, the lesions are on the soft palate but can occur anywhere on the oral cavity. The typical lesion is a fluid-filled blister; these rapidly burst leaving painful ulcerations, which typically heal very slowly. Distal involvement of the pharynx, larynx, and esophagus is possible and may account for the dysphagia noted by some patients.

Treatment of pemphigus is primarily with corticosteroids (prednisone 1.0-2.5 mg/kg/day). Adjuvant therapy includes cyclosporine, methotrexate, gold, azathioprine, cyclophosphamide, and plasmapheresis. Dehydration is common because of skin blistering and inadequate oral intake secondary to pain; this may necessitate hospitalization and admission to a burn unit for wound care and monitoring of electrolytes.[16] Topical anesthetic agents may help improve oral intake.

2. Cicatricial Pemphigoid

Cicatricial pemphigoid is a chronic blistering disease that affects the oral mucosa in up to 100% of cases. There is smooth-bordered erosion of the gingiva and buccal mucosa that tend not to be as painful as those in pemphigus. As the targeted proteins are found in the basement-membrane zone (bullous pemphigoid antigen 2 and epiligrin), the lesions heal with scarring. Ocular lesions are also very common. The disease is quite refractory to therapy, which includes systemic corticosteroids and, in some cases, cyclophosphamide.[17]

3. Epidermolysis Bullosa Acquisita

Epidermolysis bullosa acquisita is a rare disorder with variable onset and no racial or gender predilection. The antigen targeted is type VII collagen. The skin is fragile and blisters form on the dorsal hands and feet, knees and elbows. The oral cavity, larynx, and esophagus may be severely affected, resulting in severe dysphagia and nutrition problems including protein-energy malnutrition, anemia, and vitamin/mineral deficiency. Esophageal webs have been reported necessitating direct gastrostomy feeding.[18] The disease is often refractory to standard therapy using corticosteroids and dapsone. Other therapies have included colchicine, immunoglobulin, and extracorporeal photochemotherapy.

4. Others

Bullous systemic lupus erythematosus occurs with active systemic lupus erythematosus, most commonly in African American women, and is discussed further elsewhere in the chapter. Adult and childhood linear IgA bullous dermatosis is a rare, subepidermal vesiculobullous disease in which there is deposition of IgA along the basement membrane. Mucosal involvement

is common and requires high doses of dapsone; resistant cases require corticosteroids.

I. Wegener's Granulomatosis

Wegener's granulomatosis is a disease characterized by a granulomatous arteritis involving the upper and lower respiratory tracts, progressive glomerulonephritis, and extrarespiratory symptoms attributable to systemic small vessel arteritis.[19] Upper and lower respiratory tract symptoms are found in over 90% of patients. Other manifestations include weight loss, fatigue, fever, ocular symptoms, neuropathies, dermatologic, and musculoskeletal findings. Gastrointestinal manifestations are rare. Case reports describe small intestine disease, colonic involvement, pancreatitis, and esophageal involvement. Laryngeal involvement is also rare and is usually subglottic. Oral lesions are more common and include hyperplastic gingivitis, ulcerations, and soft tissue masses especially on the hard and soft palate; this accounts for most of the swallowing abnormalities encountered. Treatment consists of systemic corticosteroids, as well as cyclophosphamide.

J. Sarcoidosis

Sarcoidosis is a chronic multi-system disorder of unknown etiology; it is presumed to have an autoimmune basis, although this has not yet been elucidated. The pharynx and esophagus are rarely involved; the larynx is involved in 5% of cases, most often supraglottically.[20] Causes of dysphagia include laryngeal involvement, extrinsic compression of the esophagus by mediastinal adenopathy, dysmotility from myopathy, infiltration of Auerbach's plexus, or granulomatous infiltration of the esophageal wall producing long esophageal strictures (Fig 29-2).[21] Esophageal manometry may aid in quantifying the degree of dysphagia, as well as in determining efficacy of therapy. Treatment consists primarily of corticosteroids systemically and intralesionally. Dilatation or surgical correction of esophageal strictures may be necessary.

K. Crohn's Disease

Although it most often involves the terminal ileum, Crohn's disease may additionally involve the oropharynx and esophagus. The pathogenesis has not been fully elucidated but immune complex deposition into vessel walls has been proposed as the cause of the spectrum of the disease. The oral lesions of Crohn's disease vary in appearance. Macroscopically, they may resemble apthous ulcers or cheilitis. Differential diagnosis includes neoplasia, sarcoidosis, tuberculosis, syphilis,

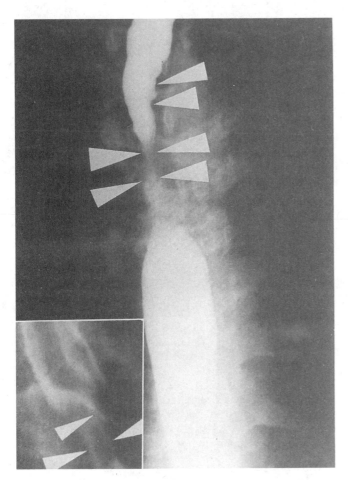

Fig 29-2. An upper gastrointestinal series in the patient with dysphagia associated with chronic sarcoid revealed narrowing of the esophageal lumen and transient hang-up of the barium column at the level of the carina (*arrowheads*). The esophageal mucosa appears smooth at the point of narrowing (*opposing arrowheads*). A spot radiograph (*inset*) shows multiple smooth indentations of the barium column in the midesophagus from external compression (*arrowheads*). (From Cappell MS. Endoscopic, radiographic, and manometric findings in dysphagia associated with sarcoid due to extrinsic esophageal compression from subcarinal lymphadenopathy. *American Journal of Gastroenterology.* 1995;90:489-492. Used with permission.)

berylliosis, as well as folate, B12, and iron deficiency.[22] Histologically, lesions contain epithelioid cells, lymphocytic and perivascular infiltrates with lymphohistiocytic cells, neuronal hyperplasia, and lymphangiectasia.

Dysphagia is the most common presenting symptom of esophageal Crohn's disease; patients may also have weight loss, odynophagia, epigastric pain, and chest discomfort.[23] The most frequent radiologic findings include esophageal strictures and fistulous tracts. Endoscopically, there is hyperemia, inflammation, friability, nodular thickening, cobblestoning, ulcerations, and stricturing. The precise diagnosis may not be possible without full thickness biopsy, but may be suspected based on the presence of Crohn's disease in other areas of the gastrointestinal tract.[24]

The clinical course of Crohn's disease is variable and includes some remissions. Patients with primary oropharyngeal involvement need regular follow-up for the possible development of intestinal disease. Painful oral lesions may be treated with topical steroids and analgesics. Intralesional injection of triamcinolone acetonide has been reported as effective as well. Esophageal disease usually responds equivocally to systemic corticosteroids, azathioprine, metronidazole, and sulfasalazine. Esophagectomy is required in 40%-50% of cases.

III. CONCLUSION

The autoimmune disorders encompass a wide variety of diseases. In some of these conditions the precise "self" antigen has been elucidated; in others the autoimmune etiology is still a matter of debate. As a group, the connective tissue diseases and the collagen-vascular diseases, are well represented among the autoimmune disorders. It is doubtful that the concepts of autoimmune diseases and dysphagia are closely linked in the minds of most health care professionals, yet there is strong association. In patients known to suffer from autoimmune disorders, a history of swallowing difficulties should be sought. With dysphagia so common in some of the autoimmune disorders, it behooves health professionals to be aware of the association and to include it in the differential diagnosis of individuals with swallowing complaints.

Frequently Asked Questions

1. Why do people with Sjögren's syndrome develop swallowing disorders?
   A. A systemic autoimmune process results in lymphocytic infiltration of the lacrimal and salivary glands. The latter are consequently unable to provide normal salivary flow rates. When the flow rate decreases by one third or more, swallowing difficulties ensue because of insufficient lubrication of the food bolus. Saliva also acts as an alkaline buffer and deficiency in this role can result in reflux esophagitis. Recently, evidence has emerged that patients who have severe dysphagia are probably experiencing defective peristalsis in addition to poor bolus lubrication.
2. What therapeutic options exist for swallowing disorders secondary to Sjögren's syndrome?
   A. Many symptomatic therapies are available. To improve bolus lubrication, the patient can drink fluids frequently, use artificial saliva prepara-

tions, stimulate salivary flow with pilocarpine, and anticholinergics drugs can be avoided. Gastro-esophageal reflux can be treated with antacids, H2 blockers (eg, ranitidine), proton pump inhibitors (eg, omeprazole), and prokinetic agents (eg, cis-apride). Corticosteroids and cytotoxic drugs are not used for the treatment of dysphagia.

3. Which autoimmune disease is most commonly associated with esophageal abnormalities?

A. Systemic sclerosis (scleroderma or CREST syndrome) is associated with an 80% prevalence of esophageal hypomotility. Only half of those with hypomotility will subjectively experience dysphagia.

4. How does one evaluate esophageal dysmotility in scleroderma?

A. The best modality is esophageal manometry, but cineradiography and radionuclide scintigraphy may also be utilized. The hallmark findings are poor motility in the inferior two thirds of the esophagus and lower esophageal sphincter incompetence.

5. Is systemic lupus erythematosus (SLE) associated with dysphagia?

A. SLE is most prevalent in African American women between the ages of 20 and 64 (1 in 250). Swallowing disorders are uncommon and only occur in 2% to 12% of patients. When it does occur the underlying pathophysiology mimics diffuse esophageal spasm.

6. What swallowing disorders can be anticipated in a patient with rheumatoid arthritis?

A. Approximately one in four patients will complain of dysphagia but the pathophysiology is very varied from case to case. In some it will be secondary to xerostomia (such as in secondary Sjögren's syndrome); in others it could be related to arthritis of the temporomandibular joint. Pain or fixation associated with cricoarytenoid joint arthritis can manifest as dysphagia and dysphonia.

7. Which autoimmune disease is well known to cause swallowing difficulties as a result of painful oral ulcers?

A. Pemphigus vulgaris is a rare muco-cutaneous bullous disease that results from production of IgG against skin and mucosal desmosomes. Oral lesions occur without any skin manifestations in 50% of cases and the oral cavity is the initial site of lesions in 70% of cases. Typically, the soft palate is affected by fluid-filled blisters that burst, leaving painful ulcers. Less commonly, the process can extend distally to involve the pharynx and the esophagus. Most cases are treated with corticosteroids.

References

1. Houck JR. Immunology. In: Lee KJ, ed. *Essential Otolaryngology Head & Neck Surgery.* 6th ed. Norwalk, CT: Appleton & Lange; 1995:289-318.

2. Fox RI. Sjögren's syndrome. In: Kelley WN, Harris ED, Ruddy S, Sledge CB, eds. *Textbook of Rheumatology.* Philadelphia, Pa: WB Saunders Company; 1997:955-968.

3. Anselmino M, Zaninotto G, Costantini M, et al. Esophageal motor function in primary Sjögren's syndrome: correlation with dysphagia and xerostomia. *Dig Dis Sci.* 1997;42:113-118.

4. Condemi JJ. The autoimmune diseases [review]. *JAMA.* 1992;268:2882-2892.

5. Geterud A, Bake B, Bjelle A, Jonsson R, Sandberg N, Ejnell H. Swallowing problems in rheumatoid arthritis. *Acta Otolaryngol Stockh.* 1991;111:1153-1161.

6. Kaye SA, Siraj QH, Agnew J, Hilson A, Black CM. Detection of early asymptomatic esophageal dysfunction in systemic sclerosis using a new scintigraphic grading method. *J of Rheumatol.* 1996;23:297-301.

7. Witt P, Thomas E. Transfer dysphagia in a patient with the rare combination of scleroderma and ankylosing spondylitis. *J Nat Med Assoc.* 1987;79:993-994, 996.

8. Goyal RK. Diseases of the esophagus. In: Fauci AS, ed. *Harrison's Principles of Internal Medicine.* 14th ed. New York, NY: McGraw-Hill; 1998:1588-1596.

9. Waszczykowska E, Kukulski K, Sysa-Jedrzejowska A. Evaluation of esophageal passage in selected connective tissue diseases. *J of Med.* 1997;28:163-174.

10. Seibold JR. Scleroderma. In: Kelley WN, Harris ED, Ruddy S, Sledge CB, eds. *Textbook of Rheumatology.* 5th ed. Philadelphia: WB Saunders Company; 1997:1133-1162.

11. Wang SJ, Lin WY, Hsu CY, Kao CH, Chang CP, Lan JL. Solid phase radionuclide esophageal motility in polymyositis and dermatomyositis. *Kao-Hsiung i Hsueh Ko Hsueh Tsa Chih [Kaohsiung Journal of Medical Sciences].* 1993;9:338-342.

12. Shapiro J, Martin S, DeGirolami U, Goyal R. Inflammatory myopathy causing pharyngeal dysphagia: a new entity. *Ann Otol, Rhinol Laryngol.* 1996;105:331-335.

13. Hunder GG. Giant cell arteritis and polymyalgia rheumatica. In: Kelley WN, ed. *Textbook of Rheumatology.* 5th ed. Philadelphia, Pa: WB Saunders Company; 1997:1123-1132.

14. Huston KA, Hunder GG, Lie JT, Kennedy RH, Elveback LR. Temporal arteritis: a 25-year epidemiologic, clinical, and pathologic study. *Ann Intern Med.* 1978;88:162-167.

15. Watson P. Temporal arteritis—dysphagia and a normal ESR [letter]. *JAMA.* 1984;252:1280-1281.

16. Mignogna MD, Lo Muzio L, Galloro G, Satriano RA, Ruocco V, Bucci E. Oral pemphigus: clinical significance of esophageal involvement: report of eight cases. *Oral Surg, Oral Med, Oral Pathol, Oral Radiol, Endod.* 1997;84:179-184.

17. Rye B, Webb JM. Autoimmune bullous diseases. *Am Fam Physician.* 1997;55:2709-2718.

18. Amarapurkar DN, Amarapurkar AD, Vora IM. Epidermolysis bullosa with esophageal web. *J Assoc Physicians India.* 1996;44:347.

19. Spiera RF, Filippa DA, Bains MS, Paget SA. Esophageal involvement in Wegener's granulomatosis. *Arthritis Rheum.* 1994;37:1404-1407.

20. Cappell MS. Endoscopic, radiographic, and manometric findings in dysphagia associated with sarcoid due to extrinsic esophageal compression from subcarinal lymphadenopathy. *Am J Gastroenterol.* 1995;90:489-492.

21. Geissinger BW, Sharkey MF, Criss DG, Wu WC. Reversible esophageal motility disorder in a patient with sarcoidosis [review]. *American Journal of Gastroenterology.* 1996;91:1423-1426.

22. Johnson DA, Cattau EL Jr, Hancock JE. Primary Crohn's disease of the oropharynx. *Ear Nose Throat J.* 1985;64:534-536.

23. Borum ML, Albert MB. An unusual case of esophageal Crohn's disease and a review of the literature [letter]. *Dig Dis Sci.* 1997;42:424-426.

24. Gaskins RD, Pasquale DN. Granulomatous diseases of the pharynx and esophagus. [review]. *Otolaryngol Clin North Am.* 1982;15:533-538.

25. Weitoft T. Occurrence of polymyositis in the county of Gavelborg Sweden. *Scand J Rheumatol.* 1997;26:104-106.

26. Marshall JB, etal. Gastrointestinal manifestations of mixed connective tissue disease. *Gastroenterology.* 1990;98(5 Pt 1):1232-1238.

CHAPTER 30

■ ■ ■

Neoplasia of the Upper Aerodigestive Tract: Primary Tumors and Secondary Involvement

Johannes J. Fagan, M.B., Ch.B., F.C.S.(SA), M.Med.(Otol)

I. INTRODUCTION

A history of dysphagia or odynophagia should alert the physician to the possibility that a patient might be harboring a neoplasm. These symptoms may also be associated with aspiration, pulmonary infection, dehydration, electrolyte abnormalities, and malnutrition. Such problems may delay treatment of the neoplasm and increase the incidence of postoperative complications.

II. PATHOPHYSIOLOGY

Normal swallowing involves oral preparation of food; propagation of the bolus through the oral cavity, pharynx and esophagus; velopharyngeal competence to prevent nasal reflux and direct the bolus; patency of the upper aerodigestive tract; and protection of the airway from aspiration. Neoplasia may affect any of these components of swallowing by causing distortion, obstruction, reduced mobility, or neuromuscular and sensory dysfunction of the upper aerodigestive tract. Additional factors that might affect swallowing are a reduced appetite, odynophagia, the presence of a tracheostomy or a nasogastric feeding tube, and a poor cough. Patients who experience pain or aspirate may also develop a psychological fear of swallowing.

Squamous cell carcinoma accounts for more than 90% of malignancy encountered in the upper aerodi-

gestive tract and is associated with smoking and alcohol abuse. Other tumors include minor salivary gland tumors; melanoma; lymphoma; Kaposi's sarcoma (associated with AIDS); and sarcomas arising from bone, muscle, fat, or nerve.

Neoplasms may have an exophytic or an endophytic (infiltrating growth) pattern (Table 30-1). Exophytic tumors interfere with swallowing principally by distorting or obstructing the aerodigestive tract. Tumors with an infiltrating growth pattern may cause reduced mobility or fixation of the tongue, soft palate, pharynx, or larynx. Advanced infiltrative tumors may reduce lymphatic and venous drainage, with resulting edema and obstruction of the upper aerodigestive tract. Tumors also affect swallowing by interfering with the afferent fibers (sensory input) from the mucosa of the upper aerodigestive tract by invasion and destruction of mucosal nerve endings, or sensory nerves such as the trigeminal (V), glossopharyngeal (IX), and vagus (X), cranial nerves and their branches. Involvement of motor cranial nerves V (trigeminal), VII (facial, IX (glossopharyngeal), X (vagal), and XII (hypoglossal) also affects swallowing (Table 30-2). Similarly, extrinsic tumors (not arising from the lining of the upper aerodigestive tract) interfere with swallowing by distorting or obstructing the lumen of the aerodigestive tract or by causing sensory or motor dysfunction by invading or stretching cranial nerves. Examples of extrinsic tumors

Table 30-1. *Pathophysiology of Swallowing in Accordance with Tumor Origin and Growth Pattern*

Tumor	Swallowing Pathophysiology
Intrinsic tumor	
• Exophytic growth	Obstruction
	Distortion
	Anesthesia/hypesthesia
• Infiltrating growth	Fixation
	Pain
	Trismus
	Cranial nerve deficits
Extrinsic tumor	
	Compression
	• Obstruction
	• Distortion
	Cranial nerve deficits
	Fixation

Table 30-2. *Clinical Manifestations of Cranial Nerve Deficits*

Dysfunctional Cranial Nerve	Clinical Manifestations
V	Impaired oral preparation and transport
VII	Drooling
	Impaired oral preparation
	Retention in gingivobuccal sulcus
IX & X	Delayed initiation of pharyngeal phase
	Nasal reflux
	Pharyngeal stasis & pooling
	Aspiration
XII	Impaired oral preparation
	Impaired oral transport

include tumors at the skull base, including nerve sheath tumors, paragangliomas, meningiomas, chordomas, or chondrosarcomas, and tumors occurring in the neck, such as cervical lymph node metastasis from malignancy in the head and neck, thyroid and parathyroid neoplasms, lymphoma, and sarcoma. Mediastinal tumors may also affect swallowing by stretching or invading the left recurrent laryngeal nerve (RLN).

A more detailed account of how neoplasms of the head and neck affect swallowing is next detailed in the phases of swallowing (ie, oral phases of bolus preparation and transport, pharyngeal phase, and esophageal phase).[1]

A. Bolus Preparation

Food is fragmented and mixed with saliva into a form and consistency suitable for swallowing. At the end of this phase the tongue gathers the food into a single bolus, and holds it against the anterior palate. Neoplasms may affect cranial nerves that are involved with this phase of swallowing: salivation (VII, IX); lip seal and buccal tone (VII); movement of the jaw (V), tongue (XII), and floor of mouth (V, VII); mucosal sensation (V); and anterior displacement of the soft palate by contraction of the palatoglossus muscle (X). Impaired lip closure causes drooling of oral contents, and reduced buccal tone causes pooling in the gingivobuccal sulcus. Impaired function of the muscles of mastication affects a patient's ability to chew and hypoglossal (XII) paralysis affects the ability of the tongue to manipulate food. Impairment of palatal movement, either by vagal (X) dysfunction or by tumor invasion of the palate, may cause premature and uncontrolled spillage of food into the oropharynx. Neoplasms of the floor of mouth, tongue, or buccal mucosa may by mass effect or by restricting mobility of the tongue and floor of mouth impair a patient's ability to interpose food between the teeth. This may be compounded by reduced sensory input from the oral cavity from mucosal destruction, or invasion of branches of the second or third division of the trigeminal nerve (V2, V3). The ability to chew or to open the mouth may be further impaired by pain or by tumor infiltration of the temporomandibular joint or of the muscles of mastication. Trismus affects the introduction of solid food into the mouth and may restrict the diet to liquids.

B. Oral Transport

Food is propelled towards the oropharynx by the approximation of the tongue against the hard palate in an antero-posterior, wavelike action. Hypoglossal (XII) nerve dysfunction or tumor infiltration of the tongue or muscles of the floor of the mouth may reduce tongue movement and the ability to approximate the tongue to the palate. Tumor invasion of the dorsum of the tongue or involvement of the lingual nerve (V3) may affect sensory input causing premature spillage of the bolus into the pharynx, and, consequently, aspiration.

C. Pharyngeal Phase

Initiation of the pharyngeal phase is dependent on the afferent (sensory) input of the glossopharyngeal (IX) and vagal (X) nerves. Food is propelled across the base of tongue and valleculae and directed by the epiglottis to the pyriform sinuses. Laryngeal protection consists of approximation of the vocal folds, assisted by the epiglottis, aryepiglottic folds, and false folds, and by elevation and anterior displacement of the larynx beneath the base of tongue. Peristaltic contraction of the pharyngeal constrictors, as well the tongue base pump action and larynx elevation, propels the bolus along the hypopharynx through a relaxed cricopharyngeal sphincter and into the proximal esophagus. The pharyngeal phase is dependent on the cranial nerves: velopharyngeal closure (IX, X), pharyngeal peristalsis (X), cricopharyngeus relaxation (X), laryngeal closure (X), pharyngeal sensation (IX, X), and laryngeal sensation (X). Abnormality of the pharyngeal phase may manifest as delayed initiation, nasal reflux, stasis and pooling of food at the level of the pharynx, or aspiration.

Tumors of the base of tongue may reduce sensory input and delay initiation of the swallow. Such patients may aspirate because of leakage of food or liquid into the pharynx prior to closure of the laryngeal inlet (early spillage). Velopharyngeal incompetence (VPI) may result from involvement of the glossopharyngeal (IX) and vagal nerves (X) by tumors at the base of the skull, or by tumor infiltration or destruction of the soft palate. Involvement of cranial nerves IX and X also impairs pharyngeal sensation and pharyngeal constrictor function. Involvement of the recurrent or superior laryngeal nerve by tumors of the pyriform sinus, postcricoid region, esophagus, thyroid gland, or mediastinum may cause both motor and sensory denervation of the hypopharynx and larynx. Denervation of the pharynx also occurs with tumor invasion of pharyngeal mucosa or the pharyngeal nerve plexus.

Tumors of the pharynx may cause an adynamic segment that interferes with peristalsis or laryngeal elevation or may cause mechanical obstruction. Tumor invading or destroying the larynx may cause either an incompetent laryngeal sphincter or sensory denervation of the larynx. The squamous carcinoma in Fig 30-1 caused dysphagia, odynophagia, and aspiration due to invasion and destruction of the base of tongue and epiglottis. The carcinoma of the hypopharynx in Fig 30-2 caused constriction, denervation, and an adynamic pharyngeal segment, as well as recurrent laryngeal nerve paralysis. This caused dysphagia, aspiration (Fig 30-3), and hoarseness.

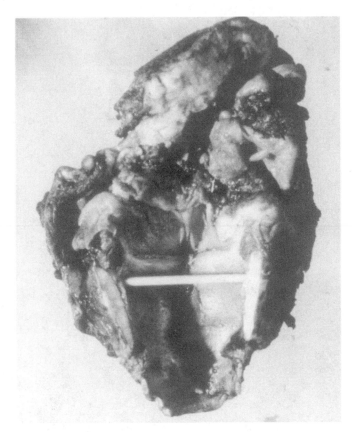

Fig 30-1. Squamous carcinoma invading the base of tongue and destroying the epiglottis.

D. Esophageal Phase

The esophageal phase is characterized by primary and secondary peristalsis and relaxation of the lower esophageal sphincter. Swallowing may be impaired by both intrinsic esophageal neoplasms and extrinsic compression by primary or metastatic tumors of the neck and mediastinum.

Additional factors, such as the presence of a tracheotomy or a nasogastric tube, and the inability to cough (respiratory function) may affect swallowing in patients with neoplasia of the head and neck. Tracheotomy may be required to secure an airway or for pulmonary toilet. Tracheotomy does not guarantee protection from aspiration, but paradoxically may aggravate both dysphagia and aspiration. (See Chapter 20.) It causes tethering of the larynx and trachea and interferes with hyolaryngeal excursion, resulting in aspiration during the pharyngeal phase of swallowing. An inflated tracheotomy cuff may obstruct and cause pooling of food and saliva in the proximal esophagus and cause aspiration. Tracheotomy may also desensitize the larynx and interfere with normal laryngeal protective

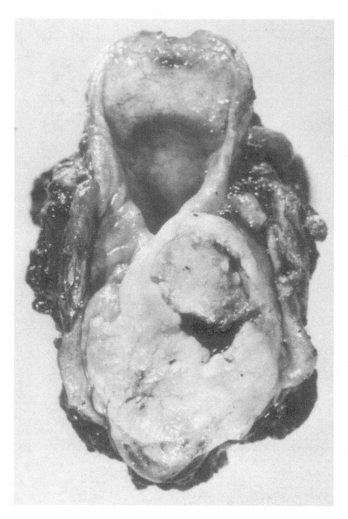

FIG 30-2. Squamous carcinoma of the hypopharynx.

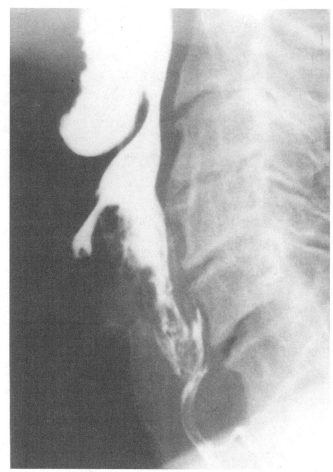

FIG 30-3. Videofluoroscopy demonstrating tumor in the hypopharynx and aspiration.

reflexes.[2] Tracheotomized patients cannot generate high subglottic pressures and, therefore, have an ineffective cough.

The ability to clear aspirated food from the airway may be an additional impairment in patients with diaphragmatic paralysis secondary to neoplastic involvement of the phrenic nerve in the lower neck, or when tumor invasion of the larynx or recurrent laryngeal nerve paralysis prevents forceful glottic closure.

A nasogastric tube may be required to ensure adequate nutrition in patients with tumors of the head and neck but causes incompetence of the upper and lower esophageal sphincters (gastroesophageal reflux), and may aggravate dysphagia. Likewise, gastrostomy tubes facilitate gastroesophageal reflux by causing relaxation of the lower esophageal sphincter and delayed gastric emptying.

III. DIAGNOSIS

In the setting of neoplasia of the head and neck, the cause of dysphagia or odynophagia is usually apparent following a detailed history and examination. The duration and nature of the swallowing disorder, the presence of aspiration, the degree of weight loss, and evidence of malnutrition should be noted. Serum electrolyte and liver function tests may reveal evidence of dehydration, electrolyte abnormality, and malnutrition. Videofluoroscopy may demonstrate mechanical obstruction or incoordination of swallowing, and may delineate the tumor extent and demonstrate aspiration (see Fig 30-3). Chest radiograms may reveal radiological features consistent with aspiration or a mediastinal tumor causing RLN paralysis. The larynx and pharynx is examined by indirect or flexible laryngoscopy (with or without videostroboscopy) or by rigid laryngoscopy. This may reveal superior or recurrent laryngeal nerve dysfunction (X), fixation or ulceration of the larynx, aspiration, or pooling of saliva or food in the hypopharynx. Palpation of the oropharynx with a tongue depressor, or of the hypopharynx and larynx with a flexible nasopharyngoscope, may reveal mucosal hypesthesia or anesthesia. Paralysis of cranial nerves IX, X, or XII necessitates CT scan and/or MRI of the skull base and posterior cranial fossa to determine if there is a tumor.

IV. TREATMENT

The aims of treatment of neoplasia of the head and neck are to cure or palliate the neoplastic process, as well as to preserve or restore swallowing, respiratory function, and speech. Initial treatment is directed at establishing and maintaining an airway; correcting fluid, electrolyte, and nutritional abnormalities; making a pathological diagnosis; and staging the neoplastic process.

Swallowing may be improved by providing analgesia, dietary manipulation, and/or antibiotic therapy if there is associated infection. Swallowing may deteriorate during the course of irradiation therapy because of pain, inflammation, or loss of appetite, and following irradiation, because of fibrosis, scarring, and lack of saliva. Patients who cannot maintain an adequate oral intake are fed by enteral or parenteral routes.

V. PEDIATRIC NEOPLASMS

Neoplasia of the head and neck presents less commonly in the pediatric age group. Examples of malignant tumors include sarcoma, lymphoma, and tumors of the thyroid gland and thyroglossal duct remnants. Hamartomas such as hemangiomas and lymphangiomas may also cause mechanical obstruction of the upper aerodigestive tract. Because infants are obligate nose breathers, tumors causing obstruction of the nose or nasopharynx may cause significant airway obstruction and interfere with feeding.

VI. CONTROVERSIES

The principal controversy relating to swallowing abnormality secondary to neoplasia is on the method of feeding and depends on the anticipated duration of swallowing difficulty and if it is possible to pass a nasogastric feeding tube. Patients who have a prospect of having improved swallowing following treatment are best managed by nasogastric feeding tube. Failure to pass a nasogastric tube beyond a tumor situated in the pharynx or esophagus may be overcome by passage of a feeding tube with rigid esophagoscopy under general anesthesia. When enteral feeding is likely to be prolonged, then a feeding tube may be inserted either by endoscopic or open gastrostomy, or a jejunostomy feeding tube may be placed. (See Chapter 45.) Total parenteral nutrition is reserved for patients who cannot be fed enterally.

Frequently Asked Questions

1. What is the most common malignancy of the upper aerodigestive tract in adults?
   A. Squamous carcinoma
2. In a patient with a neoplasm of the pharynx, a nasogastric feeding tube accomplishes what?
   A. Enteral nutrition
3. The pharyngeal phase of swallowing may commonly be impaired by what?
   A. A neoplasm of the base of the tongue

References

1. Logemann JA. Swallowing physiology and pathophysiology. *Otolaryngol Clin North Am.* 1988;21:613-623.
2. Nash M. Swallowing problems in tracheotomized patients. *Otolaryngol Clin North Am.* 1988;21:701-709.

CHAPTER 31

■ ■ ■

Benign Esophageal Webs and Strictures

Peter F. Ferson, M.D.

I. INTRODUCTION

Swallowing disorders can occur because of benign esophageal strictures. These strictures can occur at any level of the esophagus and from a variety of causes. Appropriate evaluation of these abnormalities is necessary for correct diagnosis. Selection of the best treatment option requires an understanding of the natural history of the abnormality and the expected treatment outcome.

II. HISTORY

As with most surgical intervention, major advances in methods and technology have occurred in the past century. Sporadic reports of earlier attempts to deal with esophageal obstruction, or stricture, do exist, however. Fabricius ab Acquapendente (1537-1619) has been credited with the first effort to dislodge an esophageal foreign body by pushing it with a thin wax taper into the stomach.[1] Boughinhay, an Algerian town that was a medieval center of the wax candle trade, prompted use of to the words "bougie" for the device, "bougienage" for the technique.[1] According to Brown Kelly, other devices developed to impel an impacted bolus of food into the stomach included lead weights and sounds of whalebone or silver tipped with ivory.[2] Several types of dilators have been developed in this century. They are discussed in the section on treatment.

Inspection of the esophagus was first attempted by Bozzini, who had reported examining various body orifices with light transmitted through a hollow tube. Using a wax candle and a mirror as a light source, he performed vaginal and rectal examinations, and in 1806 used his device to inspect the pharynx and possibly the upper esophagus.[3-5] Kussmal recruited a sword swallower as a subject and, in Freiberg in 1868, successfully visualized the esophagus and stomach using a lighted tube designed by Desormeaux for urethroscopy.[4,5]

During the first half of the 20th century, refinements in technique and equipment for rigid esophagoscopy occurred. Many of these refinements can be credited to Chevalier Jackson, whose clinics in Pittsburgh and Philadelphia became world-recognized centers of broncho-esophagology. His descriptions of technique are classics for students of upper aerodigestive disorders.[6] Hirschowitz and colleagues described the use of a flexible fiberoptic gastroscope in 1957.[7] Because of the ease of use of fiberoptic instruments, upper gastrointestinal endoscopy has become a frequently performed procedure that is safe.

III. ETIOLOGY

The causes of esophageal stricture are numerous. They can be grouped into a few general categories—congenital, inflammatory, traumatic, reflux induced, and postsurgical.

Congenital strictures are rare[8-10] and are often go unrecognized during early infancy. They are thought to occur either from incomplete vacuolation[11] or from tracheal remnants, the latter usually causing stricture in the distal esophagus.[12] The actual incidence of congenital esophageal strictures is unclear as many such abnormalities remain relatively asymptomatic until after infancy. Murphy and collegues noted young children and adolescents who presented with late onset of symptoms from congenital strictures.[8] Buse and colleagues noted a patch of congenital heterotopic gastric mucosa as the cause of a cervical esophageal web in a 48-year-old man.[13]

A number of inflammatory disorders have been described in association with upper esophageal stricture. In 1919,[1,13] Brown Kelly and Patterson described upper esophageal stricture in association with glossitis and microcytic anemia.[14,15] This association, which is known in the United Stated as the Plummer-Vinson syndrome, appears most commonly in women[15]; however, it's occurrence in men is described.[17] Other types of inflammatory disorders associated with esophageal stricture include pemphigus, epidermolysis, and rheumatological abnormalities.[2,18-20]

Although penetrating and severe blunt injuries of the neck can damage the cervical esophagus, delayed stricture after such injuries is quite rare. Severe fibrotic stricture has been noted due to injury from foreign bodies lodged in the upper esophagus.[21,22] Lye ingestion has certainly been a relatively frequent cause of extensive stricture of the entire esophagus.[23]

Gastroesophageal reflux (GER) accounts for the majority of benign strictures in the distal esophagus. Patients with reflux-induced stricture nearly always have a history of preceding symptoms of reflux esophagitis. The degree of such stricture can vary greatly. It may appear as a discrete, focal ring immediately above the gastroesophageal junction, as described by Schatski in 1953,[24] or as a longer segment of severe fibrosis. As chronic reflux esophagitis can be accompanied by dysplasia or carcinoma, careful endoscopic evaluation and biopsy are essential when evaluating suspected reflux-induced stricture.

The most common cause of benign narrowing in the upper esophagus is anastomotic stricture following esophageal surgery. In the pediatric population, this occurs following repair of esophageal atresia.[25] In adults, cervical anastomotic stricture follows esophagectomy and reconstruction with gastric or colonic interposition.[26,27] The incidence of anastomotic stricture following esophagectomy is higher with a cervical anastomosis than with an intrathoracic anastomosis, occurring in up to 30% of patients with a cervical procedure.[27] The cause of these strictures is attributed to ischemia in the conduit due to its extended blood supply. Anastomotic leak, which itself may be due to ischemia, is also thought to be a contributing factor to developing a stricture.[27,28]

IV. PATHOLOGIC FINDINGS

Because of the diverse causes of benign esophageal strictures, the pathologic findings are equally varied. In congenital lesions aberrant cartilage may be seen.[8] Devitt describes a "diaphanous" membrane or web as a result of incomplete vacuolation.[11] Pearson notes peptic strictures varying from changes limited to the submucosa to full thickness fibrosis and even extension into the surrounding tissue.[29] Only a surgical resection of the stricture will provide a complete specimen for pathological analysis, and as dilation is the most common treatment, such information is rare.

V. SYMPTOMS

Dysphagia, with or without regurgitation, is the typical clinical manifestation of esophageal stricture. Frequently the patient can identify the level of the stenosis by pointing to where food gets stuck; however, this is not uniformly accurate. In patients with reflux-induced esophagitis with stricture, there may be a history of reflux symptoms; however, they may be only noted as historical symptoms that subsided as fibrosis developed. Symptoms are not always present. In a review of 1000 consecutive cineradiographs of the hypopharynx and cervical esophagus, Nosher and associates found webs in 55 patients, but only 11 patients complained of dysphagia.[30]

VI. EVALUATION

The essential diagnostic procedures to investigate esophageal strictures are radiographic evaluation and esophagoscopy. When reflux disorders are suspected, motility studies are necessary for a complete analysis.

Radiographic analysis is the first method to be employed in evaluation of a suspected esophageal stricture. The progress of contrast medium, either barium or soluble contrast, is observed and recorded as it passes during active swallowing. Individually exposed still images are necessary for reference and comparison during invasive procedures such as endoscopy or surgery. Live fluoroscopic viewing and cineradiographic recording are vital, however, for a proper assessment of the severity of a stricture and the dynamic function of the esophagus. When the exact degree of narrowing is unclear using liquid contrast, the patient may be given a barium-impregnated wafer. This bolus of semi-solid opaque material will more clearly outline the diameter of a stricture than will liquid barium. A measured barium tablet is of significant help in evaluating an eccentric stricture. The diameter of the swallowed tablet which lodges in the stricture will provide an estimate of the maximum size of the narrowing.

Endoscopic evaluation can be performed either with a rigid esophagoscope or, more commonly, with a flexible instrument. Although inspection with a rigid esophagoscope can be performed under local anesthesia, general anesthesia is preferred. The ability to use local anesthesia and the relative ease of passage requiring less technical skill combine to make flexible esophagoscopy more popular. When the stenosis is high in the cervical esophagus, however, rigid esophagoscopy becomes essential to carefully examine the area immediately distal to the cricopharyngeal sphincter.

Proper assessment requires noting the location and severity of the narrow segment. If the involved area can be passed with the esophagoscope, the total length of the abnormality should be noted and then a thorough inspection of the distal esophagus and stomach performed. In the presence of reflux disorders, biopsies to rule out malignancy are crucial.

VII. TREATMENT

Several surgical methods are available for dealing with strictures and webs of the esophagus. Dilation of the stricture is the most common treatment; however, segmental resection[28] for localized narrowing and esophageal bypass, with or without resection for extensive involvement, are also possible. Although endoscopic laser excision has been described,[31] this technique adds little to mechanical bougienage, except complexity and risk.

Dilation of esophageal narrowing is accomplished either by passing serial bougies or by hydrostatic balloon dilation. Both of these techniques can be performed with either local or general anesthesia; but for severe narrowing or during the initial endoscopic evaluation of cervical strictures, general anesthesia is preferred.

Each of the techniques of balloon dilation and bougienage have specific advantages and disadvantages. Balloon dilators can be passed through the working channel of the flexible esophagoscope (Fig 31-1). This allows the procedure to be performed under direct vision with positioning of the balloon directly within the stricture. Once the balloon is inflated, however, the immediate effect cannot be seen, as the partially dis-

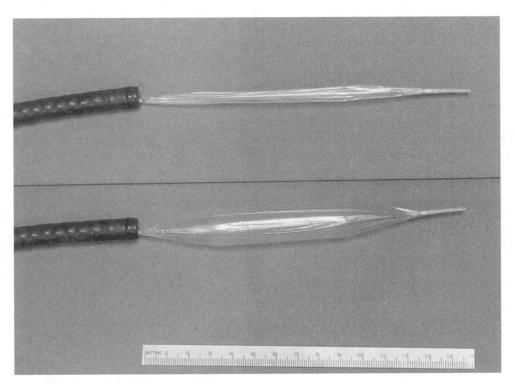

FIG 31-1. This shows a balloon dilation catheter inserted through the working channel of a gastroscope. The top view shows the balloon collapsed and the bottom distended. Note that with the distention of the balloon, the view through the gastroscope would be lost.

tended balloon obscures the view. Although it is not always necessary, fluoroscopy with distention of the balloon using a dilute contrast medium will demonstrate the balloon narrowed into a waist by the stricture (Fig 31-2A). The expansion of this waist gives evidence of a successful dilation (Fig 31-2B).

A number of devices have been used for bougienage, but currently three types of dilators are commonly employed (Fig 31-3). Jackson dilators consist of blunt, tapered flexible tips placed on the end of thin metal shafts, appearing like bananas on a stick. These are passed through a rigid esophagoscope and are only useful for very tight strictures or for gently probing to find the lumen. They are inserted under direct vision, and the maximum diameter is limited by the size of the esophagoscope tube. Maloney mercury weighted, tapered bougies are probably most commonly used. For patients with moderate stricture or for patients requiring chronic repeat dilations, passage of Maloney dilators can be performed rapidly and safely.

Although mercury-weighted bougies can be passed without any adjuncts, fluoroscopic guidance has been variably advocated.[2,32-34] Smaller diameter Maloney dilators, such as might be used to dilate a severe narrowing, are overly flexible and will curl up frequently if passed without fluoroscopic guidance. When a severe narrowing is encountered, wire-guided bougies are more effective. Savory dilators can be serially advanced over a guide wire that has been passed under

direct vision through an esophagoscope. Fluoroscopy is a necessary adjunct to such a procedures. One advantage of the use of bougies over balloon dilation is the ability to directly feel the amount of pressure being applied.

The success of dilation will depend greatly on the nature of the lesion. When there is a thin membrane, a single dilation may be sufficient; however, for fibrotic strictures, particularly anastomotic strictures, repeat dilations are typically necessary. With a very tight fibrotic stricture, it is unwise to attempt to fully expand the luminal diameter at one setting. The risk of rupture or injury, which will result in more significant stenosis, is unacceptably high. The need for multiple dilations is well recognized.[27,35,36] In some patients, chronic repeat interventions are necessary. We have successfully managed a few patients with postesophagectomy anastomotic stricture by teaching them to pass a dilator at home. The technique for swallowing a #38 or #42 Maloney dilator is easily taught and requires no topical anesthesia once the patient is comfortable and familiar with the technique. Passage of a dilator once or twice a week is sufficient to maintain an adequate lumen.

When dilation is performed for a stricture with a treatable cause, such as iron deficiency anemia or acid reflux, correction of the underlying process following dilation is essential. With acid reflux, intense management, frequently by antireflux surgery, is necessary to prevent recurrence of the stricture.

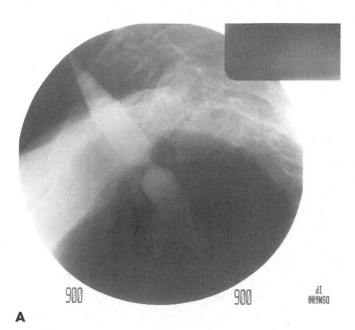

A

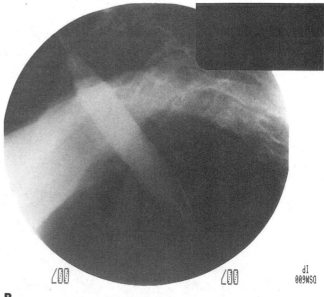

B

FIG 31-2. A. The fluoroscopic image of a balloon catheter across an upper esophageal stricture. The contrast medium within the balloon clearly demonstrating the waist of the balloon where it sits in the stricture. **B.** The stricture now dilated, and smooth contour of the balloon with no remaining stricture. In this instance, fluoroscopy allows visualization of the dilatation process, as the balloon would obscure the visibility through the esophascope.

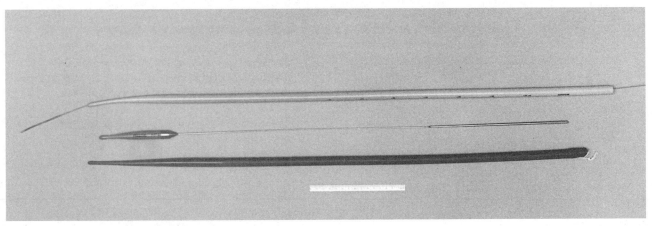

A

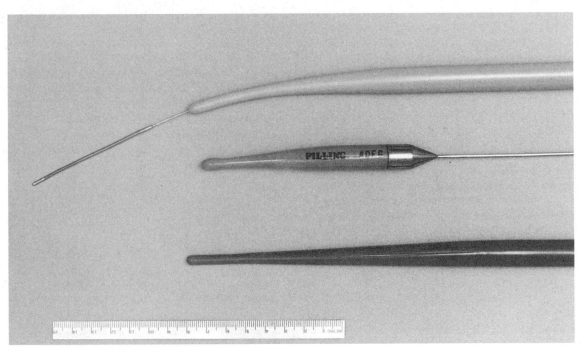

B

Fɪɢ 31-3. **A.** Three bougie type esophageal dilators are shown. At the top is a Savory dilator with a guide wire inserted through it, in the middle is a Jackson dilator, and at the bottom is a mercury-weighted Maloney dilator. **B.** A close-up of the tips of these three dilators, again showing the Savory dilator on top threaded over guide wire, the Jackson dilator in the middle, and the mercury-weighted Maloney dilator on the bottom.

VIII. SUMMARY

A wide variety of abnormalities can result in benign esophageal strictures. When symptoms of dysphagia interfere with normal dietary intake, therapeutic intervention is necessary. Aggressive surgical intervention is rarely needed, as most symptoms can be relieved by dilation. Associated abnormalities such as GER, or iron deficiency anemia, must be corrected to prevent recurrence of symptoms.

Frequently Asked Questions

1. When a benign esophageal stricture is present, is surgical resection necessary?

A. Usually a benign esophageal stricture can be managed by dilation.
2. What is the proper treatment for reflux-induced esophageal stricture?
    A. Patients with benign stricture of the esophagus due to chronic reflux esophagitis can usually be managed by dilation of the structure and control of the acid reflux. If there has been no preceding treatment, intensive medical therapy may be effective in preventing continued reflux and recurrent stricture. More commonly dilation is followed by antireflux surgery.

References

1. Kelly Brown HD. Origins of esophagology, section of laryngology. *Proceedings of the Royal Society of Medicine.* 1969;62:781-786.
2. Nostrant TT. Esophageal dilatation, *Dig Dis.* 1995;13:337-355.
3. Stock CR. Esophagoscopy. *Ear Nose Throat J.* 1985;64:502-503.
4. Berci G. History of endoscopy. In: Berci, G, ed. *Endoscopy.* New York, NY: Appleton-Century-Crofts; 1976:19-23.
5. Grant AK. A century of upper gastrointestinal tract endoscopy. *Med J Aust.* 1973;2:903-906.
6. Jackson C, Jackson CL. *Bronchoesophagology.* Philadelphia, Pa. WB Saunders; 1950:40-67.
7. Hirschowitz BI, Curtiss LE, Peters CW, Pollard HM. Demonstration of a New Gastroscope, the "Fiberscop" Presented at the Annual Meeting of the American Gastroscopic Society, May 16, 1957, Colorado Springs, Colo.
8. Murphy SG, Yazbeck S, Russo P. Isolated congenital esophageal stenosis. *J Pediatr Surg.* 1995;30:1238-1241.
9. Bluestone CD, Kerry R, Sieber WK. Congenital esophageal stenosis. *Laryngoscope.* 1969;79:1095-1103.
10. Postlethwait RW. Other congenital anomalies. In: Postlethwait RW, ed. *Surgery of the Esophagus.* Norwalk Conn: Appleton-Century-Crofts; 1986:39-82.
11. Devitt PG. Oesophageal webs. In: Jamieson GG, ed. *Surgery of the oesophagus.* New York, NY: Churchill Livingstone; 1988:515-518.
12. Foker JE, Boyle EM. Congenital anomalies: other disorders in children. In: Pearson FG, ed. *Esophageal Surgery.* New York, NY: Churchill Livingstone; 1995:184-198.
13. Buse PE, Zuckerman GR, Balfe DM. Cervical esophageal web associated with a patch of heterotopic gastric mucosa. *Abdom Imaging.* 1993;18:227-228.
14. Patterson DR. A clinical type of dysphagia. *J Laryngol.* 1919; August: 289-291.
15. Brown-Kelly A. Spasm at the entrance to the oesophagus. *Laryngol Otol.* 1919;34:285-289.
16. Okamura H, Tsutsumi S, Inaki S, Mori T. Esophageal web in Plummer-Vinson syndrome. *Laryngoscope.* 1988;98:994-998.
17. Miller JDR, Lewis RB. Esophageal webs in men. *Radiology.* 1963;81:498-501.
18. Shamma'a MH, Benedict EB. Esophageal webs: a report of 58 cases and an attempt at classification. *New Eng J Med.* 1958;259:378-384.
19. Sehgal VN, Jain JK, Bhattacharya SN, Broor SL, Mukherjee AK. Esophageal web in generalized epidermolysis bullosa. *Int J Dermatol.* 1991;30:51-52.
20. Seaman WB. The significance of webs in the hypopharynx and upper esophagus. *Radiology.* 1967;89:32-38.
21. Sheen TS, Lee SY. Complete esophageal stricture resulting from a neglected foreign body. *Am J Otolaryngol.* 1996; 17:272-275.
22. Doolin EJ. Esophageal stricture: an uncommon complication of foreign bodies. *Ann Otol Rhinol Laryngol.* 1993;102:863-866.
23. Broor SL, Lahoti D, Bose PP, Ramesh GN, Raju GS, Kumar A. Benign esophageal strictures in children and adolescents: etiology, clinical profile, and results of endoscopic dilation. *Gastrointest Endosc.* 1996;43:474-477.
24. Schatzki R, Gary JE. Dysphagia due to a diaphram-like localized narrowing in the lower esophagus. *Am J Roentgenol.* 1953;70:911-22.
25. Benjamin B, Robb P, Glasson M. Esophageal stricture following esophageal atresia repair: endoscopic assessment and dilation. *Ann Otol Rhinol Laryngol.* 1993;102:332-336.
26. Honkoop P, Siersema PD, Tilanus HW, Stassen LP, Hop HC, van Blankenstein M. Benign anastomotic strictures after transhiatal esophagectomy and cervical esophagogastrostomy: risk factors and management. *J Thorac Cardiovasc Surg.* 1996;111:1141-1146.
27. Pierie JP, de Graaf PW, Poen H, van der Tweel I, Obertop H. Incidence and management of benign anastomotic stricture after cervical oesophagogastrostomy. *Br J Surg.* 1993; 80:471-474.
28. Wu MH, Lai WW, Wu WL, Lin MY, Chou NS. Prevention and management of strictures after hypopharyngocolostomy or esophagocolostomy. *Ann Thorac Surg.* 1994;58:108-111.
29. Pearson FG. Peptic esophagitis stricture, and short esophagus. In: Griffith PF, ed. *Esophageal Surgery.* New York, NY: Churchill Livingstone; 1995:253-265.
30. Nosher JL, Campbell WL, Seaman WB. The clinical significance of cervical esophageal and hypopharyngeal webs. *Radiology.* 1975;117:45-47.
31. Roy GT, Cohen RC, Williams SJ. Endoscopic laser division of an esophageal web in a child. *J Ped Surg.* 1996;31:439-440.
32. Webb WA. Technique of esophageal dilation. *Chest Surg Clin No Am.* 1995;5:471-479.
33. McClave SA, Brady PG, Wright RA, Goldschmid S, Minocha A. Does fluoroscopic guidance for maloney esophageal dilation impact on the clinical endpoint of therapy: relief of dysphagia and achievement of luminal patency. *Gastrointest Endosc.* 1996;43:93-97.
34. Ho SB, Cass O, Katsman RJ, et al. Fluoroscopy is not necessary for Maloney dilation of chronic esophageal strictures. *Gastrointest Endosc.* 1995;41:11-14.
35. Agnew SR, Pandya SP, Reynolds RP, Preiksaitis HG. Predictors for frequent esophageal dilations of benign peptic strictures. *Dig Dis Sci.* 1996;41:931-936.
36. Allmendinger N, Hallisey MJ, Markowitz SK, Hight D, Weiss R. Balloon dilation of esophageal strictures in children. *J Ped Surg.* 1996;31:334-336.

CHAPTER 32

∎ ∎ ∎

Cardiopulmonary Disorders

Robert J. Keenan, M.D., F.R.C.S.(C.)

I. INTRODUCTION

Esophageal disorders, in particular gastroesophageal reflux (GER) disease, may present with atypical signs and symptoms, such as asthma and chronic cough, pneumonitis, interstitial fibrosis, and noncardiac chest pain. Patients may seek advice from primary care physicians, pulmonologists, otolaryngologists, and cardiologists, possibly seeing several physicians before the true nature of their complaint is known. In this chapter, the relationship between these disorders and their presentations are discussed and treatment strategies reviewed.

II. PATHOPHYSIOLOGY

A. Gastroesophageal Reflux Disease

1. Asthma

Gastroesophageal reflux (GER) disease is common among persons with asthma, with a reported prevalence ranging from 34% to 89% .[1] The relationship between GER disease and asthma is complex; GER disease may trigger an asthmatic attack or, alternatively, symptoms of GER disease may worsen during bronchospastic episodes as a result of airway obstruction and transient hyperinflation. Over time, these cycles of reflux and asthma may lead to progressive pulmonary dysfunction.

Two major mechanisms have been proposed by which GER disease may trigger asthmatic reactions. The first is a vagal reflex based on the common embryonic origins of the esophagus and the bronchial tree.[2] Acid in the esophagus could stimulate acid-sensitive receptors and initiate this reflex through shared channels of autonomic innervation. Support for this hypothesis comes from experimental and clinical data. In a canine model, instillation of acid into the distal esophagus produced a measurable increase in airway resistance.[2] This response was ablated after vagotomy. Patients with asthma, other than those with chronic bronchitis, were noted to demonstrate significant reductions in maximum expiratory flow rates following intraesophageal instillation of acid.[3] Other investigators, however, have failed to produce bronchospasm under similar conditions. More recently it has been suggested that the bronchoconstriction response may be a normal protective mechanism in which patients with asthma show a delayed recovery of pulmonary function after stimulation by intraesophageal acid.[4]

Microaspiration of gastric contents has been proposed as a second mechanism by which GER disease triggers asthmatic reactions and was first reported after observations of acute bronchospasm following induction of general anesthesia. Again, experimental and clinical evidence support a role for aspiration. In an anesthetized feline model, intratracheal injection of hydrochloric acid produced a 5-fold increase in inspiratory and expiratory flow resistance.[5] Simultaneous recording of intraesophageal and intratracheal pH demonstrated a decline in tracheal pH associated with reflux events in 3 patients with asthma.[6] Supportive evidence comes from the high prevalence rate of GER disease in patients with pulmonary fibrosis and in adults and children with asthma.[7]

Asthma may also induce or worsen episodes of reflux. Flattening of the diaphragm due to hyperinflation may reduce lower esophageal sphincter (LES) pressure.[8] Treatment of asthma may also impair LES tone. An increase in reported symptoms of heartburn and regurgitation has been described among patients receiving theophylline and systemic beta-agonists. Conversely, bronchodilators have not been found to significantly affect symptomatic reflux in persons with asthma.[1]

A patient's history is critical to establishing a link between GER disease and asthma. All persons with asthma should be questioned about heartburn, dysphagia, regurgitation, or choking. It must be remembered, however, that up to one third of persons with asthma with esophageal dysfunction have been found to have no reflux symptoms. Careful attention should be paid to the factors listed in Table 32-1.

2. Chronic Cough

A variety of ear, nose, and throat problems have been linked with GER disease. They include hoarseness, laryngitis, globus sensation, chronic cough, ulcerations, and carcinoma. Of these, only chronic cough is covered

Table 32-1. *The Varied Presentations of Gastroesophageal Reflux Disease*

A. Typical symptoms of GER disease

　Heartburn
　Regurgitation

Dysphagia

　Water brash

B. Atypical symptoms of GER disease

　Hoarseness
　Chronic cough
　Choking
　Laryngitis

C. Potential symptoms of GER disease in asthma

　Nocturnal cough
　Worsening of asthma:
　After large meals
　In recumbent position
　After alcohol ingestion
　Adult-onset asthma
　Failure to respond to bronchodilator therapy

D. Clinically silent

in this chapter; the other manifestations are discussed in other chapters. (See Chapters 7 and 26.)

Reflux disease is the third leading cause of chronic cough, after sinusitis and asthma. The incidence ranges from 10% to 75% when patients were carefully questioned about symptoms of GER disease. Even without classic symptoms, the association may be identified by esophageal testing. In one study of patients with unexplained chronic cough, intraesophageal pH testing was performed. Eleven of 23 patients had coughing episodes within 3 minutes of acidification of the esophagus.[9] This finding supported the concept of aspiration-induced cough. Other evidence suggests that distal esophageal acidification is the basis of reflux-induced coughing, and there is data to indicate that distension of the distal esophagus, rather than simple acidification, is the responsible mechanism.

3. Atypical Chest Pain

Up to one third of patients with chest pain are found to have nonsignificant coronary artery disease on cardiac catheterization. Early reports suggested that motility disorders such as diffuse esophageal spasm were the most common cause of atypical chest pain. More recently, studies indicate that 25% to 50% of these patients are experiencing symptoms of GER disease.[10,12] In one report, patients who were known to have normal coronary arteries and who had angina-like chest pains underwent ambulatory esophageal pH testing. In 23 of the 50 patients, reflux was demonstrated. Thirteen of the 23 subjects had chest pain during the monitoring and in 12, the onset of chest pain coincided with a reflux episode.[10] The significant contribution of GER disease to atypical chest pain has been confirmed by others.

A particularly difficult problem exists when there is reflux-induced chest pain in patients with known coronary artery disease. Compounding the problem is that medical therapies for angina, such as nitrates or calcium-channel blockers, may reduce LES tone and induce reflux, which can then trigger chest pain episodes. Simultaneous Holter and esophageal pH monitoring can be used to determine the true etiology of chest pain events. In a series of 34 patients, 4 patients had chest pain associated with ischemia. Of the remaining 30 patients, 20 had chest pain in association with reflux episodes.[12] More recently, 45 patients with coronary artery disease and angina-like symptoms at rest were studied. Eighteen patients had pain that could not be attributed to myocardial ischemia and was refractory to aggressive cardiac therapy. The eventual cause was identified as panic disorder in 50%, GER disease in 33%, esophageal dysmotility in 11%, and cholelithiasis in 6%.[13]

The clinical presentation of GER disease-related chest pain may mimic typical angina. It is often substernal and may radiate to the jaw, back, or arms. The pain is usually burning, but may also be characterized as squeezing. Typically, reflux-induced pain lasts from minutes to hours and resolves spontaneously or with the use of antacids. Episodes are frequently nocturnal or postprandial. Unfortunately, none of these characteristics can reliably distinguish reflux-induced pain from myocardial ischemia and both may be found in the same patient. Careful history and diagnostic testing are often necessary to determine the true etiology.

B. Esophageal Testing for Cardiopulmonary Disorders Associated with GER Disease

The choice of esophageal tests will depend on the nature of the cardiopulmonary symptom that is suspected to be related to a swallowing disorder. In some cases, none of the tests conclusively establish the likely etiology; for these patients, an empiric trial of aggressive antireflux therapy may be necessary.

1. Barium Esophagram

Demonstration of free reflux or the presence of a hiatus hernia is important but not conclusive information. The reported sensitivity is only 40%-50%,[8] and among persons with asthma, reflux was demonstrated in only 46% in one series.[1] Barium studies are not helpful, except for screening, in patients with atypical chest pain as they do not establish if reflux is the cause of the patient's complaints.

2. Upper Gastrointestinal Endoscopy

Documentation of esophagitis at endoscopy is useful, but again, not diagnostic of an association between cardiopulmonary symptoms and an esophageal disorder. The prevalence of esophagitis appears to be more common in children[7] than among adults.[14]

3. Esophageal Manometry

Measurement of esophageal motility is an important diagnostic tool. Several studies have documented the presence of an abnormally low LES pressure in persons with asthma. In addition, demonstration of abnormal peristaltic function may be an important indicator of cause and effect in asthma. It has been shown that a direct relationship exists between the number of respiratory symptoms experienced by patients and the preva-

lence of esophageal motility disorders.[10] From that same study, the best surgical results were obtained in persons with asthma who had normal motility.

The use of ambulatory 24-hour esophageal manometry has been promoted as a diagnostic tool to document the association of motility disorders with atypical chest pain. Recent studies in larger numbers of unselected patients have shown that many patients do not have spontaneous chest pain during the 24-hour monitoring period and that motor abnormalities were rarely identified in those who did experience pain.[15] The presence of certain underlying motility disorders can, however, be highly correlated with chest pain. Between 75% and 80% of patients whose underlying disorder was diffuse esophageal spasm, or nutcracker esophagus, have been shown to exhibit an even more severe esophageal motor disturbance in association with chest pain than when they are asymptomatic.[16]

4. Esophageal pH Monitoring

When GER disease is suspected, esophageal pH monitoring is the most important diagnostic tool in that it allows for direct correlation between acid reflux and the presence of cardiopulmonary symptoms. Up to 80% of adults with asthma have been shown to demonstrate an abnormal incidence of acid reflux.[2] These patients have been found to have a greater frequency of reflux episodes and greater acid exposure times when compared with healthy subjects.[2]

For patients with atypical chest pain, ambulatory 24-hour pH monitoring should be performed early in the diagnostic period. Unlike conditions for patients with typical GER disease, patients suspected of having atypical chest pain should not modify their diets, medications, smoking habits, or other daily regimens during the 24-hour test. The test is most reliable when patients have a number of chest pain episodes within the 24 hours. Correlation of these episodes to periods of acid reflux lends confidence to the diagnosis, whereas, the absence of reflux, despite a number of episodes of chest pain, excludes GER disease as the inciting factor.

C. Symptoms and Signs Associated with Other Esophageal Motility Disorders

In patients with achalasia, failure of relaxation of the lower esophageal sphincter can lead to accumulation of food proximal to the sphincter that, in turn, can cause aspiration or airway obstruction. Aspiration may cause chronic cough, asthma, or recurrent pneumonitis. Airway obstruction is rare and usually results from compression by a "megaesophagus."

Manometric studies have documented the presence of peristaltic esophageal contractions of very high magnitude in some patients with noncardiac chest pain. This condition, termed nutcracker esophagus, is characterized by peristaltic contractions whose amplitude exceeds that 95th percentile for normal patients. Nutcracker esophagus is thought to be the most common primary esophageal disorder associated with chest pain.

D. Congenital Conditions Causing Swallowing Disorders

These abnormalities will be described in detail elsewhere in this book. A brief summary will be provided here for completeness.

1. Esophageal Atresia and Tracheoesophageal Fistula

Congenital malformations in the development of the trachea and esophagus produce a wide spectrum of defects. A blind upper esophageal pouch with a distal tracheoesophageal fistula (type III) is the most common abnormality, accounting for over 85% of cases. Multiple abnormalities may be present in affected individuals, including vertebral defects, anorectal malformations, and renal anomalies, which, together, comprise the VATER association acronym.

Polyhydramnios may be identified in the prenatal period and suggest the possibility of esophageal atresia. In the early postnatal period, the diagnosis may be suggested by the finding of excessive salivation, with choking and cyanosis being seen when feeding is attempted. A feeding tube can only be passed a short distance. Radiography of the chest and abdomen usually demonstrates a distended, air-filled stomach and intestines, with signs of compressive atelectasis.

Repair by primary anastomosis should be performed when the infant is stabilized and may need to be staged if the infant is at high risk. Length of the gap between esophageal segments is the primary determinant for success because of tension on the repair.

2. Cysts and Duplications

Esophageal cysts (often referred to as duplications) are rare, but are part of a group of foregut cysts that include bronchogenic, neurenteric, and inclusion cysts. The lesions are thought to arise from seeding of cells in the esophageal wall or surrounding tissues at the gestational time of separation of the pulmonary tree and esophagus. Between 10% and 30% of mediastinal masses discovered in infants and children will be foregut cysts. The age of the patient and the type of mucosal lining are important in determining the presentation. Large cysts may cause bronchial obstruction, atelectasis, or be the cause of persistent cough or recurrent pneumonia. Intramural lesions in the wall of the esophagus can cause dysphagia that may not become apparent until later in life. These abnormalities are often found when a chest radiograph is taken for other reasons and a mediastinal mass is identified. These lesions should be excised when found, as they have a tendency to enlarge over time and become increasingly symptomatic. The rare risk of malignant transformation is also reason for elective resection.

3. Congenital Stenosis and Webs

Congenital stenoses may be the result of fibromuscular hypertrophy, intramural rests of bronchial tissue, and membranous webs. More commonly, stenoses are the result of acquired conditions, such as reflux esophagitis, chemical burns, or anastomotic complication after repair of esophageal atresia. The degree of stenosis determines the severity of symptoms and the timing of presentation. Esophageal dilation is usually the first form of therapy and works best for webs and mild stenoses. Resection may be required for high-grade lesions.

4. Vascular Rings

Vascular rings result from the abnormal development of the primitive aortic arches. The term applies strictly to a complete circle around the trachea or esophagus, but has also been applied to partial rings as well. The most common anomaly is the double aortic arch; others include right aortic arch, with left ligamentum arteriosum, left aortic arch, and pulmonary artery slings. Compression causes varying degrees of dysphagia (dysphagia lusoria) and airway obstruction. Most patients present in infancy, although some with mild compression are not identified until adulthood, and symptoms may even resolve with age. Surgical correction involves division of the ring, adequate mobilization of the tracheobronchial tree and esophagus and preservation of circulation to the aortic branches.

III. TREATMENT OPTIONS

If GER disease is responsible for asthma, adequate antireflux therapy should improve symptoms. Empiric therapy may be necessary when diagnostic tests are inconclusive. Surgical therapy (see Chapter 50) can be considered, if medical regimens are ineffective and

GER disease continues as the most likely etiology.[14] For patients with atypical chest pain, aggressive medical therapy with proton pump inhibitors should be instituted when 24-hour pH monitoring suggests the diagnosis of GER disease.

IV. SUMMARY

Esophageal disorders, in particular GER disease, may present with atypical signs and symptoms, such as asthma and chronic cough, pneumonitis, interstitial fibrosis, and noncardiac chest pain. The patient history is critical to establishing a link between GER disease and asthma. Up to one third of persons having asthma with esophageal dysfunction have been found to have no reflux symptoms. The clinical presentation of GER disease-related chest pain may mimic typical angina. Unfortunately, there are no characteristics that can reliably distinguish reflux-induced pain from myocardial ischemia and both may be found in the same patient. Careful history and diagnostic testing is often necessary to determine a true etiology.

Esophageal pH monitoring is the most important diagnostic tool, in that it allows for direct correlation between acid reflux and the presence of cardiopulmonary symptoms. Measurement of esophageal motility can document the association of motility disorders, such as diffuse spasm or nutcracker esophagus, with atypical chest pain. Aggressive medical therapy should be instituted when a diagnosis is established and should also be considered when GER disease is suspected but not proven.

Frequently Asked Questions

1. Does gastroesophageal reflux cause asthma or the reverse?
   A. The relationship between GER disease and asthma is complex; GER disease may trigger an asthmatic attack, or, alternatively, symptoms of GER disease may worsen during bronchospastic episodes as a result of airway obstruction and transient hyperinflation. Over time, these cycles of reflux and asthma may lead to progressive pulmonary dysfunction.
2. How can one distinguish between cardiac and noncardiac causes of chest pain?
   A. Up to one third of patients with chest pain are found to have nonsignificant coronary artery disease on cardiac catheterization. Studies indicate that 25% to 50% of these patients are experiencing symptoms of GER disease. A particu-

larly difficult problem exists when there is reflux-induced chest pain in patients with known coronary artery disease. Simultaneous Holter and esophageal pH monitoring can be used to determine the true etiology of chest pain events.

3. What are the most important diagnostic tests for GER disease?
   A. When GER disease is suspected, esophageal pH monitoring is the most important diagnostic tool in that it allows for direct correlation between acid reflux and the presence of cardiopulmonary symptoms. Measurement of esophageal motility is also an important diagnostic tool. Documentation of esophagitis at endoscopy is useful, but not diagnostic of an association between cardiopulmonary symptoms and an esophageal disorder.

References

1. Sontag SJ, O'Connell S, Khandewal S, et al. Most asthmatics have gastroesophageal reflux with or without bronchodilator therapy. *Gastroenterology*. 1990;99:613-620.
2. Mansfield LE, Stein MR. Gastroesophageal reflux and asthma: a possible reflux mechanism. *Ann Allergy*. 1978;41:224-226.
3. Ducolon A, Vandevenne A, Jouin H, et al. Gastroesophageal reflux in patients with asthma and chronic bronchitis. *Am Rev Respir Dis*. 1987;135:327-332.
4. Schan CA, Harding SM, Haile JM, Bradley LA, Richter JE. Gastroesophageal reflux-induced bronchoconstriction: an intraesophageal acid infusion study using state-of-the-art technology. *Chest*. 1994;106:731-737.
5. Tuchman DN, Boyle JT, Pack AI, et al. Comparison of airway responses following tracheal or esophageal acidification in the cat. *Gastroenterology*. 1984;87:872-881.
6. Donnelly RJ, Berrisford RG, Jack CI, Tran JA, Evans CC. Simultaneous tracheal and esophageal pH monitoring: investigating reflux-associated asthma. *Ann Thorac Surg*. 1993;56:1029-1033.
7. Fernando del Rosario J, Orenstein SR. Evaluation and management of gastroesophageal reflux and pulmonary disease. *Curr Opin Pediatr*. 1996;8:209-215.
8. Harding SM, Richter JE. Gastroesophageal reflux disease and asthma. *Semin Gastrointest Dis*. 1992;3:139-150.
9. Patti MG, Debas HT, Pellegrini CA. Esophageal manometry and 24-hour pH monitoring in the diagnosis of pulmonary aspiration secondary to gastroesophageal reflux. *Am J Surg*. 1992;163:401-406.
10. DeMeester TR, Bonavina L, Iascone C, Courtney JV, Skinner PB. Chronic respiratory symptoms and occult gastroesophageal reflux: a prospective clinical study and results of surgical therapy. *Ann Surg*. 1990;21:237-345.

11. Voskuil JH, Cramer MJ, Breumelhof R, Timmer R, Smout AJ. Prevalence of esophageal disorders in patients with chest pain newly referred to the cardiologist. *Chest.* 1996;109:5,1210-1214.

12. Singh S, Richter JE, Bradley LA, et al. The symptom index: differential usefulness in suspected acid-related complaints of heartburn and chest pain. *Dig Dis Sci.* 1993;38:1402-1408.

13. Ros E, Armengol X, Grande L, Toledo-Pimentel V, Lacima G, Sanz G. Chest pain at rest in patients with coronary artery disease. *Dig Dis Sci.* 1997;42:1344-1353.

14. Larrain A, Carrasco E, Galleguillos F, Sepulveda R, Pope CE 2d. Medical and surgical treatment of nonallergic asthma associated with gastroesophageal reflux. *Chest.* 1991;99:1330-1335.

15. Breumelhof R, Nadorp JH, Akkermans LM, Smout AJ. Analysis of 24-hour esophageal pressure and pH data in unselected patients with noncardiac chest pain. *Gastroenterology.* 1990;99:1257-1264.

16. Stein HJ, DeMeester TR, Eypasch EP, Klingman RR: Ambulatory 24-hour esophageal manometry in the evaluation of esophageal motor disorders and noncardiac chest pain. *Surgery.* 1991;110:753-761.

CHAPTER 33

■ ■ ■

Infectious Diseases

Jennifer Rubin Grandis, M.D., F.A.C.S.

I. INTRODUCTION

Infections of the upper aerodigestive tract and surrounding structures often present with dysphagia and/or odynophagia. Specific signs and symptoms may indicate the precise anatomic location of the infectious process. Although individuals with normal immune systems develop head and neck infections that result in swallowing difficulty, the most frequently and severely afflicted are those with compromised immunity.

II. ORAL CAVITY AND OROPHARYNGEAL INFECTIONS

A. Microbiology

Candida albicans, a yeast found in normal oral flora, is frequently isolated from the mouth, yet few carriers develop clinical signs of candidiasis. Oral thrush (candidiasis) serves as a marker for immunodeficiency. Infections associated with human immunodeficiency virus (HIV) infection include oral "hairy" leukoplakia due to Epstein-Barr virus (EBV), herpes zoster infection, histoplasmosis, and major aphthous stomatitis. In addition, viral warts induced by human papilloma virus (HPV) may occur in the mouth and molluscum contagiosum can arise on the lips in AIDS patients. Primary herpes simplex virus (HSV) gingivostomatitis is a common, self-limited illness that characteristically af-

flicts young children. Acute infection is followed by latency in nerve ganglion cells. Reactivation of HSV is determined by host-virus interactions and is more common than exogenous reinfection. Sexually transmitted diseases, such as gonorrhea, chlamydia, and syphilis, may also manifest with oral lesions and dysphagia. When suspected, appropriate culture and serology facilitate the diagnosis. Mucormycosis may involve the oral cavity in persons with diabetes or patients with hematologic malignancies.

Infections of the oropharynx that result in dysphagia include tonsillitis, pharyngitis, and purulent collections that may be associated with primary mucosal or lymphoid inflammation. Group A beta hemolytic streptococci (GABHS) commonly cause acute pharyngotonsillitis. Less frequent organisms include Groups A, C, and G streptococci and mycobacteria, to name a few. Bacteriologic analysis of peritonsillar abscesses demonstrates a high incidence of polymicrobial infections with a predominance of anaerobes.[1] *Candida* infection may also involve the oropharynx in both immunocompetent and immunocompromised individuals.

B. Pathophysiology

The oral cavity and oropharynx are colonized with numerous bacteria and fungi. Microbial infection may result from an alteration in endogenous flora, immune dysfunction, or the introduction of pathogenic organisms. Ludwig's angina is an infection of the floor of the mouth that is generally associated with dental caries and poor oral hygiene. Abscesses of the peritonsillar space are thought to result from acute tonsillitis, although it has been postulated that obstruction of Weber's glands (a small group of salivary glands located in the superior pole of the tonsillar fossa) predispose to spread of infection outside the tonsils.[2]

The retropharyngeal space is a potential space bounded anteriorly by the pharyngeal musculature and its investing fascia, posteriorly by the alar layer of prevertebral fascia, superiorly by the skull base, inferiorly by fascia at C7 or T1, and laterally by the carotid sheath. Lymph nodes in this space generally regress by the age of 6. Infection of the retropharyngeal space may occur as a complication of intraoral procedures, blunt trauma to the neck, or spread of infection from adjacent foci. Although rare, Lemierre syndrome is characterized by acute oropharyngeal infection, suppurative thrombophlebitis of the internal jugular vein, anaerobic sepsis, and metastatic infection.[3]

C. Clinical Presentation

Oral ulcers in AIDS patients are not routinely infectious. Typical vesicular lesions suggest HSV, but lesions may not be present.

Physical examination is notoriously inaccurate in predicting GABHS, although the presence of a scarlatiniform rash, pharyngotonsillitis, and tender cervical lymphadenopathy may support the diagnosis. Patients with a peritonsillar abscess will typically complain of unilateral throat pain and the soft palate will appear asymmetric on exam with deviation of the uvula. Patients with Ludwig's angina (submandibular abscess) present with the inability to tolerate secretions, elevation and protrusion of the tongue, and progressive airway compromise.

D. Diagnosis

The etiology of oral ulcers may be determined by a combination of histologic examination and culture. The diagnosis of GABHS is typically made on the basis of culture that requires 24 to 48 hours to evaluate. "Rapid strep" kits that detect antigen are gaining in popularity and provide a diagnosis at the time of the initial evaluation. However, the lack of sensitivity and specificity of these rapid tests precludes their use without a backup culture.[4] Although the diagnosis of peritonsillar abscess can generally be made on the basis of physical examination, children may require a CT scan if there is significant trismus or lack of cooperation.

E. Treatment

Early initiation of acyclovir therapy is effective in hastening lesion and pain resolution for recurrent labial HSV. Thalidomide has recently been reported to be an effective treatment for major oral aphthous ulcers in AIDS patients.[5]

Despite numerous studies reporting higher bacteriologic cure rates with broad-spectrum antimicrobial agents such as cephalosporins or clindamycin, penicillin remains the drug of choice in nonallergic individuals presenting with GABHS.[6] Although treatment of GABHS pharyngitis will not prevent acute glomerulonephritis, it will protect against the development of rheumatic fever.

Peritonsillar abscess is effectively treated by incision and drainage or needle aspiration under local anesthesia in the outpatient setting, in addition to systemic antibiotics, although children may require sedation in an operating room to drain the abscess.

III. DEEP NECK INFECTIONS

Microbial infection of the upper aerodigestive tract (generally oral cavity or oropharynx) may spread to the lateral and/or retropharyngeal spaces. The absence of fascial barriers in the neck facilitates continued spread of an infectious process to the mediastinum, resulting in life-threatening mediastinitis and necrotizing fasciitis. Polymicrobial infection is typical and, in addition to symptoms of the primary infection site, patients may present with fever, chills, neck stiffness, and swelling. Individuals who develop infections of the deep neck spaces often display some degree of immunocompromise. Emphysema of the soft tissues of the neck may result from infection with gas-producing anaerobic organisms. Radiography, particularly anatomic imaging modalities such as computed tomography (CT) and magnetic resonance imaging (MRI), can be helpful in localizing the fluid collection. Treatment includes empiric therapy with broad-spectrum agents, airway protection, and, often, surgical intervention. Incision and drainage may include debridement of necrotic tissues and closure by secondary intention. Even with extensive surgical debridement, necrotizing cervical cellulitis is often fatal.

IV. LARYNGEAL INFECTION

Epiglottitis (supraglottitis) is the most common manifestation of primary laryngeal infection of the larynx, although it is increasingly rare since the advent of routine immunization for *Haemophilus influenzae* in childhood. Adult epiglottitis may be life-threatening most likely due to a delay in diagnosis and treatment.[7] Common symptoms of supraglottic infection include sore throat that is out of proportion to results of a pharyngeal exam, dysphagia, and odynophagia. Diagnosis is generally made on the basis of a lateral soft tissue x-ray of the neck and may be confirmed by physical exam. Treatment includes appropriate antibiotic therapy and close observation for airway compromise.

Rare organisms reported to cause laryngeal infection, primarily in immunocompromised hosts, include cytomegalovirus (CMV), *Mycobacterium tuberculosis*, *Cryptococcus neoformans*, leishmaniasis, *Aspergillus*, and *Histoplasmosis capsulatum*. Although they typically result in hoarseness, patients with laryngeal papillomas, associated with HPV types 6 and 11, may present with dysphagia.

V. ESOPHAGEAL INFECTIONS

A. Microbiology

Primary esophageal infections are unusual in the general population. When they arise, these are typically due to *Candida* or HSV. However, esophagitis is a major cause of morbidity in individuals with impaired immunity caused by HIV infection, chemotherapy, or solid organ or bone marrow transplantation. *C. albicans* is the predominant cause of fungal esophagitis. Other *Candida* species, such as *C. tropicalis, C. galbrata, C. parapsilosis,* and *C. krusei,* are occasionally pathogenic. HIV infection is the most significant risk factor for the development of esophageal infection. Although the most common offending pathogens include *Candida*, HSV, and CMV, less commonly reported pathogens in AIDS patients include *Mycobacterium tuberculosis, M. avium* intracellulare complex (MAC), *Pneumocystis carinii, Cryptosporidia, Aspergillus,* EBV, *Nocardia* species, and *Leishmania donovani.* In South America, Chagas' disease caused by *Trypanosoma cruzi* can cause achalasia and, in severe cases, result in megaesophagus as a result of destruction of parasympathetic innervation.

B. Pathophysiology

Chronic mucocutaneous candidiasis is the only congenital immunodeficiency syndrome in which the esophagus is frequently involved. Acquired compromise of the immune system may result from the chronic use of corticosteroids, which generally manifests as superficial mucosal *Candida* infection or, more rarely, HSV and CMV. Aerosolized beclomethasone has been associated with *Candida*-induced esophagitis in an otherwise healthy adult, which suggests that corticosteroid therapy need not be systemically administered to increase the risk for esophageal infection; and bacterial esophagitis has been reported following corticosteroid therapy associated with CD4+ T-lymphocytopenia.[8] Cancer patients, particularly individuals with hematologic malignancies, have a high prevalence of esophageal infections. Radiation and chemotherapy treatments serve to further compromise the immune defense against bacteria and fungi as well as contribute to loss of normal esophageal mucosal integrity. Infectious esophagitis is occasionally encountered in the initial postoperative period following solid organ transplantation (approximately 6% in several large series). There is a higher incidence of *Candida* infection following renal transplantation compared with liver or heart transplant, which is generally attributed to the higher incidence of diabetes mellitus in renal transplant recipients. Although uncommon, when routine fungal and viral prophylaxis is employed, CMV- and HSV-associated esophagitis may present several weeks after transplantation because of either reactivation of latent virus or primary viral infection from transfused blood products or transplanted organs. Patients with diabetes mellitus are susceptible to *Candida* esophagitis, which may be due to persistent hyperglycemia resulting in granulocyte dysfunction. Alcoholism has been implicated in CMV esophagitis in otherwise immunocompetent individuals. Hypochloridia secondary to the use of H_2 receptor antagonists, omeprazole, gastric surgery, or AIDS-associated gastropathy, is also associated with increased risk of *Candida* esophagitis.

A small number of *C. albicans* organisms are generally present in normal oral flora. Antibiotic therapy may alter the normal balance between bacteria and fungi, allowing for overgrowth and colonization with *Candida*. Although it is generally asymptomatic, colonization may progress to infection if concurrent risk factors are present. Lack of normal esophageal motility predisposes to colonization and infection with *Candida*. Patients with progressive systemic sclerosis (PSS/scleroderma) demonstrate a high incidence of fungal esophagitis that can be reduced with antacid therapy. Less common causes of *Candida* esophagitis include achalasia, stricture, esophageal diverticula, and esophageal burns secondary to caustic ingestion. Reactivation of latent infection is responsible for the increased incidence of mycobacterial esophageal infections among immunocompromised patients.

C. Clinical Presentation

Certain presenting signs and symptoms may be characteristic of esophagitis from varying infecting organisms. HIV-infected patients are susceptible to idiopathic esophageal ulcers as well as unusual bacteria and parasites. Dysphagia and odynophagia are reported in the vast majority of patients with HIV-associated idiopathic ulcers, but are only present in little more than half of the individuals with infectious esophagitis.[8] Oral cavity lesions (eg, thrush) are present in about one third of patients with documented *Candida* (eg, thrush), HSV, and HIV-associated esophagitis, but are not reported in association with CMV or tuberculous esophageal infection. Nausea and vomiting are present in about 40% of reported patients with CMV esophagitis.[8] Abdominal pain with esophagitis is less common (reported incidence of 2%-19%) and may be due to intra-abdominal extension of the infection.

Weight loss may be a result of debilitation from reduced oral intake or the associated systemic illness (eg, HIV) and is reported in 22%-35% of cases. Fever is unusual, but if present is more indicative of CMV or mycobacterial infection, with cough exclusively reported in cases of mycobacterial esophagitis.[9] Fistulization, although rare, is a major complication of tuberculous esophagitis.

As *Candida* esophagitis is frequently asymptomatic, the true prevalence of this condition is unknown. CMV infections in immunosuppressed individuals tend to be more severe than in hosts with normal immune function. Primary CMV esophagitis differs in its clinical presentation from other viral and fungal infections, with a gradual onset of symptoms reflecting that CMV infection is systemic, involving multiple organs in addition to the esophagus. However, in transplant recipients and AIDS patients, CMV esophagitis may coexist with HSV and *Candida* infection.

D. Diagnosis

The frequency of *Candida* esophagitis in AIDS patients has led to the recommendation for empiric antifungal therapy in HIV-infected patients who present with esophageal symptoms. Radiologic studies are of limited value in the diagnosis of esophageal infection. Endoscopy with brushings and biopsy is the standard method of obtaining a definitive diagnosis of esophagitis. Transoral or transnasal blind brush cytology may provide sufficient material for diagnosis and preclude the need for endoscopy and biopsy. When mycobacteria are suspected, operating personnel should take extra precautions, as there is a risk of tubercle bacilli infection via aerosolized dispersion of the organisms. Pathologists should be alerted to a patient's history and endoscopic findings, so that each specimen is appropriately processed. Cultures are notoriously difficult to interpret because of the inability to differentiate infection from colonization or normal flora. However, if a resistant or atypical species is suspected from the clinical history, cultures can be useful. Viral culture is more sensitive than microscopic examination when HSV is suspected.[8] Characteristic histologic features of CMV infection include intranuclear and cytoplasmic inclusions. Immunochemical staining for antigens and in situ hybridization for CMV DNA can confirm the diagnosis. CMV was found in 22% of transplant recipients who had no gross lesions on endoscopy, which suggests that random biopsies are warranted in the setting of a normal endoscopic exam.[10]

E. Treatment

Treatment of *Candida* esophagitis is determined by the severity of the infection and the degree of immune compromise. Topical antifungal agents are effective in most patients (eg, clotrimazole, a nonabsorbable imidazole, delivered as a 10 mg buccal troche 5 times daily).[8] In patients who have anatomic or motility defects that predispose to colonization, *Candida* may be difficult to eradicate. HIV-infected patients can be treated with nonabsorbable imidazoles or a systemically absorbed triazole (eg, fluconazole). Chronic antifungal therapy (for treatment or prophylaxis) in patients with immune defects may lead to the emergence of resistant organisms and adverse systemic reactions. Patients with granulocytopenia should be treated aggressively with amphotericin B, as they are at high risk for disseminated fungal disease. Amphotericin B is also the treatment for esophagitis caused by *Aspergillus* or *Histoplasma* species. Supportive care is generally sufficient for HSV esophagitis in the immunocompetent patient. Acyclovir prophylaxis has almost eliminated HSV esophagitis among solid organ and bone marrow transplant recipients. Gancyclovir and foscarnet are both effective agents in the treatment of CMV infection. Achalasia caused by Chagas' disease may be treated with isosorbide dinitrate although preventive efforts aimed at eradicating the insects that carry the trypanosome in South America are more effective.

V. SUMMARY

Swallowing dysfunction frequently accompanies microbial infection of upper aerodigestive tract sites. The oral cavity and oropharynx are colonized by bacteria in healthy individuals. Alteration of normal flora, immune compromise, or introduction of pathogenic organisms may contribute to the development of an infection. Specific signs and symptoms generally help to identify the infected site. Therapy is often empiric if cultures are problematic to acquire or interpret. A fluid collection in the potential spaces of the head and neck generally requires surgical drainage.

VI. CONTROVERSIES

The decision to proceed with a diagnostic work-up versus instituting empiric therapy depends, in part, on the available resources, the experience of the clinician, and the cost of potential diagnostic studies. Surgical intervention is generally reserved for cases that present with a fluid collection or when the patient demonstrates signs and symptoms of systemic toxicity.

Frequently Asked Questions

1. How are peritonsillar abscesses managed?
   A. Much attention has focused on comparing incision and drainage with needle aspiration. It is critical to adequately drain the fluid collection, regardless of the technique employed.
2. What is the drug of choice for GABHS pharyngitis?
   A. Despite large-scale clinical trials that demonstrate improved efficacy with broader spectrum antibiotics, penicillin remains the drug of choice in this common infection.

References

1. Prior A, Montgomery P, Mitchelmore I, Tabaqchali S. The microbiology and antibiotic treatment of peritonsillar abscesses. *Clin Otolayrngol.* 1995; 20:219-223.
2. Passy V. Pathogenesis of peritonsillar abscess. *Laryngoscope.* 1994;104:185-190.
3. Weesner CL, Cisek JE. Lemierre syndrome: the forgotten disease. *Ann Emerg Med.* 1993;22:256-258.
4. Shulman ST. Streptococcal pharyngitis: diagnostic considerations. *Pediatr Infect Dis J.* 1994;13:567-571.
5. Jacobson JM, Greenspan JS, Spritzler J. Thalidomide for the treatment of oral aphthous ulcers in patients with human immunodeficiency virus infection. *N Engl J Med.* 1997;336: 1487-1493.
6. Pichichero ME, Margolis PA. A comparison of cephalosporins and penicillins in the treatment of group A beta-homolytic streptococcal pharyngitis: a meta-analysis supporting the concept of microbial copathogenicity. *Pediatr Infect Dis J.* 1991;10:275-281.
7. Dort JC, Frohlich AM, Tate RB. Acute epiglottitis in adults: diagnosis and treatment in 43 patients. *J Otolaryngol.* 1994;23:281-285.
8. Nseher PH, McDonald GB. Esophageal infections: risk factors, presentation, diagnosis, and treatment. *Gastroenterology.* 1994;106:509-532.
9. Allen CM, Craze J, Grundy A. Tuberculous broncho-oesophageal fistula in the acquired immunodeficiency syndrome. *Clin Radiol.* 1991;43:60-62.
10. Graham SM, Flowers JL, Schweitzer E, Bartlett ST, Imbembo AL. Opportunistic upper gastrointestinal infection in transplant recipients. *Surg Endosc.* 1995; 9:146-150.

PART V

NONSURGICAL TREATMENT OF SWALLOWING DISORDERS

Effective treatment of swallowing disorders relies on specialists who have a broad knowledge of nutrition and dentition and understand the significance of these when treating swallowing disorders. The importance of nutrition for recovering and maintaining total body health must be individualized based on the origin of the disorder. We give special emphasis on the care of the tracheotomized patient, including decannulation, since it affects both the short-term and long-term outcomes of recovery. In this section, the interactions of specialists who treat swallowing disorders using nonsurgical approaches is evident from each author's perspective.

CHAPTER 34

■ ■ ■

Diet Modification

Laura Molseed, M.S., R.D.

I. INTRODUCTION

The importance of providing adequate and appropriate nutrition support to individuals with dysphagia is one of the most important aspects of their care. Many of these individuals have difficulty consuming adequate food and fluids and are at high risk for protein-calorie malnutrition and dehydration. Providing adequate calories, protein, vitamins, minerals, and fluids in the consistency best tolerated by a patient is the primary goal for the nutritional management of an individual with dysphagia.[1,2]

Once an individual has been diagnosed with dysphagia, the registered dietitian should work closely with the speech-language pathologist or dysphagia therapist to determine the most appropriate method of nutritional support and the consistency of the diet. This chapter reviews the types of diet modifications commonly prescribed, consistency modifications, appropriate food choices, methods to adjust food consistency, monitoring techniques, and other available options for nutritional support when oral intake is minimal or unsafe.

II. PHASES OF SWALLOWING

Dysphagia may be the result of an impairment during the swallowing process. Neurological impairments, congenital abnormalities, surgery, various medications, and prolonged orotracheal intubation may cause impairment during one of the phases of swallowing.[2-4] Swallowing is normally described in three or four phases. (See Chapter 3.) In this chapter, four phases of swallowing, potential nutrition problems encountered during each phase, and appropriate diet modifications (see Table 34-1) are discussed.[2,3,5] It is important to remember that individual swallowing ability and tolerance will vary and the diet must be individualized for each person.

A. Oral Preparatory Phase

The mouth accepts food and holds it in preparation for swallowing. The teeth grind the food and mix it with saliva. Poor lip closure, inability to chew, and diminished saliva production will result in difficulty during this phase of swallowing. Alterations in this phase may require a pureed diet with thickened liquid; very soft, easily chewed foods; adaptive eating utensils (long-handled spoon, syringe), and/or body positioning while eating.

B. Oral Phase

The tongue moves food to the back of the mouth by pushing it up against the hard palate. The swallowing reflex is normally initiated during this phase. Individuals with decreased tongue mobility, decreased bolus control, or palatal alterations may have difficulty dur-

Table 34-1. *Consistency Modifications*

Solid Food Modification

Pureed/Liquified: Regular food may be blenderized with added liquid as needed to form a smooth consistency. The consistency may vary from a thick liquid consistency to a paste-like consistency. The consistency of baby food is often best tolerated; however, it should be adjusted to meet each individual's needs.

Mechanically Altered: Chopped and ground foods, very soft foods such as pasta and casseroles, foods that easily form a cohesive bolus are included in this diet.

Soft: Naturally soft foods that require a minimal amount of chewing are found on this diet. Meat may need to be cut in small pieces and rough food, such as nuts, popcorn, raw vegetables, and salads are avoided.

Liquid Modification

Thin: Clear liquids, milk, coffee, and tea, plus strained broth-based soups
Thick: Milkshakes, strained cream soups, nectars
Thickened: Thin or thick liquids may require thickening agents to achieve the appropriate consistency. (See Table 34-6 for thickening agents.) Nectar, honey and pudding consistencies are commonly ordered.

---

ing this phase. Swallowing may occur prior to laryngeal closure, causing aspiration or nasal regurgitation. Very soft food that forms a cohesive bolus and thick liquids are normally prescribed for individuals with alterations during this phase.[1,2]

C. Pharyngeal Phase

During this phase, the palate elevates, pharyngeal constrictors squeeze food through the pharynx, and the larynx elevates, protecting the airway. Alterations during this phase may cause an inability to protect the airway and an incomplete swallow that increases the risk of delayed aspiration and may be due to deconditioning. Potential diet modifications include thickened liquids; pureed, moist foods; and avoidance of "crumbly" foods and foods that do not form a cohesive bolus.[1,2]

D. Esophageal Phase

During this phase, esophageal peristalsis moves food from the esophagus into the stomach. Potential diet modifications to assist during this phase of swallowing include soft, moist foods and avoidance of sticky, dry foods.[1,2]

III. DYSPHAGIA DIETS

A diet to treat dysphagia adjusts food and fluid consistency for adaptation with an individual's ability to

swallow and the specific area in which they are having a swallowing difficulty (see Table 34-1, Consistency Modifications). These diets provide a stepwise approach to eating. Individuals begin with the most easily handled foods and progress to more difficult items. Dysphagia diets are normally separated into phases starting with Level I and advancing to Level IV. Clinicians working with individuals with dysphagia must remember that these are guidelines and the diet should be adjusted and altered according to each individual's needs.[1,2,6] Tables 34-2, 34-3, and 34-4 list categories of foods that are often not tolerated by individuals with dysphagia and that should not be included on dysphagia diets.

A. Level I

This is a level of pureed food and thickened liquids and is the most conservative level, commonly prescribed for individuals just beginning to eat. It is also appropriate for individuals with severe oral preparatory and oral phase dysphagia and pharyngeal dysphagia.

Table 34-2. *Crumbly and Noncohesive Foods*

Plain ground meat	Peas, corn, or legumes
Scrambled eggs	Cornbread
Rice	Cottage cheese
Jello	Coconut
Crackers	Nuts and seeds

Table 34-3. *Mixed Consistency Foods*

Vegetable Soup	Salad with dressing
Soup with large pieces or chunks of food	Canned fruit
Cold cereal with milk	Gelatin with fruit
Citrus fruit	Yogurt with fruit

Table 34-4. *Foods*

Dry mashed potatoes
Peanut butter
Fresh white or refined wheat bread
Fudge or butterscotch sauce/caramel
Bagels or soft rolls

Table 34-5. *Thinning Agents/Blenderizing Agents*

Milk	Gravy
Juice	Tomato juice

Table 34-6. *Thickening Agents*

- Commercial (ie, "Thick It," "Thick and Easy")
- Cornstarch
- Baby cereal (or other dehydrated baby food)
- Mashed potato flakes
- Instant pudding
- Unflavored gelatin

B. Level II

This phase consists of pureed and mechanically altered foods, plus thick or thickened liquids. Very soft foods that require minimal chewing may be included (ie, cottage cheese, macaroni and cheese, and pancakes with syrup). Individuals with alterations in the oral preparatory phase or decreased pharyngeal peristalsis and muscle dysfunction may tolerate this phase.

C. Level III

Mechanically altered and soft foods are provided in this phase. Liquids are allowed as tolerated. (Liquids may need to be advanced more slowly.) Individuals who are beginning to chew or who have difficulty tolerating coarse, rough textures are prescribed this phase.

D. Level IV

This diet includes soft foods and all liquids. Any rough or coarse texture food is avoided. From this phase, individuals may be advanced to a regular diet.

Dysphagia diet considerations include:

- Menus should follow guidelines for meeting nutritional adequacy and variety.
- Efforts should be made to use nutrient-dense foods and liquids to help meet nutritional needs. (See Tables 34-5 and 34-6 for thinning and thickening agents that are nutritionally dense.)
- The diet should be individualized according to patient tolerance and preference.
- The individual tolerance should be monitored closely and the diet should be adjusted regularly.
- Efforts should be made to enhance the visual appeal and flavor of the food. A variety of differently colored foods should be used for each meal. Seasoning should be used and, for some individuals, flavor may need to be enhanced to stimulate their taste buds.
- Beverages should be offered frequently (prepared according to thickening guidelines) to help meet fluid requirements.
- Liquids and solids may progress separately through the diet levels.
- Nutritional supplements should be employed to meet an individual's nutrient needs. A variety of supplements are commercially available. Thickening agents should be utilized. (See Table 34-6.) In addition, many companies provide puddings, soups and cereal bars.[2,4,6]

IV. ALTERNATIVE METHODS OF NUTRITIONAL SUPPORT

Patients diagnosed with dysphagia often have difficulty meeting nutritional needs through diet alone. Maintaining or improving a patient's nutritional status may help build strength and improve swallowing safety. Enteral nutrition support may be required in conjunction with oral nutrition or may be required prior to allowing an individual to begin swallowing. Options for enteral nutritional support include nasogastric tube, gastrostomy tube, or enteric tube. Patients may be fed around the clock, only at night (nocturnally), or periodically (intermittently) during the day.

The best method of enteral nutrition should be determined on an individual basis. Health care providers must realize that individuals who are maintained on enteral nutrition continue to be at-risk for aspiration. Critically ill and neurologically impaired individuals seem to be at the greatest risk. Although the cause of aspiration remains controversial, the following guidelines should be followed to minimize risk.[7,8]

- Utilize a small-bore, flexible feeding tube.
- Consider feeding tube placement postpylorically or having an enteric tube (nasojejunal or jejunostomy).
- Keep the head of the bed elevated at least 45° during the feeding and at least 1 hour after the feeding has stopped.
- Small volume, continuous feedings may be better tolerated by some individuals.

V. MONITORING

Individuals with dysphagia should be reassessed frequently to determine changes in their ability to swallow and obtain adequate nutrition. Swallowing function may improve rapidly or deteriorate. Alterations in the diet and/or enteral feeding program may be frequently needed. Close monitoring of the patient's nutritional status is also essential. Mealtime observations (observe length of time taken to eat, food eaten, interest in eating, fluid intake), calorie counts, body weights, tolerance to consistency modifications and periodic swallowing evaluations using modified-barium swallow (MBS) or FEES exams will help judge how best to maintain their nutrition and provide better diet acceptance.

Individuals who are maintained on both enteral and oral nutrition should be monitored closely for their tolerance of the diet, enteral feeding regime, and their nutritional and fluid status. Close monitoring will assist in transitioning off enteral nutrition to an oral diet alone while assuring adequate nutritional intake.

Regular monitoring includes:

Body weight	Calorie counts
Fluid Status	Gastrointestinal function
Swallowing function	

VI. EDUCATION

Individuals and their family members should be educated on the signs and symptoms of aspiration, dehydration, and malnutrition. Emphasizing the importance of early identification of potential problems is essential to avoiding costly hospitalizations and complications.

Establishing nutritional goals and reviewing them with each individual allows the patient to take control of his or her nutritional intake and determine how to meet the goals each day. Many individuals like to track their daily intake as a method of self-monitoring improvement.

Most food items can be mechanically altered to fit into a dysphagia diet. Knowing an individual's preferences and cooking ability helps the clinician in discussing food preparation methods. Encouraging individuals to experiment with various foods once they know the consistency they can tolerate helps promote variety in their diet.

Individuals receiving enteral nutrition, in addition to oral intake, should have their enteral feeding schedule arranged to enhance their appetite. Allow at least 2 hours off the feeding tube prior to each meal. This should maximize their oral nutrition and fluid intake.

Frequently Asked Questions

1. The presence of a gag reflex indicates an individual will be able to swallow safely?
   True or false?
   A. False. A gag reflex does not indicate that an individual is safe to swallow. Many individuals with a gag reflex continue to be at risk for aspirating.
2. What is the most conservative diet order for an individual with potential dysphagia?
   A. A pureed diet with thickened liquids is the easiest for most individuals to control and swallow.
3. Continuous enteral feedings pose the least risk of aspiration. True or false?
   A. Neither. The best method of providing enteral nutrition for an individual at-risk for aspiration is controversial. The best preventative measures are to keep the head of the bed elevated at least 45° during the feeding and at least 1 hour after the feeding... duals every 4 hours. If double the rate of feeding is withdrawn from the stomach, hold the feeding for 1 hour and recheck. Check the placement of the feeding tube before starting any feeding.

4. Individuals who are eating but require supplemental nutrition should receive what form?
   A. Nocturnal enteral feedings, intermittent enteral feedings, oral nutritional supplements, total parenteral nutrition. Each individual must be evaluated and the most appropriate method of providing nutritional support provided. In most cases, if the individual is able to eat and utilize his or her gastrointestinal tract, total parenteral nutrition should be avoided.

References

1. Curran J, Groher ME. Development and dissemination of an aspiration risk reduction diet. *Dysphagia.* 1990;5:6-12.
2. Nutrition Management of Dysphagia. In: *Manual of Clinical Dietetics.* 5th ed. Chicago: American Dietetic Association; 1996:145-163.
3. Devita MA, Spierer-Rundback L. Swallowing disorders in patients with prolonged orotracheal intubation or tracheostomy tubes. *Crit Care Med.* 1990;18:1328-1330.
4. Lewis MM, Kidder JA. *Nutrition Practice Guidelines for Dysphagia.* Chicago: American Dietetic Association; 1996.
5. Tripp F, Cordero O. Dysphagia and nutrition in the acute care geriatric patient. *Top Clin Nutr.* 1991;6:60-69.
6. Pardoe EM. Development of a multistage diet for dysphagia. *J Am Diet Assoc.* 1993;93:568-571.
7. Elpern EH. Pulmonary aspiration in hospitalized adults. *Nutr Clin Prac.* 1997;12:5-13.
8. Schwartz DB, Dominguez-Gasson L. Aspiration in a patient receiving enteral nutrition. *Nutr Clin Prac.* 1997;12: 14-19.

CHAPTER 35

■ ■ ■

Therapeutic Intervention for Swallowing Disorders

Thomas Murry, Ph.D.

I. INTRODUCTION

The treatment of swallowing disorders presents a unique challenge to rehabilitation specialists. Whether it is the speech-language pathologist, occupational therapist, or other rehabilitation specialist involved in the treatment of swallowing disorders, each must be aware of the anatomical changes, if any, and functional status of each patient's swallowing mechanism. In addition, factors such as cognitive level, environment, and psychosocial aspects involved with eating and swallowing must be considered. All attempts to treat a swallowing disorder must begin with a thorough understanding of the test results obtained from the evaluation of a patient. The clinician must understand the implications of all findings and be able to explain to the patient and caregivers the findings and their implications for nutrition, aspiration, and psychosocial aspects of swallowing. Once testing is completed and a thorough understanding of the dysphagia problem has been obtained, swallowing therapy may begin.

There are four major therapeutic approaches that a rehabilitation specialist may take when treating the organs of swallowing: (a) sensory behavioral techniques, (b) motor behavioral techniques, (c) postural compensations, and (d) facilitating maneuvers. In this chapter, behavioral management of swallowing is addressed and compensatory postures and facilitating maneuvers, along with oral motor exercises and sensory stimulation, are considered. The speech-language pathologist directs the behavioral management of treating

dysphagia; however, as dysphagia is usually the result of some other medical condition, it is imperative that the speech-language pathologist maintains active communication with all members of the treatment team. Changes in patient status and environment may require modification of the treatment program. In this chapter, specific exercises and procedures are presented according to the phase of swallowing that is being addressed.

II. SENSORY AND MOTOR BEHAVIORAL TECHNIQUES

A. Oral Phase

The oral phase of swallowing begins with an awareness that food or liquid is in the oral cavity and ready to be manipulated. Thus, it is important to have normal sensory stimulation to avoid oral phase problems. Although the oral phase problems may also be managed with prosthetic appliances, the speech-language pathologist will still participate actively in oral phase management once the prosthetic appliance is fitted.

In Chapters 2 and 3, the sensory systems of the normal swallow are presented. Although it is common to experience sensory dysfunction due to neurological disorders and postoperative conditions, the impact of these sensory aspects is often overlooked in the diagnosis and subsequent treatment of swallowing.[1,2] If the patient is going to swallow successfully, he or she must achieve functional control of lip closure. This includes sensory awareness of lip position, as well as motor control of lip closure to prevent drooling and initiate bolus transport. Sensory awareness may be attempted through pressure and temperature stimulation as well as bolus size and texture manipulation. To improve awareness and control of the lips the exercises in Table 35-1 may be used.

Oral preparatory phase exercises may be done in front of a mirror. For patients with cognitive defects, the clinician should repeat the exercises many times, keeping distracting objects out of the working area. Patients should be encouraged to watch the maneuvers in a mirror. If the therapist demonstrates these maneuvers, it is best to sit alongside the patient rather than across a table.

Oral exercises are especially important to initiate early in treatment. The patient is not required to swallow in the majority of the exercises, and the exercises are highly visible.

B. Sensory and Motor Exercises for the Tongue, Palate, and Mandible

Exercises for the tongue are used to improve tongue movement to increase tongue speed of movement and to strengthen the tongue so that food may be guided and propelled sufficiently to the oropharynx. When there is reduced tongue strength or movement because of neurological insult, surgical excision, or high-dose radiation, oral intake is slowed and food may become "pocketed" in the oral cavity. This may lead to delayed aspiration. Equally important is the problem of pre-swallow aspiration because the tongue failed to maintain bolus control.

Tongue exercises should also be continued once an oral prosthesis is fitted.[3] Tongue exercises with the oral prosthesis in place allow the patient to accommodate to the device for both swallowing and speech production.[4] The exercises in Table 35-2 are suggested for tongue strength and movement.

Table 35-1. *Labial Exercises to Improve Strength and Awareness of Control*

1. Rapid labial opening and closing using the consonants /p, b/.

2. Extended lip squeeze followed by lip retraction.

3. Repeating the vowels /u, i/ with increased lip movement. Vocalization provides additional stimulation and awareness.

4. Thermal stimulation of the lips with ice. Movement of the ice may be medial-lateral or more focal if drooling on one side is prevalent.

5. Holding different objects between the lips such as a straw, tongue blade, plastic spoon, etc, to improve sensory awareness. Objects may be of different sizes, shapes, and weights.

6. Apply various foods, such as yogurt and peanut butter, to lips and encourage the patient to massage the lips together.

7. Use the index finger to apply a sudden or quick stretch to the edges of the upper and lower lips.

8. Practice humming. Cue patient to start and stop humming. When humming stops, the patient should open the lips, then close again.

9. Have patient close the lips. Ask him or her to keep them closed while you try gently to break the lip seal.

10. Practice a "facial squeeze" by squeezing lips together. While keeping lips closed, alternately bring the teeth together and separate them. This mimics chewing activity.

11. Practice inhaling and exhaling through the nose rather than mouth. The patient may want to watch this activity with a mirror.

12. Prior to swallowing, the patient should hold a glass or cup to the lips. Practice the timing of opening the lips once the cup is placed on the lower lip.

13. Hold small objects such as a button (connected to a string) and place it between the lips and teeth. The clinician can put a gentle pull on the string to improve lip strength.

14. Intraoral stimulation of cheeks with a brush, cold object, or fingers.

15. Resistive exercises. *Example:* Have the patient push the upper lip down while the clinician resists the movement with a tongue blade. Have the patient push the tongue against the cheek while the clinician resists against the outside of the cheek.

Table 35-2. *Exercises for Tongue Strength and Movement*

1. Tongue tip elevation. Place tongue tip on alveolar ridge. Hold it for 2 seconds.

2. Tongue tip sweep. After holding the tongue on the alveolar ridge, sweep posteriorly against the palate.

3. Use the phonemes, /t, d/ for rapid contact and release of the tongue tip to the alveolar ridge.

4. Use the *ch* sound to improve tongue contact to the middle of the soft palate. Similarly, the sounds *s* and *sh* help with lateral contact of tongue to palate as well as help to groove the tongue.

5. The /k, g/ phonemes are used to increase posterior tongue to soft palate contact. Combining syllables into quick movements such as "ta-ka" or "cha-ka" is helpful to improve the sweeping motion of the tongue.

6. Range of motion exercises can be done by chewing on gauze, initially then adding small amounts of food when it is safe.[5]

7. To improve sensory awareness, use pressure and temperature stimulation.[6-8]

   a. A cold spoon may be placed on the tip, blade, or back of tongue. Light pressure is applied and the patient is asked to lift the spoon.

   b. The palate is touched with tongue blade or cotton and the patient is asked to touch the area with the tongue.

   c. Cold or sour materials are given to the patient. They may be frozen on a stick if the patient is not yet cleared to swallow.

   d. Various sizes and textures of bolus may be given to identify the size and texture most easily transported by the tongue.

8. Mandible movement. Patients with reduced mandible movement may want to use a device such as Therabite® to increase mouth opening.

9. Resistive exercises to the mandible such as lowering or closing the mandible against the pressure applied by the therapist on the chin.

10. Sucking exercises increase tongue-palate contact and help the patient to manage saliva. Sucking may be done with the tongue tip against the alveolar ridge with lips and teeth slightly apart or with teeth closed using a "slurping" or "suctioning" pull of the tongue to the mid-palate area. The patient should try to do this with as much sound as possible to increase sensory feedback.

C. Laryngeal Exercises

Elevation of the larynx and closure of the vocal folds prevent food and liquid from entering the trachea and causing aspiration. The lips, tongue, palate, and mandible may be thought of as facilitating organs of swallow, with the larynx considered as the final prevention against aspiration. Vocal fold closure exercises are shown in Table 35-3. The goals of these exercises are to increase the degree and speed of vocal fold closure, to sustain vocal fold closure, and to aid in laryngeal elevation. Sustaining vocal fold closure is especially important in patients who have a slow or delayed swallow or in those where there is residual material in the valleculae or pyriform sinuses after the first swallow and the risk of aspiration is high if the vocal folds open.

III. FACILITATING SWALLOWING POSTURES

Changes in head or body position have been demonstrated to improve bolus movement and reduce aspiration.[10-14] The use of postural techniques compensate for anatomic deficiencies, sensory loss, or the inability to move the bolus with sufficient speed and pressure to obtain a satisfactory swallow. Postural techniques are first observed during the evaluation of a patient with either flexible endoscopy or videofluoroscopy. The best posture is one that reduces aspiration maximally. Additional postural benefits include the speed and volume of bolus transit. This is especially important when the oral phase of swallowing has been severely affected either because of surgical excision or severe neurological dysfunction.

Recently, Logemann outlined the postures to eliminate aspiration or residue.[15] These are shown in Table 35-4. The clinician normally tries the appropriate technique when conducting the modified barium swallow (MBS) or the FEES. By maintaining proper records of the swallow examination, the clinician can use the facilitating postures in treatment with confidence. The effect of the chin tuck postural technique is to push the tongue back, widen the valleculae, and place the epiglottis in a more protective position, preventing the bolus from going into the endolarynx. Turning the head to one side or the other helps to direct the bolus to the stronger side. When these techniques are combined, the laryngeal entrance is narrowed and the bolus is directed to the stronger or nondamaged side.

Table 35-3. *Vocal Fold Closure and Laryngeal Elevation Technique*

1. Practice coughing.
2. Increase the loudness of the voice.
3. Initiate voice with a hard glottal onset.
4. Produce sustained phonation. Try to increase the duration while maintaining consistent voice quality.
5. Sustain phonation at various pitches. This helps with anterior vocal fold closure as well as laryngeal elevation.
6. An excellent program of laryngeal exercises has been developed by Ramig and her colleagues.[9] Although this program is primarily to increase vocal effectiveness, it also offers promise to those who require vocal fold closure improvement to reduce the risk of aspiration.

Table 35-4. *Postural Techniques to Eliminate Aspiration or Residue*

Disorder Observed on Fluoroscopy	Posture Applied	Rationale
Inefficient oral transit (Reduced posterior propulsion of bolus by tongue)	Head back	Uses gravity to clear oral cavity
Delay in triggering the pharyngeal swallow (bolus past ramus of mandible but pharyngeal swallow is not triggered)	Chin down	Widens valleculae to prevent bolus from entering airway; narrows airway entrance, reducing risk of aspiration
Reduced posterior motion of tongue-base (Residue in valleculae)	Chin down	Pushes tongue-base backward toward pharyngeal wall
Unilateral vocal fold paralysis or surgical removal (Aspiration during the swallow)	Head rotated to damaged side	Places extrinsic pressure on thyroid cartilage, improving vocal fold approximation, and directs bolus down stronger side
Reduced closure of laryngeal entrance and vocal folds (Aspiration during the swallow)	Chin down; head rotated to damaged side	Puts epiglottis in more protective position; narrows laryngeal entrance; improves vocal fold closure by applying extrinsic pressure
Reduced pharyngeal contraction (Residue spread throughout pharynx)	Lying down on one side	Eliminates gravitational effect on pharyngeal residue
Unilateral pharyngeal paresis (Residue on one side of pharynx)	Head rotated to damaged side	Eliminates damaged side of pharynx from bolus path
Unilateral oral and pharyngeal weakness on same side (Residue in mouth and pharynx on same side)	Head tilt to stronger side	Directs bolus down stronger side by gravity
Cricopharyngeal dysfunction (Residue in pyriform sinuses)	Head rotated	Pulls cricoid cartilage away from posterior pharyngeal wall, reducing resting pressure in cricopharyngeal sphincter

Source: From Logemann JA. Therapy for oropharyngeal swallowing disorders.[15] Reprinted with permission.

For patients with neurological disorders, such as CVA or head trauma, these techniques must be continually reinforced until the patient uses them automatically. Swallowing in front of a mirror may be helpful. Alternatively using a simple diagram on paper showing the chin tuck, head tilt, or head rotation may be helpful.

IV. SWALLOW MANEUVERS

Swallow maneuvers were reported as early as 1973 and 1977 in studies of the effects of tracheostomy on laryngeal closure.[16,17] These studies pointed out the need to increase the speed and timing (and, therefore, the force) when transporting the bolus through the oropharynx into the esophagus.

More recently, Logemann has expanded on these maneuvers and identified specific problems for which these maneuvers are useful in treating swallowing disorders.[15] The major maneuvers for gaining control over the pharyngeal swallow are: (1) supraglottic swallow; (2) super-supraglottic swallow, (3) effortful swallow, and (4) Mendelsohn maneuver. Although described elsewhere, a brief review of each is provided.

The **supraglottic** swallow is a 4-step maneuver: (1) inhale and hold breath, (2) place bolus in swallow position, (3) swallow while holding breath, and (4) cough after swallow before inhaling. The effect of this maneuver is to close the vocal folds (breath hold) and clear any residue that may have entered the laryngeal vestibule (cough) before breathing again.

The **super-supraglottic** swallow is similar to the supraglottic swallow, with the addition of the instruction to bear down once the breath is being held. The effect of bearing down is either to increase false vocal fold closure or assist in closing the posterior glottis.

The **effortful swallow** is simply a squeeze. The patient is told or shown to squeeze hard with all of his or her muscles. This maneuver may be the easiest for patients who have trouble with multiple-stage commands, for children, or for patients with significant sensory loss. A picture showing someone squeezing may be helpful.

The **Mendelsohn maneuver** as described by Cook is a technique to open the upper esophageal sphincter.[18] In this maneuver, the patient initiates several dry swallows while trying to feel the thyroid prominence lift. Then, the instruction is to hold the thyroid up for several seconds. By keeping the larynx tilted and elevated, the upper esophageal sphincter relaxes to allow food to pass, leaving less residual material in the area.

These maneuvers are of significant value to the clinician because: (1) they can be done without any foods or liquids, (2) their effects can be seen during FEES or ultrasound examinations, and (3) they can be done at bedside prior to objective testing to determine a patient's ability to follow directions.

V. SUMMARY

Rademaker and colleagues report that behavioral techniques that include sensory and motor oromotor techniques, swallowing maneuvers, and compensatory strategies are successful in returning more than 80% of patients with oropharyngeal dysphagia to an oral diet.[19] Although other more invasive procedures may be more conducive to improving laryngeal closure (see Chapters 40-42 and 45-46), behavioral techniques should be tried as the first steps for treating laryngeal closure problems that affect swallowing.

Communication with caregivers is critically important for patients undergoing swallowing therapy. All caregivers, from the attending physician to the family, must understand the significance of the treatment and the problems that may occur if the techniques are not done as instructed.

Frequently Asked Questions

1. What four approaches may be used to stimulate sensory awareness in the oral phase of swallowing?
   A. Pressure stimulatation, temperature stimulation, bolus sizes, textures.
2. What is a major risk of aspiration due to weakness of the tongue that may not be identified on swallow examination?
   A. Delayed aspiration due to "pocketing" of food.
3. How does the larynx help to prevent aspiration?
   A. Elevation of the larynx and closure of the vocal folds prevents food and liquid from entering the trachea.
4. When is the most appropriate time to select a facilitating posture for swallowing?
   A. During the modified barium swallow or FEES examination.
5. What are the two contributions of the super-supraglottic swallow?
   A. Increased false vocal fold closure and closure of the posterior glottis.

References

1. Aviv JE, Sacco RL, Mohr J, et al. Laryngopharyngeal sensory testing with modified barium swallow as predictors of aspiration pneumonia after stroke. *Laryngoscope.* 1997; 107:1254-1260.
2. Aviv JE, Martin JH, Sacco RL. Supraglottic and pharyngeal sensory abnormalities in stroke patients with dysphagia. *Ann Otolaryngol Rhinol Laryngol.* 1996,105:92-97.
3. Logemann J. Speech and swallowing rehabilitation for head and neck tumor patients. In: Myers EN, Suen J, eds. *Cancer of the Head and Neck.* 2nd ed. New York, NY: Churchill Livingston; 1997:1021-1043.
4. Leonard R, Gillis R. Effects of a prosthetic tongue on vowel intelligibility and food management in a patient with total glossectomy. *J Speech Hear Disord.* 1982;47:25-29.
5. Logemann J. *Evaluation and Treatment of Swallowing Disorders.* San Diego, Calif: College-Hill Press; 1983.
6. Lazarus C, Logemann JA, Rademaker AW, et al. Effects of bolus volume, viscosity, and repeated swallows in non-stroke subjects and stroke patients. *Arch Phys Med Rehabil.* 1993;74:1066-1070.
7. Lazzara C, Lazarus R, Logemann J. Impact of thermal stimulation on the triggering of the swallowing reflex. *Dysphagia.* 1986;1:73

8. Logemann J, Paulowski BR, Colagnelo L, Lazarus C, Fujiu M, Kahrilas PJ. Effects of a sour bolus on oropharyngeal swallowing measures in patients with neurogenic dysphagia. *J Speech Hearing Res.* 1995;38:556-563.

9. Ramig LO. Speech therapy for patients with Parkinson's disease. In: Koller W, Paulson G, eds. *Therapy of Parkinson's Disease.* New York, NY: Marcel Dekker; 1995;539-50.

10. Logemann J, Kahrilas PJ, Kobara M, Vakil N. The benefit of head rotation on pharyngoesophageal dysphagia. *Arch Phys Med Rehab.* 1989;70:767-771.

11. Logemann JA, Rademaker AW, Paulowski BR, Kahrilas P. Effects of postural change on aspiration in head and neck surgical patients. *Otolaryngol Head Neck Surg.* 1994;110:222-227.

12. Welch M, Logemann JA, Rademaker AW, Kahrilas P. Change in pharyngeal dimensions effected by chin tuck. *Arch Phys Med Rehab.* 1993;74:178-181.

13. Shanahan TK, Logemann JA, Rademaker AW, Pauloski B, Kahrilas P. Chin down posture effects on aspiration in dysphagic patients. *Arch Phys Med Rehab.* 1993;74:736-739.

14. Rasley A, Logemann JA, Kahrilas P, Rademaker AW, Pauloski B, Dodds WJ. Prevention of barium aspiration during videoflouroscopic swallowing studies: value of postural change. *Am J Roentgenol.* 1993;160:1005-1009.

15. Logemann JA. Therapy for oropharyngeal swallowing disorders. In: Perlman AL, Schulze-Delrieu K, eds. *Deglution and Its Disorders.* San Diego, Calif: Singular Publishing Group; 1997:449-462.

16. Cameron JL, Reynolds J, Zuidema GD. Aspiration in patients with tracheostomies. *Surg Gynecol Obstet.* 1973;136: 68-75.

17. Sasaki CT, Suzuki M, Horiuchi M, Kirchner JA. The effect of tracheostomy in the laryngeal closure reflux. *Laryngoscope.* 1977;87:1428-1433.

18. Cook IJ, Dodds WJ, Dantas RO. Opening mechanism of the human upper esophageal sphincter. *Am J Physiology.* 1989;257:G748-G759.

19. Rademaker AW, Logemann JA, Pauloski BR et al. Recovery of postoperative swallowing patients undergoing partial laryngectomy. *Head Neck.* 1993;15:325-334.

CHAPTER 36

■ ■ ■

Dental Prosthetics

Hussein S. Zaki, D.D.S., M.Sc.

I. INTRODUCTION: NONSURGICAL PROSTHETICS

There are two main etiologic factors for defects of the oral cavity: congenital and acquired. Defects of the oral cavity will affect normal swallowing directly or indirectly. Acquired defects are the results of surgical intervention to eradicate tumors, trauma, pathological changes, or burns. Cleft palate, cleft mandible, tongue-tie, or bifid tongue are examples of congenital defects that can affect swallowing.

A. Restoration of Acquired Defects of the Hard and Soft Palate

1. Soft Palate Defects

Prosthetic restoration of soft palate defects vary according to the site and extent of those defects. The defects may fall into one of the following groups:

- Large defects involving the posterior border of the soft palate,
- Defects confined to the soft palate with either a nonfunctional or functional tissue band posteriorly,
- Lateral defects of the soft palate.

The objective of treating patients with oronasal communications is to return the physiologic function of

mastication, deglutition, and speech. If these are accomplished, seepage of nasal fluids into the oral cavity and escape of food into the sinonasal tract will normally be corrected.

In general, all soft palate defects can be reconstructed with a prosthesis that relies on the functional movements of the surrounding structures for effective obturation. Large defects involving the posterior border of the soft palate require a speech aid that extends posteriorly into the pharyngeal region. This extension facilitates the sphincteric closure of the lateral and posterior pharyngeal wall, along with the remnants of the soft palate (Fig 36-1). If a nonfunctional band remains, it is best to remove this band for the posterior and lateral pharyngeal walls to be efficiently utilized. If a functional posterior band is left, the prosthesis should be extended into the defect to utilize the sphincteric action of the remaining soft palate (Fig 36-2). In this case, there is no need to extend the prosthesis to the posterior or lateral pharyngeal walls.

If the defect occurs laterally, the prosthesis should extend through the defect and behind the soft palate. The velopharyngeal closure is attained by the action of the pharyngeal muscles and the nasal surface of the remaining soft palate against the speech aid.

2. Hard Palate Defects

Prosthetic rehabilitation of hard palate defects is simple, predictable, immediate, and gratifying to the patient and the prosthodontist. Success of prosthetic rehabilitation

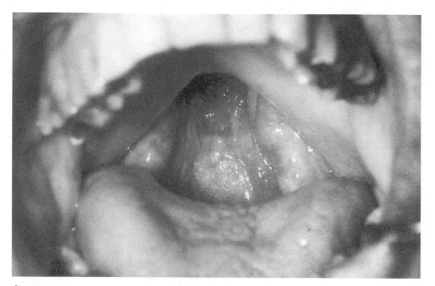

A

FIG 36-1. A. Soft palate defect involving the posterior border. **B.** Speech aid obturator in soft palate defect.

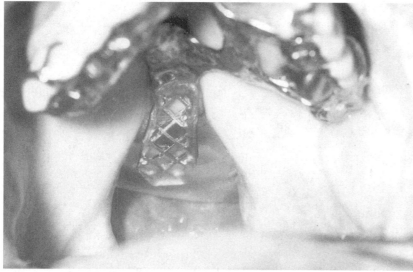

B

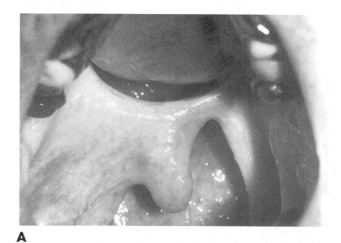

A

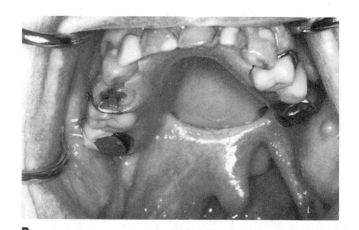

B

FIG 36-2. A. Soft palate defect leaving a functional posterior band. At rest there is a space between the prosthesis and the band. **B.** At function, the space between the mobile posterior band and the prosthesis is obturated.

of hard palate defects is greatly enhanced if the surgeon can create a defect that is well-suited for obturation without compromising tumor removal.

Preservation of the greatest possible portion of the maxilla, especially the premaxilla and the tuberosity areas, will create a tripod effect to help stabilize and improve the retention of an obturator. Retaining important teeth, like cuspids and first molars, will preserve the sense of proprioception and improve the stability, retention, and support of an obturator. The use of a split-thickness skin graft to line the cheek flap will enhance tolerance of the prosthesis by creating a sizable undercut superior and lateral to the scar band, thus enhancing mechanical retention (Fig 36-3).

Immediate surgical obturation is obtained with an acrylic resin wafer that is constructed on the preoperation cast. This surgical obturator is secured in place by screws to help maintain the surgical packing in close coaptation to the wound and the skin graft (Fig 36-4). It provides immediate oronasal separation; thus the patient can swallow and speak effectively in the immediate postoperative period. Among other benefits, the surgical obturator improves the psychological well-being of the patient and reduces communication between the oral cavity and the surgical site, thus reducing the chance of wound infection.

It is customary to remove the surgical obturator and packing 5-7 days after surgery. At this stage, the surgical obturator is altered by selective grinding, addition of retentive wires in the presence of teeth, and use of chairside relines to render the obturator independently retentive and stable. After these adjustments, the obturator should be tested for swallowing and speech and should demonstrate reasonable retention. Instructions are given to the patient on the care of the prosthesis.

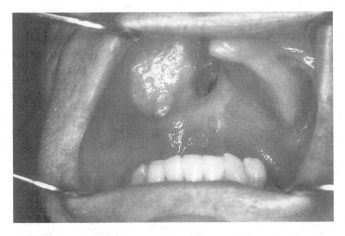

FIG 36-3. Split-thickness skin graft lining the cheek flap will create a sizable superior lateral undercut to enhance retention of the obturator.

The patient is scheduled for weekly lining changes to promote tissue healing.

After an adequate healing period of 3 to 4 months after surgery, a definitive obturator is considered. The remaining structures should be restored and maintained in optimal condition before constructing the definitive obturator. All teeth, if present, should be free of caries or periodontal disease and soft flabby ridges should be treated by frequent use of soft relines, good home care, and possibly minor surgery.

In constructing the definitive obturator, the operator should consider aggressively engaging the soft tissue undercut especially above the scar band and increasing the height of the lateral wall of the obturator.[1,2] The use of openface custom trays will help the operator to best achieve these end results.[3]

Retention and stability are critical factors for success of the obturator. In an attempt to enhance retention, several prosthetic innovations have been attempted, such as making the obturator hollow or topless or using a two-part obturator with magnets.[4-6] The use of osseointegrated implants in the residual ridge following maxillectomy have been tried successfully.[7,8]

B. Prosthetic Rehabilitation of Tongue Defects

Tongue defects due to tumor removal can result in either total or partial glossectomy. Because of the complex role the tongue plays in the oral physiology, its prosthetic rehabilitation is a difficult challenge for both the prosthodontist and the patient. The tongue is mainly involved during both the oral and pharyngeal phase of swallowing. The tongue aids in pushing the food against the palate, helps to reposition the bolus on the occlusal table after each chewing stroke, and clears the buccal vestibule and floor of the mouth.

1. Total Glossectomy

Total glossectomy will create a large oral cavity that results in pooling of saliva and liquids. These liquids tend to seep around the epiglottis, leading to aspiration. Surgical closure[9] of the laryngeal opening may reduce the incidence of aspiration and aid the patient in swallowing liquids.

With our present knowledge, it is impossible to recreate the original function of the mobile tongue either surgically or prosthetically, but it is possible to optimize the function and esthetics of the remaining tissues. The total glossectomy patient is best treated with a mandibular tongue prosthesis that helps the patient to

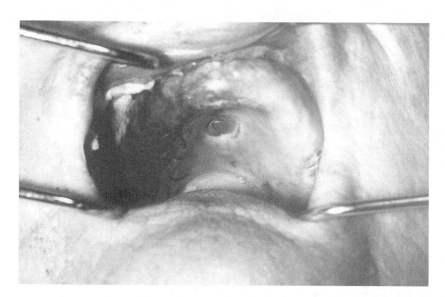

FIG 36-4. Surgical obturator is secured in place to the remaining hard palate by a screw.

articulate better and aids in swallowing. This contributes to the psychological well-being of the patient and the social acceptance of this severe handicap.

The success of prosthetic rehabilitation of tongue defects, depends primarily on the presence or absence of teeth and secondarily on the patient's motivation. The major goals in prosthetic rehabilitation after total glossectomy are:

a. To reduce the size of the oral cavity, which will minimize the degree of pooling of saliva and improve resonance;
b. To develop surface contact with the surrounding structures during speech and swallowing;
c. To protect the underlying fragile mucosa if skin flaps were not used;
d. To help direct the food bolus into the oropharynx with the aid of a trough carved into the dorsum of the prosthetic tongue; and
e. To improve appearance and psychosocial adjustment.

It has been suggested that two prosthetic tongues be made, one for speech (Fig 36-5) and one for swallowing (Fig 36-6). The prosthetic tongue for speech has anterior and posterior elevations. The anterior elevation is for the production of the anterior linguoalveolar phonemes /t/ and /d/ and posterior elevation is for the production of the posterior linguoalveolar phonemes /k/ and /g/. The prosthetic tongue for swallowing has a sloping trough-like base in the posterior aspect to help guide the food bolus into the oropharynx. Construction and final adjustment of the prosthetic tongue should be done in the presence of a speech-language pathologist. A combination tongue prosthesis can be constructed for a highly motivated patient (Fig 36-7).

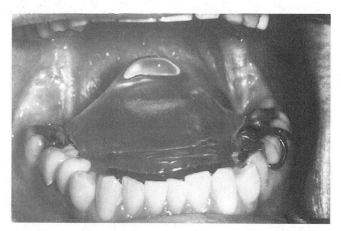

FIG 36-5. Tongue prosthesis made for speech in total glossectomy patient. Notice both the anterior and posterior lingual elevations.

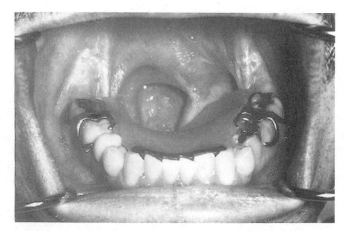

FIG 36-6. Tongue prosthesis made for swallowing in total glossectomy patient. Notice sloping trough toward the oropharynx.

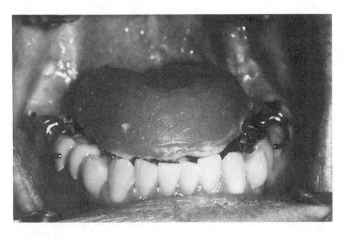

FIG 36-7. Combination tongue prosthesis for both speech and swallowing.

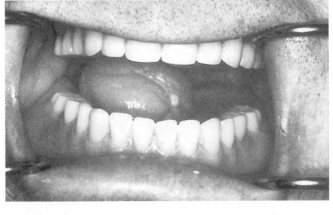

FIG 36-8. Lingual augmentation prosthesis in partial glossectomy.

2. Partial Glossectomy

In partial glossectomy, if more than 50% of the tongue is removed, prosthetic reconstruction consists of either a palatal augmentation prosthesis (Fig 36-8) or a mandibular augmentation prosthesis (Fig 36-9). The function of the augmentation prosthesis is to fill the volume deficiency created by the removal of part of the tongue. The choice between palatal and mandibular augmentation prostheses depends on the extent and site of removal and the patient's acceptance.

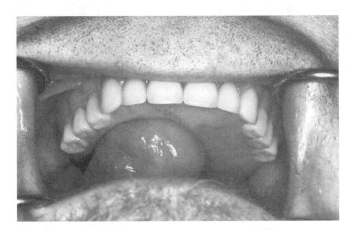

FIG 36-9. Palatal augmentation prosthesis in partial glossectomy patient.

Frequently Asked Questions

1. In restoration of soft palate defects what is critical for success?
   A. The functional movements of the residual tissues are critical for success.
2. Which factors enhance the success of a definitive obturator?
   A. Having a scar band created by a split thickness skin graft; maintenance of strong, healthy teeth; and reducing the weight of the prosthesis.
3. What is the primary function of the tongue?
   A. Swallowing.

References

1. Desjardins RP. Obturator prosthesis design for acquired maxillary defects. *J Prosthet Dent.* 1978;39:424-435.
2. Brown KE. Peripheral consideration in improving obturator retention. *J Prosthet Dent.* 1968;20:176-181.
3. Zaki HS, Aramany MA. Open-face custom tray for edentulous obturator impression. *J Prosthet Dent.* 1981;45:639-642.
4. Nidiffer TJ, Shipman TH. The hollow bulb obturator for acquired palatal opening. *J Prosthet Dent.* 1957;7:126-134.
5. Oral K, Aramany MA, McWilliams BJ. Speech intelligibility of buccal flange obturator. *J Prosthet Dent.* 1979;41:323-328.
6. Davenport J. A magnetically retained sectional prosthesis for rehabilitation of maxillectomy patients. *Quintessence Dent Tech J.* 1985;9:391.
7. Mentag PJ, Kosinski TF. Increased retention of a maxillary obturator prosthesis using osseointegrated intramobile cylinder dental implants: a clinical report. *J Prosthet Dent.* 1988;60:411.
8. Niimi A, Ueda M, Kaneda T. Maxillary obturator supported by osseointegrated implants placed in irradiated bone. *J Oral Maxillofacial Surg.* 1993;51:804-809.
9. Mitrani M, Krespi YP. Functional restoration after subtotal glossectomy and laryngectomy. *J Otolaryngol Head Neck Surg.* 1998;98:5-9.

CHAPTER 37

■ ■ ■

Passy-Muir Valve/Decannulation

Roxann Diez Gross, M.A.
David E. Eibling, M.D.

I. INTRODUCTION

Dysphagia and aspiration are commonly encountered in patients with tracheostomies. The reasons for dysphagia are multi-factorial and are discussed in detail in Chapter 20. Evidence that the presence of a tracheostomy is the cause of dysphagia and/or aspiration can be found in the long-standing clinical observation that swallowing function improves when a tracheostomy tube is capped or removed. Investigations by Sasaki et al have demonstrated significant alteration of glottic reflexes in the presence of an open tracheostomy tube, with return to normal function with closure of the tracheostomy. Although the mechanism by which this improvement occurs has not been determined,[1,2] Sasaki and colleagues have postulated that subglottic air pressure may play an important role in maintaining physiologic glottic reflexes and swallowing function. Recent reports suggest that not only laryngeal reflexes, but pharyngeal transit times are altered as well, suggesting that the presence of an open subglottic airway may affect swallowing by more than a single mechanism.[3]

Voicing requires that the column of expired air pass through the glottis, inducing a vibratory motion of the vocal folds. The presence of a tracheostomy permits some or all of this expired air to escape through the tube, bypassing the glottis and rendering the patient aphonic. This effect, obviously problematic for affected patients, varies with the size of the tube and whether or not the tube is cuffed. If there is sufficient space around the tube within the trachea and if the cuff (if present) is deflated, the patient can phonate if he or she is able to finger occlude the tube while exhaling. Early attempts to facilitate speech in patients with tracheostomies included a modification of a metal tracheostomy tube by incorporating a flipper valve within the inner cannula. The valve was opened by inhalation and then closed by the force of exhalation, redirecting expired air through the glottis. This tube was not widely accepted, as the mechanical valve tended to become encrusted with secretions.

The prototype of all removable speaking valves designed to fit disposable plastic tracheostomy tubes is the patented Passy-Muir speaking valve. This device was invented by a young patient with muscular dystrophy, David Muir, who found himself unable to speak because he could not occlude his tracheostomy tube. He, along with his father, developed and tested a removable closed position valve that opened to permit inhalation, but spontaneously closed at the end of inspiration to divert the air flow through the larynx (Figs 37-1 and 37-2). This valve, eventually marketed as the Passy-Muir valve (PMV), has been widely used by countless patients with tracheostomies to facilitate communication. Other speaking valves such as the Montgomery valve are marketed by other manufacturers, but vary in opening and closing mechanisms. Although originally intended for speech, other benefits became apparent, such

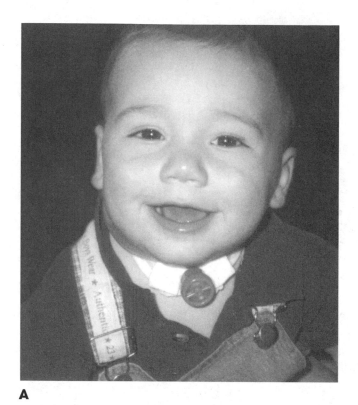

A

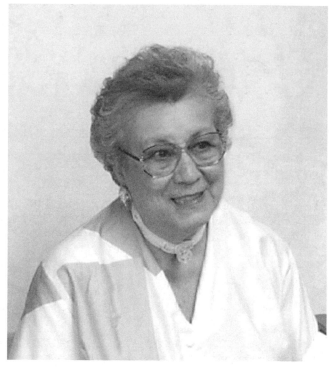

B

FIG 37-1. Photographs of Passy-Muir valves mounted on tracheostomy tubes. **A**. Child wearing model PMV2001 Passy-Muir low-profile tracheostomy and ventilator speaking valve. **B**. Adult wearing model PMV2000. (Photos courtesy of Passy-Muir, Inc., Irvine, Calif.)

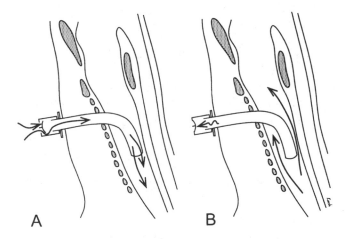

FIG 37-2. Diagram illustrating function of a speaking valve. Note that (**A**) the valve opens for inspiration to permit intake of air, and closes, and (**B**) to facilitate speech by diverting expired air through the larynx. (From Dettelbach MA, Gross RD, Mahlmann J, Eibling DE. The effect of the Passy-Muir valve on aspiration in patients with tracheotomy. *Head Neck*. 1995;17:298. Reprinted with permission.)

as facilitating cough, decreasing atelectasis, decreasing tracheal secretions, and improving swallowing function.[4] This chapter addresses the use of the Passy-Muir speak-ing valve attached to the tracheostomy tube in swallowing rehabilitation, as well as the benefit of decannulation in promoting swallowing function.

II. DECANNULATION

Elective removal of a tracheostomy tube is termed *decannulation*. Abrupt removal may be hazardous for a variety of reasons; therefore, removal of the tracheostomy tube is characteristically performed in an orderly fashion. Some estimate of a patient's ability to tolerate decannulation can usually be obtained by an estimation of the amount of oral and tracheal secretions being suctioned by nursing personnel. Cuff deflation and finger plugging of the tube will permit assessment of the adequacy of the airway with the tube in place. In many instances, patients will not be able to move air around the tube, even with the cuff deflated, because of the relative size of the tube and the deflated cuff (Fig 37-3). Most adult men can move air around a #6 Shiley or #8 Portex, whereas many women cannot. Removal of the tube and finger plugging of the stoma may provide useful information regarding the ability of the patient to move air through his or her larynx. In some centers, routine *cricothyroidotomy* is performed rather than tra-

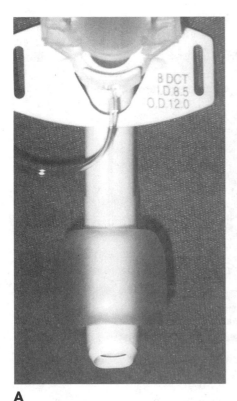
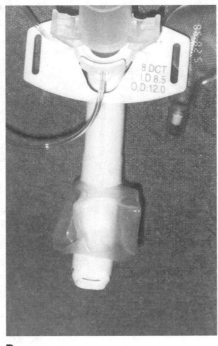
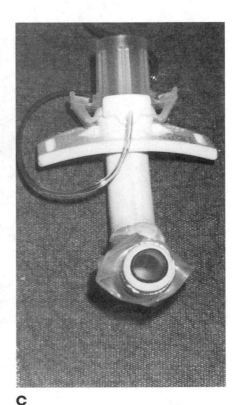

A **B** **C**

FIG 37-3. Photograph of tracheostomy tube with cuff inflated (**A**) and deflated (**B, C**). Note that even the deflated cuff results in some degree of obstruction to airflow around the tube.

cheostomy. The cricoid ring is smaller than the tracheal lumen and is inflexible. Hence, conditioning before decannulation by plugging may be impossible, and simple tube removal in an observed setting may be the only available option.

Once it has been determined that decannulation is feasible, an uncuffed tube of a smaller diameter is inserted and plugged. Men will usually tolerate a #6 uncuffed Shiley tube, whereas most women will require a #4 to permit adequate air passage (Fig 37-4). Plugging needs to occur in a carefully observed setting, especially when the patient is unable to unplug the tube if airway problems ensue. Careful observation of the airway and also the ability to handle oropharyngeal secretions is necessary. If periodic suction is necessary to assure adequate tracheal toilet, then the patient is not ready for decannulation.

The use of a *fenestrated* tracheostomy tube may facilitate the use of a larger tube during the plugging process. Unfortunately, long-term use of a fenestrated tube can induce the growth of granulation tissue through the fenestration, resulting in airway obstruction, bleeding, and other difficulties during tube removal. For these reasons, fenestrated tubes are not routinely used and the preference is to downsize to a tube size that permits air passage around the plugged tube.

Once a patient has tolerated plugging of the tracheostomy tube for more than 24 hours without requiring suction, the tube is removed. In most instances, the stoma will close in a matter of several hours to days. *It is important to recognize that for many patients with a tracheostomy, simple decannulation is the most effective single intervention to enhance swallowing.*

III. SPEAKING VALVES

Capping of the tracheostomy tube or decannulation are not always viable options because of a patient's underlying disease processes. Digital occlusion of the tracheostomy tube is beneficial for both speaking and swallowing, but requires fine motor control of at least one of the upper extremities. The dexterity required thereby eliminates use of this method by patients with quadriplegia, limb apraxia, and so on. Some patients find it a nuisance, often messy, and rather unhygienic. If this technique is utilized for swallowing improvement, precise coordination is required to close the tube during the motion induced by swallowing. It is likely that the tube is not fully occluded by the finger throughout the swallowing, although no studies have yet been performed to investigate this. Manual tube

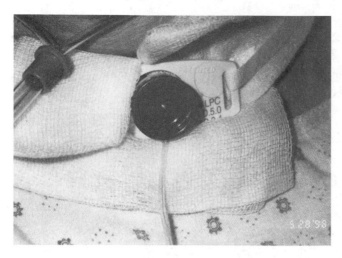

FIG 37-4. This patient has been downsized to a #4 Shiley tube, which has been plugged. If tolerated, the tube can be removed safely.

occlusion for either speech or to enhance swallowing is not feasible for ventilator patients who are ventilator-dependent.

Speaking valves permit inspired air to bypass the glottis, thereby assuring adequate inspiratory volumes. The PMV closes at the end of inspiration, redirecting expired air through the glottis and restoring subglottic air pressure to facilitate speaking and swallowing (see Fig 37-2). Restoration of subglottic pressure during swallowing by the use of a PMV valve has been demonstrated[4] (Fig 37-5). No air volume or pressure from the lungs is lost as the valve closes spontaneously at the end of the inhalatory phase and does not require expiratory air pressure to close as other available speaking valves do. This reproduces the natural closed physiology of the typical person without a tracheostomy. A column of pressurized air remains behind the valve, providing a barrier for secretions and optimizing subglottic pressure required for speech and swallowing. Because the valve does not leak air, the patient is able to use the full, inspired lung volume to cough and clear the pharynx and supraglottis following passage of the bolus (if needed). Videofluoroscopic studies of patients who continue to aspirate with a speaking valve in place often demonstrate that a valve facilitates the detection and expulsion of aspirated or penetrated bolus material that has penetrated into the airway.

A. Ventilator-Dependent Patients

A subset of patients who are ventilator-dependent can benefit from the use of an FDA-approved speaking valve positioned in-line between the ventilator and their *cuffless* (or deflated) tracheostomy tube. These patients must have compliant lungs that permit ventilation with cuff deflation. There is often a learning curve associated with the use of these in-line valves, for both the patient as well as the care team, and this strategy should be employed only in units or centers that are familiar with the technique.

B. Patient Selection

Patients who have a tracheostomy tube, none of the contraindications listed below, and require swallowing rehabilitation or are eating by mouth may benefit from the restoration of airflow through the larynx and upper airway. Although decannulation is preferable for most patients, those who cannot be decannulated should try a speaking valve. Even if decannulation is planned, many patients will benefit significantly from the interim use of a speaking valve, often as a "step" toward downsizing, plugging, and decannulation.

C. Contraindications

Speaking valves are usually very well tolerated. However, they should not be used for swallowing rehabilitation under the following circumstances:

1. Unconscious/comatose patients.
2. Severe behavior problems.
3. Severe medical instability, especially pulmonary failure.
4. Severe tracheal stenosis or edema.
5. Any airway obstruction above the tube that precludes expiration through the glottis.
6. Thick and copious secretions that persist after valve placement.
7. Foam-filled tracheostomy tube cuff (Bivona).
8. Total laryngectomy or laryngotracheal separation.
9. Insufficient passage for air around the tube, either with the cuff down or with a cuffless tube.
10. Inability to maintain adequate ventilation with cuff deflation.

D. Placement Procedure for Non-Ventilator-Dependent Patients

1. Assess tracheostomy tube to assure that *when the cuff is down air passes easily around the tube to the upper airway* (finger plug).
2. Gently, *stabilize* the tracheostomy tube with thumb and forefinger while placing the valve on the end of the tube with the other hand.

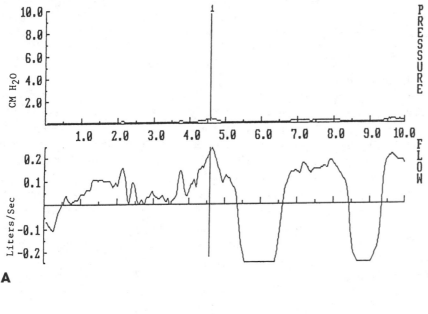

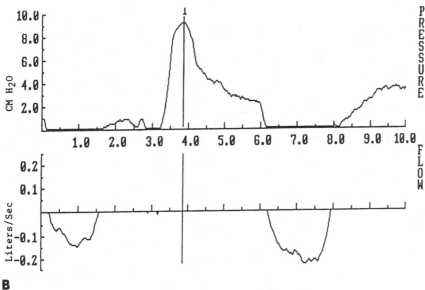

Fig 37-5. Pressure flow measurements of a subject swallowing a sip of water with a tracheostomy, without (**A**) and with (**B**) a Passy-Muir valve. Note expiratory airflow at 4.5 seconds and lack of positive pressure (**A**) without valve, and absence of expiratory flow with positive pressure measurement (**B**) with the valve plugged. (From Eibling DE, Gross, RD. Subglottic air pressure: a key component of swallowing efficiency. *Ann Otol Rhinol Laryngol.* 1996;105:256. Reprinted with permission.)

3. Because the valve does not lock, screw, or snap on, a slight *twist* is used to secure the fit.
4. Ask for patient to *phonate* (if able) to assess glottic airflow
5. Assess for valve *tolerance* using pulse oximetry, heart rate and patient report.
6. *Observe closely* for a period of time to assess patient comfort.

E. Placement Procedure for In-Line Ventilator-Dependent Patients

This procedure should only be performed when the care team is familiar with indications, risks, and technique.

1. Turn off volume alarm on ventilator. *Remember to turn back on completion of the trial.*
2. While maintaining continuous pulse oximetry, deflate cuff and suction trachea.
3. Increase volume of inspired air to compensate for the air lost through open glottis—usually about 0-200 cc, based on peak inspiratory pressure.
4. Place valve in line, observing patient and monitoring oximetry and vitals carefully for adequate ventilation.
5. Remove valve immediately if dyspnea ensues. The most common problem is inadequate space around tube for diverted air to escape through glottis. If speaking valve removal does not immediately resolve difficulty, reinflate tube cuff.
6. Encourage phonation.

F. Evaluation of Swallowing

Plugging the tracheostomy tube or use of a PMV will often dramatically improve swallowing function during radiographic or endoscopic evaluation. Several investigations have shown that swallowing function was optimized when the subglottic airway closed to restore subglottic pressure (Fig 37-5). These studies have demonstrated that use of the PMV has reduced and/or eliminated aspiration in the majority of patients studied.[3-6]

Currently it is not possible to accurately predict which patients will benefit, therefore a real-time trial with the speaking valve should be done during the evaluation. If decannulation is planned in the near future, it is probably best to delay the formal evaluation until after decannulation and the stoma has closed. During evaluation with videofluoroscopy or videoendoscopy, the patient will benefit by trial of use of the speaking valve for some of the swallows tested to determine if there is swallowing improvement. As there is a learning curve for the use of the valve, it is best that the patient have some experience with the valve prior to the evaluation.

For patients who demonstrate acceptable swallowing function both with and without the valve, we recommend that the speaking valve be used while eating and drinking to facilitate coughing. The cuff of the tracheostomy tube *must* be deflated prior to placement of the valve. Changing the tube to a cuffless model will eliminate the possibility of care providers inadvertently placing the valve with the cuff inflated.

G. Rehabilitation

Anecdotal reports and studies have suggested that restoration of airflow enhances laryngo-pharyngeal rehabilitation (Figs 37-1 and 37-2). Reflexes can be normalized over time if stimulation, such as is provided by airflow through the larynx, is increased. Clinically, one should attempt not only to improve function, but to *maintain* function in patients with a tracheostomy. Even though no clinical trials have been performed, we and others believe that facilitating glottic air flow and restoring subglottic pressure periodically each day may help to maintain function in the tracheotomized patient and reduce the chances of difficulties during decannulation. Hence, daily use of a speaking valve may be worthwhile even for those patients who must remain NPO for a time, those for whom aspiration is not a problem, and even for patients that can tolerate valve usage for only limited time periods.

Incorporating the speaking valve into swallowing therapy has three primary advantages:

1. The patient can communicate more easily with the therapist, providing verbal feedback in relation to what the patient is feeling, experiencing, and thinking. Verbal communication will also assist the therapist in making adjustments to exercises, directions, and the overall therapeutic plan.
2. Airflow through the upper airway may improve pharyngeal sensation and provide the patient with proprioceptive cues during swallowing exercises and acquisition of maneuvers. The patient may also be more sensitive to residue, premature spillage, and aspiration, allowing them to spontaneously produce a clearing swallow, catch a bolus flowing into the oropharynx, or cough in response to aspiration.
3. True vocal fold adduction exercises will be maximized because of subglottic air pressure buildup and increased sensation.

IV. PEDIATRIC PATIENTS

To date, no studies have directly compared pediatric swallowing function under open and closed tracheostomy tube conditions. Nonetheless, experienced clinicians have often observed improved feeding in children after decannulation. Pediatric patients are often very sensitive to subtle changes, and improvement may be due to improved smell and taste when the upper airway is returned to its normally closed status. As with adults, decannulation and/or capping may not be feasible, and the use of a speaking valve provides a viable alternative for many patients.

The pediatric airway is smaller and more fragile than the adult's trachea. Tubes are smaller, and there is less room for air to bypass around a plugged or closed tube. However, the reduction of airflow and pressure may play even more significant roles in swallowing function and feeding behavior in children than adults. Thus, use of a PMV may assist with facilitating improvements in swallowing function.

A. Patient Selection

The PMV can be used on infants as young as 1 month old. Contraindications for infants and children are:

1. Severe upper airway obstruction due to subglottic and glottic stenosis, edema, granulation tissue, copious secretions, or bilateral true vocal fold paralysis in the adducted position.
2. Severe medical instability.
3. Severely reduced lung compliance.

B. Placement Procedure for Non-Ventilator-Dependent Pediatric Patients

Valve placement for pediatric patients is no different from placement for adults. However, a child may not fully understand the process and may react negatively. For some, education using visual aids works best; for others, *distraction* may be required. Signs and symptoms of difficulty tolerating the valve are:

1. Increasing respiratory rate over time with or without nasal flaring, head bobbing.
2. Increased irritability with or without restlessness, stridor, grunting, fear, anxiety.
3. Decreased chest movement
4. Skin color changes such as pallor, cyanosis, mottling.

C. Placement Procedure for Ventilator-Dependent Pediatric Patients

As for adults, placement should only be performed when care team is familiar with indications, risks, and technique. Placement of the PMV in-line requires essentially the same methodology as described for adults; however, there are a few special considerations:

1. Never assume that the tube is cuffless. Although it is far more common for pediatric tubes to be cuffless, cuffed neonatal and pediatric tracheostomy tubes do exist. The cuff must be deflated prior to valve placement.
2. Ensure that the child has good airway patency and is able to pass air around the tube. Possible positive indicators include audible crying and phonation or air leakage heard around the tube with a stethoscope. Cross-checking the tube's outer diameter with the child's age is also beneficial for determining the safety of valve placement.
3. If peak inspiratory pressure rises above the normal limit for the patient, remove the valve immediately and reassess airway patency.

D. Speaking Valve Use in Therapy with Children

If no adverse signs are observed, engaging the child in blowing activities using bubbles, pinwheels, and so on is often helpful in inducing a young patient to tolerate airflow through the upper airway. Phonation exercises using visual feedback such as the Speechviewer, Visi-

pitch, or audio feedback using a tape recorder or video camera may also be helpful in gaining laryngeal control.

Feeding problems may initially occur because smell and taste can be heightened by the speaking valve. Some children are hypersensitive or may experience dysesthesia (an altered interpretation of sensation). A systematic therapeutic program addressing the heightened or altered sensitivity must ensue. Conversely, feeding improvement may result from improved taste and smell.

V. CONCLUSIONS

Swallowing function is often adversely affected by the presence of a tracheostomy. Decannulation, usually following plugging, is often the single most important intervention for rehabilitation of swallowing function. Use of a Passy-Muir speaking valve in patients who are not candidates for decannulation or who are ventilator-dependent often can provide significant improvement in swallowing function, probably through physiologic changes attending the restoration of subglottic pressure.

Frequently Asked Questions

1. How important is valve "resistance"?
   A. Slight variations in valve opening resistance are inconsequential. The mechanism of valve closure is significant. The Passy-Muir valve is the only valve that requires no force or effort from the patient to close and remain closed during the swallow. Also, the PMV does not leak air.
2. If I deflate the cuff to use the Passy-Muir valve, won't my patient be more likely to aspirate? (ie, doesn't the cuff prevent aspiration?)
   A. No. The cuff is not intended to prevent aspiration. The definition of aspiration requires that food or drink pass below the true vocal cords. Any material that reaches the cuff has already been aspirated, therefore the cuff does not prevent aspiration.
3. I've seen the Passy-Muir valve used during the course of decannulation. Why is this done?
   A. Use of the PMV as a transition step toward plugging allows the patient to adjust to airflow through the upper airway while maintaining good inspiratory volume. Patients are generally more accepting of a gradual process.
4. Can the Passy-Muir ventilator valve be used for swallowing if my patient is still on the ventilator?
   A. Yes, although comparisons of swallowing function with and without the valve have not been

made on ventilator patients, multiple anecdotal reports describe improved swallowing. Also, the patient will have improved airway clearance because his or her cough will be more forceful. Oropharyngeal sensation will also be maximized by the return of airflow through the upper airway.

References

1. Sasaki CT, Suzuki M. Horiuchi M, Kirchner JA. The effect of tracheostomy on the laryngeal closure reflex. *Laryngoscope.* 1977;87:1428-1433.

2. Buckwalter JA, Sasaki CT. Effect of tracheostomy on laryngeal function. *Otolaryngol Clin North Am.* 1984;17:41-48.

3. Eibling DE, Gross RD. Subglottic air pressure: a key component of swallowing efficiency. *Ann Otol Rhinol Laryngol.* 1996;105:253-258.

4. Gross RD, Dettelbach MA, Zajac DJ, Eibling DE. Measurement of subglottic air pressure during swallowing in a patient with tracheostomy. *Otolaryngol Head Neck Surg.* 1994;111:133.

5. Dettelbach MA, Gross RD, Mahlmann J. Eibling DE. The effect of the Passy-Muir valve on aspiration in patients with tracheostomy. *Head Neck.* 1995;17:297-302.

6. Stachler RJ, Hamlet SL, Choi J, Fleming S. Scintigraphic quantification of aspiration reduction with the Passy-Muir valve. *Laryngoscope.* 1996;106:231-234.

PART VI

SURGICAL TREATMENT OF SWALLOWING DISORDERS

Selected patients who fail conservative treatment of swallowing disorders may benefit from a variety of surgeries. Procedures such as tracheotomy or gastrostomy serve as temporizing measures, while the patient recovers his or her swallowing function. Specific deficiencies of the laryngeal sphincter can be addressed using vocal fold injections or laryngeal framework surgery that complements compensatory mechanisms offered by other nonsurgical methods. Other specific pharyngeal and esophageal conditions, such as uncontrolled gastroesophageal reflux or Zenker's diverticulum, are better addressed with primary surgery. This section provides a discussion of the historical background, indications, patient selection, surgical techniques, and possible complications of the most common surgical procedures used for the treatment of swallowing disorders.

CHAPTER 38

■ ■ ■

Tracheotomy

David E. Eibling, M.D.
Ricardo L. Carrau, M.D.

I. HISTORICAL PERSPECTIVE

Tracheotomy for the surgical management of airway obstruction has been reported since antiquity. Legend has it that Alexander the Great performed a tracheotomy in the 4th century BC.[1] Gayland and Aretaeus alleged that Aslepiades performed a successful tracheotomy, and other writings of this era suggest that tracheotomy was performed on rare occasions. The oldest known reference, however, is from religious Hindu writings approximately 4000 years ago.

The first report of a successful tracheotomy is attributed to Brasavola, who performed the procedure in 1546. Tracheotomy was performed rarely over the next two centuries until 1825, when Bretonneau successfully treated the airway obstruction associated with diphtheria by performing a tracheotomy.[2] During the early 1900s, Chevalier Jackson described the technique of tracheotomy as is performed today and established guidelines for its postoperative management, leading to a significant decrease of its morbidity and mortality.[3]

II. SURGICAL INDICATIONS

A. Mechanical Ventilation

The most common indication for the performance of a tracheotomy is prolonged mechanical ventilation. The length of time that oral or nasal endotracheal intubation can be tolerated is controversial and is influenced by a vast number of factors (Table 38-1). Physicians use different criteria regarding this issue; however, most experts acknowledge that guidelines based solely on duration of orotracheal or nasotracheal intubation are inappropriate. For example, a review of the events that precipitated the initial intubation of a chronically intubated patient may, in fact, indicate that aspiration played a significant role in the patient requiring intubation. Hence, in this population of patients, a tracheotomy may be required for the management of aspiration (tracheal suctioning).

B. Head and Neck Surgery

Tracheotomy provides access to the airway not only for the duration of the surgical procedure, but also in the postoperative period, when swelling, anatomic alterations, and oropharyngeal secretions jeopardize the airway. Surgical procedures that alter the anatomy of the upper aerodigestive tract or impair its function may result in significant aspiration, and the presence of a tracheotomy permits suctioning of the aspirated secretions (see Chapter 20, Tracheotomy/Endotracheal Intubation).

C. Airway Obstruction

A number of acute medical and surgical illnesses require a tracheotomy for the relief of airway obstruction. These include infections of the upper aerodigestive

Table 38-1. *Factors Influencing the Decision for Tracheotomy in Chronic Ventilator-Dependent Patients*

1. Primary diagnosis
2. Comorbidities
3. Nasal versus oral tube
4. Patient comfort
5. Ease of endotracheal suction
6. Expected duration of ventilator support
7. Effect of reducing "dead space"
8. Patient motion
9. Nasal tube or oral complications of endotracheal tube
10. Perceived risk of laryngeal complications

Table 38-2. *Indications for Tracheotomy*

I. Airway Obstruction
   A. Congenital abnormality
      Laryngeal Web
      Agenesis
      Vocal fold paralysis
      Cysts
   B. Infection
      Supraglottitis
      Deep neck abscess/cellulitis
      Ludwig's angina
   C. Bilateral vocal fold paralysis
      Postsurgical
      Viral
      Toxic
      CNS disorders
   D. Trauma
      Laryngeal injury
      Unstable mandible fracture
   E. Neoplasms
      Upper aerodigestive tract
      Thyroid
      Upper-mediastinum
      Lymphatic metastasis
   F. Surgery
      Head and neck surgery
      Intraoperative airway management

II. Chronic Ventilator Support

III. Pulmonary Hygiene

tract such as supraglottitis, illnesses associated with acute laryngeal and pharyngeal swelling such as angioneurotic edema, tumors of the upper aerodigestive tract or neck, bilateral vocal fold paralysis, or congenital abnormalities of the larynx that may present as life-threatening airway obstruction at birth (Table 38-2).

D. Aspiration

A wide variety of disorders of the upper aerodigestive tract result in swallowing dysfunction and aspiration (refer to Chapter 20). Many patients may ultimately adjust to their disability. Nonetheless, when arising acutely and in patients who are unable to compensate, aspiration may result in significant pulmonary morbidity and even death. In some cases, the urgent performance of a tracheotomy during morbid aspiration may be life-saving in that it facilitates access to the tracheobronchial tree for suctioning of aspirated secretions. It must be noted, however, that the presence of a tracheotomy does not enhance the ability of a patient to swallow and, in fact, will result in possible greater swallowing dysfunction and aspiration (Chapter 20). Removal of the tube or valving will often correct the dysphagia associated with a tracheotomy (Chapter 37).

III. PREOPERATIVE ASSESSMENT

In most instances, a tracheotomy is requested when it is expected that the pulmonary status of a patient who requires ventilatory support is unlikely to improve enough for extubation to be feasible in the near future. Nevertheless, it behooves the surgeon to inquire about the duration of intubation and the expectations of the primary service. In some instances, the performance of

a tracheotomy facilitates weaning a patient from mechanical ventilation through cessation of sedatives (required to tolerate the presence of the endotracheal tube), reducing the "dead space" of the ventilator circuit, and easing tracheobronchial suctioning. As a result, the surgeon and other care providers should not assume that a tracheotomy had not been required, if weaning occurs more rapidly than expected following a tracheotomy.

There is a subset of chronic ventilator patients who require high pressure for maintenance of oxygenation, often with high levels of positive end-expiratory pressure (PEEP). The required high pressures may prevent these patients from being adequately ventilated following tracheotomy, as the distensibility of the trachea may prevent an adequate seal between the tracheostomy tube cuff and tracheal wall. In these cases, it may be best to delay tracheotomy until the pulmonary status has stabilized to the extent that lower pressures may be tolerated and ventilation can be more easily maintained or to use tracheotomy tubes with "oversize" low-pressure cuffs (Bivona foam cuff).

The performance of a tracheotomy to facilitate major extirpative head and neck surgery has been previously discussed. Nevertheless, it must be noted that, in well selected patients, a tracheotomy can be avoided by using nasal or oral endotracheal intubation until extubation can be safely achieved. This strategy, which is most commonly used in the pediatric population, requires an intensive care team familiar with the management of these cases and capable of reestablishing the airway in an emergency.

IV. SURGICAL TECHNIQUE[4]

A. Location of Procedure

Many patients who require tracheotomy are dependent on mechanical ventilation for which they are admitted to intensive care units. The decision as to whether the procedure should be performed in the intensive care unit (ICU) or in an operating theater is a decision best made by the surgeon and the critical care medical specialist in the context of the overall facilities of their institution and their experience. Nevertheless, it must be noted that the performance of a tracheotomy with inadequate instrumentation or anesthesia can be challenging, at best, and life-threatening at worst. Essential equipment, such as a surgical tray with adequate retractors, head light, electrocautery, and suction, must be available.

B. Patient Position

The earliest reports of tracheotomy noted the need for tilting the chin back to elevate the trachea up into the neck. Although there is wide individual variability, in nearly all cases, the use of a shoulder roll facilitates access to the trachea inferior to the cricoid cartilage. The value of this simple maneuver cannot be overemphasized. Inability to extend the neck, such as for a patient who has undergone cervical fusion or is in a halo frame, will usually make the procedure more difficult.

C. Anesthesia

Performance of a tracheotomy under local anesthesia is inherently more difficult than under general anesthesia. The airway is unprotected and discomfort occurring during the course of the procedure can result in significant difficulties due to the patient's swallowing, difficulty breathing, or even agitation. As a result, many surgeons elect to perform nearly all tracheotomies under general anesthesia. Patients who have been intubated for some time often require minimal additional sedation and paralysis to induce a state of general anesthesia. However, even in these instances, the use of local anesthesia may be beneficial by reducing the level of required general anesthesia, with the local injection of a vasoconstrictor (epinephrine) helping with hemostasis.

Local anesthesia is infiltrated sequentially. Typically, the skin and the subcutaneous tissues are injected first, with the deeper tissues injected later in the surgical procedure. Tracheal injection can result in great apprehension by the patient with a compromised airway because of the cough reflex and the loss of airway proprioception. It may even precipitate an acute airway obstruction due to increased agitation and resultant forced inspiration and should therefore be delayed until just before entering the trachea.

D. Surgical Landmarks

Palpation of the neck should clearly identify the position of the cricoid cartilage and the cricothyroid membrane, as well as the sternal notch. If the patient has kyphosis or limited extension of the cervical spine or in patients with chronic obstructive pulmonary disease (COPD), the cricoid may not be palpated above the sternal notch.

E. Skin Incision

Some have suggested that a vertical skin incision may be more physiologic than a horizontal incision in that it permits the tracheostomy tube to move up and down and seek the optimal position, avoiding placing the tube under tension in a manner that may press the tip of the tube against the posterior or anterior tracheal walls. Conversely, a horizontal incision is parallel to the tension lines of the neck and, thus, more cosmetic. Most commonly, we use a horizontal incision placed between the cricoid and the sternal notch, although this position may vary slightly depending on the anatomy of the patient.

The skin incision should be approximately 2 cm in length and can be easily widened during the dissection of the subcutaneous tissue. Debulking of the subcutaneous fat in patients with an excess amount of adipose tissue simplifies the procedure and facilitates tube changes. Debulking, however, can lead to an unsightly scar in some patients and is not advised, if a short-term tracheostomy is anticipated. Inferior and superior skin flaps are elevated to gain wider access to the anterior neck.

F. Dissection of Strap Muscles

Fascial layers over the midline of the strap muscles are sequentially divided from superficial to deep planes (Fig 38-1A). The divided tissues are divided laterally to expose the deeper tissues. In instances in which the

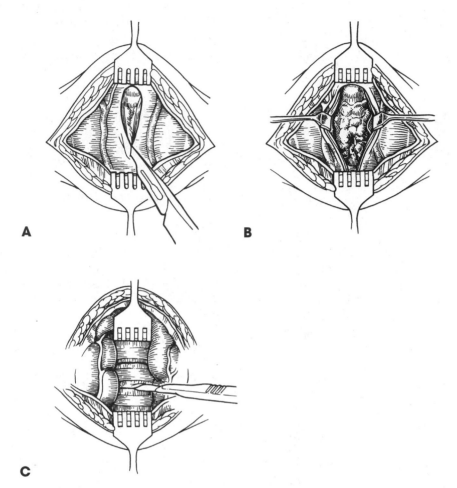

FIG 38-1. Technique of tracheotomy. **A.** Division of strap muscles. The key in this step is to stay directly in the midline and avoid the anterior jugular vein, which can become quite problematic if injured. If identification of the midline raphe is difficult, inferior dissection will often reveal its position. Straying laterally at this step will result in significant difficulties in identifying the proper location for entering the trachea. **B.** The thyroid isthmus is identified and usually retracted superiorly. A convenient way of doing this is by placing two Senn reactors under the isthmus and then dissecting it superiorly, exposing the tracheal wall. **C.** The trachea is open in a transverse direction between two tracheal rings, usually the second and third in an adult. Some surgeons create an inferiorly based flap or remove a segment of it at the vecheal ring.

midline is not easily identified, the dissection is extended inferiorly to identify where the strap muscles separate at their origin. Care must be taken to avoid injury to the anterior jugular veins, which usually course approximately 1 or 2 cm lateral and parallel to the midline.

G. Management of Thyroid Isthmus

The thyroid isthmus is usually directly over the site of the tracheotomy and must be displaced superiorly to access the anterior trachea (Fig 38-1B). This maneuver is easily accomplished by placing two Senn retractors on the inferior aspect of the isthmus or grabbing the entire isthmus with an Allis clamp and then retracting it in a superior direction.

Inferior displacement of the thyroid isthmus is more difficult due to the tethering effect of the superior thyroid vascular pedicles. Thus, the mobilization is usually not sufficient to avoid entering the trachea in the immediate subcricoid region. As a result, we prefer to either retract the thyroid isthmus superiorly or divide the isthmus.

Division of the thyroid isthmus is best accomplished using electrocautery, avoiding major vessels as the isthmus is vertically divided. The two "stumps" of the divided isthmus are then dissected from the anterior trachea. Alternatively, the fascia anterior and superior to the thyroid isthmus is incised, freeing the isthmus from the cricoid cartilage and permitting entry to the pretracheal space with a Crile hemostat or Kelly clamp. The thyroid isthmus is then clamped with two clamps and then divided and suture ligated. This maneuver, however, is cumbersome to perform through a small skin incision, and we reserve its use for an isthmus that contains major vessels that are not amenable to electrocauterization.

H. Tracheal Entry

If the cricoid cartilage is positioned low in the neck, a tracheal hook is used to retract the trachea up into the surgical field. Care must be taken during the insertion of the hook to place it immediately inferior to the cricoid and not into the thyroid isthmus. It must be noted that this maneuver is uncomfortable for the patient, so it should be delayed as long as possible.

In adults, the trachea is opened using a transverse incision between two tracheal rings (Fig 38-1C). Some surgeons routinely remove a window of cartilage, but we have not found this to be necessary. It is usually best to use the second or third inter-space in the average adult, and the fourth or fifth inter-space in the infant or young child. In general, the first inter-space is avoided, as injury to the cricoid cartilage can result from tube pressure. Nevertheless, in elderly patients with thoracocervical deformities, it is often impossible to place the tracheostomy lower than the first inter-space because of the low position of the cricoid cartilage. In infants and children, the trachea is divided between stay sutures in a vertical fashion.

There is significant controversy regarding the use of a flap of anterior tracheal wall because of the effect of the flap on stabilizing the trachea, potentially leading to greater postoperative swallowing difficulties. Nevertheless, many surgeons routinely create an inferiorly based flap, which is then tagged with a suture or sutured to the skin to assure a safe postoperative airway.

The anterior tracheal wall should be opened carefully, avoiding the cuff of the endotracheal tube. This is particularly important in patients who require high ventilatory pressures. Deflating the cuff briefly prior to entering the trachea or moving the endotracheal tube distally helps avoid the balloon. It is important to remember that in the oxygen-enriched environment, the endotracheal tube can be ignited by electrocautery. As a result, it is probably best to enter the trachea via sharp dissection or decrease the inspired oxygen concentration before entering the trachea. To ease the placement of the tracheostomy tube as well as to facilitate its replacement should inadvertent decannulation occur postoperatively, stay sutures should be routinely placed (Fig 38-2).

I. Insertion of Tracheostomy Tube

Maneuvers that ease the tracheotomy tube insertion include deflating the cuff of the tracheostomy tube and retracting the edges of the cuff and holding the tracheotomy tube at right angles to the neck with the tip of the tube directed into the trachea between the stay sutures. Once the tip is within the tracheal lumen, the

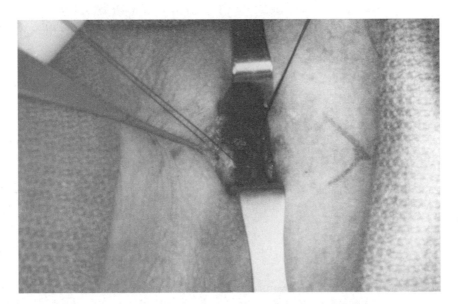

FIG 38-2. Stay sutures are placed around the superior and inferior rings to preclude inadvertent loss of the trachea lumen in the immediate postoperative period.

These sutures assist in placing or replacing the tube in the immediate postoperative period and are routinely removed in approximately 1 week.

tube is rotated and pressed into position. The obturator is removed, the inner cannula placed (if required), the cuff inflated, the airway tubing connected, and the tube secured.

The tracheotomy tube should be secured to prevent inadvertent decannulation in the postoperative period. We use sutures around the tube flange, as well as straps, to secure the tube in place. The presence of sutures (typically removed 4-5 days later) indicates to the care providers that the tracheotomy has been recently performed and that tracheotomy tube removal may result in loss of the tract.

J. Percutaneous Tracheotomy

Recently the technique of percutaneous tracheotomy has been adopted in a wide variety of settings. This technique entails the penetration of the tracheal lumen via a large bore needle, through which a guide wire is introduced. Sequential dilators are guided by the wire through the soft tissue and tracheal wall, thus creating a stoma. Once the tract is sufficiently widened, a specially designed tube is inserted into the trachea. The technique facilitates the performance of tracheotomy by the nonsurgeon.[5]

Experience with this technique has been highly variable. Reported complications include bleeding, creation of a false tract, or laceration of the posterior tracheal wall. Some surgeons suggest that the performance of percutaneous tracheotomy under direct endoscopic visualization (utilizing a flexible fiberoptic bronchoscope placed through the vocal folds to visualize the lumen of the trachea during the procedure) facilitates the safe performance of the procedure by verifying the presence of the instrumentation within the tracheal lumen.

A significant disadvantage of the technique is that the surgeon cannot place stay sutures, and that the tract collapses quickly if accidental decannulation occurs in the early postoperative period. Thus, if inadvertent decannulation occurs in the immediate postoperative period, the tube cannot be easily replaced. Moreover, the surgical time is not less than that of a formal tracheotomy. For these reasons, we have elected to continue to perform standard surgical tracheotomy rather than percutaneous tracheotomy.

K. Cricothyroidotomy

The easiest route to the subglottic airway is through the cricothyroid membrane. The airway is closest to the skin at this point and there are no large vessels overlying the airway. As a result, cricothyroidotomy is the procedure of choice when an emergent surgical airway is required.

In some institutions, the cricothyroidotomy is routinely employed in lieu of a formal tracheotomy. This strategy is most often utilized when a surgical airway is required by patients who have undergone a midline sternotomy. The performance of a cricothyroidotomy avoids placing a contaminated wound low in the neck, where it may infect the sternotomy wound.

One of the main problems with cricothyroidotomy is the limited height of the cricothyroid membrane and the lack of tubes designed for this specific procedure. The membrane is 7-9 mm high for most patients, which is smaller than the diameter of a #6 Shiley tube (10 mm). A cricothyroidotomy places the "tracheotomy tube" immediately inferior to the anterior commissure of the vocal folds, and almost invariably results in some edema of the subglottic airway and dysfunction of the vocal folds (Fig 38-3A, 38-3B). This edema, when coupled with the presence of a tube within the lumen of the cricoid cartilage, makes decannulation by routine downsizing difficult. In addition, there are reports of chronic changes in the glottis in some of these patients following decannulation. Thus, we do not perform a cricothyroidotomy in nonurgent settings, except for the subset of patients previously mentioned.

V. Pitfalls and Complications

Although a straightforward operative procedure, tracheotomy is not without risk and complications are commonly encountered (Table 38-3). These may be of minor "nuisance," quality, or severe and deadly for the patient. Complications may occur early or weeks after the tracheostomy procedure. Early complications occur

Table 38-3. *Complications of Tracheotomy*

Early complications
  Displaced tracheostomy tube
  Misplaced tracheostomy tube
  Mucous plug
  Pneumomediastinum
  Pneumothorax
  Postoperative bleeding
    Thyroid isthmus
    Anterior jugular veins
  Postobstructive pulmonary edema
  Hypoventilation due to loss of hypoxia drive
  Infection: soft tissue or trachea

Late complications
  Innominate artery erosion
  Granulation tissue
  Tracheal stenosis
  Mucous plug
  Tube disconnect (in chronic ventilator-dependent patients)

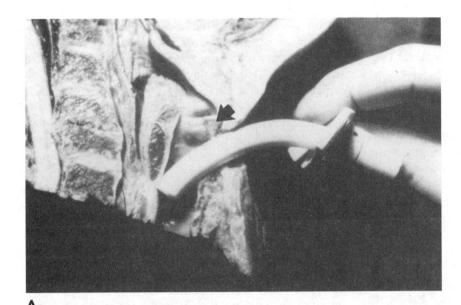

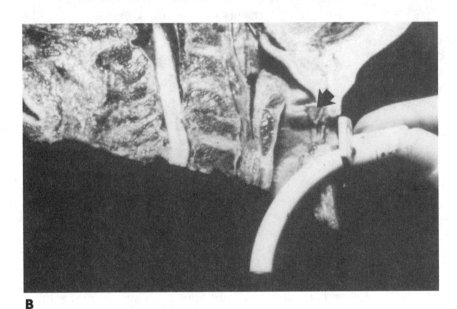

FIG 38-3. Cricothyroidotomy **(A)** and tracheotomy **(B)**. Note the proximity of the tube to the true vocal folds (*arrow*) in the cricothyroidotomy. In addition, the space between the cricoid and thyroid cartilages is limited, precluding easy tube insertion. (From Rood SR. Anatomy of Tracheotomy. In: Myers EN, Stool SE, Johnson JT, eds. *Tracheotomy.* New York, NY: Churchill Livingstone; 1985:91. Reprinted with permission.

because of difficulties that arise during the course of the procedure, the lack of a formed tract between the trachea and the skin, or due to disordered respiratory physiology of the patient that existed prior to the procedure.[6] Late complications generally occur from the presence of the foreign body (tracheotomy tube) in the lumen of the airway. Some complications, such as mucous plug, can occur at any time.

A. Displaced or Misplaced Tracheostomy Tube

The tip of the tracheostomy tube must be within the lumen of the trachea to assure uninterrupted gas exchange. The tube may be inadvertently misplaced into the soft tissues anterior to the trachea rather than into the lumen proper (false tract), or it may be placed in the correct location and then become displaced by movement or coughing. Displacement may seem easy to verify, but actual visualization may be problematic in obese patients, those with disordered anatomy because of a cervical mass displacing the trachea, or in cases where the tracheostomy had to be placed low in the neck.

This complication is far better dealt with by prevention or immediate recognition than by assuming that it either will not or has not occurred. Preventive measures include selection of a tube of sufficient length that has been secured with straps and stitches. Traction on the stay sutures during tube insertion ensures that the tip of the tube is placed within the lumen. If there is question of tube displacement, traction on the stay sutures may permit visual verification of tube position.

Tube position can also be verified by checking the gas spectrography (CO_2), air exchange by passing a suction catheter, or, ideally, a flexible fiberoptic laryngoscope to document the position of the tube. The latter is particularly valuable when the adequacy of the length of the tracheotomy tube is in question. In these instances, the position of the tube tip should be verified after the shoulder roll has been removed and the neck flexed, as this may move the trachea sufficiently lower in the neck as to displace it out of the lumen. Gentle traction on the tube while visualizing the lumen through the broncho-scope may provide some indication of the length of tube left within the lumen. Tracheotomy tubes that can be adjusted to the required length (Bivona, Rousch) are extremely useful under these circumstances.

Early tube replacement (less than 5 days) should be performed with the patient in the same position as for the initial tracheotomy—that is, with the neck extended over a shoulder roll. Instruments for retraction, adequate illumination, and suction are required. Digital palpation of the tract may assist in assessing the relative position of the skin incision and the fenestration in the trachea.

B. Bleeding

Postoperative bleeding occurs primarily from errors in surgical technique (unrecognized anterior jugular vein injury that may not be identified until the patient coughs or strains at the completion of the procedure). Another common source of bleeding is the thyroid isthmus. Typically, this type of bleeding can usually be managed at the bedside, although at times a return to the operating suite for management is required. Replacing the tracheostomy tube with an endotracheal tube often assists in exposure. Erosion of a major vessel, such as the innominate artery, is rare. Massive bleeding can be preceded by more limited "red herring" hemorrhage, which should be suspected in debilitated patients with chronic tracheotomies performed lower than the fourth tracheal ring.

C. Respiratory Dysfunction

Several physiologic events may compromise patient ventilation following relief of airway obstruction. An uncommon, but life-threatening problem is the development of postobstructive pulmonary edema. This usually occurs following the relief of a severe obstruction in which high negative intrathoracic pressures have been generated. The onset is manifested by copious pink frothy secretions and pulmonary rales on ascultation. There is usually the rapid development of hypoxemia and high ventilation pressures shortly after the airway has been opened. Chest radiograms reveal a characteristic butterfly pattern. Treatment is via ventilatory support with PEEP.

Patients who have had long-standing low-grade obstruction often become very fatigued and have blunting of their central oxygen drive. When the airway is opened, the obstruction is relieved, and their drive to breathe is reduced, leading to hypoventilation to the extent that they retain sufficient carbon dioxide to become acidotic. This is enhanced by the use of respiratory depressants such as narcotics or benzodiazepines. As a result, patients who have had long-standing obstruction should be observed closely in the perioperative period, remembering that pulse oximetry may not demonstrate hypoxemia until near to cardiac collapse.

D. Mucous Plug

Mucous plugging of the tracheostomy tube is rare during the early positive period, but can occur if inadequate nursing care is available to suction the tracheostomy, clean or replace the inner cannula, and assure adequate humidification (Fig 38-4). In almost all instances, mucous plugging can be readily corrected by removal and cleaning or replacement of the inner cannula. Occasionally the entire tube must be replaced due to ball-valve tenacious mucous hanging from the tip that cannot be removed by suction and irrigation.

VI. CONCLUSION

Tracheotomy is a valuable interventional procedure that is often very beneficial to the patient with airway obstruction or other disease processes effecting the upper airway. The procedure can be performed safely and quickly by experienced surgeons. Although rare, complications can occur, usually within the first hours to days. Prompt recognition and management can be life-saving for the patient.

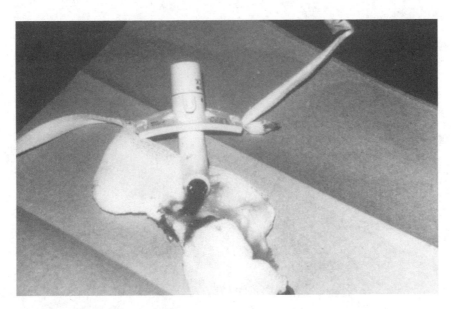

FIG 38-4. Mucous plug occluding the end of a tracheostomy tube. This complication can best be avoided by humidification and routine tracheostomy tube cleaning. Often, tube removal is life-saving in instances of severe plugging.

References

1. Frost EAM. Tracing the tracheostomy. *Ann Otolaryngol.* 1976;85:618.
2. Eavey R.D. The evolution of tracheotomy. In: Myers EN, Stool SE, Johnson JT, eds. *Tracheotomy.* New York, NY: Churchill Livingstone; 1985:1-11.
3. Jackson C. High tracheotomy and other errors—chief causes of chronic laryngeal stenosis. *Surg Gynecol Obstet.* 1923; 32:392.
4. Myers EN. Tracheostomy. In: Myers EN ed. *Operative Otolaryngology—Head and Neck Surgery.* Philadelphia, Pa: WB Saunders; 1997:575-585.
5. Carrillo EH, Spain DA, Bumpous JM, Schmieg RE, Miller FB, Richardson JD. Percutaneous dilational tracheostomy for airway control. *Am J Surg.* 1997;174:469-473.
6. McHenry CR, Raeburn CD, Lange RL, Priebe PP. Percutaneous tracheostomy: a cost-effective alternative to standard open tracheostomy. *Am Surg.* 1997;63:646-651.
7. Myers EN, Carrau RL. Early complications of tracheotomy: incidence and management. *Clin Chest Med.* 1991;12:589-595.

CHAPTER 39

■ ■ ■

Percutaneous Tracheotomy

Karen M. Kost, M.D., F.R.C.S.(C)

I. INTRODUCTION

Tracheotomy is a frequently performed procedure as part of the management of patients with swallowing disorders, particularly those with severe or intractable aspiration. Indeed, many of these patients are critically ill, intubated intensive care unit (ICU) patients with complex multi-system disorders. More than half of modern day tracheotomies are performed on such patients,[1] who by virtue of their severe illnesses, are at higher risk for complications. Stauffer et al[2] noted a 66% complication rate in tracheotomies performed on ICU patients; Zeitouni and Kost[1] noted a 30% complication rate in ICU patients undergoing tracheotomy compared to a 17% rate in non-ICU patients.

Traditionally these patients are taken to the operating room for a "standard" open tracheotomy, which is usually a variation of Chevalier Jackson's technique involving sharp dissection. With few exceptions, these patients are already intubated, the procedure is considered semiselective, and they are given a low surgical priority. Operating room time is expensive, in high demand, and often in short supply. Consequently, the procedure may be performed late at night 1 or more days after the initial consultation. Transporting these critically ill patients with their monitors requires additional personnel and carries a number of inherent risks, including accidental extubation and vital sign changes requiring pharmacological intervention.[3] These factors have led to interest in developing a safe, convenient, and cost-effective bedside procedure.

Standard tracheotomy at the bedside is often inconvenient and requires importing instrument trays, ade-

quate suction, extra lighting, and electrocautery from the surgical department. The procedure may be further compromised by the lack of trained operating room nurses and assistants. Risks include inadequate visualization and spontaneous ignition with the use of electrocautery in the presence of $\geq 30\%$ oxygen.

Several percutaneous techniques have been introduced as a means of simplifying, increasing the efficiency, and decreasing the cost of the procedure. The Seldinger technique is based on progressive dilatation of an initial tracheal puncture and has been recommended particularly for the ICU population. There have been concerns over safety, because the procedure, as originally described, is blind. With the notable addition of endoscopic guidance, first reported in 61 patients by Marelli et al,[4] the "blind" aspect has been addressed. This author's experience with more than 150 cases to date has demonstrated that, with bronchoscopic visualization and attention to technical detail, percutaneous tracheotomy (PCT) is a safe, cost-effective alternative to standard open tracheotomy in the operating room with complication rates comparable to or lower than standard open tracheotomy.

II. PREOPERATIVE EVALUATION

A. Patient Selection

PCT should be considered only for adult intubated patients (Table 39-1). This patient population accounts for

Table 39-1. *Indications and Contraindications for Percutaneous Tracheostomy*

Indications

- Adult intubated ICU patients

Contraindications

- Inability to palpate cricoid
- Midline neck mass
- High innominate artery
- Uncorrected coagulopathy
- Unprotected airway
- Children
- PEEP ≥20 cm H_2O

close to two thirds of all tracheotomies performed today.[1] The more common indications include:

1. Removing the endotracheal tube
2. As an aid in weaning from mechanical ventilation
3. For pulmonary toilet
4. To alleviate upper airway obstruction

Anatomic suitability must be determined preoperatively with the neck extended. As a minimum, the cricoid cartilage must be palpable above the sternal notch. Inability to do so constitutes a contraindication to the procedure. Similarly, the patient with a midline neck mass, high innominate artery or large thyroid gland should undergo standard open tracheotomy in the operating room. Coagulopathies are common in this patient population and should be corrected preoperatively. Platelets should be ≥ 50,000 and the international normalized ratio (INR) corrected to ≤ 1.5. Patients requiring an elevated positive end-expiratory pressure (PEEP) of ≥ 20 cm H_2O are at high risk for complications such as subcutaneous emphysema and pneumothorax and should undergo standard open tracheotomy in the operating room.

There is no place for PCT in nonintubated patients with acute airway compromise. The procedure is too lengthy and requires bronchoscopic visualization through an endotracheal tube.

Although there is little experience with PCT in the pediatric population, it is this author's opinion that the procedure is contraindicated in this age group for a number of reasons. These include the different airway anatomy and dimensions in children, as well as the technical difficulties of maintaining adequate ventilation with a bronchoscope within a small endotracheal tube (Table 39-1).

B. Laboratory Testing

Preoperative testing for PCT is minimal and includes a recent chest radiograph as well as serum determination of hemoglobin, prothrombin time, partial thromboplastin time, and platelets. Cross-matching is not necessary. A fully equipped intubation cart should be available near the bedside in the event of accidental extubation during the procedure. In patients with short thick necks, consideration should be given to placement of an extra long tracheotomy tube to prevent accidental decannulation or displacement into the pretracheal soft tissues.

III. SURGICAL PROCEDURE

A. Personnel

A minimum of 4 people is required, including the attending staff surgeon, a resident or critical care colleague to perform the bronchoscopy, a respiratory technician to assist in adjusting ventilator settings and to firmly hold the endotracheal tube in position, and a nurse to administer medication, monitor vital signs, and aid in obtaining necessary materials or instruments. The surgeon and necessary instruments are positioned to the patient's right, the respiratory technician to the left, and the bronchoscopist at the head of the bed.

B. Instruments

At present, two kits are commercially available for the procedure. Both are based on the use of graduated tapered dilators to allow placement of an appropriately sized tracheotomy tube. The only significant difference between the two units lies in the curved versus straight shape of the dilators. The curved dilators have the empiric advantage of conforming to the anatomical arc of the surgically created tract. Other differences between the kits are principally cosmetic and this author has found them both equally simple to use.

The Cook kit in its present form includes seven curved dilators increasing in size from 12 French to 36 French. A 38 French dilator is available separately and is highly recommended for routine use. The 24 French dilator can be used to insert a #6 Shiley or #9 Portex tracheotomy tube, with a 28 French dilator appropriate for inserting a #8 Shiley or #11 Portex tracheotomy tube. In practice with this kit, an appropriate dilator can be found to fit and allow insertion of most types of tracheotomy tubes. The size of the tube can be determined at the time of the procedure (Fig 39-1).

The technology and instrumentation associated with this technique are continually evolving and subject to refinement. Cook has recently introduced a kit containing a single, acutely angled dilator tapered from 12 French to 38 French. This dilator is designed to enlarge the tracheal aperture in a single maneuver, thus eliminating the need for multiple dilations and further simplifying the procedure.

The Sims kit contains three straight dilators (17, 25, and 37 French), along with a specially marked obturator/dilator and Portex tracheotomy tube. With this kit, the size of the tracheotomy tube must therefore be determined before commencing the procedure (Fig 39-2).

Although the kits are designed for single use, this author has found that the guiding catheter and dilators can be safely reused 10-15 times, provided that they are closely inspected for integrity, cleaned, and gas sterilized after each use. Instruments that are kinked or otherwise deformed should be discarded and replaced or purchased individually as needed.

Other required instruments include a scalpel, curved hemostat, straight scissors, needle driver, nonresorbable sutures, water-based lubricant, two 10-cc syringes, and an appropriately sized tracheotomy tube (tube included in the Sims kit). The instruments should be placed on an instrument stand over the patient's bed and in the order in which they are to be used (Figs 39-3 and 39-4). An appropriately sized bronchoscope with a suction port must be chosen to fit within the endotracheal tube, while allowing adequate ventilation. This is difficult, if not impossible, when the endotracheal tube is <7 mm. A video monitor, if available, may be connected to the bronchoscope allowing full visualization of the intratracheal portion of the procedure by the operating surgeon and staff.

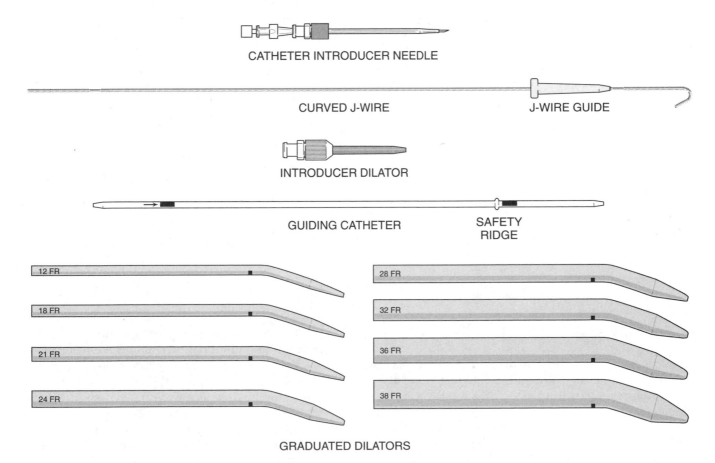

CATHETER INTRODUCER NEEDLE

CURVED J-WIRE   J-WIRE GUIDE

INTRODUCER DILATOR

GUIDING CATHETER   SAFETY RIDGE

12 FR   28 FR

18 FR   32 FR

21 FR   36 FR

24 FR   38 FR

GRADUATED DILATORS

FIG 39-1. Ciaglia Percutaneous Tracheotomy Set by Cook. The #38 French dilator is not part of the kit but is available separately. It is highly recommended for routine use.

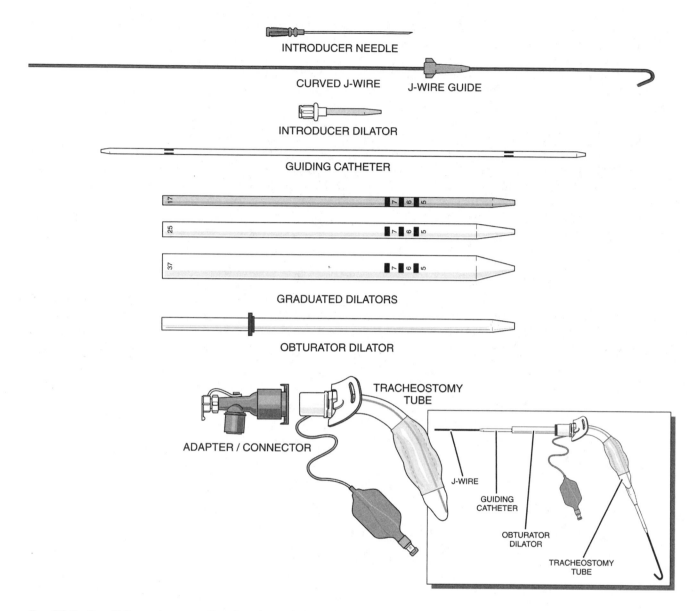

INTRODUCER NEEDLE

CURVED J-WIRE J-WIRE GUIDE

INTRODUCER DILATOR

GUIDING CATHETER

GRADUATED DILATORS

OBTURATOR DILATOR

ADAPTER / CONNECTOR

TRACHEOSTOMY TUBE

J-WIRE

GUIDING CATHETER

OBTURATOR DILATOR

TRACHEOSTOMY TUBE

FIG 39-2. Per-fit Percutaneous Tracheotomy Introducer Set by Sims. Inset: Note assembly of obturator dilator and tracheotomy tube.

C. Anesthesia

Any procedure involving manipulation of the trachea is highly stimulating and requires adequate local anesthesia augmented by intravenous sedation. Local anesthesia, consisting of 1% or 2% lidocaine with 1:100,000 epinephrine, is used for generous infiltration of the incision site down to the level of the trachea. Topical anesthesia in the form of 2%-4% lidocaine may be injected through the bronchoscope and is useful in decreasing the cough reflex. Intravenous sedation is also required, with the particular drug combination dependent on the individual patient and the institution. Frequently used medications include morphine, midazolam, sublimaze, and propofol. Short-acting muscle relaxants may be used as an adjunct in cases in which agitation is a problem. The presence of an anesthesiologist is optional and may depend on hospital policy. Care should be exercised in administering these medications, particularly in elderly patients, as large fluctuations in blood pressure and heart rate may occur even with small doses.

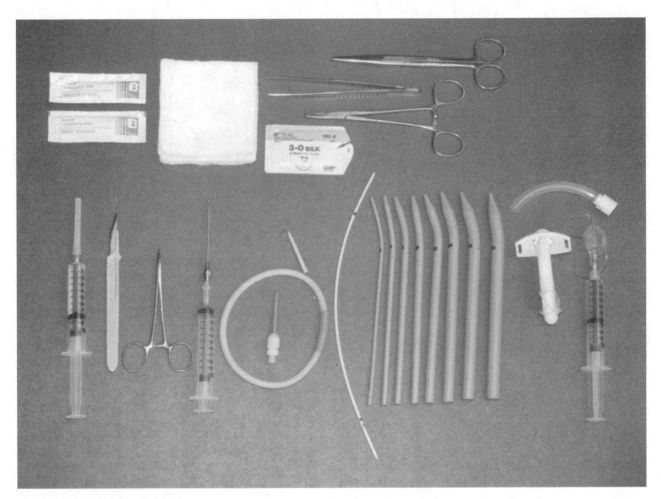

FIG 39-3. Cook kit: Top: water-based lubricant, gauze, silk suture, straight scissors, toothed forceps, and needle driver. Left to right (instruments arranged in order of use): (1) syringe with local anesthesia, (2) scalpel, (3) hemostat, (4) syringe with #14 Teflon catheter introducer needle, (5) J-wire, (6) introducer dilator, (7) guiding catheter, (8) dilators, (9) tracheotomy tube.

D. Technique

Following appropriate sedation, the patient is positioned as for conventional tracheotomy, with the neck extended provided there is no contraindication (eg, cervical spine fracture). In cases where sand and flexi-care beds are used, it may be necessary to place a rigid support under the head, shoulders, and chest. Ventilator settings are adjusted to allow for the presence of the bronchoscope and deliver 100% O_2. Vital signs, including heart rate, blood pressure, and oxygen saturation, are continuously monitored. Important anatomical landmarks including the thyroid and cricoid cartilages, 1st tracheal ring, and sternal notch are palpated. The patient's neck and upper chest are then prepped and draped in a standard fashion and the incision site (approximately 1 finger breadth above the sternal notch) is infiltrated with 1% lidocaine with 1:100000 epinephrine.

A 1.5 cm-2 cm skin incision, just long enough to allow insertion of a tracheotomy tube, is made at the level of the 1st and 2nd tracheal rings. The subcutaneous tissues are gently separated horizontally and vertically with a curved hemostat to allow accurate palpation of the cricoid cartilage and tracheal rings and to allow clear visualization of the bronchoscope light. No attempt is made to divide or otherwise manipulate the thyroid gland.

The flexible bronchoscope is inserted through the appropriate adapter into the endotracheal tube and any tapes or ties securing the latter are loosened or cut. From this point on, the endotracheal tube is securely held by the respiratory technician to prevent accidental extubation. The bronchoscope is advanced through the endotracheal tube until its tip is aligned with the end of the tube. The endotracheal tube (with the cuff momentarily deflated) and bronchoscope are slowly with-

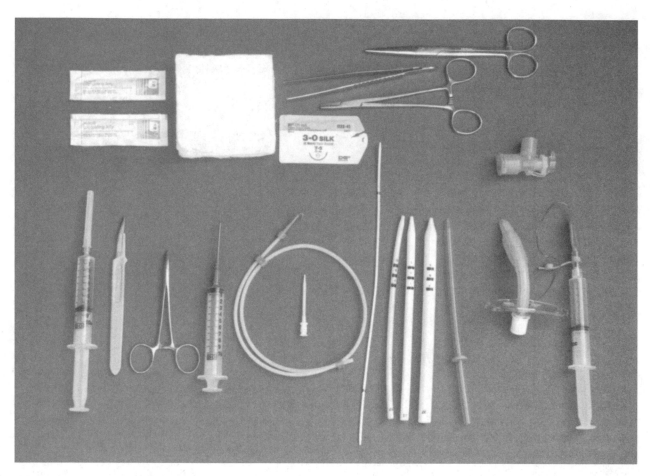

FIG 39-4. Sims kit: Instruments arranged in order of use.

drawn as a unit to a level just below the vocal folds or until the light can be easily visualized through the incision. Reducing the ambient light in the room facilitates this maneuver. In a patient with a short thick neck, it is recommended to precede this maneuver by first withdrawing the bronchoscope only to allow for inspection of the brightness of the light through the incision. With the endotracheal tube and bronchoscope properly positioned, the tracheal rings are palpated and a #14 or #16 Teflon catheter introducer needle is inserted between the 1st and 2nd (or 2nd and 3rd) tracheal rings. Needle location is verified endoscopically and modified until a midline intercartilaginous position is achieved. Care is taken not to puncture the posterior tracheal wall. Approximately 2-3 ml of 2%-4% lidocaine may then be injected into the trachea either through the needle or through the bronchoscope. The needle is removed and a J-tipped guidewire is threaded through the remaining catheter into the trachea (Fig 39-5). This catheter is removed and replaced by the introducer dilator (Fig 39-6), which facilitates passage of the #8 French guiding catheter. The guiding catheter and J-wire then form a unit (Fig 39-7) over which serial dilations are carried out beginning with a #12 or #16 French dilator and pro-

gressing to a #38 French dilator (Fig 39-8); all maneuvers are verified through the bronchoscope. Some collapse of the anterior tracheal wall will occur with the larger dilators. As the final step, a #6 or #8 Shiley cuffed tracheotomy tube with the inner cannula replaced by a snugly fitting dilator is inserted into the trachea (Fig 39-9); the dilator, guiding catheter, and J-wire are removed and replaced with the inner cannula. The cuff is inflated and the appropriate adapter fitted to the ventilator tubing. The tracheotomy tube is secured with tracheotomy tapes and 4 corner sutures. The trachea is suctioned for any blood or secretions. The endotracheal tube is not removed until the integrity of the tracheotomy tube is verified for a good seal and adequate ventilation is established. The vocal folds are inspected as the bronchoscope and endotracheal tube are withdrawn. In a patient with a short, thick neck, a longer tracheotomy tube should be used to prevent accidental displacement of the tube into the pretracheal soft tissue (Fig 39-10). In the event of accidental decannulation within 5 days of the procedure, the ICU staff is advised to reintubate the patient orally rather than attempt to reinsert the tracheotomy tube through a tight, immature tract.

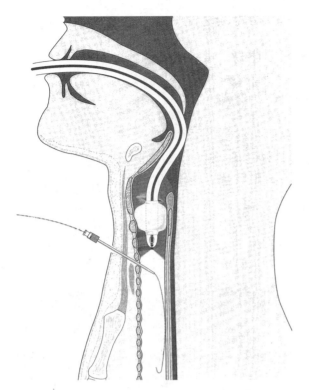

FIG 39-5. Introducer needle is removed. J-tipped guidewire is threaded through the remaining catheter. Note the position of the endotracheal tube with the cuff just below the vocal folds. The bronchoscope projects a short distance beyond the tip of the endotracheal tube.

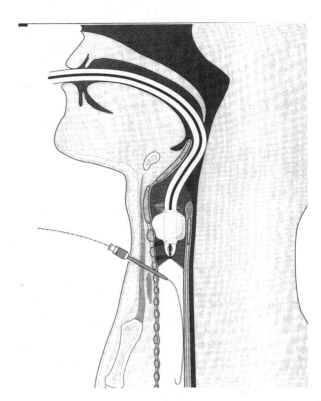

FIG 39-6. Introducer dilator inserted over the J-tipped guidewire.

This author's preliminary experience thus far with the new Cook kit containing a single dilator has translated into a simpler, more rapid procedure.

IV. POSTOPERATIVE CONSIDERATIONS

Particular care is taken in monitoring for changes in vital signs such as hypotension, tachycardia, or O_2 desaturation. With the termination of the intense stimulation produced by the procedure, the effects of the sedation may become more pronounced, resulting in hypotension requiring pharmacologic correction. Excess secretions or blood may compromise ventilation and result in an O_2 saturation drop requiring suctioning. A postoperative chest radiograph is required to ensure the absence of pneumothorax and pneumomediastinum.

Many of these patients have copious secretions from the tracheotomy site from their associated pulmonary conditions. A tracheotomy tube with an inner cannula facilitates care and hygiene and ensures added safety by easy removal, should obstruction from secretions occur. The PCT technique is primarily dilational, with minimal tissue dissection, resulting in a tighter tract and a very snugly fitting tracheotomy tube. The technique does not allow placement of traction sutures at the level of the trachea. Because of these factors, the patient should be reintubated orally in the event of accidental decannulation within the first 5 days of the procedure, when the tract is still relatively immature. Although not specifically reported, attempts at replacing the tracheotomy tube in an emergent situation could result in bleeding, the creation of a false passage, pneumomediastinum, hypoxia, and even death.

V. COMPLICATIONS

Possible complications with PCT are the same as those discussed for standard open tracheotomy and need not be repeated here. Discussion is centered on the incidence and type of complications and how these compare with standard open tracheotomy. Although this author has experienced over 150 PCTs, results have been compiled for the first 75 patients and are highlighted here. Complications occurred in 16% (12 of 75) of patients and most were minor (Table 39-2). Eight complications occurred intraoperatively. There were two instances of desaturation: one female patient with severe

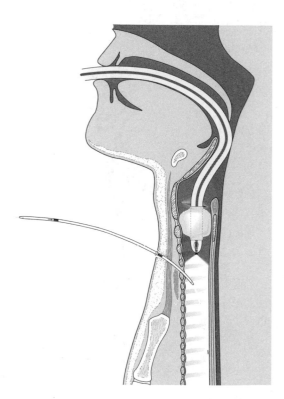

Fig 39-7. #8 French guiding catheter is introduced over the J-wire, forming a unit for subsequent dilations.

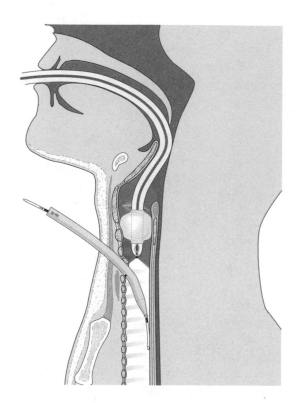

Fig 39-8. Serial dilations are carried out over the J-tipped guidewire/catheter unit, ending with a #38 French dilator. Note the proper position of the dilator with respect to the guiding catheter.

adult respiratory distress syndrome and known periods of bradycardia had a brief (15 sec) fall in saturation from 90% to 85% and heart rate from 80 to 40 during insertion of the tracheotomy tube. In the second case, the patient bled 60 ml during the procedure, a small amount of which was intratracheal. A clot partially occluding the left mainstem bronchus resulted in a brief fall in oxygen saturation to 68% for 1 to 2 minutes. The clot was suctioned through the bronchoscope and the procedure completed uneventfully. In two cases, the initial needle puncture penetrated the posterior tracheal wall; the bronchoscopist alerted the surgeon, the needle was repositioned, and the procedure completed. In two patients with large tracheas, the cuff of a #6 tracheotomy tube did not adequately seal the airway. The tube was changed by reinserting the J-wire and #8 French guiding catheter, removing the #6 tracheotomy tube and repositioning a #8 Shiley tube over the appropriate dilator. Two patients were inadvertently extubated early in the procedure as the endotracheal tube ties were loosened. These patients were reintubated without difficulty and the procedure successfully completed.

Postoperative complications (4 of 12) consisted of persistent oozing around the tracheotomy tube for 24 hours in two cases. This was managed with an application of silver nitrate to the bleeding site in one patient and with a small Surgicel packing in the other. In addition, two patients developed peristomal cellulitis that was successfully treated with aggressive wound care and intravenous antibiotics. There were no instances of pneumothorax, pneumomediastinum, subcutaneous emphysema, or false passage.

A comprehensive study between PCT and standard open tracheotomy by Kost and Zeitouni (unpublished data) assessed the complications from 75 prospective, endoscopically guided PCTs in intubated ICU patients to complications from 157 retrospectively reviewed standard open tracheotomies performed in intubated ICU patients. The total complication rate in the PCT group was 16% compared to 30% in the standard open tracheotomy group (Fig 39-11). The striking findings included:

1. Very low incidence of intraoperative and postoperative bleeding with PCT compared to standard open tracheotomy. Intraoperative bleeding was defined as blood loss ≥100 ml. Postoperative bleeding was considered significant, if medical intervention was required.

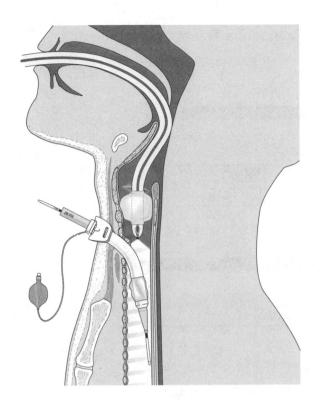

Fig 39-9. #8 cuffed Shiley tracheotomy tube with #28 French dilator is inserted over the J-tipped guidewire/catheter unit.

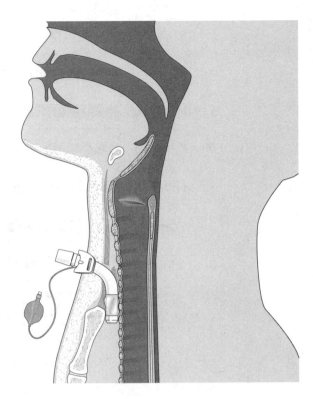

Fig 39-10. Displacement of tracheotomy tube out of the trachea and into the soft tissues in a patient with exceptionally thick pretracheal tissues. Extra-long tracheotomy tubes should be used in these situations.

2. Low incidence of stomal infection (erythema/cellulitis ≥2 cm from the wound edges) with PCT (3%) compared to standard open tracheotomy (10%).
3. Absence of pneumothorax and false passage in the PCT group, which is attributed to the addition of bronchoscopy.

Several authors have substantiated the reduced incidence of bleeding and stomal infections with PCT compared to standard open tracheotomy.[5-8] The low incidence of bleeding is related probably to technical factors, such as the short skin incision, the progressive blunt dilatation, and the tamponading effect of a tight tract. The much smaller wound reduces the surface area for bacterial colonization and translates into decreased infection.

The importance of bronchoscopic visualization with PCT is highlighted by the incidence of serious complications such as pneumothorax, false passage, and subcutaneous emphysema when the procedure is done blindly. In a review and compilation of the literature to date, there have been 634 PCTs performed with endoscopic guidance [1,4,8-10] and 690 PCTs performed without endoscopic guidance.[5-7, 11-15] The collective incidence of pneumothorax, false passage, and subcutaneous em-

Table 39-2. *Perioperative Complications of Percutaneous Tracheostomy**

Complications	No.
Intraoperative	
Desaturation	2
Posterior Wall Injury	2
Cuff Leak	2
Exubation	2
Postoperative	
Oozing	2
Cellulitus	2

* Complications derived from a total of 75 procedures

physema is nil in the 634 endoscopically guided cases, compared to 2.3 % in the 690 cases performed blindly (see Fig 39-11).

In summary, endoscopically guided percutaneous tracheotomy in adult intubated patients is a technically simple procedure that offers an attractive alternative to

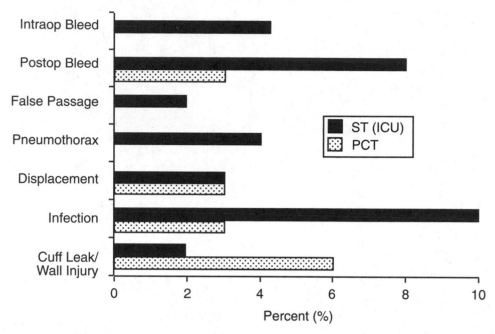

FIG 39-11. Complications of a standard surgical tracheotomy (*ST*) compared to percutaneous tracheotomy (*PCT*). (Inclu des data from Zeitouni and Kost[1] as well as unpublished data.)

standard tracheotomy in the operating room with comparable or lower complication rates.

References

1. Zeitouni A, Kost K. Tracheotomy: a retrospective review of 281 patients. *J Otolaryngol.* 1994;23:61-66.
2. Stauffer JN, Olsen DE, Petty TL. Complications and consequences of endotracheal intubation and tracheotomy: a prospective study of 150 critically ill adult patients. *Am J Med.* 1981;70:65-76.
3. Indeck M, Peterson S, Smith J, Brotman S. Risk, cost, and benefit of transporting ICU patients for special studies. *J Trauma.* 1988;28:1020-1025.
4. Marelli D, Paul A, Manolidis S, et al. Endoscopic guided percutaneous tracheotomy: early results of a consecutive trial. *J Trauma.* 1990;30:433-435.
5. Hazard PB, Garret HE Jr, Adams JW, Robbins ET, Aguillard RN. Bedside percutaneous tracheotomy: Experience with 55 elective procedures. *Am Thorac Surg.* 1988;46: 63-67.
6. Hazard PB, Jones C, Benitone J. Comparative clinical trial of standard operative tracheotomy with percutaneous tracheotomy. *Crit Care Med.* 1991;19:1018-1024.
7. Friedman Y, Fildes J, Mizock B, et al. Comparison of percutaneous and surgical tracheotomies. *Chest.* 1996;110:480-485.
8. Winkler WB, Karnik R, Seelmann O, Havlicek J, Slany J. Bedside tracheotomy with endoscopic guidance: experience with 71 ICU patients. *Intensive Care Med.* 1994;20: 476-479.
9. Schrager JB, Sing RF, Anderson HL, et al. Percutaneous dialational tracheotomy. *Surg Rounds.* 1994;681-685.
10. Baba CA, Angood PB, Kauder DR, et al. Bronchoscopic guidance makes percutaneous tracheotomy a safe, cost-effective, and easy-to-teach procedure. *Surgery.* 1995;118: 879-883.
11. Griggs WM, Myburgh JA, Wothley LI. A prospective comparison of a percutaneous tracheotomy technique with standard surgical tracheotomy. *Intensive Care Med.* 1991;17:161-163.
12. Toursarkissian B, Zweng T, Kearney P, Pofahl WE, Johnson SB, Barker DE. Percutaneous dialational tracheotomy: report of 141 cases. *Ann Thorac Surg.* 1994;57:862-867.
13. Ciaglia P, Graniero KD. Percutaneous dialational tracheotomy: results and long-term follow-up. *Chest.* 1992; 101:464-467.
14. Wang MB, Berke GS, Ward PH, Calcaterra TC, Watts D. Early experience with percutaneous tracheotomy. *Laryngoscope.* 1992;102:157-162.
15. Bodenham A, Diament R, Cohen A, Webster N. Percutaneous dialational tracheotomy: a bedside procedure in the intensive care unit. *Anesthesia.* 1991;46:570-572 .

CHAPTER 40

■ ■ ■

Vocal Fold Injection

Clark A. Rosen, M.D.

I. HISTORICAL PERSPECTIVE

Vocal fold injection has been used for over 100 years utilizing a variety of materials, such as paraffin, silicone, and bone pate.[1-3] Vocal fold injection (VFI) techniques can be divided by location of injected material into either the medial or the lateral region of the vocal fold. Medial VFI is done in a superficial location of the vocal fold typically using collagen and is done primarily to improve voice. Medial VFI has a limited role for the treatment of swallowing disorders. The experimental findings of Ford demonstrated a rapid absorption of collagen in the lateral (deep) position precluding the use of collagen as a lateral VFI material.[4] Lateral VFI (deep) medializes the vocal fold, improving the closure of the glottis, thus improving swallowing efficiency and safety. The most common materials injected during lateral VFI are Teflon, Gelfoam, and fat.

II. SURGICAL INDICATIONS FOR VOCAL FOLD INJECTION

Indications for vocal fold injection include dysphonia and dysphagia due to glottal incompetence (Table 40-1). Incompetence of vocal fold adduction can occur from a variety of causes, the most common of which are unilateral vocal fold paralysis, vocal fold atrophy (unilateral or bilateral), or vocal fold scar. Symptoms of glottal incompetence typically range from vocal fatigue to a breathy, weak voice to coughing with swallowing (ie, aspiration). Dysphagia associated with glottal in-

competence is frequently seen in patients with a history of weight loss and/or aspiration pneumonia. Improvement of glottal competence following vocal fold injection leads to an improvement in the swallowing function and a more effective clearance of materials that "penetrate" the endolarynx (saliva, liquid, food).[5,6]

Contraindications for vocal fold injection include a compromised airway and/or lack of clear evidence that the dysphagia is secondary to glottal incompetence. Patients with a compromised airway (bilateral vocal fold motion deficit, glottal web, tracheal stenosis) are poor candidates for vocal fold injection, as the VFI narrows the glottic airway. One should also be concerned about patients who present with a unilateral recurrent laryngeal nerve (RLN) paralysis and who are at significant risk for future contralateral paralysis (eg, pending thyroid surgery, aggressive esophageal carcinoma, or bilateral glomus vagale).

When assessing a patient for vocal fold injection, the exact cause(s) of dysphagia must be elucidated. This is to prevent persistent dysphagia following correction of

---

Table 40-1. *Highlights—Vocal Fold Injection*

- Aspiration associated with glottal incompetence can be helped with vocal fold injection

- Vocal fold paralysis is the most common cause of dysphagia related to glottal incompetence

- Other symptoms of glottal incompetence include dysphonia, vocal fatigue, cough associated with eating.

---

a glottal incompetence due to difficulties produced by other swallowing deficits, such as bolus control or pharyngeal anesthesia. For this reason, preoperative evaluation of patients with dysphagia in preparation for vocal fold injection requires a careful evaluation of all stages of swallowing. A complete head and neck examination and functional evaluation of swallowing (functional endoscopic evaluation of swallowing [FEES] or modified barium swallow[MBS]) must be a part of the preoperative assessment (see Chapters 11 and 12).

III. PREOPERATIVE ASSESSMENT

Evaluation of the cause and severity of the dysphagia associated with glottal incompetence is a critical component of the preoperative assessment. Clinical evaluation should include posing questions to the patient and/or family regarding coughing while eating, recent weight loss, history of head and neck surgery and/or radiation treatment, and present diet status (see Chapters 4-10).

The head and neck examination should specifically address the oral cavity and larynx, including a detailed sensory and motor examination of these areas. The laryngeal examination should involve particular attention to vocal fold morphology and motion, glottal closure during cough, and laryngeal sensation. This examination is best done with a flexible nasopharyngoscope with or without videostroboscopy. Flexible nasopharyngoscopy allows an assessment of the patient's pharynx and laryngeal mucosa.[7] Sensory function of these areas can be evaluated by observing the tolerance to endoscopy as well as pooling of secretions and recently swallowed materials. Rosen and Murry have reviewed the details of this examination in a recently released videotape.[8]

Determination of the cause for a unilateral immobile vocal fold and its prognosis is paramount in the evaluation process. Differentiation between a vocal fold paralysis and pathology of the cricoarytenoid joint, either dislocation or fixation, is required. This can be accomplished by history (known RLN section during neck or chest surgery), laryngeal EMG, and arytenoid palpation, the latter during direct laryngoscopy. These investigations will determine subsequent management decisions regarding the treatment of laryngeal lesions, as well as comprehensive planning for the treatment of the patient's dysphagia. Laryngeal electromyography can differentiate between a vocal fold paralysis and cricoarytenoid joint disease. Laryngeal EMG may also assist to determine prognosis for recovery of an unilateral vocal fold paralysis.[9]

IV. SURGICAL TECHNIQUE

A. Vocal Fold Injection Material Options

Teflon was the first reliable injection material to be used for the successful treatment of both swallowing and voice problems.[10] Teflon is well tolerated initially and has no significant decrease in volume over time. Over time, a foreign body reaction to the injected Teflon can lead to the formation of an inflammatory mass named Teflon granuloma that severely disrupts the shape and function of the injected vocal fold. Dedo and colleagues argue that a Teflon granuloma occurs from either overinjection or misplacement of the Teflon.[11] These factors clearly increase the risk of the formation of a Teflon granuloma; however, some patients have developed a Teflon granuloma many years after a VFI with excellent initial postoperative results, suggesting that in these individuals the Teflon was in the right location and not overinjected. Thus Teflon is associated with a significant risk for the development of a granuloma.[12]

Schramm et al popularized vocal fold injection using Gelfoam as a temporary treatment of vocal fold paralysis.[13] The injection involves mixing gelatin powder with a buffered saline solution to form a paste that is then used for a lateral vocal fold injection. Gelatin is naturally degraded in the body, with the medialization obtained with a Gelfoam injection of the vocal fold lasting 6 to 8 weeks. Gelfoam injection of the vocal fold can result in improved swallowing and is an excellent option for the treatment of dysphagia due to vocal fold paralysis when the possibility for vocal fold recovery is uncertain.

Autologous fat injection has been used as lateral VFI material for the treatment of both voice and swallowing disorders. Fat is harvested from the patient at the time of the VFI via liposuction or a small incision in the abdominal skin to expose subcutaneous fat. The harvested fat is copiously rinsed to remove free fatty acids around the lipocytes, dried, and then loaded into the injection device. The advantages of lipoinjection of the vocal fold include ease of harvest, availability of material and the advantages of being autologous. The limiting factor of this technique is the initial absorption of 30%-50% of the injected material within the first month following the injection. This has lead most surgeons to overinject the vocal fold by 30%-50% to account for this resorption. Excellent long-term results of lipoinjection of the vocal fold have been demonstrated in several independent studies.[14-16] In my 3-year experience with lipoinjections, there has been no change in the injected volume of fat that persists 1 month after injection.

B. Vocal Fold Injection Technique

Methods of vocal fold injection include transoral via indirect laryngoscopy or direct laryngoscopy or percutaneous using transnasal fiber optic guidance. The majority of the vocal fold injections are done transorally. The advantage of VFI done via indirect laryngoscopy in a sitting position is the ability to titrate the injection in the most natural position. This advantage is less significant if VFI is done for the treatment of dysphagia. In addition, many patients, especially those presenting with aspiration, do not tolerate this approach. The most frequently used VFI method is transoral via direct laryngoscopy, done using either general or local anesthesia with sedation. The advantage of the former is the improved visualization of the larynx using suspension microlaryngoscopy. The disadvantage of general anesthesia for VFI is the loss of the ability of the surgeon to visualize the glottic deficit during vocal fold adduction and thus monitor the adequacy of the injection. For Teflon and Gelfoam injections, the use of local anesthesia instead of a general anesthetic allows "real-time" monitoring of the glottal deficit and its correction. For lipoinjection, the advantage of a VFI done under local anesthesia is negligible, as the vocal fold is purposely overinjected.

C. Endoscopic Vocal Fold Injection

At the University of Pittsburgh Voice Center, VFI is usually performed under local anesthesia via endo-scopic direct laryngoscopy. This technique avoids the risks and limitations of a procedure done under general anesthesia and provides magnified, well-illuminated visualization of the larynx during VFI.

This technique is used in a similar manner for Gelfoam, Teflon, and fat injection of the vocal fold. Prior to entering the operating room, the patient receives a small amount of IV sedation and nebulized lidocaine (pontocaine for lipoinjection) to provide anesthesia to the oropharynx, larynx, and trachea. Preoperative intravenous glycopyrolate and solumedrol are also administered.

The patient is in the supine position with the neck flexed and head extended. Additional topical anesthesia of 10% lidocaine is administered via spray to the oropharynx and larynx. Direct laryngoscopy is performed using a slotted anterior commissure laryngoscope (Figure 40-1). The side of the laryngoscope slot, as seen from behind the laryngoscope, should be opposite to the intended vocal fold to be injected. During the initial direct laryngoscopy, additional 10% lidocaine is sprayed onto the larynx if needed and the glottal pathology is confirmed (unilateral vocal fold paralysis, vocal fold atrophy, and so on). If a presumptive diagnosis of a unilateral vocal fold paralysis has been made (without laryngeal electromyography), the suspected paralyzed arytenoid is palpated to rule out cricoarytenoid joint fixation. Anesthesia is monitored by touching an instrument to the vocal fold injection site to ensure that there is adequate anesthesia prior to proceeding with the vocal fold injection. The laryngoscope is then positioned over the affected vocal fold to be injected in a manner that the distal tip of the laryn-

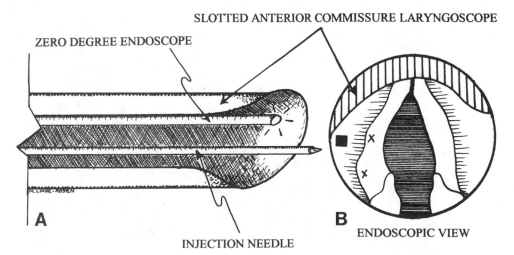

Fig 40-1. A. Demonstrates zero-degree endoscope and injection in slotted anterior commissure laryngoscope. **B.** Endoscopic view during vocal fold injection. "X" marks typical injection sites. "■" marks false vocal retraction from the distal tip of the laryngoscope.

goscope retracts the false vocal fold exposing the laryngeal ventricle, the membranous vocal fold, and the vocal process. This position is then maintained with the nondominant hand suspending and positioning the laryngoscope throughout the procedure (see Figure 40-1**A**). A zero-degree rigid telescope of 4 mm diameter and 30 cm length coupled with a video camera, such as used in endoscopic sinus surgery or laparoscopy, is then passed down the laryngoscope by an assistant. The injection needle attached to the loaded Bruening injection gun (Storz, St. Louis, MO) is then passed through the laryngoscope under direct endoscopic guidance by the surgeon's dominant hand. The injection needle is then placed at the junction at the superior surface of the vocal fold and laryngeal ventricle at the level of the vocal process of the arytenoid (see Fig 40-2). The injection is placed deep into the vocal fold (approximately 4-5 mm) and is done incrementally, observing the vocal fold from the endoscopic image. Typically, 2 to 3 clicks of Gelfoam or Teflon are required at this location to adequately medialize the vocal fold. Often 1

or 2 additional click of material is injected at the midpoint of the membranous vocal fold at the same depth and lateral vocal fold position (see Fig 40-1**B**). The injection needle is retracted into the laryngoscope and glottic closure while phonation is observed from the endoscopic image.

V. PITFALLS AND COMPLICATIONS

Complications of vocal fold injection are summarized in Table 40-2.

A. Overinjection of the Vocal Fold

Overinjection of the vocal fold can result in dysphagia, as well as dysphonia secondary to glottal incompetence. The overinjected vocal fold typically will not allow adequate glottic closure and subsequently will not improve the patient's dysphagia. Also, an overinjected

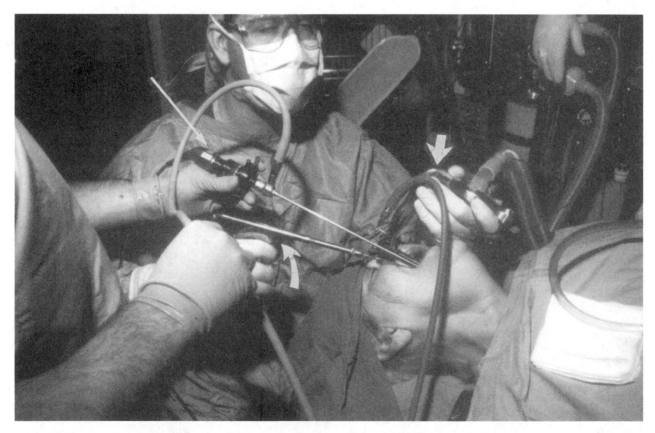

FIG 40-2. Surgeon and assistant performing endoscopic vocal fold injection. Short arrow shows the slotted anterior commissure laryngoscope held in the surgeon's nondominant hand . The curved arrow is at the surgeon's dominant hand holding the injection device. The long arrows demonstrate the assistant holding the video camera attached to the zero-degree endoscope. Note that the stem of the endoscope is rotated upward to avoid contact with the injection device.

Table 40-2. *Complications of Vocal Fold Injection*

- Vocal fold injection, temporary or permanent, can result in airway obstruction.
- Lipoinjection resorption may occur within the first month following surgery.
- Teflon granuloma, overinjection, and misplaced injection of Teflon usually results in severe dysphonia and dysphagia.

vocal fold frequently will result in dysphonia that can be quite troubling to the patient.

B. Airway Obstruction

Airway obstruction is the most serious complication following a vocal fold injection. Fortunately, this is quite rare. Airway obstruction can be temporary or permanent. Temporary airway obstruction most typically occurs from extensive manipulation of the larynx during the vocal fold injection procedure and subsequent significant supraglottic edema. The edema complication can be prevented by minimizing direct laryngoscopy manipulation of the supraglottis and perioperative steroid administration. Permanent airway obstruction following vocal fold injection is extremely rare and only occurs when the contralateral vocal fold becomes immobile secondary to RLN paralysis or cricoarytenoid joint fixation, dislocation, or extreme vocal fold overinjection.

C. Resorption of Fat Following Lipoinjection

Incomplete medialization of the injected vocal fold following lipoinjection is considered a complication. Such resorption occurs within the first 3 to 4 weeks following surgery. Inadequate medialization secondary to lipoinjection resorption occurs from either insufficient lipoinjection, poor processing of the injected material, or unknown reasons. This may be considered a complication because of the need for further treatment of the patient's dysphagia. A repeat lipoinjection is frequently the most reasonable course of action following this complication; however, laryngeal framework surgery to medialize the vocal fold(s) is also a reasonable treatment option.[17] (See Chapter 41.)

D. Teflon Granulomas/Overinjection

A Teflon granuloma or overinjection to a vocal fold is a major complication of vocal fold injection utilizing Teflon. The patient typically presents with both dys-

phagia and dysphonia secondary to glottal incompetence caused by the inflammatory Teflon granuloma or the excessive injected material within the vocal fold. A Teflon granuloma can also present with airway symptoms. This unfortunate condition can be remedied via endoscopic laser ablation of the Teflon granuloma.[18] This is a tedious operation that leads to scarring of the vocal fold and may result in a need for an alternative vocal fold medialization procedure, which can be quite difficult because of the stiffness of the scar tissue. Vocal fold injection or laryngeal framework surgery can be done following removal of overinjected Teflon material or a Teflon granuloma. An alternative method of Teflon removal from the paraglottic space and vocal fold region uses an external approach via a thyroplasty window or from a posterior approach to the thyroid cartilage (personal communication, JL Netterville).

E. Impaired Vocal Fold Vibration

Care must be taken to perform all lateral (deep) vocal fold injections at the depth of the thyroarytenoid muscle and not too superficial. Injection of Gelfoam, Teflon, or fat into the superficial portion of the vocal fold will result in impaired vocal fold vibration, distortion of the membranous vocal fold free edge, and tracking of the injected material into the laryngeal ventricle. The latter results in a loss of the flat contour of the superior surface of the vocal fold and effacement of the laryngeal ventricle. This complication can be prevented by careful observation of the depth of the injection needle and observation of the response of the vocal fold during the injection. The appropriate response of the vocal fold during injection is a medial displacement of the free edge without change to the contour of the superior surface of the vocal fold. If any indication of laryngeal ventricle swelling or ballooning of the superior surface of the vocal fold is seen during the injection, the injection should be stopped and the needle advanced to a deeper tissue plane.

References

1. Bruening W. Über eine neue Behandlungsmethode der Rekurrenslahmung. *Berh Dtsch Laryng.* 1911;18:230.
2. Arnold GE. Vocal rehabilitation of paralytic dysphonia: cartilage injection into a paralyzed vocal cord. *Arch Otolaryngol.* 1955;62:593.
3. Hirano M, Mori K, Tanaka S, Fujita M. Vocal function in patients with unilateral vocal fold paralysis before and after silicone injection. *Acta Otolaryngol (Stock).* 1995;115:553-559.
4. Ford CN. Histologic studies on the fate of soluble collagen injected into canine vocal folds. *Laryngoscope.* 1986;96:1248-1257.

5. Rontal E, Rontal M, Morse G, Brown EM. Vocal cord injection in the treatment of acute and chronic aspiration. *Laryngoscope.* 1976;86:625-634.

6. Griffin SM, Chung SC, van Hasselt CA, Li AK. Late swallowing and aspiration problems after esophagectomy for cancer: malignant infiltration of the recurrent laryngeal nerves and its management. *Surgery.* 1992;112:533-535.

7. Aviv JE, Sacco RL, Thomson J, et al. Silent laryngopharyngeal sensory deficits after stroke. *Ann Otol Rhinol Laryngol.* 1997;106:87-93.

8. Rosen CA, Murry T: *Dynamic Voice Evaluation: Nasoendoscopic Techniques and Applications.* [Videotape], San Diego, Calif: Singular Publishing; 1997.

9. Min YB, Finnegan EM, Hoffman HT, Luschei ES, McCulloch TM. A preliminary study of the prognostic role of electromyography in laryngeal paralysis. *Otolaryngol Head Neck Surg.* 1994;111:770-775.

10. Dedo HH, Urrea RD, Lawson L. Intracordal injection of Teflon in the treatment of 135 patients with dysphonia. *Ann Otol Rhinol Laryngol.* 1973;82:661-667.

11. Dedo HH. Injection and removal of Teflon for unilateral vocal cord paralysis. *Ann Otol Rhinol Laryngol.* 1992;101:81-86.

12. Nakayama M, Ford CN, Bless DM. Teflon vocal fold augmentation: failures and management in 28 cases. *Otolaryngol Head Neck Surg.* 1993;109:493-498.

13. Schramm VL, May M, Lavorato AS. Gelfoam paste injection for vocal cord paralysis: temporary rehabilitation of glottic incompetence. *Laryngoscope.* 1978;88:1268-1273.

14. Brandenberg JH, Unger JM, Koschkee D. Vocal cord injection with autogenous fat: a long-term magnetic resonance imaging evaluation. *Laryngoscope.* 1996;106:174-180.

15. Shaw GY, Szewczyk MA, Searle J, Woodroof J. Autologous fat injection into the vocal folds: technical considerations and long-term follow up. *Laryngoscope.* 1997;107:100-186.

16. Mikaelian DO, Lowry LD, Sataloff RT. Lipoinjection for unilateral vocal cord paralysis. *Laryngoscope.* 1991;101:465-468.

17. Pou AM, Carrau RL, Eibling DE, Murry T. Laryngeal framework surgery for the management of aspiration in high vagal lesions. *Am J Otolaryngol.* 1998;19:1-7.

18. Ossoff RH, Koriwchak MJ, Netterville JL, Duncavage JA. Difficulties in endoscopic removal of Teflon granulomas of the vocal fold. *Ann Otol Rhinol Laryngol.* 1993;102:405-412.

CHAPTER 41

■ ■ ■

Laryngeal Framework Surgery: Medialization Laryngoplasty

Robert J. Andrews, M.D.
James L. Netterville, M.D.
Albert L. Mercati, M.D.

I. HISTORICAL PERSPECTIVE

The major purpose of the larynx is to regulate swallowing and prevent aspiration during food and liquid intake. Vocal fold paralysis, especially in combination with deficits of cranial nerves IX and XII, often results in mild to severe aspiration. From the closure of the lips to the relaxation of the upper esophageal sphincter there are approximately 10 steps in the swallowing process. Closure of the laryngeal valve at the level of the vocal folds is the single most critical step in preventing aspiration.

Recent advancements in laryngeal framework surgery and arytenoid adduction have significantly improved the care of patients with glottal insufficiency due to paralysis, scarring, or bowing of the true vocal folds. A review by Koufman and Isaacson[1] provides an excellent description of the historical background of medialization laryngoplasty. The following is a brief synopsis of the major developments in this field.

In 1911, Brunings[2] described intracordal injection of paraffin for the treatment of glottic insufficiency. The paraffin resulted in a foreign body reaction. In 1915, Payr[3] described the first laryngeal framework procedure for vocal fold medialization using an anteriorly based rectangular thyroid cartilage flap. This alone did not provide adequate displacement of the vocal fold. For many years afterward, both intracordal injection and laryngeal framework surgery were discarded in the rehabilitation of glottal incompetence.

In the 1960s and 1970s, intracordal injection of Teflon, popularized by Arnold,[4] Arnold and Stephens,[5] and Dedo and Colleagues,[6] became the standard of therapy. There are, however, several limitations of this technique that when compared to current methods make it a poor choice for rehabilitation of vocal fold paralysis (Table 41-1).

In the 1950s to early 1970s, several procedures for medialization laryngoplasty were described. Yet, it was not until Isshiki and other colleagues[7,8] published his methods using Silastic as the implant material that laryngeal framework surgery became widely accepted. Koufman[1,9,10] and Netterville and coworkers[11-14] have helped to popularize and refine this technique in the United States.

Table 41-1. *Problems and Complications of Intracordal Teflon Injection*

- Difficult surgical exposure under local/topical anesthesia
- Nonreversible, nonadjustable
- Technically challenging
- Does not close posterior glottic gap
- Teflon migration is unpredictable
- Teflon diffusion, soft tissue scar/fibrosis, and severe dysphonia will result if vocal fold function returns after Teflon injection
- Teflon granuloma

II. SURGICAL INDICATIONS

Medialization laryngoplasty with Silastic has several distinct advantages when compared to other methods of treating glottic insufficiency (Table 41-2). The primary indication is glottic incompetence secondary to unilateral vocal fold paralysis. Other indications include incomplete closure secondary to unilateral vocal fold paresis and selected traumatic defects. Patients with symptomatic senile bowing and atrophy or presbylaryngis are candidates for bilateral medialization laryngoplasty.

Contraindications to this technique include previous Teflon injection and impairment or compromise of contralateral vocal fold abduction where medialization could limit the size of airway. Relative contraindications include previous laryngeal radiation and post-operative laryngeal defects following procedures such as vertical partial laryngectomy (Table 41-3).

III. PREOPERATIVE ASSESSMENT

All patients need to undergo an extensive preoperative evaluation to determine the etiology and characteristics of their vocal fold paralysis as well as to document the degree of aspiration. This includes a complete head and neck examination by an otolaryngologist and a functional voice assessment by a speech-language pathologist. If severe, aspiration is assessed by performing a modified barium swallowing (MBS).

The voice assessment consists of a complete battery of perceptual, acoustic, and aerodynamic studies. This includes videolaryngoscopy and stroboscopy. A preoperative video shows the position of the immobile vocal fold. If there is a posterior glottal gap, with the vocal process widely spaced during phonation, then the addition of arytenoid adduction may be necessary to obtain complete closure and therefore produce an optimal vocal result.

In the case of idiopathic vocal fold paralysis, the entire course of the ipsilateral vagus nerve is radiographically evaluated with either a CT or magnetic resonance imaging (MRI) scan. These studies have revealed etiologic lesions such as paragangliomas and schwannomas.

IV. SURGICAL TECHNIQUE

Medialization laryngoplasty can be accomplished with a variety of implants. The most commonly used is silicone elastomer; however, the use of Gortex and Hydroxyapatite has been well described. Each of the implant materials has strengths and weaknesses. It is not the choice of the implant material that predicts good results, but a basic understanding of the physiologic phonating position of the true vocal fold and how to position the paralyzed vocal fold into that position. With this understanding, one can achieve good results with any implant. In view of this we will describe our technique using silicone elastomer—other implant material may be substituted.

In recent years, modifications to the surgical technique used at Vanderbilt University for the treatment of glottic incompetence have included, in the vast majority of cases, the addition of arytenoid adduction to medialization laryngoplasty. The adduction of the arytenoid plays a significant role in bringing the true vocal cord into the physiologic phonating position. As a separate chapter is devoted to arytenoid adduction, medialization laryngoplasty alone is discussed in this section.

The procedure is performed under local anesthesia supplemented by intravenous sedation. The endolarynx is monitored during the entire operation with a nasopharyngoscope attached to a video camera system. This arrangement allows simultaneous monitoring of the voice and glottal closure.

After exposure of the thyroid cartilage, the window that is at least 6 mm tall, ranging from 12 to 15 mm in length, is outlined using a window template. It is very important to make a window large enough to work gently to prevent injury to the thyroarytenoid muscle. In the larynx with a more obtuse angle, as often seen in women, the window is placed closer to the anterior commissure (approximately 5 mm); while in the larynx

Table 41-2. *Advantages of Silastic Medialization Laryngoplasty*

- Well tolerated by patient under local anesthesia
- Both reversible and adjustable
- Clearly defined surgical technique
- Reproducible vocal results
- Can be performed in conjunction with arytenoid adduction
- Implant does not migrate, change shape, or produce a foreign body reaction

Table 41-3. *Indications and Contraindications of Silastic Medialization Laryngoplasty*

Indications
- Glottic incompetence secondary to unilateral vocal fold paralysis
- Loss or sacrifice of cranial nerve X during neurotologic skull base surgery
- Incomplete glottic closure secondary to unilateral vocal fold paresis
- Selected traumatic defects

Contraindications
- Scarring from laryngeal radiation or trauma
- Loss of ipsilateral thyroid cartilage (ie, airway limitation)
- Prior Teflon injection

with a more acute angle, noted more often in men, the window is positioned farther posteriorly (approximately 7 mm). Care must be taken to prevent overmedialization of the anterior third of the vocal fold, even if the posterior glottis does not close well; otherwise, a strained quality to the voice results. The lower edge of the window lies parallel to the lower border of the thyroid cartilage, leaving a 3-mm strut along the lower border.

The cartilage island is removed under magnification from the outlined window using an otologic drill with a 2-3 mm cutting burr. This has two distinct advantages over medialization of the mobilized cartilage island. First, the position of the window on the lateral surface of the thyroid cartilage is no longer critical. The point of maximum medialization is seldom in the central plane of the window, but rather is usually near its lower edge. The shape of the implant can be carved to yield medialization in this plane. If the entire cartilage island is medialized, one does not have this level of accuracy.

Second, it is easier to produce maximum medialization at the posterior aspect of the window with only 1 to 2 mm of anterior medialization using the carved implant than by medialization of the entire cartilage island. The thyroid cartilage is 3 to 4 mm thick at the anterior aspect of the window. Medialization of the island with a Silastic T to stabilize it into position will often result in overmedialization of the anterior commissure.

While removing the thyroid cartilage window, the inner perichondrium is left intact. The perichondrium is then incised at the superior, inferior, and posterior margins of the window, making it a flap. The long laryngeal elevator is used to gently separate the thyroarytenoid fascia from the inner perichondrium in the same direction as the perichondrial incisions. At the anterior aspect of the window, where the ventricle is only 1 to 2 mm from the plane of dissection, elevation is often not needed. Violation of the ventricle will result in implant contamination, which may lead to extrusion. Care must be taken to avoid violating the thyroarytenoid fascia, below which are the distal superior laryngeal vessels. Trauma at this level may result in intracordal hemorrhage and/or edema.

At this point, the patient is asked to phonate and the larynx is viewed on the video monitor. The depth gauge is used to gently medialize the soft tissues of the endolarynx at various locations in the window (Fig 41-1). This step enables determination of the relationship of the window to the level of the true and false vocal folds and the location and depth of medialization necessary for glottic closure. The plane of maximal medialization usually corresponds to the lower edge of the window in men; in women it typically is in the lower half of the window.

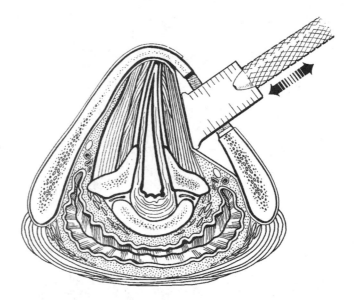

FIG 41-1. Voice quality is assessed using a depth gauge that simulates the medialization acquired with the implant. This prevents the need to place and remove many different implant sizes, which may lead to trauma of the paraglottic muscles.

The anterior and posterior dimensions of the implant are measured with the depth gauge. This step is important, as the depth gauge simulates the medialization of the implant, accurately predicting the voice results. This prevents the need of adjusting voice quality by placement and removal of multiple different implant sizes. Vocal fold edema results from multiple manipulations of the implant obscuring the intraoperative results.

After the dimensions have been acquired, the implant is carved from the Silastic block as outlined in previous publications.[12,13] Softer grades of Silastic are now available and allows the implant to be placed through the window in one piece. The final position of the implant should medialize the vocal process, but not impinge on the muscular process of the arytenoid (Fig 41-2). Contact at that point could block the adduction of the vocal process. To prevent this, the implant is tapered as it extends posterior to the thyroid window.

If the quality of the voice is not as good as expected, then the implant can be removed with two small skin hooks and adjusted appropriately. The time from intralaryngeal elevation to final placement of the implant should be as short as possible to prevent intralaryngeal edema from influencinge interpretation of the voice result.

If the voice is still breathy or the posterior glottic gap cannot be closed with the implant alone, then the addition of arytenoid adduction is important to acquire closure and improve voice quality. Before removing the nasopharyngoscope, one needs to observe the larynx

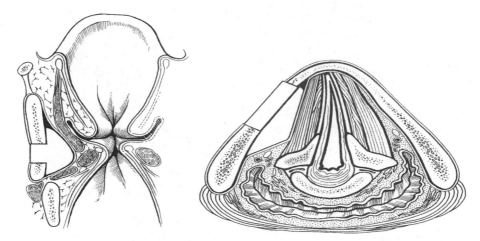

FIG 41-2. The implant should have smooth contours that gently displace the entire paraglottic space as needed. The maximum plane of medialization can be placed at any level, either within the window or below the level of the window, as determined by the depth gauge. Here the maximum plane of medialization is at the lower border of the window, with the implant tapered posterior to the window to prevent contact with the muscular process of the arytenoid.

for evidence of hematoma or airway obstruction. The patient is admitted overnight for observation and discharged the following morning after removal of the drain.

V. PITFALLS AND COMPLICATIONS

There are several problems that can be encountered with this technique.[1,11-15] Undermedialization may result if significant intraoperative vocal fold edema develops prior to placement of the Silastic implant.

Care must be taken to avoid perforation of the laryngeal ventricle. This can lead to implant contamination, infection, and the need for implant removal. Injury to the distal superior laryngeal vessels may result in intracordal hemorrhage. Transient postoperative stridor from laryngeal edema is treated with racemic epinephrine and systemic steroids. A strained voice will ensue if there is overmedialization of the anterior one third of the true vocal fold.

The major drawback of this procedures the inexperience of the surgeon. Table 41-4 outlines some of the pitfalls seen in performing medialization laryngoplasty. As one can see, with moderate experience, most of this points will only rarely occur (Table 41-4). To obtain optimal results one must be ready to perform arytenoid adduction as needed.

Table 41-4. *Complications and Limitations of Medialization Laryngoplasty*

- Undermedialization secondary to intraoperative vocal fold edema
- Implant contamination from injury to the ventricle
- Intracordal hemorrhage from injury to the distal superior laryngeal vessels
- Transient stridor from postoperative edema
- Overmedialization of anterior one third of the true vocal fold resulting in a strained voice
- Posterior glottic gap requiring addition of arytenoid adduction for closure
- Expectation of modest improvement with bilateral medialization for presbylaryngitis

References

1. Koufman JA, Isaacson G. Laryngoplastic phonosurgery. *Otolaryngol Clin North Am.* 1991;24:1151-1177.

2. Brunings W. Ueber eine neue Behandlungsmethode der Rekurrenslahmung. *Verhandl Ver Deutsch Laryngol* 1911; 18:93.

3. Payr A. Plastic am Schildknorpel zur Behebung der Folgen einseitiger Stimmbandlahmung. *Deut Med Wochenschr (Stuttgart).* 1915;41:1265-1270.

4. Arnold GE. Vocal rehabilitation of paralytic dysphonia. IX. technique of intracordal injection. *Arch Otolaryngol.* 1962; 76:358-368.

5. Arnold GE, Stephens CB. Laryngeal injections with poltef paste. *Ear Nose Throat J.* 1980;59:415-418.

6. Dedo HH, Urrea RD, Lawson L. Intracordal injection of Teflon in the treatment of 135 patients with dysphonia. *Ann Otol Rhinol Laryngol.* 1988;97:234-238.

7. Isshiki N, Morita H, Okamura H, Hiramoto M. Thyroplasty as a new phonosurgical technique. *Acta Otolaryngol (Stockh).* 1974;78:451-453.

8. Isshiki N. Recent advances in phonosurgery. *Folia Phoniatr (Basel).* 1980;32:119-134.

9. Koufman JA. Laryngoplasty for vocal fold medialization: an alternative to Teflon. *Laryngoscope.* 1986;96:726-730.

10. Koufman JA. Laryngoplastic phonosurgery. In: Johnson JT, ed. *Instructional courses. American Academy of Otolaryngology—Head and Neck Surgery.* St. Louis, Mo: CV Mosby; 1988:339-350.

11. Netterville JL, Aly A, Ossoff RH. Evaluation and treatment of complications of thyroid and parathyroid surgery. *Otolaryngol Clinics North Am.* 1990;23(3):529-552.

12. Netterville JL, Stone RE, Luken ES, Civantos FJ, Ossoff RH. Silastic medialization and arytenoid adduction, a review of 116 procedures: the Vanderbilt experience. *Ann Otol Rhinol Laryngol.* 1993;102:413-424.

13. Wanamaker JR, Netterville JL, Ossoff RH. Phonosurgery: silastic medialization for unilateral vocal fold paralysis. *Op Tech Otolaryngol Head Neck Surg.* 1993;4:207-217.

14. Netterville JL, Jackson CG, Civantos FJ. Thyroplasty in the functional rehabilitation of neurotologic skull base surgery patients. *Am J Otolaryngol.* 1993;14:460-464.

15. Maves MD, McCabe BF, Gray S. Phonosurgery: indications and pitfalls. *Ann Otol Rhinol Laryngol.* 1989;98:577-580.

CHAPTER 42

■ ■ ■

Treating Swallowing Disorders: Arytenoid Adduction

Gayle E. Woodson, M.D.

I. HISTORICAL PERSPECTIVE

The development of mirror laryngoscopy during the last century made it possible to diagnose laryngeal paralysis.[1] Ever since, it has been recognized that the symptoms of laryngeal paralysis are highly variable. Some patients have no symptoms, others have mild to moderate vocal impairment, while others have extreme hoarseness and suffer from aspiration during swallowing. The severity of symptoms has been observed to correlate with the position assumed by the paralyzed vocal fold. Symptoms are least severe when the vocal fold lies nearest the midline (paramedian) and are worse with a more lateral (cadaveric) position.[2]

For the first half of this century, laryngeal paralysis was regarded as an untreatable condition.[3] However, surgeons explored various ways of moving the paralyzed vocal fold to the midline to improve function. In the 1960s, injection of Teflon into the unilaterally paralyzed vocal fold gained wide acceptance as a treatment for laryngeal paralysis.[4] Teflon injection is frequently effective in improving vocal function, particularly when the vocal fold is not too far from the midline. However, Teflon is not very effective in treating aspiration and vocal results are poor when the paralyzed vocal fold is in the cadaveric position.[5] In such patients, a large "posterior gap" persists after Teflon injection, even when there appears to be adequate closure of the anterior glottis. Additionally, Teflon has lost favor as an injectable material for the larynx, because of the occurrence of Teflon granuloma.[6] In 1975, thyroplasty was reported as a means of medializing the paralyzed vocal fold.[7] This operation gained popularity in the United States during the last decade, and some authors have reported successful closure of the posterior glottis with thyroplasty.[8] However, many find thyroplasty to be inadequate in closing the posterior glottis or in treating aspiration.

In 1978, Isshiki introduced arytenoid adduction, a novel procedure designed specifically to close the posterior portion of the glottis in patients with laryngeal paralysis.[9] For nearly a decade, the procedure received little attention in the United States. But in recent years, several authors have reported good results with arytenoid adduction.[10-12]

II. SURGICAL INDICATIONS

Arytenoid adduction is indicated in patients who have symptoms of significant glottic incompetence and in whom physical examination reveals unilateral laryngeal paralysis with a large posterior gap during phonation. Many patients with laryngeal paralysis are asymptomatic and most do not aspirate during swallowing. Even if the glottis cannot close completely during swallowing, other protective mechanisms, such as laryngeal elevation and epiglottic folding, usually prevent laryngeal penetration. Factors associated with an increased risk of aspiration are a very wide glottal gap, impairment of pharyngeal motor function, and sensory deficit. This clinical scenario is frequently observed in patients with lesions of the vagus nerve. However, not all patients with vagus nerve paralysis need surgical rehabilitation. A slowly progressive lesion of the vagus nerve, such as in glomus tumors, sometimes allows time for gradual development of compensation, so that no therapy is needed.[13]

The "posterior" gap in patients with laryngeal paralysis represents inability to approximate the vocal processes of the arytenoid cartilages. Thus the gap is not truly posterior, but extends throughout the length of the glottis and is maximal at the junction of the membranous and cartilaginous portions of the vocal fold. Abduction of the vocal fold involves rotation of the arytenoid, creating an angle between the membranous and cartilaginous portions of the vocal fold. This angle prevents approximation of the vocal processes, even with vigorous hyper-adduction of the mobile vocal fold (Fig 42-1).[14]

Arytenoid adduction is the only vocal fold medialization procedure that specifically addresses the posterior gap by rotating the arytenoid to achieve a favorable position of the vocal process. This is very important in patients in whom the vocal fold is paralyzed in a lateral, or "cadaveric," position. When the paralyzed vocal fold is near the midline, the vocal process is very near to the physiologic position for glottic closure and aspiration is rare. In such cases, vocal symptoms are due to incompetence of only the anterior glottis and procedures that medialize the membranous portion are sufficient.

Patients with laryngeal paralysis due to pathology of the central nervous system or vagus nerve lesions frequently have associated impairment of pharyngeal motor and sensory function that contributes to a swallowing impairment. In these patients, restoration of glottic closure may not be sufficient to correct the dysphagia and aspiration. In unilateral pharyngeal paresis, pharyngeal propulsion is often inadequate to propel the bolus past the cricopharyngeal sphincter, which retains significant tone because of its bilateral innervation. In such patients, cricopharyngeal myotomy is a useful adjunct to arytenoid adduction.[15]

Sensory impairment can severely impair swallowing function, by interfering with the afferent limb of swallowing reflexes. It can also reduce or abolish a patient's sensations of secretions or ingested material in the pharynx. Thus, a patient may not respond to and clear matter in the hypopharynx, such as pooled secretions or residue from an inadequate swallow. Sensory impairment reduces the likelihood of substantial improvement in swallowing after arytenoid adduction, but is not an absolute contraindication to the procedure.

III. PREOPERATIVE ASSESSMENT

It is very important to establish the etiology and duration of a problem. If the recurrent laryngeal or vagus nerve has been disrupted by surgical resection or by tumor, then surgery may be indicated right away. However, if the nerve was traumatized but not transected or if paralysis is idiopathic, recovery of function

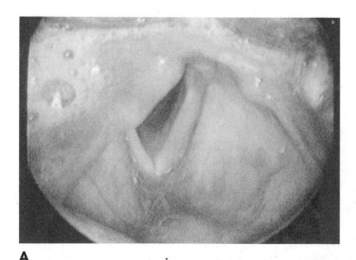

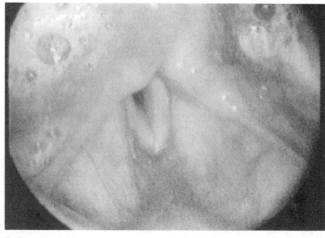

A **B**

FIG 42-1. Larynx of a patient with laryngeal paralysis due to a vagus nerve injury. **A**. Inspiration **B**. Phonation. *Note.* From Woodson GE. Configuration of the glottis in laryngeal paralysis I: Clinical study. *Laryngoscope.* 1993;103:1231. Reprinted with permission.

is possible and permanent alteration of the glottis should be deferred for at least 6 months.[16]

The presence and severity of aspiration are determined by the history, physical examination, and modified barium swallow (MBS). Patients should be questioned specifically as to whether or not they "choke" during swallowing or have significant coughing associated with eating or drinking. Not all patients are aware of aspiration; some have such profound sensory impairment that aspiration does not provoke a cough. Pneumonia may be the first clinical symptom of aspiration. Thus, all patients diagnosed with laryngeal paralysis must be considered as possible "silent aspirators," with a low threshold for performing modified barium swallow (MBS).

Mirror laryngoscopy is only a screening examination for detecting laryngeal paralysis. Adequate evaluation of these patients requires flexible laryngoscopy, preferably with video recording of the examination. A vocal fold that appears completely paralyzed on mirror examination may actually have significant residual or regenerating function. The first signs of recovery are usually seen within 2 months, with slight twitching movements of the arytenoid occurring synchronously with appropriate motions in the normal vocal fold. A vocal fold that remains flaccid at 6 months is extremely unlikely to recover.

The configuration of a paralyzed vocal fold is very important in planning surgical rehabilitation. A vocal fold positioned near the midline is nearly straight, with an angle of almost 180° between the cartilaginous and membranous portions of the vocal fold. Thus, the normal vocal process is able to approximate the paralyzed vocal process, resulting in no glottal gap or only a slit-like gap during phonation (Fig 42-2A). In such patients, only the membranous portions of the vocal folds need be medialized. However, when the vocal fold lies in a more lateral position, the vocal process is displaced laterally, so that the edges of the cartilaginous and membranous portions of the vocal fold form an obtuse angle approaching 90°. The normal vocal process cannot approximate the vocal process on the paralyzed side[15] (Fig 42-2B). This situation can only be corrected by moving the vocal process into a phonatory position, which can be accomplished by arytenoid adduction.

In patients with unilateral laryngeal paralysis, the paralyzed vocal fold appears shorter than the mobile side.[17] Studies indicate that the paralyzed fold is not really shorter, but only appears so because the vocal process moves upward as it moves laterally.[18] The normal side attempts to compensate for this spatial difference, resulting in foreshortening of the normal vocal fold as well[15] (Fig 42-3). Successful arytenoid adduction moves the vocal process caudally, reversing foreshortening of the paralyzed vocal fold.[14,18] Thus, foreshort-

ening of the paralyzed vocal fold is an indication for arytenoid adduction.

The shape of the membranous vocal fold should also be evaluated. If the fold is atrophic and bowed, then a thyroplasty may be required in conjunction with the arytenoid adduction.

Another characteristic distortion of the larynx in laryngeal paralysis is anterior tilting of the arytenoid, which obscures the vocal fold to varying degrees. The severity of anterior tilting has been correlated to the degree of denervation.[19] Tilting is most severe in patients with complete denervation, and a more erect posture of the arytenoid is seen in patients with high levels of EMG activity in laryngeal muscles on the immobile side. The anterior tilting probably represents loss of support by the posterior cricoarytenoid muscle and may contribute to the flaccidity of the paralyzed fold. This feature of laryngeal paralysis is not directly addressed by arytenoid adduction. Recent research suggests that the addition of a posterior suspension suture can correct this arytenoid "sagging" to some degree and may restore some tension to the fold.[20]

Flexible endoscopy should also be used to evaluate palate and pharyngeal function. Palate motion and com-

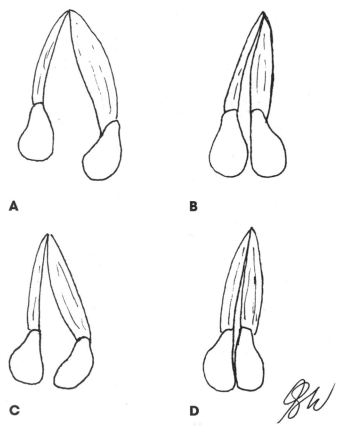

FIG 42-2. Diagramatic representation of vocal fold configuration in laryngeal paralysis with the vocal fold (**A, B**), near the midline and in the cadaveric location (**C, D**), in inspiration (**A, C**), and phonation (**B, D**).

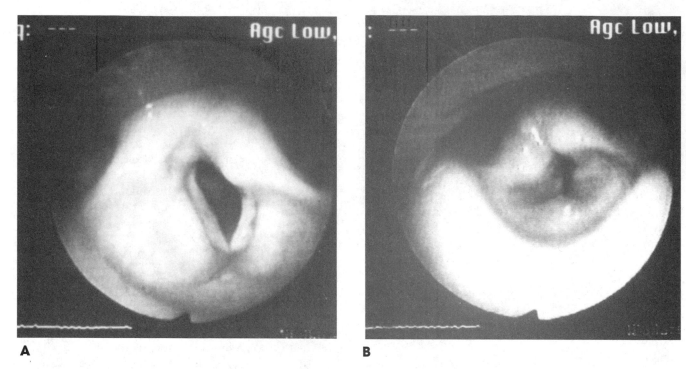

A

B

FIG 42-3. Compensatory hyperfunction in laryngeal paralysis. **A**. Inspiration, **B**. Phonation.

petence can be assessed with the scope positioned at the back of the nose. Patients with vagus nerve injury may have impairment of palatal motion with velopharyngeal incompetence that may need to be addressed surgically. The pharynx should be observed during a swallow. In a normal swallow, the pharynx collapses completely, resulting in a "white out" on videoendoscopy. However, in unilateral pharyngeal paralysis, the pharynx usually does not close completely, with the lumen visualized throughout the swallow and asymmetry of movement of the palatal walls able to be observed. Pooling of secretions in the vallecula and pyriform sinuses indicates impaired swallowing due to motor dysfunction or sensory impairment. The presence of secretions within the glottis itself is strong evidence of sensory impairment (see Chapter 12).

Clinical assessment of pharyngeal sensation is difficult to perform. The posterior pharyngeal wall can be stimulated to observe motion of the palate during a gag reflex. Laryngeal sensation can be assessed during flexible endoscopy by using the tip of the scope to contact the epiglottis, arytenoids, or vocal folds. Normally such contact results in vigorous coughing and, sometimes, laryngospasm. An objective protocol has recently been described for quantifying laryngeal sensation using calibrated puffs of air; however, this system is not in widespread use.[21]

Modified barium swallow (MBS) is indicated in patients who are extremely hoarse, have a large glottal gap, and those with pooling of secretions, pharyngeal weakness, or decreased sensation. The study is important for detecting aspiration and, if aspiration is present, determing the cause (see Chapter 11). Scintigraphy can be quite sensitive in detecting aspiration and providing quantitative information about swallowing efficiency. Manometry may be helpful in assessing pharyngeal function and for determining the possible need for simultaneous arytenoid adduction and cricopharyngeal myotomy. If studies indicate incomplete relaxation of the upper esophageal sphincter, cricopharyngeal myotomy is indicated in combination with the arytenoid adduction. On the other hand, if studies indicate delayed or absent swallow reflex or if laryngeal elevation is impaired, arytenoid adduction and cricopharyngeal myotomy are not likely to be sufficient to restore swallowing.

IV. SURGICAL TECHNIQUE

The goal of the arytenoid adduction procedure is to place anterior traction on the muscular process of the arytenoid, mimicking the activity of the lateral cricoarytenoid muscle. The arytenoid is rotated internally, about an oblique axis, displacing the vocal process medially and caudally, thereby adducting the vocal fold (Fig 42-4).[22]

Arytenoid adduction is best performed under local anesthesia to allow intraoperative monitoring of voice

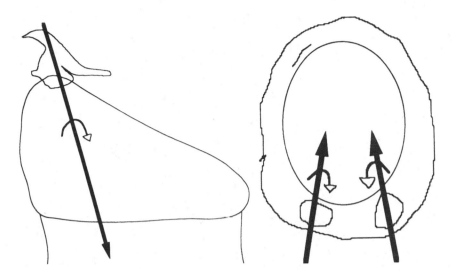

FIG 42-4. Axis of rotation in arytenoid adduction. *Note.* From Neuman TR, Hengesteg A, Lepage RP, Kaufman KR, Woodson GE. Three dimensional motion of the arytenoid adduction procedure in cadaver larynges. *Ann Otol Rhinol Laryngol.* 1994;103:269. Reprinted with permission.

and glottic configuration and to avoid the constraint of the endotracheal tube. Additionally, local anesthesia has less risk and morbidity than general anesthesia. Although the procedure requires rotation of the larynx more than 90°, it does not produce significant constriction of the airway. Cricopharyngeal myotomy can also be easily performed under local anesthesia in many patients. However, general anesthesia is preferable in patients with a tracheotomy in place, as the presence of the tracheotomy makes the dissection more difficult and can interfere with local anesthesia. General anesthesia is also a good option in uncooperative patients or those who need concomitant palate surgery, such as an adhesion procedure.

A horizontal skin incision is made at about the level of the cricothyroid membrane and superior and inferior flaps are elevated. The posterior larynx is approached by dissection lateral, rather than medial, to the cervical strap muscles, so that the hyoid, thyroid cartilage, cricoid, and trachea all rotate as a unit. This rotation reduces the risk of carotid artery injury. Alternatively, one may transect the strap muscles to maximize exposure.

A sturdy hook on the superior cornu of the thyroid cartilage is used to rotate the larynx (Fig 42-5) and the thyroid gland is displaced laterally. The inferior constrictor muscle is identified and is transected from the posterior border of the thyroid cartilage. The pyriform fossa mucosa is then elevated from the inner surface of the thyroid cartilage, leaving perichondrium in situ, and elevating mucosa out of the fossa and off of the posterior cricoarytenoid muscle. This portion of the procedure should be performed cautiously and meticulously to avoid entry into the pharynx and a potential

risk of fistula. Dissection should then carry anteriorly, elevating soft tissues away from the inner surface of the thyroid cartilage, preserving perichondrium, and creating a tunnel for passage of the suture.

The next step is to identify the muscular process. The posterior cricoarytenoid muscle serves as a reliable guide to the muscular process. Its fibers can be easily seen converging to insert on the arytenoid, even in patients with long-standing atrophy from paralysis of as long as 25 years[15] (Fig 42-6). As originally described, arytenoid adduction includes opening the cricoarytenoid joint; however, this can destabilize the larynx, allowing the arytenoid to be displaced anteriorly. By utilizing a lateral approach or division of the strap muscles, there is usually sufficient exposure to locate the muscular process without disruption of the cricoarytenoid joint. If necessary, the thyrohyoid ligament may be divided or a segment of cartilage removed from the posterior thyroid ala.

A sturdy, nonabsorbable suture is placed through the vocal process, and traction is applied to the suture while palpating the arytenoid to judge the adequacy of the suture placement. This author prefers a 4-0 Tevdek on a cardiac valve needle. If the suture placement is unsatisfactory (eg, only passing through soft tissue), tension on that suture can stabilize the arytenoid to permit more accurate placement of a second suture. Once a satisfactory placement is confirmed, the suture is tied, leaving 2 long ends.

One of the more difficult steps in arytenoid adduction is passing the 2 ends of the suture through the correct locations in the anterior larynx. Ideally, the 2 sutures should pass through the anterior thyroid carti-

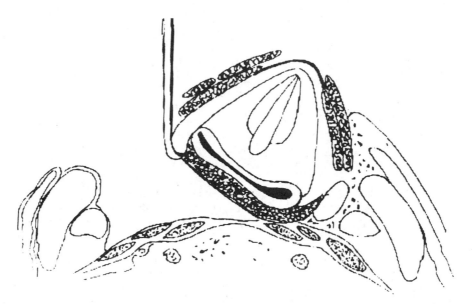

FIG 42-5. Technique of surgical exposure for arytenoid adduction. *Note.* From Woodson GE. Cricopharyngeal myotomy and arytenoid adduction in the management of combined laryngeal and pharyngeal paralysis. *Otolaryngol Head Neck Surg.* 1997;116: 341. Reprinted with permission.

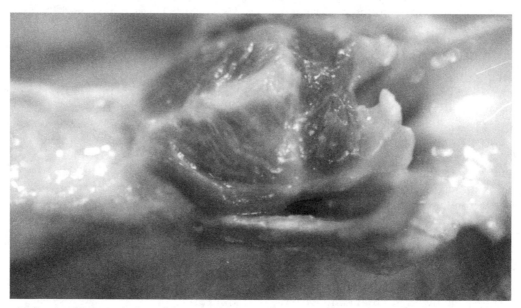

FIG 42-6. Muscle fibers of the posterior cricoarytenoid muscle converging at the muscular process of the arytenoid.

lage, approximately 5 mm above the inferior rim and at least 1 centimeter lateral to the midline and separated from each other by approximately 5 mm. If the thyroid cartilage is not very ossified and if thyroplasty is not being performed simultaneously, the suture can be placed using a large straight needle, passing from posterior to anterior. This is similar to playing pool. It is also impossible to pass the needle through a heavily laryngeal cartilage. Another approach that has been suggested is to drill holes in the appropriate places in the thyroid cartilage and then pass a spinal needle ret-

rograde, so that the suture may be threaded through the lumen of the needle. This approach is not recommended, as it can result in trauma of the paraglottic tissue, potentially resulting in bleeding that has potential for obstructing the airway. The placement of sutures is greatly facilitated by the use of a thyroplasty window, even if a thyroplasty is not performed. At least one end of the suture should be passed through a hole separate from the window, to assure a sufficiently anterior vector of force.

Once the sutures are in place, traction should be applied while listening to the patient phonate and observing vocal fold position endoscopically to assure optimal position. Then the sutures are securely tied. If a thyroplasty is to be performed, the implant should be in place before tying the AA suture.

If a cricopharyngeal myotomy is indicated, it can be easily added to the arytenoid adduction procedure, adding only a few minutes. After transection of the inferior constrictor muscle, the fibers of the cricopharyngeus can be identified and followed to their insertion on the cricoid cartilage. The muscle is then bluntly elevated from the underlying cartilage and esophagus, and a 1- to 2-cm segment is removed. Addressing the cricothyroid muscle at its attachment facilitates identification of all muscle fibers, while diminishing the risk of violating esophageal mucosa. As the recurrent laryngeal nerve is nonfunctional in these patients, the consequences of this nerve are negligible in most patients.

V. PITFALLS AND COMPLICATIONS

Arytenoid adduction carries the risk of pyriform sinus injury with possible fistula and carotid injury.[23] These complications are most effectively avoided by obtaining adequate surgical exposure and by employing careful dissection. The risk of carotid injury is greatest in patients who have had previous surgery in the area, such as thyroidectomy or neck dissection. Pyriform sinus fistula is more likely to occur in patients with prior radiotherapy. If the pyriform is entered, it should be immediately repaired and a nasogastric tube should be placed for feeding during healing. It is best to proceed with the adduction if possible, as a second surgery would not be advisable. However, the resulting contamination would preclude placement of a thyroplasty implant.

In the postoperative period, bleeding and swelling can lead to airway obstruction, sometimes occurring suddenly. Therefore, outpatient surgery is not recommended and patients should be observed at least overnight.

Prior Teflon injection does not preclude arytenoid adduction, although rotation of the arytenoid can be constrained by scarring and fibrosis around a Teflon implant. If there is a large granuloma, management may dictate its removal via a thyroid cartilage window.[24]

In most cases, arytenoid adduction for management of aspiration should be performed in conjunction with cricopharyngeal myotomy. This is particularly true when there is ipsilateral pharyngeal paresis or paralysis.[8,13,15]

The presence of other neurological deficits reduces the chance for successful control of aspiration.[15] Hypoglossal nerve injury and sensory impairment are two deficits that can profoundly impair swallowing. In such cases, aspiration frequently persists, despite correction of the glottal gap.

References

1. Garcia M. Physiological observations on the human voice. *Proc R Soc Lond.* 1855;7:399.
2. Arnold GE. Vocal rehabilitation of paralytic dysphonia: III. present concepts of laryngeal paralysis. *Arch Otol.* 1932; 65:317-336.
3. Jackson C, Jackson CL. *Diseases and Injuries of the Larynx.* New York, NY: Macmillan; 1942:330.
4. Arnold GE. Vocal rehabilitation of paralytic dysphonia. IX: technique of intracordal injection. *Arch Otolaryngol.* 1992;76:358-368.
5. Miller RH, Duplechain JK. Hoarseness and vocal cord paralysis. In: Gailey GJ, ed. *Head and Neck Surgery—Otolaryngology.* Philadelphia, Pa: Lippincott; 1993:626-627.
6. Varvares MA, Montgomery WW, Hillman RE. Teflon granuloma of the larynx: etiology, pathophysiology, and management. *Ann Otol Rhinol Laryngol.* 1995;104:511-515.
7. Isshiki N, Morita H, Okamura H, Hiramoto M. Thyroplasty type I for dysphonia due to vocal cord paralysis or atrophy. *Arch Otolaryngol.* 1975;80:465-473.
8. Montgomery WW, Hillman RE, Varvares MA. Combined thyroplasty type I and inferior constrictor myotomy. *Ann Otol Rhinol Laryngol.* 1994;103:858-862.
9. Isshiki N, Tanabe M, Sawada M. Arytenoid adduction for unilateral vocal cord paralysis. *Arch Otolaryngol.* 1978;104: 555-558.
10. Slavit DH, Maragos NE. Physiologic assessment of arytenoid adduction. *Ann Otol Rhinol Laryngol.* 1992;101:321-327.
11. Woodson GE, Murry T. Glottic configuration after arytenoid adduction. *Laryngoscope.* 1994;104:965-969.
12. Bielamowicz S, Berke GS, Gerratt BR. A comparison of type I thyroplasty and arytenoid adduction. *J Voice.* 1995; 9:466-472.
13. Biller HF, Lawson W, Som P, Rosenfeld R. Glomus vagale tumors. *Ann Otol Rhinol Laryngol.* 1989;98:21-26.
14. Woodson GE. Configuration of the glottis in laryngeal paralysis I: clinical study. *Laryngoscope.* 1993;103:1227-1234.
15. Woodson GE. Cricopharyngeal myotomy and arytenoid adduction in the management of combined laryngeal and pharyngeal paralysis. *Otolaryngol Head Neck Surg.* 1997;116: 339-343.
16. Woodson GE, Miller RH. Timing of surgical intervention in patients with recurrent laryngeal nerve paralysis. *Otolaryngol Head Neck Surg.* 1981;89:264-267.
17. Brewer DW, Woo P, Casper JK, Colton RH. Unilateral recurrent laryngeal nerve paralysis: a re-examination. *J Voice.* 1991;5:178-185.
18. Woodson GE, Hengesteg A, Rosen CA, Yeung D, Chen N. Changes in length and spatial orientation of the vocal fold with arytenoid adduction in cadaver larynges. *Ann Otol Rhinol Laryngol.* 1997;106:552-555.
19. Blitzer A, Jahn AF, Keidar A. Semon's law revisited: an electromyographic analysis of laryngeal synkinesis. *Ann Otol Rhinol Laryngol.* 1996;105:764-769.
20. Woodson GE, Pacero D, Hengesteg A, Yeung D. Modification of the arytenoid adduction procedure. Paper presented at the ALA annual meeting; May 1998; Orlando, Fla.

21. Aviv JE, Sacco RL, Mohr JP, et al. Laryngopharyngeal sensory testing with modified barium swallow as predictors of aspiration pneumonia after stroke. *Laryngoscope.* 1997; 107:1254-1260.

22. Neuman TR, Hengesteg A, Lepage RP, Kaufman KR, Woodson GE. Three-dimensional motion of the arytenoid adduction procedure in cadaver larynges. *Ann Otol Rhinol Laryngol.* 1994;103:265-270.

23. Koufman JA, Isaacson G. Laryngoplastic phonosurgery. *Otolaryngol Clin North Am.* 1991;24:1151-1177.

24. Coleman JR, Netterville JL, Chang SL, Rainey CL. Lateral laryngotomy for the removal of Teflon granuloma. Paper presented at the ALA annual meeting; May 1997; Palm Springs, Ca.

CHAPTER 43

■ ■ ■

Surgical Treatment of Swallowing Disorders: Cricopharyngeal Myotomy

Anna M. Pou, M.D.

I. HISTORICAL PERSPECTIVE

The cricopharyngeus muscle is the major component of the upper esophageal sphincter (UES), which is also composed of the distal inferior constrictor muscle and the proximal circular esophageal muscle. The cricopharyngeus muscle is in continuous tonic contraction, mediated by the sympathetic plexus; the pharyngeal plexus (vagal and glossopharyngeal nerve fibers) causes its relaxation. Advancements in radiologic techniques, as well as expanding knowledge of the anatomy and function of the cricopharyngeus muscle, have aided in the treatment of its dysfunction.

The cricopharyngeus muscle was first described by Valsalva in 1717.[1] Its distinction from the other muscles of the UES was clarified by Jackson in 1914[2]; nevertheless, the term UES is often used interchangeably with the cricopharyngeus. In 1926, Jackson and Shallow[2] proposed that pulsion diverticula result from incoordination of the "cricopharyngeal pinchock," and in 1946, Lahey[3] proposed cricopharyngeus dilatation in treating this condition. The first cricopharyngeal myotomy was performed by Kaplan in 1951,[4] who successfully treated dysphagia in a patient with polio. It was not until 1955 that Fyke and Code systematically analyzed pressure changes at the pharyngoesophageal region, discovering the biphasic nature of pressure changes that occur during swallowing.[5] This led to a greater understanding of the swallowing act, which led to a greater understanding and treatment of dysphagia. Cricopharyngeal myotomy has been used to treat a variety of swallowing disorders in the past decade.

II. SURGICAL INDICATIONS

When the swallow occurs, the cricopharyngeus muscle relaxes during pharyngeal contraction, permitting the bolus to pass into the esophagus. If the relaxation fails or there is incoordination of the cricopharyngeus, dysphagia results. Cricopharyngeal myotomy is the most reliable surgical means to improve bolus transit.

Cricopharyngeal myotomy has been used to treat dysfunction of the cricopharyngeus muscle secondary to lesions of the central and peripheral nervous systems, diseases affecting muscular activity, laryngeal and pharyngeal paralysis, idiopathic discoordination, and postsurgical dysphagia (Table 43-1). Although the surgical indications and postoperative results are controversial, a cricopharyngeal myotomy is most successful in treating patients with normal or near normal pharyngeal function, which is needed to propel the bolus. Cricopharyngeal myotomy, however, may be successful in treating patients with weakened pharyngeal function because of the relief of the "relative obstacle" presented by the cricopharyngeus muscle in these patients.[6] This procedure is contraindicated in those with severely impaired propulsion due to weakened pha-

Table 43-1. *Indications and Contraindications of Cricopharyngeal Myotomy*

Indications: Dysphagia secondary to:

Central nervous system disorders
    Parkinsonism
    Cerebrovascular vascular accident
    Multiple sclerosis (MS)
    Amyotrophic lateral sclerosis (ALS)

Peripheral nervous system
    Vagal injury (laryngeal/pharyngeal paralysis)
    Diabetic/peripheral neuropathy

Muscular disease
    Oculopharyngeal dystrophy
    Steinert myotonic dystrophy
    Polymyositis
    Myasthenia gravis

Hyperthyroidism/hypothyroidism

Postsurgical
    Supraglottic laryngectomy
    Total laryngectomy
    Oral cavity/oropharyngeal resection

Tracheoesophageal speech (spasticity)

Zenker's diverticulum

Cricopharyngeal achalasia

Contraindications

Severe weakness of the pharyngeal muscles (unable to propel bolus)
Severe/uncontrolled GER disease
Pharyngeal varices:
    Postbilateral neck dissections
    Thoracic outlet syndrome

ryngeal muscles,[6] and in those with severe, uncontrolled gastroesophageal reflux (GER) disease (Table 43-1).

III. PREOPERATIVE ASSESSMENT

A thorough history is imperative prior to surgery. One should inquire if the patient requires multiple attempts at swallowing, has a history of pneumonia, weight loss, wet-sounding voice, or choking with liquids. A history of cerebrovascular accident, neurologic or neuromuscular diseases, head trauma, and previous head and neck surgery should be ascertained. The physical exam should include a complete head and neck and neurologic exam. If dysphagia is thought to be secondary to a neurologic disease, consultation with a neurologist is warranted.

Patients with underlying medical conditions should be evaluated and treated preoperatively. If the patient has a history of GER disease, the severity of reflux should be determined and treatment should be rendered prior to cricopharyngeal myotomy.

Radiologic studies including barium swallow, modified barium swallow (MBS), and manometry are used to assess cricopharyngeus muscle dysfunction, although these exams may be normal in symptomatic patients. The MBS provides a sensitive means of visualizing pharyngeal and UES dysfunction (Logemann, 1997).[7] The presence of a horizontal bar on the posterior wall of the pharyngoesophagus occurring at the level of vertebral bodies C5 to C7 or obstruction of the bolus indicates incomplete cricopharyngeus relaxation. The role of manometry is controversial (Kelly, 1997),[8] but simultaneous use of this and videofluoroscopy may provide more definitive information about the UES.

IV. SURGICAL TECHNIQUE

The patient is placed in a supine position with the neck extended by a shoulder roll (Table 43-2). Rigid esophagoscopy is performed to rule out neoplasms and inflammatory diseases. A No. 40-44 bougie dilator is placed transorally into the esophagus. If preferred by the surgeon, a nasogastric tube can be used in place of a bougie dilator.

A horizontal skin incision is made 2 finger breaths above the clavicle in a natural skin crease near the level of the cricoid cartilage. This incision is usually made in the left neck, unless contraindicated by a right vocal fold paralysis. An alternative skin incision can be made obliquely along the anterior border of the sternocleidomastoid muscle. Subplatysmal flaps are elevated to the level of the clavicle inferiorly and to the level of the hyoid superiorly. The fascia overlying the anterior border of the sternocleidomastoid is incised along its entire length. The areolar tissue is dissected, identifying the carotid sheath and the prevertebral fascia. The omohyoid muscle is identified and retracted. If additional exposure is needed, the omohyoid muscle may be transected, tagging the ends with suture so that the muscle can be sewn together at the end of the procedure. The middle thyroid vein is also ligated if necessary to gain exposure. The sternocleidomastoid and carotid sheath are retracted laterally. The posterolateral aspect of the thyroid ala and the cricoid cartilage are identified.

The cricopharyngeus originates from the cricoid cartilage, which is the key landmark in performing this procedure. A double-pronged hook is placed on the posterolateral aspect of the thyroid ala, and it is retracted medially to expose the cricopharyngeus muscle. The surgeon should avoid retractors below the level of the inferior cornu of the thyroid cartilage, as they may cause pressure injury to the recurrent laryngeal nerve (RLN). Using a No. 15 blade, the cricopharyngeus muscle is incised, along with, fibers of the distal inferior constrictor muscle and the proximal circular esophageal muscle (Fig 43-1). This incision is approximately 3-6 cm in length. The muscle fibers are divided posteriorly to avoid injury to the RLN. The muscle fibers are cut until

Table 43-2. *Cricopharyngeal Myotomy: Surgical Technique (Highlights)*

1. Rigid esophagoscopy is performed.
2. A No. 40-44 bougie dilator is placed transorally into the esophagus prior to the start of the procedure.
3. A horizontal skin incision is made 2 finger breadths above the clavicle in a natural skin crease.
4. Subplatysmal flaps are raised to the level of the clavicle inferiorly and to the level of the hyoid bone superiorly.
5. The fascia overlying the sternocleidomastoid is incised in its entire length, and the areolar tissue is dissected identifying the carotid sheath and prevertebral fascia.
6. The omohyoid muscle and middle thyroid vein are retracted to gain exposure.
7. The sternocleidomastoid and the carotid sheath are retracted laterally.
8. The posterolateral aspect of the thyroid ala and the cricoid cartilage are identified and retracted medially using a double-pronged hook; this exposes the cricopharyngeus muscle.
9. Using a No. 15 blade, the cricopharyngeus is incised, in addition to the distal inferior constrictor muscle and the proximal circular esophageal muscle fibers (approximately 3-6 cm). The muscle fibers are divided posteriorly in the midline to avoid injury to the recurrent laryngeal nerve. The muscle fibers are incised until mucosa is identified.
10. A suction drain is placed and the incision is closed in layers.
11. A diet is started on postoperative day 1 and, if food is tolerated, the patient is discharged.

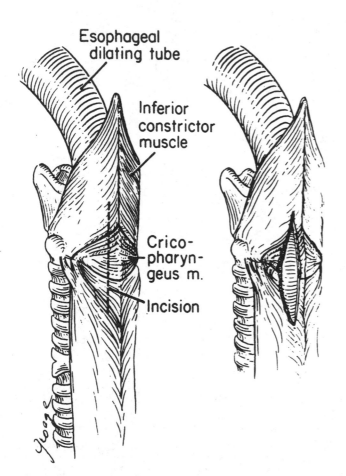

Esophageal dilating tube

Inferior constrictor muscle

Crico- pharyn- geus m.

Incision

FIG 43-1. Muscle fibers of the cricopharyngeus, inferior constrictor, and circular esophageal muscles are incised posteriorly. Note: From Calcaterra TC, Kadell BM, Ward PH. Dysphagia secondary to cricopharyngeal muscle dysfunction. *Arch Otolaryngol.* 1975;101:728. Copyright 1995, American Medical Association, reprinted with permission.

mucosa is seen over the underlying dilator (Fig 43-1). Care is taken not to injure the mucosa. If a nasogastric tube was placed in lieu of the bougie dilator, both the muscle to be incised and the tube are clasped with a Babcock clamp at both ends of the muscle. The cricopharyngeus muscle is incised until mucosa is seen, and then an additional strip of muscle is elevated and excised using scissors.[9] A third alternative requires the use of neither an nasogastric tube or bougie dilator. The muscle is identified posteriorly and is elevated from the mucosa using a hemostat. The muscle is then incised over the hemostat using a No.15 blade. This method greatly reduces the risk of inadvertent injury to the mucosa. A small suction drain is placed and the wound is closed in layers. The patient is fed a clear liquid diet, which is advanced as tolerated. The patient is discharged from the acute care setting following successful oral intake.

In patients undergoing a supraglottic or total laryngectomy, a cricopharyngeal myotomy is performed to decrease the incidence of postoperative dysphagia and cricopharyngeus spasm. In patients undergoing total laryngectomy, a finger is simply placed into the pharynx and the muscle is incised over the finger as previously described.

V. PITFALLS AND COMPLICATIONS

Pitfalls and complications of cricopharyngeal myotomy can be due to poor patient selection and/or errors in surgical technique. These are summarized in Table 43-3. Cricopharyngeal myotomy in a patient with severe, uncontrolled gastroesophageal reflux disease (GER disease) can cause worsening of this condition, leading to aspiration and subsequent pneumonia. Cricopharyngeal myotomy in a person with very poor pharyngeal muscle function will fail if the patient cannot adequately propel the bolus. A thorough preoperative history, physical examination, and appropriate testing should identify patients at-risk.

Table 43-3. *Pitfalls and Complications*

Patient Factors/Poor Patient Selection

Severe/uncontrolled GER disease resulting in postoperative aspiration and pneumonia
  Extreme pharyngeal muscle weakness with inability to propel bolus
  Complications avoided by obtaining a good history and physical exam

Surgical Errors

Injury to the recurrent laryngeal nerve
  Avoid by incising muscle fibers in the posterior midline
  Avoid retraction below the level of inferior cornu
  Treat symptomatically

Pharyngotomy
  Avoid by using extreme caution while incising muscle fibers
  Repair pharyngotomy by inverting mucosa, administering tube feeds for 5 days, and administering perioperative intravenous
  antibiotics

Fistula (see above)
  Treatment also includes local wound care and, if necessary, neck exploration and closure of fistula

Recurrence of symptoms
  Avoid by performing a complete myotomy and obtaining a good history, radiologic studies, and esophagoscopy to exclude
  other causes of cervical dysphagia

Errors in surgical technique include incomplete transection of the muscle fibers and injury to the RLN, pharyngotomy, salivary fistula formation, and failure to provide resolution of dysphagia. To avoid RLN injury, the myotomy should be performed posteriorly in the midline. To avoid a pharyngocutaneous fistula, extreme caution should be taken in performing the myotomy. The absence of a mucosal injury can be demonstrated by instilling a solution of povidone iodine periorally. Similarly, a solution of diluted methylene blue can be given to detect a fistula. If the pharynx is entered, it is repaired by inverting the mucosa using absorbable sutures. A nasogastric tube is also placed and perioperative antibiotics are given intravenously. Feedings are administered via the nasogastric tube for 5 days, allowing the mucosa to heal. If a postoperative fistula develops, it may be managed conservatively with systemic antibiotics, nasogastric feedings, and suction drainage. Local wound care is administered if an abscess forms. If conservative management is not effective, the patient is taken to the operating room for closure of the fistula. Recurrence or failure to provide resolution of dysphagia can be avoided by completely incising *all* muscle fibers of the cricopharyngeus, in addition to a portion of the inferior constrictor muscle and the fibers of the circular esophageal muscle. A thorough history, radiologic studies, and esophagoscopy should be performed to rule out other causes of cervical dysphagia that may not be corrected by this procedure.

References

1. Ross ER, Green R, Auslander MO, Biller, HF. Cricopharyngeal myotomy: management of cervical dysphagia. *Otolaryngol Head Neck Surg*. 1982;90:434-441.
2. Jackson C, Shallow TA. Diverticula of the esophagus, pulsion, traction, malignant and congenital. *Ann Surg*. 1926; 83:1-19.
3. Lahey FH. Pharyngo-esophageal diverticulum: its management and complications. *Ann Surg*. 1946; 124:617-636.
4. Kaplan S. Paralysis of deglutition, a post-poliomyelitis complication treated by section of the cricopharyngeus muscle. *Ann Surg*. 1951;133:572-573.
5. Fyke FE, Code CF. Resting and deglutition pressure in the pharyngo-esophageal region. *Gastroenterology*. 1955;29:1-19.
6. St. Guily JL, Perie S, Wilig TN, Chaussade S, Eymard B, Angelard B. Swallowing disorders in muscular diseases: functional assessment and indications of cricopharyngeal myotomy. *Ear Nose Throat J*. 1994;73:34-40.
7. Logemann J. Role of the modified barium swallow in management of patients with dysphagia. *Otolaryngol Head Neck Surg*. 1997;116:335-8.
8. Kelly JH. Use of manometry in the evaluation of dysphagia. *Otolaryngol Head Neck Surg*. 1997;116:355-357.
9. Myers EN. Cricopharyngeal myotomy. In: Myers EN, ed. *Operative Otolaryngology: Head and Neck Surgery*. Philadelphia, Pa: WB Saunders; 1997:466-471.

CHAPTER 44

■ ■ ■

Palatal Adhesion/Pharyngeal Flap

James L. Netterville, M.D.

I. INTRODUCTION

Defects of soft palate function can be either congenital or acquired. When congenital, except in some cases of complete cleft lip and palate, infants compensate and can take adequate oral intake. Even with severe cleft palate and cleft lip adequate nutrition can be acquired in most cases. The evaluation and treatment of these patients is reviewed in Chapter 36. This chapter addresses acquired palatal defects.

Acquired defects can result from (1) surgical loss of the soft palate, either partial or complete, or (2) neurogenic dysfunction of the soft palate. Neurogenic dysfunction resulting in either unilateral or bilateral paralysis of the soft palate creates varying degrees of velopharyngeal incompetence (VPI). During the process of swallowing, incompetence is manifest by regurgitation of liquids and, rarely, solids into the nasopharynx with each swallow. This liquid regurgitation can be quite severe, if the head is tilted forward to drink from a water fountain, resulting in liquids draining out of the nose with each swallow. As the head is tilted in the opposite direction to look upward, partial compensation can be accomplished decreasing the fluid reflux when swallowing. With palatal paralysis, regurgitation of solid food is less common, because of pressure of the tongue with each swallow on the weak soft palate. Fifty percent of patients with unilateral paralysis will improve over time, thus persisting with minimal complaints of swallowing dysfunction. However, on close questioning they will say they shy away from drinking from water fountains or with the head tilted forward.

Unilateral paralysis or paresis most commonly results from loss of the vagal nerve at the skull base.[1] Palatal paralysis is also common after surgery of the parapharyngeal or infratemporal space because of damage of the palatal branch of the vagal nerve. Viral polyneuropathies and idiopathic causes also lead to a patient presenting with unilateral paralysis.

Bilateral paralysis is less common and is usually caused by a stroke to the brainstem region, resulting in bulbar palsy and incoordination of the entire pharynx and larynx. Other rare causes include sarcoidosis, viral polyneuropathies, and idiopathic causes. Treatment in this group is difficult, because pharynx, tongue, and larynx are weak. Isolated treatment of the palate will provide very little benefit to such a patient.

Because of our large population of patients with unilateral paralysis resulting from lateral skull base surgery, we set out to search the literature to find a reasonable treatment for these patients.[2,3] In the mid 1980s these patients were treated with swallowing therapy, palatal lift prostheses, or, rarely, a midline pharyngeal flap. Very little improvement resulted from the first two, with the midline pharyngeal flap not an ideal solution—partially treating the paralyzed side while partially injuring the normal side. With this background, we initiated the treatment of these patients with unilateral palatal adhesion, first described in 1992 after successfully being used in 8 patients. A more extensive review of 31 patients undergoing palatal adhesion (PA) was presented in 1997, demonstrating the significant benefit to both swallowing and voice. This study demonstrated that palatal adhesion improved the postoperative vocal quality in 96% of patients. Nasopharyngeal reflux was significantly improved in 83% of patients. However, at least partial improvement in nasal reflux was seen in 100% of the patients.

II. SURGICAL INDICATIONS

Unilateral palatal adhesion is indicated for patients with unilateral palatal paralysis. Even patients with very mild liquid reflux often have moderate to severe nasal quality to their speech, which dramatically improves with palatal adhesion. In most patients with bilateral palatal paralysis, a midline pharyngeal flap is appropriate. There are no absolute contraindications to this procedure. However, relative contraindications include severe untreated sleep apnea, multiple pharyngeal polyneuropathies, history of high-dose radiation therapy to the nasopharynx, and previous resection and scarring of the palate or nasopharynx (Table 44-1).

III. PREOPERATIVE ASSESSMENT

Preoperative assessment can be very simple or complex, depending on the degree of documentation possible at different institutions. At a minimum, a complete history and exam of the head and neck is mandatory to assess the cause and the degree of the problem of each patient. If the etiology is unknown, then a thorough search, including physical exam and imaging of the skull base and nasopharynx, is necessary. With a known cause of cranial nerve loss due to previous surgical resection, then documentation of the unilateral

Table 44-1. *Palatal Adhesion: Indications and Contraindications*

Indications

1. Unilateral palatal paralysis
2. Unilateral scarring resulting in unilateral VPI
3. Unilateral partial palatal defect

Contraindications

Relative

1. Severe untreated sleep apnea
2. Multiple pharyngeal polyneuropathies
3. High-dose radiation therapy to the nasopharynx
4. Previous resection with scarring of the palate or nasopharynx

paralysis and the degree of VPI is important. On physical exam, the palatal function can be best documented with a 70° rigid Hopkins rod, viewing the nasopharynx from both the transoral and the transnasal view. If possible, this should be recorded on videotape with static pictures of the nasopharynx during ventilation and during phonation placed in the record. A rhinometer can be used to document the abnormal nasal airflow with speech; however, the use of a cold laryngeal mirror placed below the nares will also demonstrate abnormal airflow. We do not usually document the reflux of liquids into the nasopharynx by use of a videoswallow. The patient history usually provides excellent information and reflux can be well demonstrated in the office by having the patient drink in the head down position. However, if hard documentation is needed, a videoswallow will show the degree of nasal reflux. It may, however, be difficult to correlate the findings on the swallow with the degree of symptoms seen in the patients.

IV. SURGICAL TECHNIQUE

Palatal adhesion is performed under general anesthesia through a transoral approach. Wide oropharyngeal exposure is obtained with a Dingman mouth gag. The adhesion is created unilaterally at the level of Passavant's ridge, where the normal closure of the nasopharynx occurs. Lidocaine with epinephrine is instilled into the palate and the posterior pharyngeal wall. After palpation of the posterior pharyngeal wall to prevent damage to an aberrantly positioned internal carotid artery, an incision is created through the hemipalate extending from the midline to the lateral pharyngeal wall (Fig 44-1). A parallel incision is created through the posterior pharyngeal wall down to the premuscular fascia (Fig 44-2). With careful inverting sutures, the raw edge of the posterior pharyngeal wall is attached to the raw edge of the nasopharyngeal surface of the palate. A special "hooked needle" (PS4-C) on a 4-0 Vicryl is extremely helpful in creating this attachment working through the 2.5 cm incision in the palate. No sutures are tied until 7-8 sutures are placed across both the superior and the inferior aspect of the adhesion. The utility of the Dingman gag is noted here, as the untied sutures are secured to the storage springs keeping an organized surgical field until all sutures are placed. The oral surface of the palate is either closed or left open to heal by secondary intention. This results in unilateral closure of the nasopharynx on the defective side (Fig 44-3). The adhesion stretches out, allowing a normal anterior to posterior distance on the contralateral normal side of the nasopharynx, which allows adequate airflow (Fig 44-4).

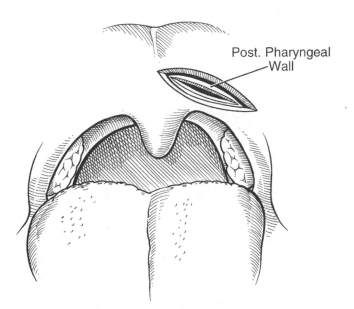

Post. Pharyngeal
Wall

FIG 44-1. The incision in the palate is created from the midline over to the lateral pharyngeal wall. It is placed 9-10 mm superior to the anterior tonsilar fold to prevent entry into the tonsilar fossa.

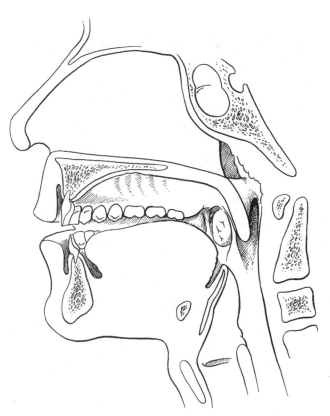

FIG. 44-3. The adhesion is at the level of Passavant's ridge to allow closure of the contralateral normal velopharynx.

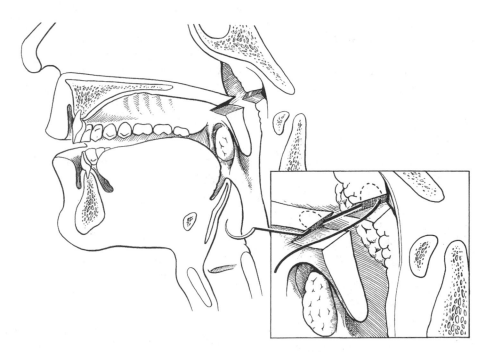

FIG. 44-2. The parallel incision into the posterior pharyngeal wall is carried down to the premuscular fascia. The inverting mattress suture is very important to approxi-mate the raw surface of each flap. Simple suture placement without eversion will close mucosa against mucosa, which will result in a high breakdown rate.

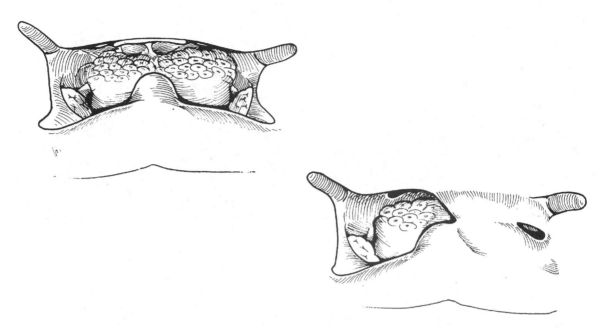

Fig. 44-4. The unilateral adhesion stretches out to allow for a normal anterior to posterior dimension of the con-

tralateral nasopharynx, allowing adequate airflow.

Patients are allowed a full liquid diet for 1 week after surgery to prevent trapping of particulate food in a partially open palatal wound. Saline oral rinses are often helpful in the postoperative care of these intraoral wounds. Pain is not a major obstacle. Most often hydrocodone and acetaminophen, either tablet or liquid form, is adequate for pain control after PA.

V. PITFALLS AND COMPLICATIONS

Pitfalls that might prevent a good outcome are listed in Table 44-2. If the palatal incision is placed too high on the palate, it is difficult to attach it to the posterior pharyngeal wall because of excessive tension. One must be very careful to not close across the midline, which might lead to decreased nasal airflow.

Table 44-2. *Potential Pitfalls and Complications*

Pitfalls

1. Performing adhesion too soon in patient who may return to function
2. Palatal incision too high on soft palate
3. Closure of nasopharynx across midline
4. Failure to adequately suture palate to the posterior pharyngeal wall

Complications

1. Breakdown of adhesion
2. Palatal fistula
3. Decreased nasal airflow

VI. OUTCOME

Of the 28 evaluable patients who underwent palatal adhesions, 24 (89%) had uncomplicated postoperative healing. Of the remaining 4 patients, 2 developed intraoral dehiscence with partial breakdown of the palatal-pharyngeal adhesion resulting in a temporary palatal fistula with marked nasality. The other 2 developed isolated superficial wound dehiscence, intraorally. All 4 patients had complete healing within 1 month, with no long-term sequelae. No other major or minor complications were encountered in these patients.

In summary, palatal adhesion provides improved voice and swallow function in those patients with unilateral palatal paralysis. For patients with nasal reflux who do not improve over time, this procedure is recommended.

References

1. Netterville JL, Civantos FJ. Rehabilitation of cranial nerve deficits after neurotologic skull base surgery. *Laryngoscope*. 1993;103:45-54.
2. Crockett DM, Bumsted RM, Van Demark DR. Experience with surgical management of velopharyngeal incompetence. *Otolaryngol Head Neck Surg*. 1988;99:1-9.
3. Bumsted RM. Velopharyngeal incompetence. In: English GM, ed. *Otolaryngology* Vol. IV. New York, NY: Lippincott-Raven; 1995:1-25.
4. Netterville JL, Vrabec JT. Unilateral palatal adhesion for paralysis after high vagal injury. *Arch Otolaryngol Head Neck Surg*. 1994;120:218-221.
5. Netterville JL, Fortune S, Stanziale S, Rainey S. Palatal adhesion: the treatment of unilateral palatal paralysis following high vagus nerve injury. *Ann Otol Laryngol Rhinol*. 1998; in press.

CHAPTER 45

■ ■ ■

Laryngeal Closure

Carl H. Snyderman, M.D.

I. HISTORICAL PERSPECTIVE

Intractable aspiration is a major cause of morbidity and mortality for patients with severe laryngeal dysfunction. It detracts greatly from a patient's quality of life and increases the costs of medical care. The treatment of chronic aspiration is dependent on the cause and severity of the aspiration. A wide variety of therapeutic interventions may be employed (Table 45-1).

Although the initial treatment of aspiration often involves a tracheotomy, it is well established that a tracheotomy does not prevent aspiration and its sequelae (see Chapter 20). In fact, a tracheotomy has multiple adverse effects on laryngeal function that may promote aspiration. An improved understanding of the physiological effects of tracheotomy on laryngeal function has resulted in the development of novel tracheostomy tube designs and speech valves to increase subglottic pressure and expel aspirated secretions.[1] In fact, placement of a speech valve in a patient with a tracheostomy may decrease aspiration and prevent the need for additional surgical interventions (see Chapter 37).

For patients with aspiration that persists despite the use of conservative measures or adjunctive surgical procedures (Table 45-1), surgical closure of the larynx is necessary to prevent aspiration.[2] Although many techniques have been reported in the medical literature, few have met with consistent success. Laryngeal closure techniques range from conservative (laryngeal stents) to radical (total laryngectomy) (Table 45-2).

Table 45-1. *Treatment of Aspiration*

Nonsurgical procedures
Nothing by mouth
Nasoenteric feeding
Videoendoscopic feedback
Swallowing therapy
Thermal stimulation technique
Nasotracheal suctioning
Pharmacologic inhibition of secretions
Nasogastric suctioning
Medical treatment of underlying gastrointestinal and esophageal disorders (gastroesophageal reflux, peptic ulcer disease)

Adjunctive surgical procedures
Tracheostomy
Cricopharyngeal myotomy
Gastrostomy/feeding jejunostomy
Pharyngotomy tube
Polytef vocal fold injection
Thyroplasty for vocal fold medialization
Laryngeal suspension
Partial cricoid resection
Tympanic and chorda tympani neurectomy
Vocal fold reinnervation

Although laryngeal stents are effective for the treatment of aspiration,[3] questions remain regarding their suitability for the long-term management of patients. The advantages of laryngeal stents are that they are easy to insert, have little morbidity, and can be removed if neurologic function improves. Newer designs, such as the Eliachar stent, are soft and compressible, mini-

Table 45-2. *Definitive Surgical Procedures*

Laryngeal stenting
Supraglottic closure
  Epiglottic closure
  Epiglottic flap
  Epiglottopexy
  Epiglottic tube laryngoplasty
Glottic closure
Subglottic closure
  Tracheoesophageal diversion
  Laryngotracheal separation
Laryngectomy

mizing the risk of pressure necrosis. Stents have been used successfully in patients for over 1 year without evidence of laryngotracheal injury.[4] In contrast, a total laryngectomy carries significant morbidity, is less acceptable to patients, and results in permanent loss of voice.

Laryngeal closure techniques can be divided into supraglottic, glottic, and subglottic surgical techniques. Supraglottic and glottic closure techniques have proven to be unreliable and may not be reversible, because of excessive scarring of the larynx. Lindeman first proposed a subglottic closure procedure, or laryngotracheal separation, in 1975.[5] As first described, the subglottic trachea was diverted by creating an anastomosis with the esophagus (Fig 45-1A). The technique was subsequently modified by Lindeman[6] and Baron and Dedo[7] to create a subglottic pouch without diversion (Fig 45-1B). In comparison to other procedures, this technique best meets the desired criteria of simplicity, reliability, and reversibility (Table 45-3). For patients who fail more conservative therapy, we have found laryngotracheal separation to be the preferred surgical option.

II. SURGICAL INDICATIONS

A wide variety of medical conditions may result in chronic aspiration (Table 45-4). The most common diagnoses are neurologic disorders such as cerebrovascular accidents (CVA) and amyotrophic lateral sclerosis (ALS). Most patients have multiple neurologic deficits in addition to laryngeal dysfunction. The management of patients with aspiration is dependent on the degree of laryngeal dysfunction. As shown in the schematic Fig 45-2, patients with abnormal laryngeal function but intact glottic sensation can often be managed medically or with adjunctive surgical procedures. If a tracheotomy is necessary or already present, the use of a Passy-Muir valve may alleviate any need for further surgical intervention.[1] If aspiration persists despite the use of a Passy-Muir valve or laryngeal function is severely compromised by the absence of glottic sensation, laryngotracheal separation is considered.

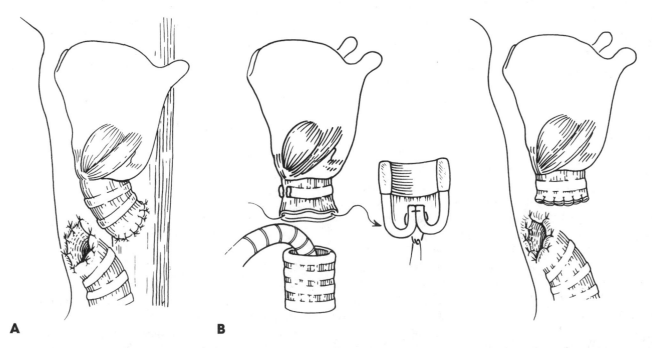

A   **B**

FIG 45-1. A. Laryngotracheal diversion (standard Lindeman procedure) involves the creation of an anastomosis between the subglottic trachea and the esophagus, and a permanent stoma from the distal trachea.

B. With laryngotracheal separation (modified Lindeman procedure), the proximal subglottic trachea is closed as a blind pouch and a permanent stoma is created from the distal trachea.

Table 45-3. *Comparison of Surgical Procedures for Aspiration*

	Control of Aspiration	Preservation of Speech	Reversibility
Tracheostomy	−	+	+
Laryngeal stent	±	±	+
Laryngotracheal separation	+	−	+
Total laryngectomy	+	−	−

Table 45-4. *Pathologic State Associated with Aspiration*

Surgical
  Skull base
  Head and neck
    Thyroid carcinoma
    Supraglottic laryngectomy
    Major oropharyngeal resection
    Carotid endarterectomy
    Anterior spinal fusion
Reduced Consciousness
  Alcohol or sedative drug overdose
  Head injury
  General anesthesia
Gastrointestinal Disease
  Zenker's diverticulum
  Esophageal neoplasm
Neurologic and Neuromuscular Disease
  Cerebrovascular accident
  Intracranial tumors
  Amyotrophic lateral sclerosis
  Parkinson's disease
  Myasthenia gravis
  Polymyositis/dermatomyositis
  Guillain-Barré syndrome
  Dystonia/tardive dyskinesia
  Vocal fold paralysis
  Progressive muscular dystrophy
  Meningitis

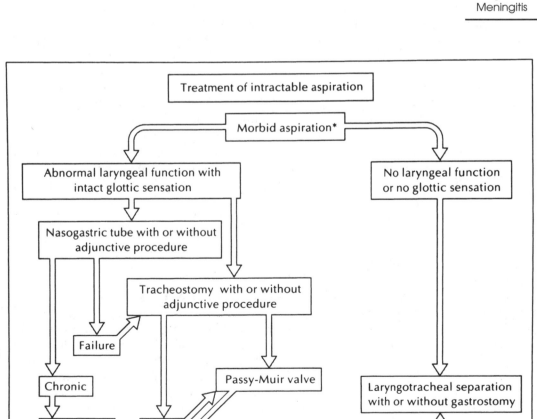

© 1994 *Curr Opin Otolaryngol Head Neck Surg*

FIG 45-2. Schematic for treatment of patients with intractable aspiration. Asterisk indicates recurrent pneumonitis or hypoxia. *Note:* From *Current Opinion in Head and Neck Surgery*, 1994; 2; Fig. 2. Reprinted with permission.

Whenever possible, laryngotracheal separation should be considered early in the management of patients with severe aspiration. It is more difficult to perform the surgery after a tracheotomy has been performed. Therefore, one should always consider laryngotracheal separation when a tracheotomy is being considered. If the need for laryngotracheal separation is unclear or if the patient is not receptive, the tracheotomy may need to be performed first. If so, the tracheotomy should be performed at a low enough level (3rd or 4th interspace) to facilitate laryngotracheal separation, if aspiration persists.

The decision to perform laryngotracheal separation is dependent on multiple factors, including medical morbidity associated with aspiration, associated medical conditions, prognosis for recovery, such social factors as level of nursing care and independence, and patient and family expectations and acceptance. If properly selected, most patients requiring laryngotracheal separation will have already lost the ability to communicate using their voice.[8] In addition to preventing aspiration and its sequelae, a frequent goal of laryngotracheal separation is the restoration of an oral diet. For many patients, the pleasure of eating outweighs the importance of minimal vocal communication. Although laryngotracheal separation may prevent aspiration, it may not allow resumption of an oral diet, depending on a patient's underlying condition and degree of swallowing dysfunction. Laryngotracheal separation also greatly simplifies the nursing care of patients with severe aspiration. In some cases, this may allow the transfer of a patient from an intensive care unit to a lesser skilled nursing facility. The care of a permanent stoma is also easier for the patient than maintaining a tracheostomy tube.

III. PREOPERATIVE ASSESSMENT

Important points to consider regarding the history of the patient's aspiration include etiology, duration, frequency, pulmonary morbidity, and prior treatment. The functioning level of the patient should be ascertained, with particular attention paid to communication abilities and deglutition. In a patient with minimal vocal communication, the relative importance of residual vocalization and resumption of an oral diet should be specifically addressed. Some consideration should be given to social support and the level of nursing care required and available.

The physical examination should include a complete assessment of the upper aerodigestive tract. Fiberoptic examination of the larynx at the bedside allows an assessment of structure and function. Pooling of secretions in the hypopharynx and the absence of a cough reflex are strong indicators of severe aspiration. The function of other cranial nerves, in particular VII, IX, X, and

XII, is also important. Patients with multiple lower cranial nerve deficits are more likely to have severe aspiration requiring surgical intervention. Swallowing function may also be impaired by prior surgery of the oral cavity, pharynx, or larynx for head and neck cancer. The anatomy of the neck should be assessed for factors that may make the surgery more difficult, including the level of the cricoid cartilage, obesity, kyphosis, or thyroid enlargement. If a tracheostomy is present, the level of the tracheotomy should be noted, as this may preclude closure of the subglottic trachea.

Although the degree of aspiration may be confirmed with a barium esophagram or scintigraphic techniques, they are usually not necessary to confirm a diagnosis. A modified barium swallow (MBS), however, may be helpful in selecting food consistencies or compensatory swallowing maneuvers designed to decrease the risk of aspiration. The chest X ray may demonstrate pneumonitis or pneumonia associated with aspiration.

Some consideration should be given to the nutritional status of the patient. If oral intake has been limited because of aspiration, a gastrostomy should be considered. In the presence of severe malnutrition, providing adequate nutritional supplementation preoperatively may avert postoperative problems with wound healing.

Preoperative informed consent includes a discussion of treatment alternatives, risks of the procedure, and expected limitations and benefits. Alternatives to laryngotracheal separation include a tracheotomy, laryngeal stent, or laryngectomy. The risks of the procedure include the risks of anesthesia as well as the risks of the surgical technique. Potential surgical complications are similar to a tracheotomy. In the event that a tracheocutaneous fistula develops, it may be necessary to perform a secondary surgery to repair the fistula. Although the reversibility of laryngotracheal separation has been successfully demonstrated, the potential difficulties in reversing the procedure should be discussed. It should also be stressed that the surgery will not correct any underlying swallowing disorders and resumption of an oral diet may not be possible.

IV. SURGICAL TECHNIQUE

Laryngotracheal separation may be performed under local anesthesia if necessary. This may be an important consideration in patients with serious comorbidities. If general anesthesia is used, oral endotracheal intubation is performed if the patient does not have a tracheostomy. Otherwise, an endotracheal or anode tube may be inserted through the tracheotomy site. Perioperative antibiotic prophylaxis is administered and continued for 24 hours postoperatively.

The patient is positioned on the operating table with the neck hyperextended. In patients without a prior tracheotomy, a transverse neck incision is made equidistant between the cricoid cartilage and the suprasternal notch. Laterally, the incision extends over the sternocleidomastoid muscles. Skin flaps are elevated superficial to the strap muscles and the strap muscles are retracted laterally. The thyroid isthmus is divided and ligated. The pretracheal fascia is incised and the tracheal rings are identified. Dissection is performed on the lateral surfaces of the trachea to mobilize the cervical trachea. By maintaining a plane of dissection on the wall of the trachea, injury to the recurrent laryngeal nerves (RLN) is avoided. Identification of the nerves is not necessary. In patients with a prior tracheotomy, the tracheotomy site is incorporated into the neck incision. An ellipse of skin is incised around the tracheostomy site and the tract is excised to the level of the tracheal wall.

The trachea is preferably transected at the 3rd or 4th interspace. If a tracheotomy is present, the trachea is transected at the level of the tracheotomy. The cut is not beveled across tracheal rings, but stays in the interspace. Care is taken to avoid injury to the esophagus posteriorly. At this point, it is helpful to replace the oral endotracheal tube with one in the distal trachea. The proximal and distal ends of the trachea are mobilized for several centimeters, maintaining a plane of dissection on the surface of the trachea to avoid injury to the RLN. The inferior edge of the distal trachea is secured to the margin of the skin flap with a 2-0 chromic suture.

The last cartilage ring of the proximal trachea is dissected free, preserving the underlying mucosa (Fig 45-3). This is best accomplished with sharp dissection scissors or a Cottle elevator. The next proximal cartilage ring is transected in the midline without violating the underlying mucosa (Fig 45-4). The mucosa of the proximal trachea is then closed in an inverting fashion with a 4-0 polyglycolic acid suture (Fig 45-5). The tracheal stump is oversewn with a 3-0 polyglycolic acid suture (Fig 45-6). This suture collapses the transected tracheal ring and prevents tension on the mucosal closure. A

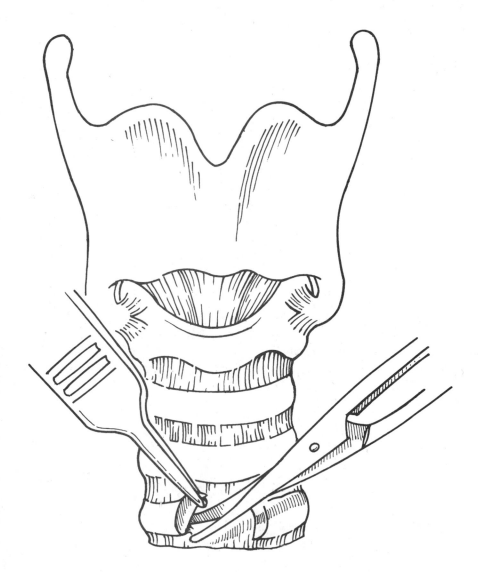

FIG 45-3. After the trachea is transected, the last tracheal ring is dissected from the underlying mucosa with preservation of the mucosa for closure. *Note:* From Eibling D, Laryngeal Separation. In Myers E, ed. *Operative Otolaryngology—Head and Neck Surgery.* Philadelphia: WB Saunders; 1987:Fig 61-4. Reprinted with permission.

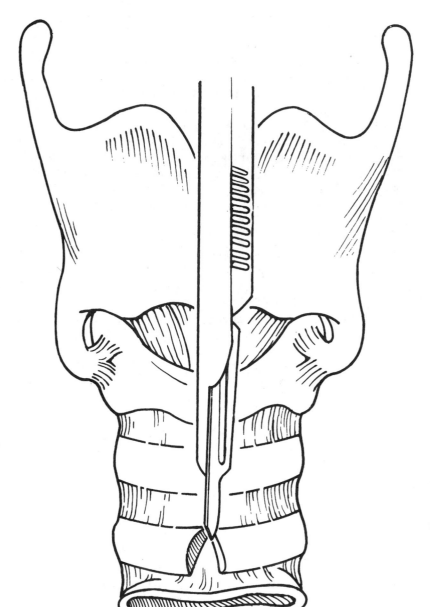

FIG 45-4. The next proximal tracheal ring is transected in the midline without violating the underlying mucosa. This allows collapse of the tracheal lumen to relieve tension on the mucosal closure. *Note:* From Eibling D, Laryngeal Separation. In Myers E, ed. *Operative Otolaryngology—Head and Neck Surgery.* Philadelphia: WB Saunders; 1987: Fig 61-5A. Reprinted with permission.

nonsuction drain is inserted and the permanent stoma is constructed with 2-0 chromic sutures. It is important to splay the cartilage rings laterally to prevent postoperative stenosis of the stoma. The skin flaps are approximated and a pressure dressing is applied.

A cuffed tracheostomy tube is used for several days to prevent aspiration of wound drainage. The drain is removed after 24-48 hours. An oral diet may be resumed on the first postoperative day in most cases, although some surgeons prefer to wait 3-5 days.

V. PITFALLS AND COMPLICATIONS

Complications have been infrequent with this procedure.[8] Patients requiring laryngotracheal separation may be at increased risk for medical complications as a result of underlying medical problems. For example, patients with ALS may have poor ventilatory function due to weakness of respiratory muscles and be susceptible to postoperative hypoventilation and pneumonia. General anesthesia may be contraindicated in such patients.

The most common wound-healing problem is a fistula from the proximal tracheal stump. Tension on the mucosal closure is the most likely precipitating factor. This can be avoided by collapsing and oversewing the proximal tracheal ring. Although local muscle flaps have been used to reinforce the closure, they do not appear to be effective in preventing fistula formation in the presence of a tenuous closure. Most fistulas can be managed conservatively with drainage of the wound,

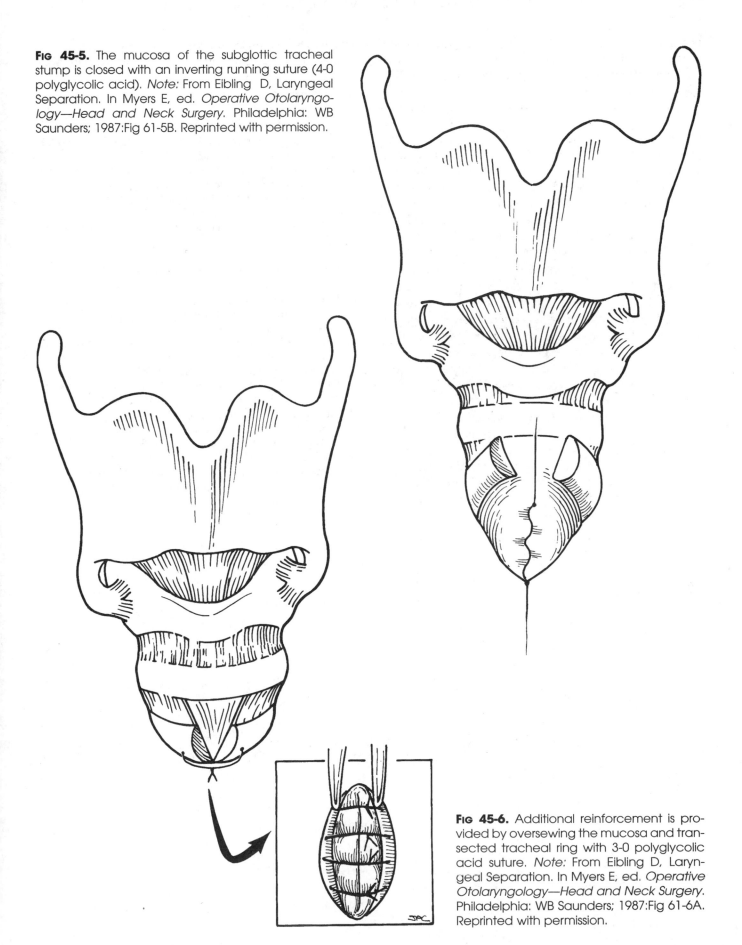

FIG 45-5. The mucosa of the subglottic tracheal stump is closed with an inverting running suture (4-0 polyglycolic acid). *Note:* From Eibling D, Laryngeal Separation. In Myers E, ed. *Operative Otolaryngology—Head and Neck Surgery.* Philadelphia: WB Saunders; 1987:Fig 61-5B. Reprinted with permission.

FIG 45-6. Additional reinforcement is provided by oversewing the mucosa and transected tracheal ring with 3-0 polyglycolic acid suture. *Note:* From Eibling D, Laryngeal Separation. In Myers E, ed. *Operative Otolaryngology—Head and Neck Surgery.* Philadelphia: WB Saunders; 1987:Fig 61-6A. Reprinted with permission.

pressure dressings, and antibiotics. The nutritional status of the patient may be an important consideration in the prevention of wound-healing problems, as well as the successful management of a complication. If the patient had a prior high tracheostomy, there may be insufficient mucosa to close the proximal trachea without tension. Options include a narrow field laryngectomy, a glottic or supraglottic closure procedure, or a subperichondrial cricoidectomy.[9,10] Subperichondrial cricoidectomy should be considered an irreversible procedure.

Because the larynx is intact, there is no excess skin on the superior skin flap and there may be increased tension on the posterior wall of the distal trachea with construction of the permanent stoma. This may result in laceration of the posterior tracheal wall, resulting in breakdown of the wound at this area. This problem can be avoided by adequate mobilization of the distal trachea.

Although there have been concerns about pooling of secretions in the proximal tracheal pouch, radiographic studies have demonstrated that there is emptying of the pouch when the patient is supine.[7] We have not observed infectious complications related to retained material in the blind pouch.

The outward appearance of a patient is not much different from a standard tracheostomy, leading others to assume that there is connection between the trachea and larynx. This can lead to inappropriate management of the airway, such as placement of an expiratory speaking valve or attempts to intubate the patient through the larynx. The altered anatomy should be clearly explained to other physicians and nurses caring for the patient.

References

1. Dettelbach MA, Gross RD, Mahlmann J, Eibling DE. Effect of the Passy-Muir valve on aspiration in patients with tracheostomy. *Head Neck.* 1995;17:297-302.
2. Eibling DE, Bacon G, Snyderman CH. Surgical management of chronic aspiration. In: *Advances in Otolaryngology Head and Neck Surgery.* Chicago: Mosby-Year Book; 1992: 93-113.
3. Miller FR, Eliachar I. Managing the aspirating patient. *Am J Otolaryngol.* 1994;15:1-17.
4. Weisberger EC. Treatment of intractable aspiration using a laryngeal stent or obturator. *Ann Otol Rhinol Laryngol.* 1991; 100:101-107.
5. Lindeman RC. Diverting the paralyzed larynx: a reversible procedure for intractable aspiration. *Laryngoscope.* 1975;85: 157-180.
6. Lindeman RC, Yarington CT Jr, Sutton D. Clinical experience with the tracheoesophageal anastomosis for intractable aspiration. *Ann Otol Rhinol.* 1976;85:609-612.
7. Baron BC, Dedo HH. Separation of the larynx and trachea for intractable aspiration. *Laryngoscope.* 1980;90:1927-1932.
8. Eibling DE, Snyderman CH, Eibling C. Laryngotracheal separation for intractable aspiration: a retrospective review of 34 patients. *Laryngoscope.* 1995;105:83-85.
9. Eisele DW, Seely DR, Flint PW, Cummings CW. Subperichondrial cricoidectomy: an alternative to laryngectomy for intractable aspiration. *Laryngoscope.* 1995;105: 322-325.

CHAPTER 46

■■■

Gastrostomy

Randy J. Woods, M.D.
Andrew B. Peitzman, M.D.

I. INTRODUCTION

Swallowing disorders requiring surgical treatment to initiate feedings have many etiologies. Frequently, a neurologic basis such as cerebral vascular accident (CVA) or amyotrophic lateral sclerosis (ALS) severely effects deglutition such that adequate nutritional intake is not feasible, because of the risk of aspiration and bronchopneumonia. As many as 30% of patients after a CVA experience dysphagia, with silent aspiration diagnosed by videofluoroscopy in another 40%.[1] Head and neck malignancies and trauma lead to the remaining patients requiring some form of nutritional support.

II. INDICATIONS

Table 46-1 presents the indications for each type of gastrostomy. In patients who are unable to take adequate nutrition by mouth but otherwise have a functioning GI tract, enteral feeding is superior to parenteral feeding. Enteral feeds should begin as soon as the GI tract is functioning. Many options are available for the delivery of an enteral formula to the absorptive surfaces of the intestine. Broken down into three main categories there are: (1) nasoenteric (nasogastric or nasoduodenal), (2) jejunostomy, and (3) gastrostomy. This chapter reviews gastrostomies.

The gastrostomy is thought to be more physiologic, compared to the jejunostomy, especially when bolus feedings are used. Nutrition by a gastric tube can also be administered by continuous feedings. The advantages are that the gastric tube is less likely to become dislodged compared to nasoenteric tubes, with patients tolerating gastric tubes better than nasal tubes. For the patient who is ambulatory, gastric tubes are easily hidden, providing more privacy in public situations. Medications are more easily administered through the larger bore gastrostomy tubes with less clogging. A gastrostomy can be created through a percutaneous endoscopic route (PEG); by surgical placement of a tube, or by creation of a stoma. The PEG has become the procedure of choice as it can be done in an intensive care unit or procedure room under local anesthesia. In general, the PEG takes less time and costs less than laparoscopic-assisted or open gastrostomies.[2]

III. CLASSIFICATION OF GASTROSTOMIES

In much of the literature, the gastrostomy is classified as either permanent or temporary. From an anatomic standpoint, the gastrostomy can be classified as either being lined with serosa (temporary) or being lined by mucosa (permanent). Functionally, choice governs not only the care of the gastrostomy site, but what is required for reversal when no longer needed.

Table 46-1. *Indications for Gastrostomy*

- Functioning gastrointestinal tract
- Unable to take adequate fluids or nutrition by mouth

Percutaneous Endoscopic Gastrostomy

- Ideal for cooperative patients—may be performed under local anesthesia with IV sedation
- Ability to perform gastrostomy mandatory—may not be feasible with some head and neck or esophageal malignancies
- Relative contraindication—degree of morbid obesity

Laparoscopic-Assisted Gastrostomy

- Must be able to perform laparoscopy
- Relative contraindications to laparoscopy:
  - Multiple prior abdominal procedures
  - Prior gastric surgery
  - Obesity
- Ideal for patients unable to undergo endoscopy.

Open Gastrostomy

- Can be performed on almost all patients
- No surgical contraindications

Serosa-lined gastrostomies include PEG, laparoscopic-assisted gastrostomy, and open (Stamm) gastrostomy. They are, in fact, serosa-lined gastrocutaneous fistulas. The lining of the tract is granulation tissue, which will quickly close if the tube is removed. Therefore, if this type of gastric tube is displaced it must be replaced within 4-6 hours, if the tract is to stay open. In a matured serosa-lined fistula (typically older than 2-3 weeks), a foley catheter can be inserted into the stomach if the original gastrostomy tube comes out. If there is any uncertainty about the tube being in the stomach, a contrast study (water soluble contrast) can be conducted by way of the gastric tube to quickly verify the tube's position prior to use for feeding.

The "permanent," or mucosa-lined gastrostomy (Janeway gastrostomy), requires a laparotomy in the operating room and is constructed by creating a tube of stomach that is brought out through the anterior abdominal wall. The mucosa-lined gastrocutaneous fistula, as opposed to the serosa-lined fistula, will not close if the feeding tube is removed. In these gastrostomies, it is not necessary to urgently replace a gastric tube, if it is inadvertently removed. Reversal of a permanent gastrostomy typically requires another laparotomy.

A. Percutaneous Endoscopic Gastrostomy (PEG)

The percutaneous endoscopic gastrostomy tube, which has been thought of as temporary, may actually be used for years and may be in place and functioning until death. Using a flexible fiberoptic gastroscope, a tube gastrostomy is created by way of a percutaneous puncture in the anterior abdominal wall (Fig 46-1).

This may be performed under local anesthesia with IV sedation in the operating room, ICU, or a procedure suite. The PEG does require the ability to pass a scope down to the stomach via the esophagus, which may be difficult in patients with head and neck or esophageal cancer. The laparoscopic-assisted gastrostomy, or open gastrostomy, may be indicated for this patient population. In obese patients, proper position of the PEG tube may be difficult because of a too thick anterior abdominal wall.

B. Laparoscopic-Assisted Gastrostomy

Under general anesthesia, a laparoscope is placed (periumbilical site) and used to direct the placement of four "T" fasteners. These approximate and secure the anterior wall of the stomach to the anterior abdominal wall. In the center of the four "T" fasteners, a tube gastrostomy is placed in a percutaneous fashion (Fig 46-2). The lack of endoscopy in this procedure may make this the ideal procedure for the patient with a nearly obstructing esophageal mass. The requirement of a general anesthetic is a disadvantage.

C. Open Gastrostomy

An open gastrostomy (eg, Stamm) can be created under a general or local anesthesia in an operating room. A laparotomy is performed and under direct vision a tube gastrostomy is created. The anterior stomach wall is sutured to the anterior abdominal wall (Fig 46-3).

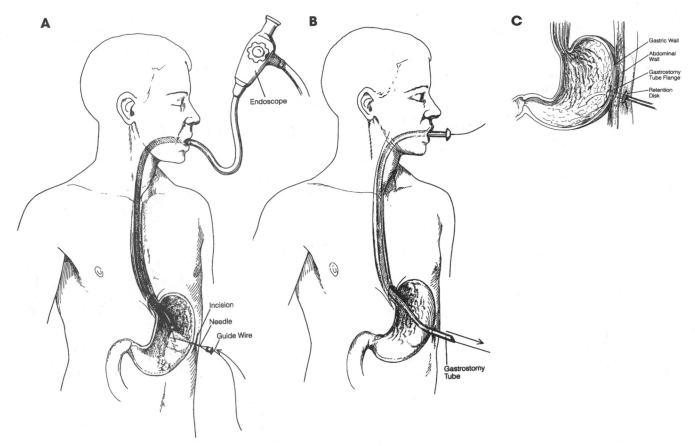

Fɪɢ 46-1. Illustration of percutaneous endoscopic gastrostomy. Under endoscopic visualization, a needle and cannula are placed through the anterior abdominal wall into the stomach. A guide wire is passed through the cannula and retrieved with the endoscope through the oropharynx. After securing the gastrostomy tube to the guide wire, the tube is passed antegrade through the oropharynx, esophagus, and into the stomach and out through the anterior abdominal wall. The endoscope should be reinserted to verify that the flange is in proper position against the gastric wall and not under too much tension. A retention disk or T-bar is used to secure the gastric tube in place. *Note:* From Daly, JM. Malnutrition. In: *American College of Surgeons Care of the Surgical Patient.* New York, NY: Scientific American Inc; 1988-1996: Section VII, Chapter 12, p. 7. Reprinted with permission.

IV. PERIOPERATIVE CARE

Perioperative antibiotics (ie, first generation cephalosporin) for 24 hours are considered adequate prophylaxis. Postoperatively, initiation of feedings via the gastrostomy tube may be initiated within 24 hours in most cases. Beginning with a solution of dextrose 5% (D5W) at 20 cc/hr for 12-24 hrs will allow the gastric residuals to be monitored and reduce the risks associated with emesis. In functional gastric outlet obstruction, a gastric tube fed beyond the pylorus into the duodenum (ie, triple lumen Moss gastrostomy tube) will usually allow feedings to resume. If there is a mechanical obstruction, then surgical revision will be needed.

Gastroesophageal reflux (GER) disease is often considered a contraindication to a gastrostomy and an indication for a jejunostomy. There is not convincing evidence in the literature that a jejunostomy results in less GER disease when compared to a gastrostomy. Medical treatment of GER disease in the dysphagic patient requiring enteral feeds may be successful. Surgical treatment of more severe GER disease with a fundoplication may be required.

The medical utility of placing a feeding gastrostomy is difficult to ascertain in a prospective manner. Reviewing the PEGs placed in a medical environment (head and neck cancer, CVA, and organic neurologic disease), nearly 24% of the patients died during the admission when the PEG was placed; the overall median survival was 7.5 months.[3] In a medical population of only CVA patients, the results were less optimistic with 57% in-hospital mortality and a median survival of 53 days.[4] Consideration must be given to a patient's expected course. If the patient is in the terminal phase of the medical illness, then the purpose of the gastric tube must be questioned. A patient in advanced stages of malignancy and anorexia-cachexia syndrome

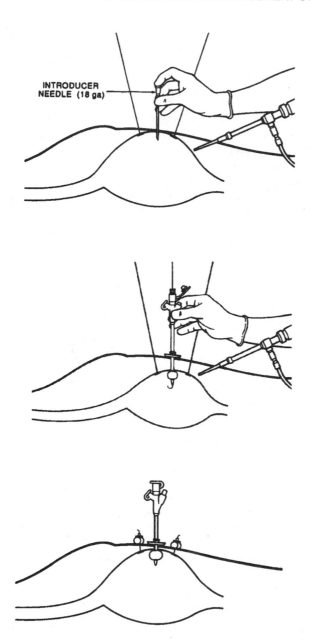

FIG 46-2. The technique of laparoscopic-assisted gastrostomy. Under endoscopic visualization, the anterior abdominal wall of the stomach is fixed to the abdominal wall with four "T" fasteners. A guide wire is placed by way of the introducer needle in the stomach and the tract is enlarged with a dilator. The gastric tube is placed via Seldinger technique under endoscopic visualization. The stomach is secured to the abdominal wall with the "T" fasteners. *Note:* Modified from Duh QY, Way LW. Laparoscopic gastrostomy using T-fasteners as retractors and anchors. *Surg Endosc.* 1993;7:60. Modified with permission.

will not be able to benefit from the nutrition delivered by the planned gastric tube, because of the change in the metabolism that is refractory to nutritional support. If the goal is nutritional support, then this proce-

dure would be contraindicated secondary to its medical futility. However, if the gastric tube is intended to supply the patient with medications to ease and comfort the patient during the remaining days, substantial benefit may be achieved.

V. COMPLICATIONS

The most common complication is the wound or exit site infection (Table 46-2). Often the surrounding skin will be escoriated from leaking gastric contents, without evidence of cellulitis. This can be treated by first stopping the leaking of gastric contents onto the skin. At times the gastric tube balloon will have separated from the stomach wall and need to be pulled up and secured to the anterior abdominal wall. If leakage persists in a matured gastrostomy (older than 3 weeks), the gastric tube can be removed and a slightly larger diameter foley catheter inserted. By filling the balloon with only 5-10 cc of water, there will be less risk of inadvertently obstructing the pylorus. The escoriated skin can be treated with any of the many enterostomal skin barriers or even a thin layer of antacid dried with a hairdryer set on mild heat.

A true cellulitis (erythema, induration, tenderness, and warmth) requires a course of antibiotics. A first generation cephalosporin or a fluoroquinolone will cover the gram-positive cocci typically resulting in the cellulitis. Abscess is infrequent, but requires adequate surgical drainage and possible revision of the gastric tube site to another location.

Diarrhea is not infrequent after initiation of enteral feeds. Any change in formula or increase in the tube feed rate can instigate loose stools. Changing the tube feed formula, decreasing the rate, or adding fiber (ie, Metamucil) to the feeds may be helpful. A change from bolus feeds to continuous may also be beneficial.

It is not uncommon for needle catheter feeding jejunostomies, PEGs, or even the larger bore Stamm gastrostomy tubes to become clogged. The smaller diameter of the needle catheter feeding jejunostomy will last longer if the tube feeding formula is limited to the elemental form. This will increase the cost of the enteral feeds in a patient who could usually tolerate the nonelemental formula. The larger PEG and open gastrostomy tubes can become clogged if medications are given through the tube or when routine flushes are omitted. An active enteral feeding nutrition service has been shown to reduce the number of readmissions or unnecessary emergency room visits secondary to tube blockage.[5]

Gastrostomy tube extrusion through the anterior abdominal wall occurs from too much tension being placed on the gastric tube. Typically this occurs when a PEG tube is found leaking and it is tightened to pre-

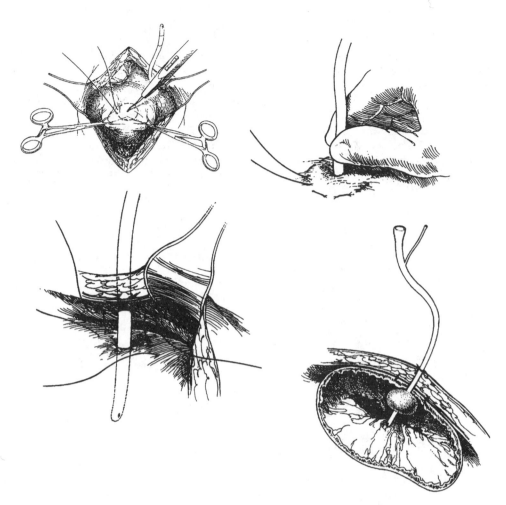

FIG 46-3. Creation of open gastrostomy. Through an upper midline abdominal incision, the stomach is grasped with two Babcock clamps. Through a separate incision in the left upper quadrant over the body of the stomach, the gastric tube is brought through the anterior abdominal wall. Two purse-string sutures of 2-0 silk are placed in the anterior wall of the stomach. Using electric cautery, the stomach is entered and the catheter is placed and secured with the purse-string sutures. The anterior wall of the stomach is secured to the parietal peritoneum with silk sutures. The gastric balloon is inflated and pulled up against the anterior abdominal wall. A stitch is used to secure the catheter to the skin. *Note:* Modified from Economou SG, *Atlas of surgical techniques*. Philadelphia, Pa: WB Saunders; 1996:245. Modified with permission.

Table 46-2. *Complications of Gastrostomy*

- Excoriated skin around gastrostomy site
- Cellulitis around gastrostomy site
- Abscess at gastrostomy site—rare
- Catheter clogging
- Gastrostomy tube extrusion

vent further leakage. This can result in ischemia and necrosis of the anterior wall of the stomach and necrosis of the fascia of the abdominal wall. Care must be taken to prevent excessive force being placed on the gastric tube. If the gastrostomy site continues to leak

after ensuring the flange of the PEG tube is seated against the stomach, then consideration should be given in a mature PEG to change the tube to a larger diameter foley catheter.

Complications can be significant, especially in severely debilitated patients. Mortality directly related to the placement of a gastric tube is between 0.4% to 2%.[3,5] However, the 30- and 90-day mortality for patients following a gastrostomy is 8% and 31%, respectively.[6] The long-term mortality is related to the underlying condition and disease process. Many elderly patients will be severely malnourished prior to being referred for gastrostomy. This, along with their underlying chronic disease, appears to predispose them to a poor outcome.

References

1. Raha SK, Woodhouse K. The use of percutaneous endoscopic gastrostomy (PEG) in 161 consecutive elderly patients. *Age Aging.* 1994:162-163.
2. Norton B, Homer-Ward M, Donnelly MT, Long RG, Holmes GK. A randomised prospective comparison of percutaneous endoscopic gastrostomy and nasogastric tube feeding after acute dysphagic stroke. *BMJ.* 1996;312:13-16.
3. Lazarus BA, Murphy JB, Culpepper L. Aspiration associated with long-term gastric versus jejunal feeding: a critical analysis of the literature. *Arch Phys Med Rehabil.* 1990; 71:46-53.
4. Jones M, Santanello SA, Falcone RE. Percutaneous endoscopic versus surgical gastrostomy. *J Parenter Enterol Nutr.* 1990;14:533-534.
5. Rabeneck L, Wray NP, Petersen NJ. Long-term outcomes of patients receiving percutaneous endoscopic gastrostomy tubes. *J Gen Intern Med.* 1996;11:287-293.
6. Hull MA, Rawlings J, Murray FE, et al. Audit of outcome of long-term enteral nutrition by percutaneous endoscopic gastrostomy. *Lancet.* 1993;341:869-872.

CHAPTER 47

■ ■ ■

Zenker's Diverticulectomy

Erica R. Thaler, M.D.
David E. Eibling, M.D.
Andrew N. Goldberg, M.D.

I. INTRODUCTION

Dysphagia is occasionally encountered in patients in association with a diverticulum of the hypopharynx immediately superior to the upper esophageal sphincter. This diverticulum, termed "Zenker's diverticulum," is a pulsion diverticulum that forms above the cricopharyngeal sphincter muscle through an area of lesser muscle strength termed "Killian's triangle." The diverticulum is created by failure of the upper esophageal sphincter to open before the peristaltic wave and by failure of active opening of the cricopharyngeal muscle through weakness of the laryngeal elevators. This chapter reviews surgical management of Zenker's diverticulum.

II. HISTORICAL PERSPECTIVE

Although there are earlier descriptions of the diverticulum, Zenker's work in 1877 was seminal in defining the anatomy and pathophysiology of its development.[1] Treatment of Zenker's diverticulum has been purely surgical and has evolved over the course of this century from more to less invasive procedures. The first successful reports of resection of the diverticula were in the late 19th century. Although diverticulopexy was also described in that era, diverticulectomy was the favored technique for the first half of the 20th century. Debate centered on whether to perform the operation in one or two stages, the latter having been developed to avoid uncontrolled pharyngocutaneous fistulae and infectious complications. Cricopharyngeal myotomy was introduced as an accompaniment to diverticulotomy by Harrison in 1958.[2] Diverticulopexy has resurfaced in more modern times, with some improvement in morbidity and mortality over diverticulectomy while maintaining efficacy.[3]

Endoscopic management in which the cricopharyngeal muscle is divided and the pharyngeal pouch is marsupialized into the pharynx was first introduced by Dohlman in 1960. He designed a specific endoscope and used diathermy electrosurgical technique to divide the party wall, including the cricopharyngeal sphincter, and create a single cavity.[4] Recent refinements include the use of a laser rather than diathermy,[5] and the use of endoscopic intestinal stapling devices that effectively seal the mucosal edges and prevent salivary leakage.[6]

III. SURGICAL INDICATIONS

As surgery is the only therapeutic option for Zenker's diverticulum, the decision to operate is driven by the degree of the patient's symptoms. Typical symptoms include: regurgitation of partially digested food, potentially foul smelling and resulting in halitosis; dysphagia; coughing and choking on swallowing; inanition and weight loss; esophageal obstruction; and recurrent aspiration pneumonia (Table·47–1). All of these symptoms represent potential indications for surgery, although clearly the severity of the symptoms drives the urgency of the procedure. It should be noted that size of the diverticulum is not related to the severity of symptoms.

Absolute contraindications to surgery include inability to tolerate general anesthesia (a significant consideration in the elderly population in which Zenker's diverticula are found) and carcinoma of the esophagus (which has been rarely reported within the actual diverticular pouch). The presence of untreated severe gastroesophageal reflux (GER) disease is a relative contraindication, as continued reflux may result in stricture formation and inhibit successful healing (Table 47–1), and a cricopharyngeal myotomy may facilitate GER.

IV. PREOPERATIVE ASSESSMENT

A careful history and barium swallow esophagogram are the fundamental diagnostic means for Zenker's diverticulum. A thorough head and neck examination is also necessary, including indirect examination of the hypopharynx and larynx, either with a mirror or preferably with a flexible fiberoptic endoscope. The results of this examination are often entirely within normal limits; however, it is important to document the findings of the hypopharynx and larynx preoperatively. If flexible endoscopy is performed with test feedings, one may occasionally visualize regurgitation of material back into the hypopharynx within seconds after it has passed through the pharynx.

A patient's complaints of dysphagia, regurgitation, halitosis, and repeated aspiration pneumonia all should trigger the physician to order a barium swallow. (Fig 47-1) The barium swallow should be both static and fluoroscopic to best visualize the diverticulum. The presence of GER disease also may be identified on this study. It is important to have a good examination of the esophagus distal to the diverticulum, so that any additional pathology that may contribute to a patient's complaints is identified prior to surgery.

An evaluation for the presence of GER disease is important before surgery as well. The gold standard for this diagnosis is a 24-hour pH probe, with both gastroesophageal and cervical pH probes. It is not critical that this examination be performed prior to surgery and, indeed, it may be technically difficult. But, if there is a significant esophageal stenosis at the mouth of the diverticulum, it is important to obtain a thorough history regarding reflux symptoms and to start antireflux therapy if the patient is not already on it. Proton-pump inhibitors are the medications of choice.

V. SURGICAL TECHNIQUE

A discussion of the surgical technique of repairing Zenker's diverticula is best divided into external and internal approaches. However, generally speaking, all patients must have a thorough endoscopic examination of the Zenker's pouch, plus cervical and, where possible, distal esophagus. This is typically performed at the same time as the definitive repair and is done with a rigid esophagoscope. Often there is significant debris present in the Zenker's pouch, which must be suctioned clear to examine its walls.

A. External Approaches

External approaches to Zenker's diverticula have been used with considerable success since the beginning of the 20th century. Diverticulectomy and diverticulopexy are both widely performed today. Diverticulectomy is performed as follows. After endoscopic examination

Table 47-1. *Surgical Indications and Contraindications*

Indications	Contraindications
Coughing and choking on swallowing	Inability to withstand general anesthesia
Recurrent aspiration pneumonia	Carcinoma of the esophagus
Regurgitation/halitosis	Untreated severe GER disease (relative)
Inanition/weight loss	
Dysphagia	
Esophageal obstruction	

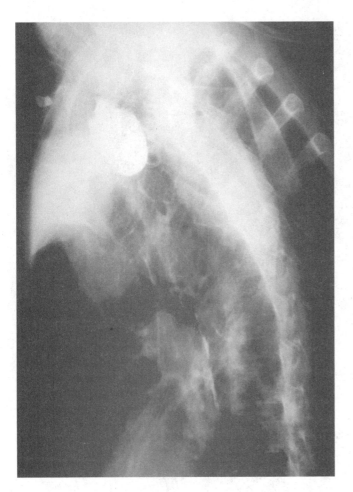

FIG 47-1. Barium swallow demonstrating a large Zenker's diverticulum.

has been performed, a nasogastric tube or esophageal bougie is passed into the cervical esophagus to facilitate transcervical identification. The diverticulum can be packed with gauze to further facilitate localization when the diverticulum is small. The approach is via a horizontal incision in the left neck, with subplatysmal skin flaps elevated superiorly to the level of the thyroid notch and inferiorly to the level of the clavicle. The sternocleidomastoid muscle and carotid sheath are identified and retracted laterally. The larynx, with overlying thyroid and strap muscles, is retracted medially.

The Zenker's diverticulum is in this location and may then be dissected free of surrounding structures (Fig 47-2). Palpation of a nasogastric tube or bougie will facilitate this portion of the procedure. If the diverticulum is not immediately identified, dissection through several layers of fascia overlying the posterior lateral aspect of the esophagus will frequently reveal its presence. Palpation of the cricoid cartilage will facilitate the identification of its superior aspect. Although the recurrent laryngeal nerve (RLN) is somewhat protected by the overlying thyroid gland, care must be taken to avoid injury through overzealous dissection in the area or by the pressure of a retractor. Once the diverticulum has been dissected to its mouth, it is clamped and the sac is excised. The mucosa is inverted and closed with 3-0 vicryl suture. Alternatively, an intestinal stapling device may be used to divide the sac and staple close the mucosa in one maneuver.

Diverticulopexy was developed to avoid the risks inherent in making an esophagotomy. The sac is dissected as just described, but instead of being excised, its fundus is inverted and sewn to the prevertebral fascia. A third external approach involves diverticular inversion into the esophagus, with imbrication of the overlying soft tissues to maintain the inversion.[7]

Cricopharyngeal myotomy is performed in conjunction with external approaches, typically prior to the removal, pexy, or imbrication of the diverticulum. The muscle fibers surrounding the esophagus are transected with a 15 blade knife for a distance of approximately 4 cm to ensure an adequate myotomy, using the cricoid cartilage as the anatomic landmark for the cricopharyngeus muscle. This is done down to the level of mucosa.

B. Endoscopic Approaches

Endoscopic approaches for the management of Zenker's diverticula have been performed successfully for the last 40 years. All such approaches require use of a bivalved endoscope, one blade of which is passed into the cervical esophagus and the other into the diverticular pouch (Fig 47-3). This is suspended either off a surgical stand or the patient's chest. The operating microscope facilitates examination of the pouch and esophagus.

The mucosa and muscle that make up the party wall between the diverticular pouch and the esophagus are then divided. This may be done with electrocautery or laser (typically CO_2, as it is readily available and can be easily managed with a micromanipulator). Recently, good results have been reported with the use of an endoscopic stapling device, which not only divides the party wall, but also provides several rows of staples on either side of the cut and a row of staples at the distal end of the incision.[6] This technique requires the use of a rigid lighted endoscope for visualization in addition to use of the suspension bivalved scope, as the width of the stapling device obstructs the surgeon's view.

C. Choice of Technique

There is little literature comparing the different techniques to address Zenker's diverticula. Laccourreye

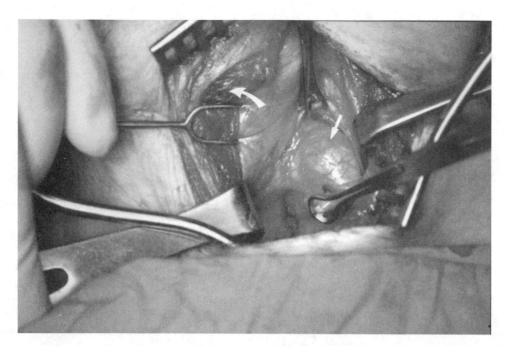

FIG 47-2. External approach through a transverse left neck incision to the Zenker's pouch (*small arrow*). A double hook around the left thyroid ala rotates the larynx to the right for improved exposure (*curved arrow*).

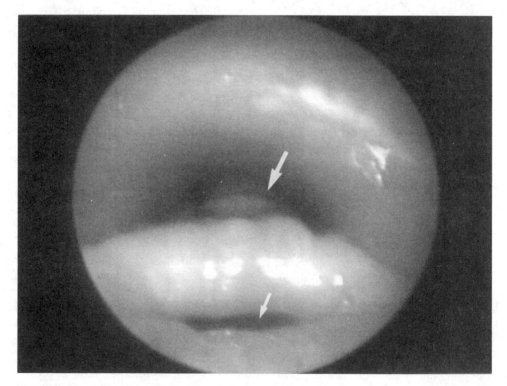

FIG 47-3. Endoscopic view of the esophagus (*large arrow*) and Zenker's diverticulum (*small arrow*).

and colleagues reported equal incidence of duration of surgery and complications in comparing diverticulectomy and diverticulotomy. Significant improvement was made in duration of nasogastric feeding and shortened length of hospital stay if diverticulopexy was performed.[3] Bonafede et al reported no statistically significant difference in complication rate when comparing diverticulopexy and diverticulectomy with and without cricopharyngeal myotomy. Myotomy alone, however, was associated with a worse outcome.[8] Wouters and Overbeek reported a large series of endoscopically repaired diverticula, finding a 92% highly satisfactory outcome with less than 0.2% mortality and an acceptably low complication rate.[9]

It is therefore prudent to select a technique with which the surgeon has experience, for which there are available resources, and that the patient can tolerate. For the elderly, debilitated patient, a shorter, less invasive procedure is preferable. In such a situation, an endoscopic technique is the method of choice.

V. PITFALLS AND COMPLICATIONS

All surgical approaches for Zenker's diverticula repair carry the risk of infection from leakage of esophageal contents into surrounding soft tissues, either from inadequate closure of an excision or from inadvertent disruption of the mucosa. This may result in esophagocutaneous fistula, neck abscess, and even mediastinitis (Table 47–2). It is best avoided by meticulous closure of any identified opening made into the esophagus. Treatment includes prompt drainage, appropriate intravenous antibiotic therapy, and no oral feeding until the mucosal break has healed.

Recurrent laryngeal nerve injury is a potential risk of all approaches, though considerably less of a risk by endoscopic means. If using the external approach, care should be taken to avoid the tracheoesophageal sulcus. Minimizing clamping and cautery of tissue in this area is also prudent. If an injury occurs, a standard allowance of 6 to 12 months is allotted for return of vocal fold mobility before definitive treatment is undertaken. Temporary measures, such as Gelfoam injection, may be appropriate. Medialization procedures for the paralyzed vocal fold are discussed in Chapters 41 and 42.

Esophageal stricture may occur from overzealous resection of a diverticular pouch. This is best avoided by careful dissection of the pouch at the initial procedure. Use of a large esophageal bougie will

Table 47-2. *Pitfalls and Complications*

Pharyngocutaneous fistula
Neck abscess
Mediastinitis
Recurrent laryngeal nerve injury
Hypopharyngeal stricture

help prevent overresection. Postoperative strictures may be treated with periodic esophageal dilation.

References

1. Zenker FA, von Ziemssen H. Krankheiten des Oesophagus. In: von Ziemssen H, ed. *Handbuch des Speziellen Pathologie und Therapie*, vol 7 (suppl). Leipzig: FC Vogel; 1877:1-87.
2. Harrison M. The etiology, diagnosis and surgical treatment of pharyngeal diverticula. *J Laryngol Otol.* 1958;72:523-534.
3. Laccourreye O, Menard M, Cauchois R, et al. Esophageal diverticulum: diverticulopexy versus diverticulectomy. *Laryngoscope.* 1994;104:889-892.
4. Dohlman G, Mattson O. The endoscopic operation for hypopharyngeal diverticula. *Arch Otolaryngol.* 1960;71:744-752.
5. Overbeek J. Upper esophageal sphincterotomy in dysphagic patients with and without a diverticulum. *Dysphagia.* 1991;6:228-234.
6. Scher R, Richtsmeier W. Endoscopic staple-assisted esophagodiverticulostomy for Zenker's diverticulum. *Laryngoscope.* 1996;106:951-956.
7. Johnson J, Weissman J. Diverticular imbrication and myotomy for Zenker's. *Laryngoscope.* 1992;102:1377-1378.
8. Bonafede J, Laverty P, Wood B, Eliachar I. Surgical outcome in 87 patients with Zenker's diverticulum. *Laryngoscope.* 1997;107:720-725.
9. Wouters B, Overbeek J. Endoscopic treatment of the hypopharyngeal (Zenker's) diverticulum. *Hepato-gastroenterology.* 1992;39:105-108.

CHAPTER 48

■ ■ ■

Esophagectomy for Swallowing Disorders

Richard Maley, M.D.
James D. Luketich, M.D.

I. HISTORICAL PERSPECTIVE

The first successful report of esophagectomy is attributed to Czerny, who in 1877 described the excision of a carcinoma of the cervical esophagus.[1] The patient survived for 1 year being nourished via a distal cervical esophagostomy. The first successful intrathoracic esophagectomy was reported in 1911, but, again, intestinal continuity was not reestablished and a cervical esophagostomy and gastrostomy were connected by an extrapleural rubber tube for feeding.[2] Attempts at reestablishing intestinal continuity were unsuccessful until Turner described a successful pull-through operation in 1931,[3] an approach that was later popularized in the United States by Orringer and Sloan[4] In 1946, Lewis introduced a two-stage, combined laparotomy and right thoracotomy for resection of midesophageal cancer that has since been popularized as a single-stage procedure.[5] More recently, minimally invasive approaches to esophagectomy have been successfully performed.[6,7]

In the past, squamous cell carcinoma of the midesophagus has been the most common histology and site of esophageal cancer. However, the National Institutes of Health has reported the incidence of adenocarcinoma of the lower one third of the esophagus is increasing at an alarming rate in the United States.[8] In large institutions, surgical resection of the esophagus can now be performed with a mortality rate of less than 5% and minimal morbidity. However in less experienced hands, the mortality can soar to 20% with major morbidity.[9]

II. SURGICAL INDICATIONS

The most common indication for esophagectomy for the treatment of a patient with a swallowing disorder is carcinoma. In the case of carcinoma, esophagectomy can be done with curative intent or for the palliation of dysphagia. In our experience, esophagectomy is rarely indicated for palliation of dysphagia, as excellent palliation can be obtained with flexible expandable metal stents or with photodynamic therapy or a combination of these treatments [10] (see Chapter 54). Esophagectomy for carcinoma most often consists of a near-total esophagectomy, which is often required to obtain negative margins because of the propensity for spread along the submucosal lymphatics. The results of surgical resection alone for cure approach a 5-year survival of only 20%-30%, depending on the stage of disease. Although in the less common situation of early stage disease (I or II), cure by esophagectomy alone can approach 90%.[11]

For low risk patients who present with dysphagia and advanced stage esophageal cancer, we recommend minimally invasive staging to allow us to better evaluate a new neoadjuvant protocol, which includes Taxol, plantinum, and 5-FU.[7,12,13] If minimally invasive staging and endoscopic ultrasound reveal a T1 or T2N0 esophageal cancer, the patient is a potential candidate for thoracoscopic and laparoscopic esophagectomy, depending on the tumor location and body habitus.[6,14]

Other indications for esophagectomy include the sigmoid-shaped megaesophagus found in end-stage achalasia, complicated esophageal perforations associated with sepsis, and a number of other rare conditions such as severe strictures associated with lye ingestion or high-dose radiotherapy that may require esophagectomy, if other interventions fail. Barrett's esophagus is a premalignant condition in which the normal squamous epithelium is replaced by a columnar-lining secondary to chronic reflux of gastric contents into the esophagus. In severe cases, when Barrett's progresses to high-grade dysplasia, esophagectomy is indicated, as between 40% to 70% of cases will already have invasive carcinoma.[15]

III. PREOPERATIVE ASSESSMENT

Preoperative assessment for esophagectomy can be classified into three basic questions: (1) Does the patient have general medical contraindications to a major surgical procedure? (2) Has the stage of esophageal cancer been accurately assessed and the appropriate treatment chosen? This is an important question if one is considering options such as immediate surgical resection, neoadjuvant therapy, or palliative measures such as photodynamic therapy or expandable metal stents. (3) Finally, is the available conduit for reconstruction of the esophagus suitable? In more than 95% of cases, we have found the gastric tube satisfactory for reconstruction. In unusual cases, we use the colon or the jejunum with satisfactory results.

General medical contraindications, such as major cardiac and/or pulmonary compromise that are not reversible, comprise the primary contraindications to esophagectomy. Advanced age can also be a relative contraindication. If staging of the patient reveals a potentially curable tumor, then aggressive approaches to medical conditions should be considered when indicated. For example, if stress testing is positive, then cardiac cath and possible coronary bypass should be considered. If pulmonary compromise is a concern, initial palliation of dysphagia with photodynamic therapy, expandable metal stent, or a feeding tube may allow nutritional repletion while smoking cessation and pulmonary rehabilitation are in progress for 3-6 weeks.

Accurate staging of esophageal cancer before beginning treatment is important. For example, we have found that patients who are staged by conventional imaging (CT scan and bone scan) will have occult metastatic spread in up to 20% of cases when studied by positron emission tomography (PET) and confirmed by minimally invasive biopsies.[16] Others have reported that minimally invasive staging changes the stage of esophageal cancer in up to 40% of cases compared to staging by conventional imaging.[17] Endoscopic ultrasound is an important staging tool to evaluate locoregional involvement. Extension into surrounding structures, such as the aorta or left main stem bronchus (T4 disease), or metastatic disease are relative contraindications to surgical resection.

Our approach is to begin with conventional imaging. Patients with obvious metastatic disease or overwhelming medical conditions are treated with nonsurgical approaches, such as photodynamic therapy or expandable metal stents.[10] Patients then undergo PET scanning to rule out occult distant metastatic disease and endoscopic ultrasound to assess local tumor extension. We then perform laparoscopic and thoracoscopic staging to confirm any PET abnormalities and to accurately assess lymph node status. Using this information, a pretreatment stage is assigned and treatment is instituted based on stage.

IV. SURGICAL TECHNIQUE

The two most commonly employed approaches to esophagectomy include the transhiatal approach and the Ivor Lewis esophagectomy. In 1993, Orringer and colleagues reported a series of transhiatal esophagectomies without thoracotomy in 583 patient; 70% for carcinoma and 30% for benign disease.[18] The overall mortality rate was 5.5%. In a recent series by Mathisen et, a 2.9% mortality and 9% leak rate were reported using the Ivor Lewis approach in 104 patients.[19]

The transhiatal esophagectomy can be used to treat both benign and malignant conditions. One advantage of this procedure is that it avoids thoractomy and, hence, the possible complications of respiratory failure and atelectasis. However, the incidence of pneumonia appears to be similar when compared to the Ivor Lewis esophagectomy. The leak rate is higher when the anastomosis is done in the neck, but the mortality associated with this complication is essentially zero. Late functional results are good and clinically significant reflux symptoms are uncommon. Transhiatal esophagectomy is performed with the patient in the supine position and has three separate phases: abdominal, transhiatal, and cervical. The procedure is concluded with cervical esophagogastric anastomosis. This procedure is most often used for benign disease and tumors involving the lower one third of the esophagus.

The Ivor Lewis esophagectomy is most often used for tumors in the lower one third of the esophagus and at the level of the gastroesophageal junction. The gastric conduit does not need to be as long as for the transhiatal esophagectomy, hence part of the proximal stomach can be resected if needed for negative margins. The leak rate is extremely low, but if it occurs, the mortality is significant. The operation has two phases. The first phase, the abdominal phase, is completed with the patient supine. The second phase, the thoracic phase, is completed with the patient in the full left lateral decubitus position.

Multiple authors have now reported using video-assisted thoracoscopy or laparoscopy to facilitate esophagectomy.[20] Most reports utilized a standard laparotomy with thoracoscopic esophageal mobilization or laparoscopy to facilitate gastric mobilization combined with a minilaparotomy to bluntly complete the esophageal dissection. Clear advantages of thoracoscopic esophageal mobilization over thoracotomy were not demonstrated in these studies. DePaula was the first to report a large series of 48 patients undergoing a total laparoscopic transhiatal esophagectomy.[21] Our initial experience using a total laparoscopic approach was reported in patients with Barrett's esophagus with high-grade dysplasia.[6]

Our approach has evolved to include thoracoscopy as the initial step for thoracic esophageal mobilization. We have now performed minimally invasive esophagectomy in 32 patients primarily for Barrett's esophagus with high-grade dysplasia or early stage adenocarcinomas of the distal esophagus confirmed by the extensive staging described above. If a T1N0 or T2N0 tumor or carcinoma in-situ is discovered, we proceed with thoracoscopic esophageal mobilization, laparoscopic gastric mobilization, and gastric tubularization with gastric pull-up. Thoracoscopy improves our ability to perform a more complete lymph node dissection and more easily complete mobilization of the intrathoracic esophagus. The neck anastomosis is performed in the standard fashion. No access thoracotomy or laparotomy is performed. Using this approach there was no operative mortality and a 10% leak rate from the neck anastomosis was observed. Three conversions were required early in our experience to complete the transhiatal mobilization.

V. PITFALLS AND COMPLICATIONS

Transhiatal esophagectomy without thoracotomy had been shown by Orringer and colleagues to be a safe and effective operation from both benign and malignant disease. In a series of 583 patients reported by Orringer and colleagues in 1993, the overall in hospital mortality was 5%.[18] Of the 27 deaths that occurred, no specific pattern of cause-of-death was obvious, but renal failure and sepsis were the most common etiology (4 cases). The most common intraoperative complication is entry into one or both pleural spaces (75%) requiring one or more chest tubes. Less common intraoperative complications include splenectomy (4%), membranous tracheal laceration (<1%), and major bleeding (<1%). Postoperative complications include bleeding, recurrent laryngeal nerve palsy, cervical leaks, and chylothorax.

One of the key technical points when comparing types of esophagectomy is the location of the esophagogastric anastomosis intrathoracic versus cervical. Intrathoracic anastomosis should have leak rates less then 2%. Large series of esophagectomies with cervical anastomoses, report leak rates of 5% to 15%. However, the mortality from a cervical leak is essentially zero and the mortality from an intrathoracic leak can be as high as 50%.[18,19]

If preoperative staging is inaccurate or incomplete, the rate of exploratory surgery with inability to resect the tumor or incomplete resection will be unacceptably high. This can be avoided by minimally invasive staging, endoscopic ultrasound, and PET. However, these approaches are associated with significant costs and are not universally available and, therefore, the ideal preoperative staging approach is still in evolution.

There are many consideration in how one can avoid the pitfalls and complications of esophageal surgery. We agree with the following observation on complications of esophageal surgery by Clement A. Hiebert "The most critical determinant of morbidity is the surgeon's proficiency based on a personal experience with the operation." Recent clinical reports support this observation that surgical experiences and volume are the most important factors in achieving a low surgical morbidity and mortality.[9]

References

1. Czerny V. Neue Operationen: Vorlauf ist Mittheilung. *Zentrable Chir.* 1877;4:433.
2. Torek F. The first successful case of resection of the thoracic portion of the esophagus for carcinoma. *Surg Gynecol Obstet.* 1913;16:614.
3. Turner GG. Some experiences in the surgery of the esophagus. *N Engl J Med.* 1931;205:657.
4. Orringer MB, Marshall B, Stirling MC. Transhiatal esophagectomy for benign and malignant disease. *J Thoracic Cardiovasc Surg.* 1993;105:265-276.
5. Lewis I. The surgical treatment of carcinoma of the esophagus with special reference to a new operation for growths of the middle third. *Br J Surg.* 1946;34:18.
6. Luketich JD, Nguyen NT, Schauer PR. Laparoscopic transhiatal esophagectomy for Barrett's esophagus with high grade dysplasia. *JSLS.* 1998;2:75-77.
7. Nguyen NT, Schauer PR, Luketich JD. Thoracoscopic and laparoscopic esophagectomy (abstract). *Can J Gastroenterol.* 1996;12(suppl B):9B.
8. Blot WJ, Deresa SS, Kneller RW, et al. Rising incidence of adenocarcinoma of the esophagus and gastric cardia. *JAMA* 1991;265:1287-1289.
9. Patti MG, Corvera CU, Glasgow RE, Way LW. A hospital's annual rate of esophagectomy influences the operative mortality rate. *J Gastrointest Surg.* 1998;2:186-192.
10. Nguyen NT, Veigel TL, Keenan RJ, et al. Photodynamic therapy for obstructing esophagus cancer: a single year experience. *Surg Endosc.* 1998;12:627. (Abstract)
11. Lerut TE, deLeya P, Cousemans W, et al. Advanced esophageal carcinoma. *World J Surg.* 1974;18:379-387.
12. Belani CP, Luketich JD, Landreneau RJ, et al. Efficacy of cisplatin, 5-Fluorouracil, and paclitaxel regimen for carcinoma of the esophagus. *Semin Oncol.* 1997;24(6, suppl 19):519-592.
13. Luketich JD, Schauer PR, Landreneau RL, et al. Minimally invasive staging is superior to endoscopic ultrasound in detecting lymph node metastases in esophageal cancer. *J Thoracic Cardiovasc Surg.* 1997;114:817-823.

14. Luketich JD, Nguyen NT, Weigel Tl, Ferson PF, Keenan RJ, Schauer PR. Minimally invasive approach to esophagectomy. *JSLS*. 1998: accepted for publication.

15. Rice TW, Falk G, Achkar E, Petras RE. Surgical management of high-grade dysplasia in Barrett's esophagus. *Am J Gastroenterol.* 1993;88:1132-1138.

16. Luketich JD, Schauer PR, Meltzer CC, et al. Role of positron emission tomography in the staging of esophageal cancer. *Ann Thorac Surg.* 1997;64:765-769.

17. Krasna MJ, Reed C, Jaklitsch MT, Cushing D. Thoracoscopic staging of esophageal cancer; a prospective multi-institutional trial. *Ann Thorac Surg.* 1995;60:1137-1340.

18. Orringer MB, Sloan H. Esophagectomy without thoracotomy. *J Thorac Cardiovasc Surg.* 1978;76:643-654.

19. Mathisen DJ, Grillo HC, Wilkins EW, Moncure AC, Hilgenberg AD. Transthoracic esophagectomy: a safe approach to carcinoma of the esophagus. *Ann Thorac Surg.* 1998;45:137-143.

20. Luketich JD, Landreneau RJ. Future directions in esophageal cancer. *Chest.* 1997;113;120S-122S.

21. DePaula AL, Hashiba K, Ferreira ERB, et al. Transhiatal approach for esophagectomy. In: Toauli S, Gossot D, Hunter SG, eds. *Endosurgery.* New York, NY: Churchill Livingstone; 1996:293-299.

CHAPTER 49

■ ■ ■

Surgery for Motility Disorders of the Esophagus

James D. Luketich, M.D.

I. HISTORICAL PERSPECTIVE

Primary motor disorders of the esophagus include achalasia, nutcracker esophagus, and diffuse esophageal spasm. Achalasia is the most common disorder and was first described and successfully treated by Thomas Willis in 1679 by dilation with a small whalebone. Balloon dilation was first described in the late 1800s and the first report of surgical management was by Mikulicz in 1904 and included laparotomy and dilation of the cardia. The first report of successful myotomy was by Heller in 1914, with a modification of this having remained the standard of surgical treatment. With the advent of minimally invasive surgery, thoracoscopic and laparoscopic approaches are now well described.[1,2]

II. SURGICAL INDICATIONS

The medical management of achalasia includes a trial of calcium channel blockers, although previous investigations have not consistently shown success. The disease often follows an indolent course, but ultimately progression of symptoms will require intervention in most cases. In less than 5% of cases, progression to squamous cell carcinoma may occur. In the past, it has been widely accepted that pneumatic dilation should be the first line of interventional management for achalasia. Satisfactory results can be seen in up to 67% of patients after a single dilation and up to 75%-80%, if multiple dilations are performed. Surgical esophagomyotomy has been shown to be more effective than pneumatic di-

lation in a prospective study.[3] In the largest series from the Mayo clinic, good to excellent results followed dilation (n = 431) in 65% compared to 85% in the surgical myotomy group (n = 468).[4] Cost and the less invasive nature continue to lead many clinicians to use pneumatic dilation as the first line treatment. In our experience, improvement following botulinum injection is limited.

Minimally invasive surgical techniques are now challenging this dogma. Reports of thoracoscopic and laparoscopic myotomy have shown similar success to open procedures.[1,2] As long-term follow-up and cost analysis data become available, minimally invasive surgical approaches could replace dilation as the first line treatment or at least be employed prior to multiple dilations. Currently, most clinicians consider recurrent symptoms after balloon dilation the most accepted surgical indication. In our practice, patients are given the option of laparoscopic myotomy or balloon dilation as the initial intervention.

III. PERIOPERATIVE ASSESSMENT

A clinical diagnosis of achalasia should be included in the differential diagnosis in patients with significant dysphagia to solids or liquids. We have found the barium swallow to be a good initial diagnostic test to rule out other causes of dysphagia such as malignancy (sometimes referred to as pseudoachalasia). In the classic case, the barium videoesophagram will demonstrate absence of peristalsis, a dilated esophageal body with a distal "bird's beak" narrowing. Manometry is the gold standard diagnostic procedure that characteristically will reveal aperistalsis, failure of LES relaxation with swallowing, and an elevated LES pressure. Aperistalsis of the esophagus is the most important and consistent manometric finding in achalasia.

IV. SURGICAL TECHNIQUE

Esophagomyotomy is the most common surgical procedure performed for achalasia. Although Heller's original operation included an anterior and posterior myotomy, this has been modified and the accepted approach is a single anterior myotomy. The myotomy is performed with a single longitudinal incision to include the outer longitudinal and inner circular muscle layers without entering the mucosa. There continue to be several controversial areas regarding surgery for achalasia, including the surgical approach, the length and distal extent of the myotomy, and whether or not an antireflux procedure should be a routine component of the operation.

The surgical approach most commonly used in the United States has been open thoracotomy with long myotomy; the abdominal approach is more common in Europe. Thoracotomy and long myotomy can be performed via left posterolateral thoracotomy, with the addition of a Belsey partial fundoplication, if an antireflux procedure is desired. We have found that left videothoracoscopy allows good exposure for a long esophageal myotomy and can be followed by a Belsey antireflux procedure.[5] We reserve the thoracoscopic approach when a long myotomy is desired such as for diffuse esophageal spasm or motility disorders associated with an intrathoracic diverticulum. Some authors advocate the thoracoscopic approach for all cases of achalasia.[1]

For routine cases of achalasia, the laparoscopic approach is the most widely reported minimally invasive procedure performed. The initial results are similar to those obtained in open operations. We have found that an 8-cm to 10-cm myotomy can be performed laparoscopically with excellent clinical results. We add a Dor or Toupet partial fundoplication routinely after laparoscopic myotomy and have had no postoperative dysphagia. In end-stage cases with a sigmoid esophagus or failed myotomies, esophagectomy may be required.

V. PITFALLS AND COMPLICATIONS

One of the major pitfalls of medical management is the reluctance to refer for surgical management after multiple failed balloon dilations. In the past, this reluctance was primarily related to the avoidance of a major surgical procedure. Multiple dilations often lead to significant scarring of the esophagus and can make subsequent surgical myotomy difficult, leading to a higher perforation rate. With the advent of minimally invasive procedures, we are hopeful that consideration of a minimally invasive surgical myotomy will avoid the pitfall of multiple failed dilations.

Complications of balloon dilations include acute perforations and, as mentioned, chronic scarring and obscuring of the myotomy surgical plane of dissection. If a perforation is recognized immediately, it is possible that immediate surgical myotomy, repair of the perforation, and partial fundoplication will yield a good result. Delayed perforations and significant local infection may require aggressive surgical debridement and esophagectomy in severe cases. In cases of small, well-drained, and localized perforations, conservative management with intravenous antibiotics and NPO may suffice.

Complications of surgical approaches include perforations of the mucosa during myotomy. If these are recognized, immediate repair and buttressing with a partial wrap is easily accomplished. Incomplete myotomies have been reported as a complication of minimally invasive procedures, but these have generally occurred in the early experience of most reports.

References

1. Arreola-Risa C, Sinanan M, Pellegrini CA. Thoracoscopic Hellers myotomy: treatment of achalasia by the videoendoscopic approach. *Chest Surg Clin N Am.* 1995;5:459-469.
2. Swanstrom LL, Pennings J. Laparoscopic esophagomyotomy for achalasia. *Surg Endos.* 1995;9:286-292.
3. Csendes A, Braghetto I, Henriquez A, Mascaro J. Late results of a prospective, randomized study comparing forceful dilation and esophagomyotomy in patients with achalasia. In: Siewert JR, Holscher AH, eds. *Diseases of the esophagus: pathophysiology, diagnosis, conservative and surgical treatment.* Berlin: Springer Verlag; 1988:957-961
4. Payne WS, King RM. Treatment of achalasia of the esophagus. *Surg Clin North Am.* 1983;63:963-970.
5. Nguyen NT, Schauer PR, Hutson W, et al. Preliminary results of thoracoscopic Belsey Mark IV antireflux procedure. *Surg Laparosc and Endos.* 1998;8:185-188.

CHAPTER 50

∎ ∎ ∎

Nissen Fundoplication

Robert J. Keenan, M.D., F.R.C.S.(C.)
Rodney J. Landreneau, M.D.

I. INTRODUCTION

Gastroesophageal reflux (GER) disease is estimated to affect more than 40 million Americans. This disease is most commonly manifested by intractable heartburn and regurgitation symptoms. Most patients control their symptoms with nonprescription drugs and lifestyle changes; many of the remainder can be helped with prescription drug regimens. For a small but significant fraction of patients, however, surgical methods offer the only effective option for long-term relief.

Surgical reconstruction of the lower esophageal sphincter (LES) has been shown to be an effective means of reversing the esophageal injury that results from reflux of gastric contents. The technical basis of fundoplication is the flap-valve mechanism created by wrapping the fundus of the stomach around the distal esophagus. As the stomach becomes distended during a meal, the fundic wrap compresses the distal esophagus, preventing reflux.

II. HISTORICAL PERSPECTIVE

Rudolph Nissen developed the technique of fundoplication in 1936 and first applied it to patients with GER disease in 1956. The original technique involved enveloping the distal esophagus with the gastric fundus by suture approximation of the fundal folds over the anterior esophagus. This total wrap was constructed over a bougie and extended for 4 to 6 cm. The technique also included an anterior gastropexy, a modification that has been eliminated. Others added modifications such as division of the short gastric vessels, anchoring the wrap to the crura or preaortic fascia, and shortening the length of the wrap to 1-2 cm. The operation is classically performed through a laparotomy incision but can also be performed through a left thoracotomy. Long-term success at achieving good to excellent control of symptoms have been reported,[1] although up to 30% of patients also report symptoms of dysphagia, gas bloat, and an inability to belch.[2]

In 1991, Dallemagne and colleagues [3] first performed a Nissen fundoplication using the laparoscopic approach. The first report from the United States was by Hinder and Filipi in 1992.[4] As experience has grown, laparoscopic fundoplications have become the procedure of choice at most institutions. Long-term follow-up is only now becoming available for comparison of the results of laparoscopy with the traditional open approach.

III. SURGICAL INDICATIONS

The defining indication for surgery is failure of medical therapy (Table 50-1). Failure may take the form of refractory symptomatology such as persistent heartburn, cough, or chest pain or it may relate to the development of complications from reflux disease. These com-

Table 50-1. *Indications for Surgical Therapy for GER Disease*

A. Failure of medical therapy
Incomplete relief of symptoms (including cough, chest pain)
Progression of symptoms
Early relapse after discontinuation of drug therapy

B. Complications of GER disease
Recurrent peptic strictures or ulcerations
Progression of Barrett's esophagitis
Development of dysplastic changes

C. Compliance
Failure to maintain prescribed medical regimen
Inability to pay drug costs
Unwillingness to persist with long-term medical therapy

plications include peptic stricture or ulceration, progression of Barrett's esophagitis, and the development of dysplastic changes within Barrett's mucosa. A lack of compliance with medical regimens or inability to pay for long-term medical therapy are also indications for surgical referral.

Contraindications for surgical reconstruction with a Nissen fundoplication primarily relate to the presence of significant esophageal motor abnormalities. Patients with primary motor disorders such as achalasia, diffuse esophageal spasm, and nutcracker esophagus or secondary motor disorders such as scleroderma, diabetic neuropathy, stroke, amyloidosis, or other motility problems of the esophagus may also have symptomatic reflux. In these situations, performance of a total fundoplication such as the Nissen repair leads to dysphagia, because the poorly peristaltic esophagus is unable to overcome the resistance of the sphincter mechanism. For these individuals, a partial wrap (eg, Dor, Belsey, or Toupet techniques) is indicated. Patients with secondary disorders may also have impairments of gastric emptying that needs to be corrected to avoid a gastric "closed loop." Occasionally patients with severe reflux esophagitis will develop an acquired shortened esophagus. To provide a tension-free repair, a gastroplasty must be added to the fundoplication. Failure to do so often results in breakdown of the repair and recurrence of symptoms.

IV. PREOPERATIVE ASSESSMENT

When patients with defective sphincter mechanisms are accurately identified, the results of surgical correction are usually gratifying. It is vital to confirm that the patient's upper gastroesophageal symptoms are truly related to reflux and that the etiology of the acid reflux comes from a defective lower esophageal sphincter mechanism before surgery is performed. A careful preoperative as-

sessment, including esophageal and gastric endoscopy, esophageal manometry, and 24-hour esophageal pH testing, is vital for proper patient selection.

The three functional variables of the LES that are important in determining its competency are lower sphincter pressure, intra-abdominal LES position, and overall sphincter length. Abnormalities in any one of these is usually related to sphincter deficiency. The method of choice for defining these issues is esophageal manometry (see Chapter 13). This procedure measures the differential pressure between two sensors approximately 5 cm apart on the manometric catheter, and so can be used both to observe lower sphincter pressure and to measure gastroesophageal compartments by mapping changes in pressure as the catheter moves through the gastroesophageal tract.

V. SURGICAL TECHNIQUE

Over the last few years, surgeons have begun to use laparoscopic approaches to repair the lower esophageal sphincter. This minimally invasive technique is similar to the video-assisted surgery usually used to perform laparoscopic cholecystectomy. Surgeons have found the laparoscopic approach to be useful for the majority of patients with uncomplicated, but refractory, GER disease requiring surgical intervention.

The primary advantage of the laparoscopic approach is the potential for reduced operative morbidity, resulting in a quicker hospital recovery and return to normal activities. Although the average hospitalization following open surgical repair is commonly 7 to 10 days, the hospital stay following laparoscopic repair is customarily 1 to 2 days. Furthermore, return to full activity usually occurs 1 to 2 weeks following most laparoscopic antireflux repairs, but often takes 4 to 6 weeks following open surgery .

Laparoscopic Nissen fundoplication requires 4 to 5 individual half-inch incisions for use of endoscopic surgical instruments and the laparoscopic camera system (Fig 50-1). The repair is essentially identical to that performed in open surgery. An initial 10-mm port is inserted to the left of midline, midway between the xiphoid and the umbilicus. This port is often placed under direct vision or with the use of a Verres needle. Additional ports are placed in the right subcostal space, to retract the liver, and in the left subcostal space for retraction of the stomach and to assist with the dissection. Two additional ports, one to the right of the xiphoid and the other to the right of the camera port, are primarily used for the dissection.

The dissection begins by dividing the gastrohepatic ligament, taking care to preserve any aberrant hepatic vessels and vagal branches to the portal structures. The right limb of the crus is then freed from the esophagus using blunt and sharp dissection. We have found that use of the ultrasonic scalpel has greatly aided in coagulation of vessels and in avoiding the problems of cautery smoke in the field. Dissection is carried over the anterior border of the esophagus to mobilize the phrenoesophageal ligament and to take the dissection laterally and caudally down the left limb of the crus. Next, the retroesophageal space is mobilized to create a posterior window through which the fundal wrap will be drawn. During this dissection, care is taken to identify and avoid injury to the vagal nerves (Fig 50-2). The esophagus must be sufficiently mobilized so that a 2-3 cm portion lies well within the abdomen without tension. We also make a point to routinely mobilize the short gastric vessels along the greater curvature of the fundus to reduce tension on the wrap. Again, we have found the ultrasonic scalpel to be quite satisfactory for division of these vessels.

The first part of the repair involves re-approximation of the crura. A 54 Fr bougie is inserted through the esophagus into the stomach and multiple 2-0 sutures are used to bring the right and left limbs of the crus together to tighten the esophageal hiatus and reduce the risk of hiatal herniation. The bougie is then withdrawn into the midesophagus to allow the leading edge of the

mobilized fundus to be brought posteriorly through the retroesophageal space (Fig 50-3). The bougie is then repositioned into the stomach to stent the wrap. A 1- to 2-cm wrap is created by stitching the left lateral fundal wall the anterior surface of the distal esophagus and then through the right lateral fundal wall (Fig 50-4). Two or three stitches are placed for this repair. We tend to anchor the wrap to the crura with additional stiches to provide further security against herniation. At the end of the procedure, the bougie is replaced with a nasogastric tube, which can be removed after several hours. Patients are then started on fluids and advanced to a soft diet as tolerated. The majority of patients can be discharged home the following day and, occasionally, we have sent people home on the evening of their surgery.

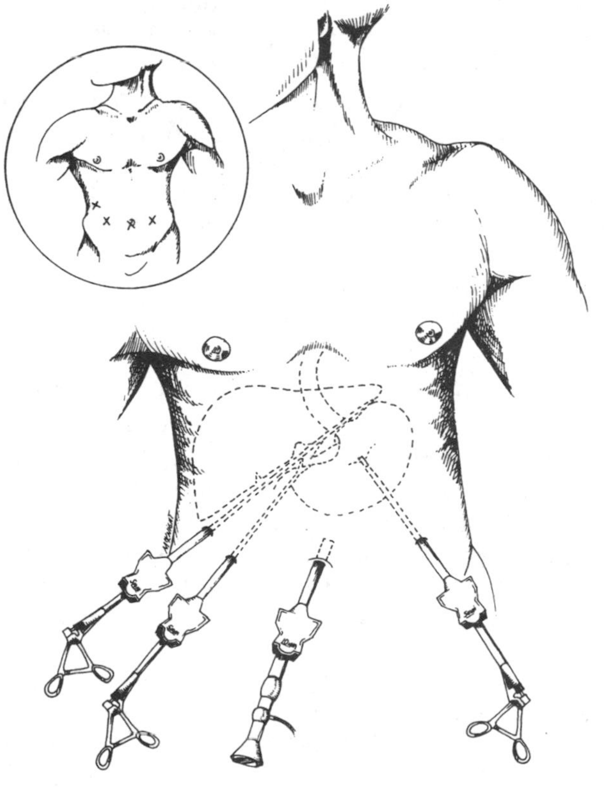

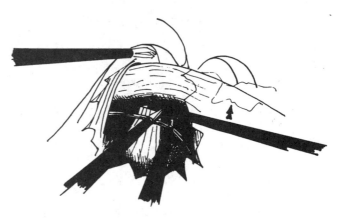

FIG 50-2. Dissection of the retroesophageal space. Care must be taken to avoid injury to the stomach, back wall of the esophagus, and posterior trunk of the vagus nerve.

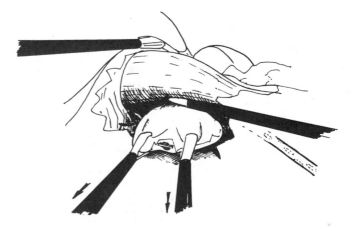

FIG 50-3. The leading edge of the fundus is brought around behind the esophagus in preparation for creating the wrap.

FIG 50-1. Placement of camera and operating ports for laparoscopic Nissen fundoplication.

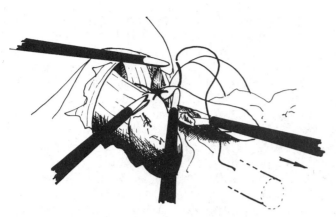

FIG 50-4. A short wrap is created by suturing the edges of the gastric fundus together. The sutures pass through the anterior wall of the distal esophagus to anchor the wrap at this location.

VI. PITTFALLS AND COMPLICATIONS

Complications associated with laparoscopic Nissen fundoplication (or any laparoscopic antireflux procedure) can be categorized into preoperative, perioperative, and postoperative problems (Table 50-2).

Not all patients with typical symptoms of heartburn will have reflux esophagitis. In the absence of endoscopic evidence of esophagitis, pH monitoring is required to document the presence of acid reflux. We use esophageal manometry extensively to document the peristaltic activity of the esophagus and to diagnose potential primary or secondary motor disorders. A barium swallow examination is occasionally useful in diagnosing a peptic stricture as the cause of dysphagia, although this is less important now with the liberal use of flexible esophagoscopy.

The antireflux operation must be tailored to the individual patient. Patients with poor peristaltic function tend to do better after partial rather than total fundoplication. Patients with severe reflux and significant esophagitis have greater relief of symptoms after total fundoplication. Patients with significant gastric or duodenal ulceration benefit from an added highly selective vagotomy. When acquired shortening of the esophagus has been documented, the addition of a gastroplasty is necessary.

As many as 40% of failed antireflux repairs may be due to technical errors during surgery. This is particularly true when a laparoscopic approach is used, as there is a temptation to bypass certain steps if they appear too difficult. Adequate mobilization with a tension-free intra-abdominal esophagus is crucial. Careful attention must be paid to the crural repair with the use of a bougie to avoid a closure that is too tight and causes dysphagia. We routinely mobilize the short gastric

Table 50-2. *Complications of Laparoscopic Nissen Fundoplication*

Preoperative
Patient selection
Perioperative
Choice of antireflux repair
Inadequate procedure
Perforation
Bleeding
Splenic injury
Pneumothorax
Wound infection
Postoperative
Periesophageal herniation
Dysphagia
Recurrent reflux
"Gas bloat" syndrome
Periesophageal hernia
Large sliding hiatal hernia

vessels to ensure that the fundal wrap is not on tension. Attention to the vagal trunks will reduce the risk of injury and gas bloat. A short wrap should be performed over a bougie of at least 51 Fr to reduce the chances of postoperative dysphagia.

Perforation of the esophagus, stomach, or duodenum has been reported in 1% to 4% of laparoscopic procedures.[5] Injury to the stomach is most common, particularly at the gastroesophageal junction during mobilization of the distal esophagus and creation of the retroesophageal window. Bleeding, severe enough to require transfusion or exploration, has been reported in less than 1% of laparoscopic cases.[4,6] A recent review indicated that the risk of splenic injury during laparoscopic Nissen fundoplication was less that 0.1%.[4] Pneumothorax is a unique complication of the laparoscopic approach and has been reported in 2% to 5% of patients.[5] Insertion of a chest tube is only rarely required.

Periesophageal herniation may occur early in the postoperative period, in which case it is usually associated with a technical problem with the crural repair. Dysphagia may be related to patient selection, but is most frequently caused by the use of small-sized bougie or failure to sufficiently mobilize the fundus, leading to a wrap with excessive tension.

Recurrent reflux is usually caused by a disruption of the wrap or by slippage of the wrap onto the stomach. Symptoms usually appear within a year of the procedure. Contributing factors include obesity, older age, steroid use, and technical errors such as inadequate mobilization of the stomach and the use of absorbable sutures.[5] The wrap may "slip" onto the stomach if not properly anchored to the distal esophagus. On occasion, the wrap may be incorrectly constructed around the proximal stomach by an inexperienced surgeon. These complications almost always require surgical correction.

We do not consider that conversion from a laparoscopic approach to an open procedure represents a complication. It is important to stress that the primary goal of obtaining long-lasting relief of a reflux problem must be given foremost priority by the surgical team. To this end, it is better to convert to an open procedure to accomplish the repair rather than compromise a good result by persisting with the laparoscopic approach.

VII. SUMMARY

The vast majority of patients with symptomatic GER disease will be capably managed by medical therapy. When surgical intervention becomes necessary, the laparoscopic approach offers distinct advantages in patient acceptance, length of hospitalization, and return to function compared with open procedures. Our experience has been that outcomes may be further optimized by a careful presurgical analysis of patient candidacy for the procedure. Attention should be paid to performing the operation in exactly the same manner as would be done in an open procedure. Surgical experience can prevent some of the more serious complications, such as perforation, vagal nerve injury, tissue ulceration or ischemia, and splenopancreatic injury.

References

1. DeMeester TR, Bonavina L, Albertucci M. Nissen fundoplication for gastroesophageal reflux disease: evaluation or primary repair in 100 consecutive patients. *Ann Surg*. 1986;204:9-16.
2. Negre JB: Post fundoplication symptoms. Do they restrict the success of Nissen fundoplication? *Ann Surg*. 1983;198:698-702.
3. Dallemagne B, Weerts JM, Jehaes C, Markiewicz S, Lombard R. Laparoscopic Nissen fundoplication: preliminary report. *Surg Laparosc Endosc*. 1991;1:138-143.
4. Hinder RA, Filipi CJ. The technique of laparoscopic Nissen fundoplication. *Surg Laparosc Endosc*. 1992;2:265-272.
5. Ferguson MK. Pitfalls and complications of antireflux surgery: Nissen and Collis-Nissen techniques. *Chest Surg Clin N Am*. 1997;7:489-509.
6. Collet, D, Cadière GB. Formation for the Development of Laparoscopic Surgery for Gastroesophageal Reflux Disease Group. Conversions and complications of laparoscopic treatment of gastroesophageal reflux disease. *Am. J Surg*. 1995;169:622-626.

PART VII

SWALLOWING DISORDERS: PREVALENCE AND MANAGEMENT IN SPECIAL POPULATIONS

Specific populations of patients present distinct challenges to the clinicians who manage their swallowing disorder. This section highlights the unique problems related to children, the elderly, and patients requiring intensive care. For infants and children, modifications to both the testing and treating of swallowing disorders are necessary. For the expanding populations of patients in critical care units, especially the elderly, the clinician must have a keen awareness of other disorders interfering with and often complicating the treatment of dysphagia. This section also addresses the palliation of the patient at the terminal stages of esophageal cancer.

CHAPTER 51

■ ■ ■

Swallowing Disorders
in the Pediatric Population

Lisa A. Newman, Sc.D.
Mario Petersen, M.D., M.S.

I. INTRODUCTION

There has been an increase in pediatric swallowing disorders as the result of improved survival rates for multiple medical conditions. The infant or child with dysphagia presents a unique challenge to the clinician because of the multiple health problems, which may include a swallowing disorder and the severe and even fatal complications that can result from dysphagia (eg, malnutrition, pneumonia, sudden infant death syndrome [SIDS]). Working with pediatric dysphagia requires a broad base of knowledge, including an understanding of the normal anatomy, physiology, and neurophysiology of a vast age spectrum from premature infant through adolescent and young adult.

The infant is born with variations in the relationship of anatomic structures and an immature neurologic system. These differences are exacerbated in premature infants. As infants grow and develop throughout childhood, there are changes in growth, relationship of anatomic structures, development of neurologic system, and cognitive development—all of which affect swallowing. Thus, there are changes in normal swallowing function as infants and children grow and develop that complicate the diagnosis and management of dysphagia.

There has been an explosion of research on adult dysphagia in the past 20 years. Research in pediatric dysphagia has been more limited. This chapter provides a basic understanding of pediatric swallowing and dysphagia. The fundamentals of infant swallowing are presented, including anatomy, developmental anatomy, neurophysiology, swallowing physiology, and feeding development. Dysphagia in the pediatric population is discussed with respect to underlying causes of dysphagia, swallowing and feeding abnormalities, and complications. Particular attention is paid to the diagnosis and management of feeding and swallowing disorders.

II. ANATOMY AND PHYSIOLOGY

A. Anatomy

The upper aerodigestive tract, consisting of the oral, pharyngeal, and nasal cavities as well as the larynx, serves three functions in the human: respiration, swallowing, and speech. The adult human is unique in that the base of the tongue makes up the anterior wall of the oropharynx and the larynx assumes a low position.[1] This anatomic configuration yields a bending of the vocal tract that is an important characteristic of the sound-producing apparatus.[2] The human infant is not born with this characteristic bending of the vocal tract.[2,3] Thus, there is a difference from adults in the configuration of anatomic structures in newborns. Furthermore, these anatomic relationships change as children grow and develop. Anatomic variations in developing infants and children directly affect physiology and must be considered when examining swallowing function.

Anatomic differences in the oral and pharyngeal cavities of infants as compared with adults include the size and shape of the oral cavity; tongue placement; vertical placement of the hyoid, larynx, laryngeal introitus, and epiglottis; sucking pads; and placement and angle of the eustachian tube. First, the size of the infant oral cavity is small in relationship to the overall size of the infant due to the small size and placement of the mandible.[1,4] More of the tongue surface is within the oral cavity and may completely fill the space.[5] In addition, the hard palate in newborns is short, wide, and only slightly arched, compared to a deeper arch in the adult. These characteristics of the oral cavity allow very little space in any direction for tongue movement in the newborn.

In the pharynx, the high position of the epiglottis, which is attached to the tongue, often allows it to make contact with the soft palate. Radiographic examination of the tip of the epiglottis, which marks the superior extent of the larynx found it to be at C2 for infants 6 months of age and under as opposed to C3 in the adult.[6] The hyoid and larynx lie at a higher level in the infant than in the adult, located almost directly beneath the base of the tongue.[1,4,7] As a result of the tongue surface within the oral cavity and the higher placement of the epiglottis, which is attached to the tongue, the opening of the larynx is just below the oral cavity. It has been suggested that the anatomy of the newborn is a more desirable arrangement for feeding, because if material lodges in the pharynx, it would not block the flow of air to the larynx as it would in the adult with a lower laryngeal position.[1]

Another difference is the presence of sucking or buccal pads. This fatty substance is a mass of adipose tissue encased in the space between the buccinator and masseter muscles in the infant's cheek and is thought to provide stability during the act of sucking.[1,4]

The final difference involves the eustachian tube. In the infant, the opening of the eustachian tube lies at the level of the floor of the nasal cavity near the junction of the hard and soft palates, as compared with adults, in whom the tube opening is shifted upward and backward so that it lies posterior to the inferior nasal concha.[1]

B. Developmental Changes in Anatomy

The relationships between anatomical structures that affect swallowing change as infants grow and develop. The period between 4 and 6 months has been noted to be a crucial stage in development of the upper respiratory/upper digestive tract.[4,8,9] It has been theorized that this period is a time of respiratory instability, either due to changes in relationship of anatomic structures, neuromuscular development, or change from obligate nasal to occasional oral respiration.

The primary changes that affect swallowing during childhood are elongation and enlargement of the pharynx, larynx, and oral cavity with growth of the mandible and face.[7,10] The changes in pharyngeal elongation are associated with differential enlargement of the cricoid and thyroid cartilages. Exact ages are not documented. As shown in Figs 51-1 and 51-2, sketches

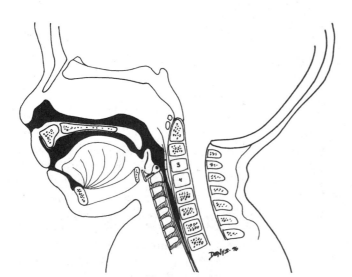

Fig 51-1. Newborn.

The tip of the epiglottis remains at C2 in the newborn and 8-month-old. As the infant matures, the larynx lengthens so that the inferior aspect of the larynx or cricoid cartilage is opposite C3-C4 in the newborn and

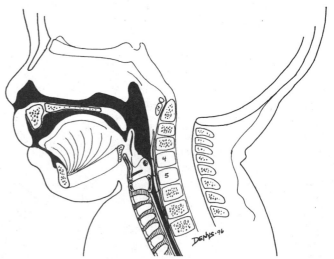

Fig 51-2. Eight-month-old infant.

C5-C6 in the older infant. As the larynx descends, the level of the cricopharyngeus muscle and superior aspect of the esophagus also descend.

drawn from magnetic resonance images (MRI) of a newborn and an 8-month-old, the tip of the epiglottis (superior aspect of the larynx) remains high approximately at the C2 level, while the inferior aspect of the larynx is opposite C5-C6 in the 8-month-old infant as compared with C3-C4 in the newborn.[6] Other developmental changes include the downward descent of the hyoid, larynx, and base of tongue. Thus, as infants mature, there is likely to be greater hyoid and laryngeal excursion and a more active role in base of tongue propulsion of the bolus.[8,10] Gradual reduction of the sucking pads will require more active movement of the check muscles.[4]

All developmental changes in the relationship of upper aerodigestive anatomic structures impact swallowing physiology. Unfortunately, there is very little developmental data on the anatomy and physiology of swallowing. Thus, the parameters that define normal swallowing in the pediatric population can be puzzling for a clinician who must diagnose and treat an abnormal swallow in an infant or child.

C. Neurophysiology

Our understanding of the infant/pediatric swallowing mechanism is further complicated by neurologic immaturity. Animal studies have shown that, although the swallow is present at a prenatal stage and developed at birth, the maturation of the control of swallowing continues postnatally.[3] As there is little information on neurological development as it affects the swallowing mechanism in humans, our information must be inferred from animal studies.[11]

Neural control of swallowing appears to involve two areas of the medulla: (1) the nucleus of the tractus solitarius and the adjacent reticular formation and (2) the nucleus ambiguus.[3,12,13] The nucleus of the tractus solitarius is composed of general visceral afferent fibers of cranial nerves VI, IX, and X, including the superior laryngeal nerve (SLN), and is the first synaptic relay for multiple inputs affecting heart rate, blood pressure, respiratory drive, taste reception, and deglutition.

The development of myelination of the vagus in human infants is not known. However, we can infer from animal studies that it may not be fully myelinated at birth. Microscopic examination of the SLN (cranial nerve X, vagus) in postnatal kittens revealed that, within the first month after birth, 75% of the fibers were unmyelinated. By 42 days, 50% of the fibers were myelinated.[14] In a study of human sudden infant death syndrome (SIDS) victims between 1 and 9 months of age, smaller and fewer large myelinated vagal fibers were found on autopsy than in age-matched controls.[15] This same study found that SIDS victims between the ages of 3 and 6 months had delayed axonal growth in

the vagus nerve. The vagus gives feedback to the nucleus of the tractus solitarius in the medulla, a synaptic relay for respiration and swallowing.

Apnea and bradycardia during feeding are complicating factors in the treatment of infants with swallowing disorders. However, it is important to be aware that there are strong neurologic relationships between swallowing, apnea, and bradycardia. This relationship has been examined in the animal model. For example, stimulation of the SLN nerve in a 5-day-old kitten produced apnea, with this same stimulation in the 28- to 30-day-old kitten evoked a swallowing response.[14] Similar apneic responses were found in young puppies under 50 days of age; whereas the laryngeal closure was evoked in the adult dog with the same stimulation.[9] The newborn lamb responded to the insertion of water into the larynx with persistent apnea, a rise in arterial pressure, bradycardia, and a reduction in cardiac output during apnea.[16]

These studies demonstrate an interdependence between swallowing, cardiac function, and respiration in young mammals, which disappears with maturation. What is not known is how this interdependence manifests itself in premature infants, newborns, and developing infants. The issues of apnea and bradycardia are additional compounding factors to be considered when evaluating an infant. Furthermore, there is little information about developmental neurophysiology and its effect on the swallowing mechanism.

III. SWALLOWING AND FEEDING

The developing fetus begins swallowing many weeks before delivery. Newborns born prematurely, 30 weeks or less gestation, already have suck and swallow reflexes; however, they lack the coordination necessary for oral feedings. Between 30-34 weeks, the preterm infant develops enough coordination of sucking, swallowing, and breathing for self-support with oral feeding.[17,18] In the full-term newborn, sucking or suckle feeding is fully developed.[7,20-22] Established reflexes allow the human infants to start breast feeding immediately and accommodate to the breast or bottle.

A. Swallowing Physiology

Swallowing has been divided into four stages: oral preparatory, oral, pharyngeal, and esophageal. In the infant, the oral preparatory stage is the suck or suckle. The suck is accomplished by placing the nipple to the mouth. The infant mouth opens and rooting for the nipple begins upon circumoral touch.[22] The suckle has been described as the acquisition of fluid from the nipple as a result of combined intraoral suction and external pressure on the nipple by the closing mandible.[21] Cinefluorographic investigations of sucking in 35 normal infants revealed that the infant narrows the neck of the nipple by closing the jaw. The tongue indents the lower surface of the nipple squeezing the contents of the nipple into the mouth and partly back into the bottle. Tongue movements during sucking have been described as a stripping action, or a lingual peristaltic motion, which squeezes fluid out of the nipple and moves it posteriorly.[6,24,25] Infants may suck one or more times per swallow, especially when swallowing barium contrast material.[6,7,23,26] When infants suck more than once per swallow, they must hold the material until they initiate the swallow. Infants may collect this material in several locations within the oral cavity and oropharynx, including between the tongue and palate, posterior tongue and soft-palate, and in the valleculae.[4,7,21,25] Unlike the adult swallow, the valleculae is an area where material can collect and from which the pharyngeal stage of swallowing can be triggered. In the adult, this same pattern would be considered a pharyngeal response delay.

The pharyngeal stage of swallowing in infants has been described as being similar to that of the adult. One difference is that the pharyngeal swallow occurs more frequently and with greater speed than that of adults.[7,25] The airway of the infants lies at a comparatively higher level than in adults, requiring less laryngeal excursion for airway protection. A small amount of residue may remain in the space between tongue and epiglottis (valleculae) in the normal infant swallow.[23,25] The mechanics of hyoid and laryngeal motion and upper esophageal opening have not been fully examined in infants.

Many clinicians believe that the infants can breathe air and swallow liquid simultaneously. This notion has been challenged by multiple research studies. Cessation of nasal airflow has been documented during nonfeeding and feeding swallows in term and preterm infants.[26,27] Many feeding swallows were initiated during intervals of absent airflow or respiratory pauses.[27,28] simultaneous ultrasound and respiratory investigation of swallowing has revealed that both term and preterm infants achieved some periods of 1:1:1 sequential linking of sucking, swallowing, and breathing.[28] The proportion of the feed in which this uniform pattern occurred increased with maturity. In more preterm infants, sucking occasionally disrupted regular, quiet breathing that was not observed in term infants.

B. Development of Normal Feeding

Feeding is a complex behavior that requires the integration of multiple physiologic systems (eg, pulmonary, gastrointestinal), parental or caregiver support

systems, and intellectual requirements. Table 51-1 shows the major systems that must be present and functional for normal feeding. The development of feeding is sustained by neurological maturation and ongoing experiences of a child. Table 51-2 demonstrates the interdependence between these systems. For example, the type of food that a child receives depends on maturation of oral-motor coordination, balance and postural control needed to keep the head straight, and fine motor coordination. The interplay of these systems allows older infants to hold a bottle and develop skills to facilitate finger feeding in the toddlers. Cognitive and socioemotional development are necessary for the normal learning of feeding. Cultural and societal factors provide the framework for the development of feeding. Societal and parental expectations not only direct the how, when, and what a child should eat, they will also shape the treatment of a child with feeding and/or swallowing disorders. Most of the development required for feeding is complete by 2 years of age. The understanding of the interaction among all systems that support feeding is fundamental for the assessment and treatment of children with swallowing and feeding disorders. In children, which is different from the adult situation, disorders in systems other than oral-motor and pharyngeal function can result in dysphagia. Tables 51-3 to 51-6 illustrate the presenting symptoms and the differential diagnosis for typical young children and for children with developmental disabilities.

Feeding is a learned skill. Development from the suck-swallow response in the newborn to the adult pattern of chewing and swallowing is not prewired. Infants need to have appropriate exposure to the increasing challenge produced in handling more difficult types of food. If a child is deprived of a normal experience during the first months of life, he or she will have long-term difficulties. Illingworth and Lister used the concept of sensitive periods developed by ethologists and applied it to feeding in children.[29] Sensitive periods are those points in time when a given learning process or experience must occur for normal development. Evidence from other studies supports the Illingworth and Lister hypothesis. Children who receive feedings through nasogastric or gastrostomy tubes for long periods will have severe difficulties initiating oral feedings.[30,31] Senez et al compared the results from weaning children from tube to oral feeding between a group of children with previous experience with oral feeding and a group without it.[31] Children without previous oral feeding took significantly more time to complete the transition to oral feeds. Dello Strologo et al examined the outcome of 12 patients with chronic renal failure who received nasogastric tube feeding for at least 9 months.[31] Three of four children who were older than 1 year at the beginning of tube feeding had no

Table 51-1. *Systems Involved in the Development of Feeding*

Systems	Required for:
Oral motor function	Sucking, munching, chewing, and movement of the bolus; also needed for speech
Respiratory system	Maintaining normal oxygen exchange, coordinating suck and swallow, coughing to protect airways
Cardiovascular system	Maintaining normal blood pressure and oxygenation of the tissues
Pharyngeal coordination	Coordinating swallowing and breathing, safely transporting the bolus to the esophagus
Gastrointestinal system	Esophageal transporting of the bolus to the stomach and lower esophageal sphincter to avoid reflux. Gastric emptying to the duodenum and transporting throughout the bowel
Gross motor	Maintaining head in midline and upright position, sitting stability on the chair
Fine motor	Finger feeding, using a spoon, holding a cup
Expressive language	Asking for more or saying no
Nonverbal communication games	Pointing for food, opening mouth to receive food, gesturing, playing
Receptive language	Comprehension of the meaning of words "food, bottle," understanding of commands
Hypothalamus	Controlling hunger and satiety
Cognitive	Recognizing foods by color, appearance, taste, and so on; learning the associations related to feeding (ie, sound of the bottle = food is coming); learning to self-serve food
Social	Giving positive feedback to the caregiver, eye contact
Caregiver (socioeconomic)	Providing appropriate amount and type of food
Caregiver (emotional)	Funneling positive emotional support of a child during the learning process, setting rules and limits

Sources: Data from Arvedson, Cloud, Gesell, Amatruda, Howard-Teplansky, Roger, & Campbell, 1993; Rudolph, 1994; Stevenson & Allaire, 1996.

problems as compared to 7 of 8 younger children who had feeding problems after reinstitution of oral feedings.

IV. CAUSES OF PEDIATRIC DYSPHAGIA

Etiologies of swallowing disorders in the pediatric population are numerous and can include neurologic disorders, anatomic anomalies, chronic diseases, gastrointestinal disorders, respiratory disorders, and psychological disorders.[32,33] Many disorders are associated with dysphagia and may either be the underlying etiology for dysphagia (eg, neurologic dysfunction), may complicate the management of an existing dysphagia (eg, bronchopulmonary dysplasia) or be a complication of dysphagia (eg, pneumonia). Table 51-3 lists associated medical disorders in approximately 100 children seen in the first year of a swallowing program at a metropolitan children's hospital. Table 51-4 is a chart of how medical conditions can affect the amount of food a child eats. Tables 51-7 and 51-8 list medical conditions

that can make a child refuse to eat. Children with dysphagia often have more than one factor interfering with feeding. For example, a child with cerebral palsy may have problems with oral dysphagia due to poor oral motor coordination, abnormal posture control, pain secondary to gingivitis (poor oral hygiene), gastroesophageal reflux (GER), delayed gastric emptying, mental retardation, or poor interaction with a caregiver because of lack of effective communication. The following sections describe three common etiologies of pediatric dysphagia that warrant special attention: prematurity, cerebral palsy, and esophageal disorders.

A. Prematurity

Preterm infants may exhibit temporary swallowing disorders that can be life-threatening and must be managed. One of the most serious problems in the treatment of dysphagia is the occurrence of apnea and bradycardia during feeding. Several studies have established a relationship between feeding and apnea or

Table 51-2. Feeding Development in Typical Children

Mo.	Feeding Skills	Oral Motor Skills	Food Type	Fine Motor Skills	Gross Motor Skills	Cognitive/ Sensory Skills	Language: Expressive/ Receptive Skills	Socioemotional Development Skills
1	Suckle swallow reflex. Starts interaction with caregivers. Pushes food out	Suck and swallow reflex, rooting reflex. Bite reflex. Suckling pattern. Extension retraction movements of the tongue.	Liquids (breast feeding, bottle)	Palmar grasp reflex	Holds head up	Visual fixation and tracking	E = Coos R = Alert to sounds	Regulation of states. Interest in the world. Can be calm. Eye contact and mutual gaze
2	when placed on tongue. Initial swallow involves posterior part of the tongue.				Holds Chest up		R = Smiles when stroked or talked	Smile. Mother child interaction
3	Anterior part of the tongue starts to be involved in initial swallow, facilitating the ingestion of semisolids.	Corners of mouth become active during sucking. Extends tongue in feeding anticipation.		Unfisted grasp		Recognition of parents		
4	Voluntary grasps with both hands. Sits with support.	Transfers bolus from anterior tongue to pharynx. Rooting reflex desappears.	Pureed food. Fed by caregiver, taken passively from spoon.	Starts reaching to objects. Objects to midline	Roll F -> B	Anticipates feeding	E = Laughs R = Orients to voice	Shows positive affect to caregivers. Displays negative affect. Responds with pleasure to social interactions.
5	Upright supported position for spoon feeding. Approximates lips to rim of the cup.	Sucking pattern		Transfers Objects	Roll B->F sits with support	Stereoscopic vision. Enjoys looking around environment	E = Razzes, blows bubbles, "Ah-goo" R = Orients to bell/keys	
6	Initiation of finger feeding. Drinks from the cup.	Chewing pattern emerges. Close of lips around spoon. Biting reflex disappears.	Pureed foods and teething crackers. Cup introduced.	Unilat reach, raking grasp	Sits	Visual interest in small objects. Oral exploration of objects	E = Babbles	Referential look. Reciprocal vowel play
7	Able to eat crackers. Starts helping spoon find mouth.	Lips begin to move while chewing		Radial grasp			R = Localizes bell indirectly	
8	Begins use of cup.	Lip closure achieved.			Come to sit/ crawl	Object permanence	E = Dadda (not specific)	Stranger anxiety
9	Pincer approach to food. Holds bottle.	Tongue lateralization of food bolus emerges.	Ground and mashed table foods	3 finger grasp	Pull to stand/ cruises		R = Understands No/ Gesture games	Plays pat a cake, Peek a boo. Interacts in a purposeful manner. Initiates interactions.

Age (mo)	Language (E/R)	Cognitive/Social	Adaptive	Gross Motor	Fine Motor	Oral Feeding	Self-Feeding
10	E = Mama/Dada R = Orients to bell directly						Finger feeding.
11	E = 1st word other than mama or dada R = 1 step command with gesture			Walks alone	Mature pincer		Drinks from cup (mother holds it)
12	E = 2 words other than mama		Help dressing. Imitates actions		Voluntary release	Soft table foods (easily chewed); Munching with improved lateralization. Licks food from lower lip	Reaches for food. Plays with food (throwing food, spoon, etc). Tries to keep spoon for self. Begins using cup.
15	E = Jargon/4-5 words R = Command no gesture	Comprehends, communicates, elaborates sequences of interactions	Use of tools	Runs, creeps up stairs	Tower 2 blocks		
18	E = Mature jargon R = Points to body parts 2 words phrase	Imitates parents in tasks	Imitates parents in tasks	Throws ball from standing	Turns pages	Mature chewing and drinking	Prefers to feed self over longer periods of time. Imitates others during feeding.
21			Asks for food or toilet	Goes up steps	Tower 5 blocks	Soft table foods (easily chewed)	Eats with spoon, but spills. Holds glass with both hands
24	E = 50 words. R = Follows 2 step command	Pretend play (representational capacity of ideas)	Help w/ undressing	up/down stairs alone	Turns 1 page		Correct use of spoon. Distinguishes between food and inedible materials
30	E = Pronouns approp R = Concept of 1			Jumps	Unbuttons	Table food. Vegetables, meat	Spear w/fork
3 y	E = Plurals / 250 words / 3-word phrase R = Concept of 12		Undresses completely	Rides tricycle, throws ball	Copies Circle		Straw drinking (3 years), can eat by himself, can serve cup

Sources: Data from Arvedson, Cloud, Gesell, Amatruda, Howard-Teplansky, Roger, & Campbell, 1993; Rudolph, 1994; Stevenson & Allaire, 1996.

Table 51-3. *Associated Medical Disorders Seen in 100 Children with Dysphagia*

Neurologic	Anoxia
	Arnold-Chiari malformation
	Arterial-venous malformation
	Brain tumors
	Cerebral palsy
	Cranial hemorrhage
	Developmental delay
	Head trauma
	Lessencephaly
	Meconium aspiration
	Meningitis
	Muscular atrophy
	Neurosurgical procedures
	Scoliosis
	Seizure disorder
	Spinal bifida
	Vocal fold paresis or paralysis
Maternal factors, including teratogens and viruses	Cytomegalovirus
	Drug substance abuse
	Fetal alcohol syndrome
	HIV
	Human papilloma virus
Pulmonary	Apnea
	Bronchopulmonary dysplasia
	Bronchospasms
	Chronic lung disease
	Chronic respiratory failure
	Laryngomalacia
	Pneumonia
	Pseudomonas tracheitis
	Tracheomalacia
	Tracheostomy
	Upper respiratory infections
	Ventilator dependent
Esophageal	Esophageal malacia
	Esophageal stricture
	Esophagitis
	GER
Genetic syndromes	CHARGE
	Cornelia de Lange
	DiGeorge
	Down
	Klippel Feil
	Noonan
	Sotos
	Pierre Robin
	VATER
Other	Cardiac anomalies
	Congestive heart failure
	Craniofacial anomalies
	Failure to thrive
	Medications that affect motor movement, sensation, or salivation
	Munchausen's by proxy
	Prematurity
	Radiation therapy
	Sepsis

bradycardia in premature infants. Bu'Lock et al examined the coordination of sucking, swallow, and breathing in preterm and full-term infants.[28] The youngest group of preterm infants (33-34 weeks gestation) exhibited apneic pauses in breathing movement during suck-

ing that occurred occasionally in the 35-36 weeks gestation infants and did not occur in the term infants. The premature infants alternated periods of apnea during feeding with breathing bursts when feeding was suspended.[28] Menon, Schefft, and Thach compared the fre-

Table 51-4. *Medical Conditions That Can Affect the Amount of Food a Child Eats. Usually the Child Will Stop Eating After Few Bites*

Clinical Condition	Symptoms	Some Specific Etiologies
Cardiac insufficiency	Cyanosis, tachypnea, edema, abnormal auscultation (gallop, murmurs)	Congenital malformations Myocarditis (infectious, autoimmune, toxic)
Respiratory insufficiency	Fast or labored breathing, cyanosis, wheezing, history of URI, bronchopulmonary dysplasia	Bronchopulmonary dysplasia Chronic aspiration Restrictive pulmonary insufficiency (severe scoliosis)
Respiratory-swallow incoordination	Apneas or bradycardia during feeding, symptoms of aspiration (choking, coughing during meals)	Malformations: choanal atresia Prematurity Neurogenic dysphagia: cerebral palsy
Hypotonia	Delay in achieving milestones, hypotonia, decreased strength, increased range of motion in joints	Cerebral Hypotonia • Chromosomal abnormalities (Prader-Willi, trisomies) • Metabolic defects • Nonprogressive encephalopathy (CP) Motor neuron disorders • Werdnig-Hoffman • Spinal cord injury (high), trauma, spina bifida • Muscular dystrophy • Metabolic myopathies
Esophageal disorders	Slow feedings, tolerates liquids better than solids	Esophageal webs Achalasia Arterial rings Stenosis posttrauma (surgery, caustic ingestion)
Slow gastric emptying	Abdominal distention, regurgitation	Cerebral palsy Cystic fibrosis, cancer: treatment and terminal stages

quency of swallowing during episodes of prolonged apnea with nonapnea control periods in preterm infants and found that 75 of 100 apneic episodes occurred during swallows.[34] During prolonged apnea, the swallow preceded bradycardia by an average of 6-7 seconds.

Tongue function, which affects the ability to propel the bolus into the pharynx, may also be altered or immature in the premature infant. Bu'Lock, Woolridge, and Baum, in their ultrasound studies, described three patterns of abnormal tongue movements seen most frequently in premature infants.[9] These movements consisted of incomplete or fragmentary peristaltic waves of tongue motion starting or finishing at abnormal regions of the tongue, purposeless nonperistaltic tongue movements, and twitching or tremulous tongue movements.

Unfortunately, there is a paucity of data of how premature infants resolve their swallowing difficulties. As younger and younger premature infants survive, the manifestation of swallowing difficulties in these younger and smaller infants will likely change.

B. Cerebral Palsy

The most frequent and challenging pediatric group with dysphagia are children with cerebral palsy. Cerebral palsy (CP) is a disorder of movement and posture resulting from a static, nonprogressive lesion of the developing brain.[36] More than 90% of the patients with CP have oral-motor problems[36] and 30%-60% have significant feeding problems.[36-38] Pelegano and Allaire in their study of 369 children with CP, found that 75% of the children with quadriplegia had at least one symptom of dysphagia.[39] Approximately 14% of the children with spastic or mixed quadriplegia had a gastrostomy and 11%-13% of children with hemiplegia or diplegia had severe symptoms of an abnormal swallow.

Cerebral palsy also affects the gastrointestinal system. Abnormal gastrointestinal function can result in esophageal dysphagia (GER, delayed gastric emptying, and constipation). Up to 70% of children with spastic quadriplegia can have GER without vomiting.[40]

Table 51-5. *Medical Conditions That Can Affect the Normal Transition to Solid Food*

Mechanism	Causal Factors or Etiology
Oral hypersensitivity	Rejects oral stimulation
	History of overstimulation (prolonged nasogastric tube feeding, oral trauma)
	History of understimulation (prolonged gastrostomy feeding without oral stimulation)
	Sensory deficits (blindness)
Developmental delay	Mental retardation
	Maltreatment/neglected child
Neurogenic dysphagia	Cerebral palsy
	Mobious syndrome
	Chiari malformations
Autism	Abnormal language development
	Abnormal social interaction
	Stereotyped behaviors

Table 51-6. *Differential Diagnosis in Children with Feeding Disorders Associated With Chronic Respiratory Problems*

Mechanism	Diagnosis or Specific Etiologies
Malformations	Tracheoesophageal fistula
	Cleft-lip-palate
	Pierre-Robin sequence
Neurogenic dysphagia	Arnold-Chiari malformation (spina bifida)
	Cerebral palsy (congenital, posttrauma, postinfectious)
	Oral motor dysfunction
	Nerve injury (trauma, surgery)
Respiratory-swallow discoordination	Prematurity
	Bronchopulmonary dysplasia
	Tracheotomy
Gastroesophageal reflux	Increased in children with CP

Abnormal tone and postural responses can also contribute to impaired feeding and to a progressive deterioration in feeding. This progression is associated with other deformities of the spine and extremities.[41] Abnormal bite has also been observed in children with CP and dysphagia. The association between bite and dysphagia suggests that the deterioration of feeding observed in some children is due to progressive retraction and sometimes luxation of the jaw resulting in limitation of movement.[42]

Swallowing disorders can have severe consequences in children with cerebral palsy—mainly respiratory infections and malnutrition. In children with CP, malnutrition can be caused by many factors. Children with CP can usually manage solid foods better than liquids and also require more time per swallow and per meal.[36,43,44] Tongue thrust, poor coordination of the tongue and mouth, and weak lip closure can result in a significant amount of food loss, thereby decreasing the amount of oral intake.[45] These problems can result in severe caloric malnutrition as well as deficits in minerals, vitamins, and trace elements.[46]

Chronic respiratory infection is the leading cause of death in children with CP. Respiratory complications can be due to food aspiration, aspiration of stomach content secondary to GER, and aspiration of secretions. Careful clinical assessment and videofluoroscopy are essential to the clinical diagnosis and development of appropriate treatment. For example, in an investigation of 90 children with CP who were seen for videofluoroscopic modified barium swallow (MBS), 97% of the children exhibited silent aspiration.[17] Thus, the necessity of an instrumental assessment in the diagnosis and treatment planning for the child with cerebral palsy is imperative.

C. Esophageal Disorders

GER is a frequent cause of dysphagia and can result in feeding resistance. Gianfrate et al studied 251 individuals with disability living in institutions of whom 107 (49%) had an abnormal Ph test.[48] The endoscopic fol-

Table 51-7. *Medical Conditions That Can Make a Child Refuse to Eat: Chronic Food Refusal (Sometimes Episodic)*

Mechanism	Causal Factors or Etiology
Food intolerance, milk allergy	History of diarrhea, patient rejects certain foods, rash, wheezing, family history of allergy
Hypersensitivity	Rejects oral stimulation History of overstimulation (prolonged nasogastric feeding, oral trauma, cleft lip and/or palate, endotracheal tube) History of understimulation (prolonged gastrostomy feeding without oral stimulation). Apneas during feeding
Loss of appetite	Medication GER Diencephalic syndrome
GER, peptic ulcer	Abdominal pain, unexplained pain or crying between meals, wakes up crying during sleep, frequent vomiting or regurgitation
Esophageal lesions	History of surgery, prolonged nasogastric tube History of GER Strictures Burns Malformations Tumors

Table 51-8. *Medical Conditions That Can Make a Child Refuse to Eat: Acute Etiologies (Can Become Chronic)*

Mechanism	Causal Factors or Etiology
Odynophagia	Oral injuries or infections (aphthous ulcers, gingivitis, oral or pharyngeal abscess) Esophageal foreign bodies (infants, toddlers, and individuals with mental retardation) Otitis media
Neurogenic dysphagia	Botulism, tetanus
Loss of appetite	Depression Posttraumatic stress disorder Anxiety Medications

low-up showed that 47% had esophagitis, 14% had Barret's esophagus, and 3.9% had peptic strictures. No similar study has yet been done in children. Surgical treatment with Nissen fundoplication can result in a new onset of dysphagia, sometimes requiring reoperation.[49,50] Foreign bodies in the esophagus should be suspected in toddlers, as well as children with mental retardation who present with acute dysphagia. Dysphagia can be one of the symptoms caused by esophageal stenosis. Esophageal stenosis may be caused by scarring after caustic ingestion or by general disorders such as Stevens Johnson syndrome or epidermolysis bullosa. Other less frequent esophageal disorders that can result in dysphagia are achalasia, sarcomas, vascular rings, esophageal duplication, congenital esophageal stenosis, cricopharyngeal rings, esophageal pseudodiverticulosis, and cricopharyngeal dysfunction.

V. SWALLOWING DISORDERS

A combined clinical examination and instrumental assessment can reveal a variety of swallowing disorders that can span the range from sensory disorders to motor disorders to behavior disorders. This section addresses oral and pharyngeal disorders that can be observed on a modified barium swallow (MBS).

Many clinicians refer to laryngeal penetration, aspiration, and material in the pharynx after the swallow (pharyngeal residue) as the swallowing disorder. Aspiration and pharyngeal residue are signs of a swallowing problem. The clinician must determine the physiologic reason for laryngeal penetration or aspiration. Furthermore, pediatric patients may not demonstrate aspiration during the instrumental assessment or MBS, yet they may be aspirating during mealtime. Therefore, swallowing abnormalities must be determined with respect to the potential for aspiration.

Swallowing disorders are discussed based on stages of swallowing: oral preparatory, oral, pharyngeal, and cervical esophageal. It should be noted that swallowing is a complex process and the disorders in one stage may effect other stages of swallowing. Specific radiographic findings during the four stages and their possible etiologies are listed in Table 51-9. Beginning with the oral preparatory stage, the grasp of a nipple by an infant or spoon by a child should be observed. When and how an infant responds to the nipple must be noted both clinically and during fluoroscopy. For a child, the ability to scrape material off a spoon with the lips must be assessed. Once food is in the oral cavity, one must observe how the infant prepares to swallow and whether he or she can form a bolus or loses material out of the mouth or to the floor of mouth.

Oral transit in the infant includes sucking and posterior propulsion of the bolus that occurs in one continuous anterior to posterior tongue motion. Often, infants will suck several times per swallow and collect the material in the oral cavity and/or valleculae before initiating the swallow.[6,25] Disorders of the oral stage will include the sucking/tongue movement and coordination and where the infant collects material before initiation of the swallow. Infants without swallowing difficulties may have multiple sucks per swallow, especially when given a foreign substance in a foreign environment. However, when sucking is excessive and lacks coordination with tongue movement and respiration, it may signal a problem for a dysphagic infant. Tongue movement in infants delivers the bolus to the pharynx by a phased application of the dorsum of the tongue to the nipple in an anterior-posterior peristaltic wave of contraction. Abnormal tongue movements have been described as incomplete or fragmentary peristaltic waves of motion starting from and finishing at abnormal regions of the tongue and may progress in a posterior-anterior direction, purposeless nonperistaltic movements, and twitching or tremulous movements.[28] In children, abnormalities of tongue movement may involve uncoordinated or repetitive movement of the posterior-anterior tongue wave that moves the bolus towards the front of the mouth. It is normal for infants to collect material in the valleculae before initiation of the swallow; however, dysphagic infants and children often collect material in the pyriform sinuses or have spillover of material into the pyriform sinuses before initiation of the pharyngeal response.[23,25] This places these children at-risk for aspiration. Nasopharyngeal backflow is observed during sucking in infants and toddlers from poor motor coordination of the oral musculature. Breathing must be observed especially in the young infant. Preterm infants may present with periods of sucking interrupted by a period of rapid breathing without sucks.

The pharyngeal phase of swallowing serves to guide the bolus through the pharynx into the esophagus without penetration into the nasopharynx or larynx. Difficulties with the pharyngeal stages can include a delayed or absent pharyngeal response, slow or uncoordinated velopharyngeal closure, slow laryngeal closure, and reduced hyoid/laryngeal excursion. These disorders may cause pharyngeal residue, laryngeal penetration, aspiration, or nasopharyngeal backflow. The response to laryngeal penetration or aspiration must be assessed. Does the child clear his or her throat, cough, and clear the airway?

The cervical esophageal stage must be evaluated for any anatomic or motility abnormalities. After the swallow, the presence of esophageal reflux may be a cause of aspiration.

VI. MANAGEMENT OF OROPHARYNGEAL DYSPHAGIA

Management or therapeutic intervention is possible only after the pathophysiology of the swallowing mechanism is diagnosed. Two important factors must be considered with the pediatric patient when managing swallowing disorders: (1) can the infant or child swallow safety with or without therapeutic intervention and (2) can the child consume adequate calories for growth and development? Management may be either surgical or behavioral. Surgical intervention may include myotomy, tracheal diversion (to manage secretions), or feeding tube placement. Behavioral treatment techniques often provide a lower risk, are less costly, and can be a more effective alternative to surgery in the treatment of dysphagia.

A variety of clinical factors may influence how a clinician approaches behavioral management. Children should be awake, alert, and clinically stable when fed. Although this may seem intuitive, many chronically ill children may have seizures or periods where alertness is diminished. Nursing staff, parents, hospital aids, or other caregivers should be instructed not to feed a patient during nonalert periods. Behavioral issues may interfere with the management of dysphagia. A child must be able to cooperate with parents and/or clinicians while being challenged with new food textures, more food, and new environments. The child must also have adequate receptive language and/or cognitive skills to perform recommended therapy techniques. Thus, therapy techniques must be tailored to a child's receptive language and/or cognitive skills. Finally, the etiology of the swallowing disorder or underlying disease process must also be considered in approaching management. For example, swallowing function may improve in a child after successful removal of a brain tumor; however, improvement is not likely in the child with a nonoperable progressive brain tumor.

Table 51-9. *Radiographic Findings and Possible Etiologies*

Radiographic (and/or Clinical) Findings	Possible Etiologies
Oral Preparatory Stage	
Oral defensiveness	Previous negative oral experiences or lack of oral/eating experiences
Poor grasp of nipple, biting on nipple, tongue placed behind nipple and not under nipple	Compliance, jaw or lip weakness, inability to organize in response to stimulus, oral defensiveness
Inability to scrape material off spoon	Jaw or lip weakness
Loss of material to floor of mouth or anterior sulci	Reduced tone, reduced tongue coordination
Drooling	Reduced lip and jaw tone, lack of sensitivity to material in the oral cavity
Oral Stage	
Excessive sucks per swallow	Uncoordinated sucking and tongue movement or suck/swallow/breath

Tongue movement
  Back to front tongue peristalsis
  Uncoordinated
  Poor tongue-to-palate contact
  Random tongue movements
	Reduced tongue coordination or strength

Spillover of material into the pyriform sinuses while sucking or moving bolus	Sensory/motor deficits
Laryngeal penetration/aspiration from spillover	
Oral residue	Reduced tongue function, reduced oral sensation
Pharyngeal Stage	
Pharyngeal response delay	Reduced sensation
Absence of pharyngeal response	Motor and/or sensory deficits
Slow laryngeal closure	Motor deficits
Laryngeal penetration/aspiration as a result of pharyngeal response delay, absent pharyngeal response, and slow laryngeal closure	
Absent cough reflex in response to aspiration	Reduced laryngeal sensation
Inability to clear airway when cough is present after aspiration	Vocal fold paresis/paralysis, laryngomalacia
Nasopharyngeal backflow	Cleft palate, velopharyngeal insufficiency, motor incoordination
Pharyngeal residue	Pharyngeal motor dysfunction including reduced laryngeal excursion, reduced base of tongue function
Aspiration from residue	
Cervical Esophageal Stage	
Esophageal stricture or narrowing	
Esophageal reflux	

Nonsurgical management techniques can be either direct or indirect. Direct intervention involves training techniques that a child performs when swallowing. Thus, direct intervention can only be employed for an the older child when there is adequate cognition, receptive language skills, and cooperation. Indirect intervention involves environmental modifications that can be controlled for the patient, such as alterations in temperature, viscosity, food texture, position, or pace of feeding by caregivers. Indirect techniques are most often employed with infants and children who have cognitive, motor, or language impairment.

The management of swallowing cannot be separated from other developmental issues, the rehabilitation process, and the entire medical picture. The team approach to habilitation of swallowing is often the most desirable requiring input from multiple disciplines including speech/language pathology, physical therapy, occupational therapy, psychology, and medical specialties.

VI. COMPLICATIONS OF OROPHARYNGAEAL DYSPHAGIA

Complications of oropharyngeal dysphagia in infants and children include respiratory disorders, malnutrition, and dehydration. These complications can cause other medical conditions and affect overall development. Respiratory complications include apnea (and bradycardia) in infants, pulmonary disorders such as respiratory infections and recurrent pneumonia, and SIDS. Pharyngeal swallowing incoordination and nasopharyngeal reflux have been shown to be associated with apnea or bradycardia.[51-53] Infants and young children with swallowing dysfunction (laryngeal penetration and aspiration) as demonstrated on videofluoroscopy has been shown to have an increased risk of pneumonia and near-miss SIDS.[54,55] Hypoxemia, as demonstrated with pulse oximetry, has been described during oral feeding in children with severe cerebral palsy.[56]

Malnutrition and dehydration are severe complications of dysphagia in developing infants and children. It is also possible that malnutrition may further impact swallowing function. Often feeding tubes are employed to deal with nutritional and fluid requirements in severely dysphagic infants and children. Children who have feeding tubes for long periods of time will have severe difficulties in initiating oral feeding. A child who has not eaten orally is often defensive about anything placed in his or her mouth. Oral defensiveness may be due to lack of experience or fear from previous negative feeding experiences or choking. Nonfeeding oral activities such as tooth brushing and oral hygiene may also be difficult for this population.

VIII. PARENT AND FAMILY INTERACTIONS

Two key dysphagia issues distinguish children from adults. Feeding is the role of the parents and for the parents to be able to feed a child, he or she must cooperate. Many parents measure themselves by the nutritional status of their child. Parents may not feel guilty if their child is not able to walk, but most of them will feel that a feeding problem is their failure.

Eating is a social event. When a child is not able to eat in public because he or she requires tube feeding or spills food during mealtime, it can be a source of embarrassment to the parents or a cause of tension with other family members. Nonoral tube feeding can be a major stress factor for parents. In the beginning, most parents are reluctant to see their child being fed in such an unnatural manner.

On the other side, there are many reasons why a child may refuse to eat. The second year of life is normally a period when food becomes a control issue between parent and child. The health professional needs to assess each situation individually. It is mandatory for the team to rule out any organic condition that may cause a child's behavior. Once organic conditions have been ruled out, the behavior can be dealt with from a psychological approach. In this case, the interaction of the parents and whole family system should be considered in assessment and treatment.

IX. CONCLUSIONS

The swallow mechanism develops and changes with growth and maturation. Infants and children are not miniature adults and the research on adult swallowing disorders may not always apply to pediatric populations. Furthermore, a variety of medical conditions can affect swallowing, and swallowing disorders can have severe and even fatal consequences. Swallowing must, therefore, be put in the context of the entire medical picture. Swallowing cannot be separated from feeding and feeding cannot be separated from development. Swallowing also has a direct impact on nutrition, and adequate nutrition is required for growth and development of every bodily system in a developing child.

New methods are being developed to diagnose and treat swallowing disorders in the pediatric population. For management and treatment to have a chance of being effective, it is of utmost importance that the entire swallow be visualized using an instrumental technique and that the pathophysiology of the swallow be determined. Our knowledge of pediatric swallowing and dysphagia is constantly growing. Diagnosis and treatment of pediatric dysphagia is both exciting and challenging. However, research is greatly needed for this vast and complex range of pediatric swallowing disorders.

Acknowledgment

Supported in part by Grant 90-DD-0364-03 from the U.S. Department of Health and Human Services, Administration for Children and Families and by Grant MCJ-479158-06 from the Health Resources and Services Administrations Maternal and Child Health Bureau.

References

1. Crelin E. *Functional Anatomy of the Newborn*. New Haven, Conn: Yale University Press; 1973.
2. Perkins WH, Kent RD. *Functional Anatomy of Speech, Language and Hearing. A Primer*. San Diego, Calif: College-Hill Press; 1986.
3. Miller A. Deglutition. *Physiol Rev*. 1982;62:129-184.
4. Morris SE. *The Normal Acquisition of Oral Feeding Skills: Implications for Assessment and Treatment*. Central Islip, NY: Therapeutic Media; 1982.
5. Bosma J. *Anatomy of the Infant Head*. Baltimore, Md: Johns Hopkins University Press; 1986.
6. Newman LA. *Oral and Pharyngeal Swallowing in Infancy* [dissertation]. Boston, Mass: Boston University; 1992.
7. Kramer S. Special swallowing problems in children. *Gastrointest Radiol*. 1985;10:241-150.
8. Laitman JT, Reidenberg JS. Specializations of the human upper respiratory and upper digestive systems as seen through comparative and developmental anatomy. *Dysphagia*. 1993;8:318-325.
9. Sasaki CT, Suzuki M, Horiuchi M. Postnatal development of laryngeal reflexes in the dog. *Arch Otolaryngol*. 1977; 103:138-171.
10. Bosma JF. Functional anatomy of the upper airway during development. In: Matthew OP, SantAmbrogio G, eds. *Respiratory Function of the Upper Airway*. New York, NY: Marcel Dekker Inc; 1988:47-86.
11. Newman LA. Infant swallowing and dysphagia. *Curr Opin Otolaryngol Head Neck Surg*. 1996;4:182-186.
12. Jean A, Car A. Inputs to the swallowing medullary neurons from the peripheral afferent fibers and the swallowing cortical area. *Brain Res*. 1979;178:567-572.
13. Miller A. Neurophysiological basis of swallowing. *Dysphagia*. 1986;1:91-100.
14. Miller A. Characterization of the postnatal development of superior laryngeal nerve fibers in the postnatal kitten. *J Neurobiol*. 1976;7:483-494.
15. Becker LE, Zhang W, Pereyra PM. Delayed maturation of the vagus nerve in sudden infant death syndrome. *Acta Neuropathol (Berl)*. 1993;86:617-622.
16. Harding R, Johnson P, Johnston B, McClelland M, Wilkinson A. Cardiovascular changes in new-born lambs during apnea induced by stimulation of laryngeal receptors with water. *J Physiol (Lond)*. 1976;256;359-369.
17. Dumont RC, Rudolph CD. Development of gastrointentinal motility in the infant and child. *Gastroenterol Clin North Am*. 1994;23:655-671.
18. Rudolph CD. Feeding disorders in infants and children. *J Pediatr*. 1994;125:5116-5124.
19. Fisher S, Painter M, Milmoe G. Swallowing disorders in infancy. *Pediatr Clin North Am*. 1981;28:845-853.
20. Herbst J. Development of suck and swallow. *J Pediatr Gastroenterol Nutr*. 1983;2(suppl 1):S131-S135.
21. Logan W, Bosma J. Oral and pharyngeal dysphagia in infancy. *Pediatr Clin North Amer*. 1967;14:47-61.
22. Doty R. Neural organization of deglutition. In Code CF, ed. *Handbook of Physiology, Alimentary Canal*. Vol IV, Section 6. Washington, DC: American Physiology Society; 1976:1861-1902).
23. Ardran G, Kemp F. Some important factors in the assessment of oropharyngeal function. *Dev Med Child Neurol*. 1970;12:158-166.
24. Weber F, Woolridge M, Baum J. A ultrasonographic study of the organization of sucking and swallowing by newborn infants. *Dev Med Child Neurol*. 1986;28:19-24.
25. Newman LA, Cleveland RH, Blickman JG, Hillman RE, Jaramillo, D. Videofluoroscopic analysis of the infant swallow. *Invest Radiol*. 1991;26:870-873.
26. Thach B, Menon A. Pulmonary protective mechanisms in human infants. *Am Rev Respir Dis*. 1985;131(suppl): S55-S58.
27. Wilson S, Thach BT, Brouilette RT, Abu-Osba YK. Coordination of breathing and swallowing in human infants. *J Appl Physiol*. 1981;50:851-858.
28. Bu'Lock F, Woolridge MW, Baum JD. Development of co-ordination of sucking, swallowing and breathing: ultrasound study of term and preterm infants. *Dev Med Child Neurol*. 1990;32:669-678.
29. Illingworth RS, Lister J. The critical or sensitive period, with special reference to certain feeding problems in infants and children. *J Pediatr*. 1964;65:840-848.
30. Dello Strologo L, Principato F, Sinibaldi D, et al. Feeding dysfunction in infants with severe chronic renal failure after long-term nasogastric tube feeding. *Pediatr Nephrol*. 1997;11:84-86.
31. Senez C, Guys JM, Mancini J, Paz Paredes A, Lena G, Choux M. Weaning children from tube to oral feeding. *Childs Nerv Syst*. 1996;12:590-594.
32. Arvedson JC, Rogers BT. Pediatric swallowing and feeding disorder. *Med Speech-Language Pathol*. 1993;1: 203-202
33. Prontniccki J. Presentation: symptomatology and etiology of dysphagia. In: Rosenthal SR, Sheppard JJ, Lotze M, eds. *Dysphagia and the Child with Developmental Disabilities: Medical, Clinical, and Family Interventions*. San Diego, Calif: Singular Publishing Group Inc; 1995:1-4.
34. Menon AP, Schefft GL, Thach BT. Frequency and significance of prolonged apnea in infants. *Am Rev Respir Dis*. 1984;130:969-973.
35. Bax M. Terminology and classification of cerebral palsy. *Dev Med Child Neurol*. 1964;6:295-307.
36. Reilly S, Skuse D, Poblete X. Prevalence of feeding problems and oral motor dysfunction in children with cerebral palsy: a community survey. *J Pediatr*. 1996;129:129: 877-882.
37. Dahl M, Thommessen M, Rasmussen M, Selberg T. Feeding and nutritional characteristics in children with moderate or severe cerebral palsy. *Acta Paediatr*. 1996; 85:697-701.
38. Waterman ET, Koltai PJ, Downey JC, Cacace AT. Swallowing disorders in a population of children with cerebral palsy. *Int J Pediatr Otorhinolaryngol*. 1992;24:63-71.
39. Pelegano J, Allaire J. Parental reports of oral motor dysfunction by type of cerebral palsy. 1998: Unpublished.
40. Booth IW. Silent gastro-oesophageal reflux: how much do we miss? [editorial]. *Arch Dis Child*. 1992;67:1325-1327.
41. Detoledo J, Icovinno J, Haddad H. Swallowing difficulties and early CNS injuries: correlation with the presence of axial skeletal deformities. *Brain Inj*. 1994;8:607-611.

42. Pelegano JP, Nowysz S, Goepferd S. Temporomandibular joint contracture in spastic quadriplegia: effect on oral-motor skills. *Dev Med Child Neurol.* 1994;36:487-494.

43. Casas M J, Kenny DJ, McPherson KA. Swallowing/ventilation interactions during oral swallow in normal children and children with cerebral palsy. *Dysphagia.* 1994; 9:40-46.

44. Gesell A, Amatruda CS. *Developmental Diagnosis: Normal and Abnormal Child Development.* 2nd ed. New York, NY: Paul H. Hoeber Inc; 1956.

45. Chigira A, Omoto K, Mukai Y, Kaneko Y. Lip closing pressure in disabled children: a comparison with normal children. *Dysphagia.* 1994:9:193-198.

46. Hals J, Ek J, Svalastog AG, Nilsen H. Studies on nutrition in severely neurologically disabled children in an institution. *Acta Paediatr.* 1996;85:1469-1575.

47. Rogers BR, Arvedson J, Buck G, Smart P, Msall, M. Characteristics of dysphagia in children with cerebral palsy. *Dysphagia.* 1994;9:69-73.

48. Gianfrate L, Bianchi C, Rota Bachetta L, et al. Gastroesophageal reflux disease in mentally retarded patients. *J Pediatr Gastroenterol Nutr.* 1997;25(suppl. 1):S43.

49. Anvari M, Allen CJ. Prospective evaluation of dysphagia before and after laparoscopic Nissen fundoplication without routine division of short gastrics. *Surg Laparosc Endosc.* 1996;6:424-429.

50. Cadiere GB, Himpens J, Rajan A, et al. Laparoscopic Nissen fundoplication: laparoscopic dissection technique and results. *Hepatogastroenterology.* 1997;44:4-10.

51. Itani Y, Fujioka M, Nishimura G, Niitsu N, Oono T. Examinations in older premature infants with persistent apnea: correlation with simultaneous cardiorespiratory monitoring. *Pediatric Radiology.* 1988;18:464-467.

52. Plaxico DT, Loughlin GM. Nasopharyngeal reflux and neonatal apnea, their relationship. *Am J Dis Child.* 1981; 135:793-794.

53. Oestreich AE, Dunbar JS. Pharyngonasal reflux: spectrum and significance in early childhood. *Am J Roentgenol.* 1984;141:923-925.

54. Kohda E, Hisazumi H, Hiramatsu K. Swallowing dysfunction and aspiration in neonates and infants. *Acta Otolaryngol (Stockh).* 1994;517(suppl):11-16.

55. Loughlin G M, Lefton-Grief M A. Dysfunctional swallowing and respiratory disease in children. *Adv Pediatr.* 1994;41:135-162.

56. Rogers BR, Arvedson JJ, Msall M, Demerath RR. Hypoxemia during oral feeding of children with severe cerebral palsy. *Dev Med Child Neurol.* 1993;35:3-10.

CHAPTER 52

■■■

Swallowing Disorders in the Critical Care Patient

Melissa A. Simonian, M.Ed., CCC-SLP
Andrew N. Goldberg, M.D.

I. INTRODUCTION

Special considerations need to be addressed in the diagnosis and management of dysphagia in the critical care patient. Multiple physicians and allied health professionals are involved in the care of a critically ill patient, and each has a slightly different perspective along with a specific responsibility to the management process. As patients in the intensive care unit are commonly subjected to multiple interventions, these patients suffer combinations of insults to the swallowing mechanism that may coalesce to produce dysphagia.

Priorities for care shift as a patient's needs and the level of illness changes; therefore, it is vital that the evaluation and management of dysphagia in this population be integrated with the overall treatment plan. Appropriate and timely diagnosis contributes to a reduction in a patient's risk for aspiration and further pulmonary compromise.

To reduce repetition of the separate conditions that exacerbate dysphagia, referral to other sections of this book that discuss specific neurologic conditions, altered mental status related to medication administration, and effects of surgery on swallowing are not repeated here. Specific procedures for identification of swallowing disorders and subsequent treatment options are provided.

II. ASSESSMENT

The evaluation of a critically ill patient should begin, as in any patient, with a comprehensive review of the medical history and hospital course. Particular attention must be paid to mechanical ventilation and respiratory status, mental status and alertness, and surgical alteration of the upper aerodigestive tract or related structures. Differentiation must be made between chronic, compensated conditions that are unlikely to change and acute insults that may be in a state of flux. The evolution of a stroke and the subsequent neurologic deficits or improvement of the dysphagia associated with postsurgical or postendotracheal dysphagia pain and edema are examples of changing conditions that alter the clinical picture. The superimposition of an acute problem on a chronic condition may be too great a challenge for a patient to compensate for, especially in the elderly where plasticity, compensation, and resiliency may be lacking.

III. CLINICAL EVALUATION

The minimum requirements for a patient to actively participate in the dysphagia evaluation process include the ability to maintain alertness, follow basic commands, and ideally be 24 hours postextubation or 48 hours posttracheotomy (Figs 52-1 and 52-2). Swallowing evaluation in orally or nasally intubated patients is usually deferred, although it is possible in selected cases (eg, young patients with an intact upper aerodigestive tract). The evaluation continues with visualization of the oral cavity. This includes oral hygiene, presence or absence of reflexes (ie, gag, cough), sensation, and movement and coordination of the lips, tongue, mandible, and palate. During the oral phase of the swallow food is masticated and propelled posteriorly. Any labial leakage, pocketing, or delay in the swallow reflex should be noted. Pharyngeal peristalsis propels the food material through the pharynx as the epiglottis inverts and the larynx elevates to close off the airway, preventing aspiration. The cricopharyngeal sphincter relaxes to allow food to enter the esophagus, completing the pharyngeal phase of the swallow. Multiple

swallows, a cough, or a wet vocal quality may be an indication that food material has been aspirated .[1] If a tracheotomy tube is present, the cuff must be deflated to fully detect aspiration. If the patient is unable to tolerate cuff deflation secondary to copious secretions or the absence of a protective cough reflex, this is an indication that it is too early to proceed and the evaluation should be deferred. It should be noted, however, that some patients require up to 12 hrs to "re-accommodate" to a deflated cuff. A period of observation is advisable, whenever possible, before testing the swallow.

The vocal folds are the last protective mechanism before material enters the airway; therefore, assessment of voice can provide clues to the competency of the swallow and potential for aspiration. For example, a wet vocal quality may be a sign that material is resting at the level of the vocal folds waiting to enter the air-

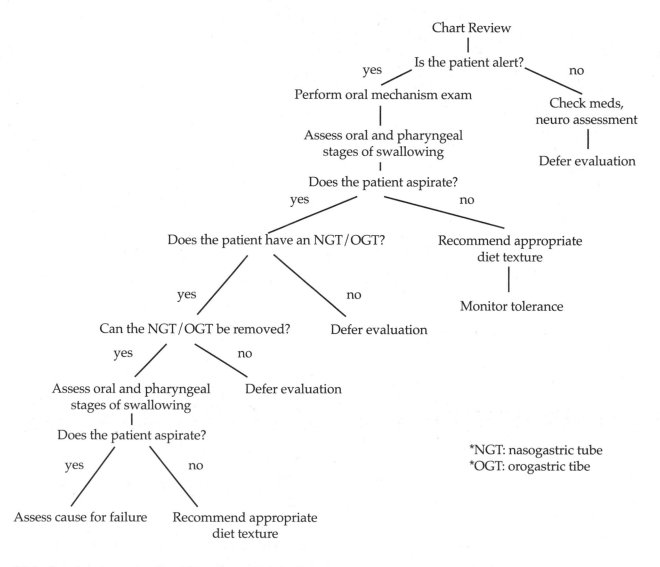

Fig 52-1. Dysphagia evaluation 24 hours postextubation.

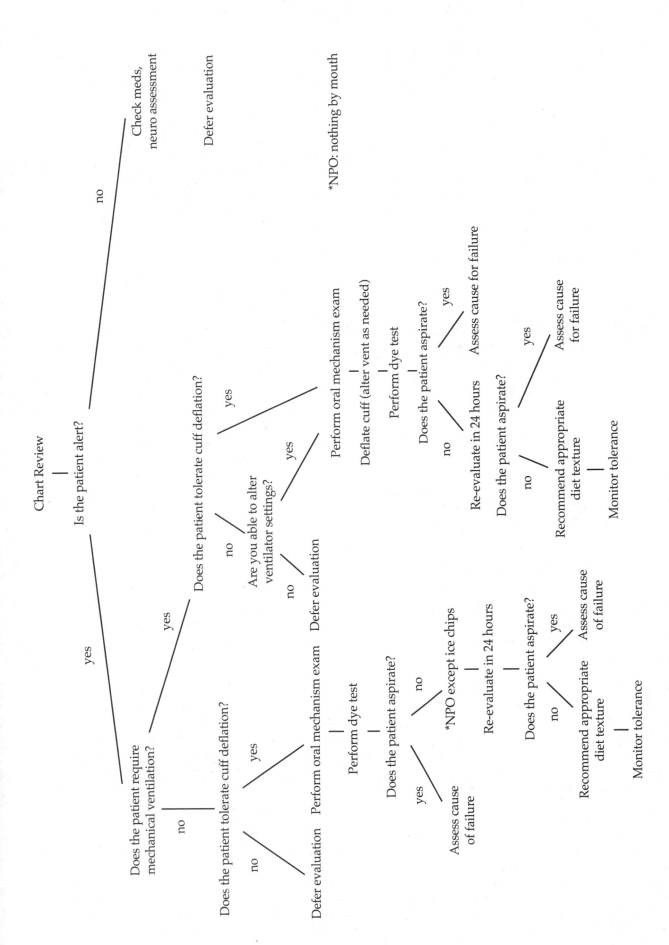

Fig 52-2. Dysphagia evaluation 48 hours posttracheostomy.

365

way. If the patient has a tracheotomy tube, the cuff is deflated and the tube digitally occluded to assess the patient's vocal quality. Some patients will be unable to phonate secondary to the size of the tube or other factors and this portion of the assessment may need to be deferred. [2]

The dye test is a useful tool in assessing the swallowing function of a tracheotomized patient. The patient's tracheotomy cuff is deflated and the tracheotomy tube is deep suctioned for secretions that may have been resting on or above the level of the cuff. Dye is added to various consistencies of food material and the oral and pharyngeal phases of the swallow are observed as during a routine swallowing evaluation. However, at the completion of the evaluation, the patient's tracheotomy tube is deep suctioned again, this time looking for evidence of dyed material in the airway. The dye test should be repeated 24 hours later and prior to the patient beginning oral feeding secondary to the risk for delayed aspiration or reflux aspiration that may not have been noted during the initial evaluation.

In the evaluation of the patient who has a tracheotomy and is mechanically ventilated, the ventilator settings and parameters of ventilation may need to be adjusted for the patient to tolerate deflation of the tracheotomy cuff.[2] The speech-language pathologist along with the respiratory therapist and physician must collaborate to provide a safe swallowing environment without respiratory compromise. The patient's ability to tolerate deflation of the tracheotomy cuff may be assisted by increasing the tidal volume and pressure support to make up for the loss of volume around the deflated tracheotomy cuff. The patient who is breathing both spontaneously and requiring mandatory breaths from the ventilator must be instructed on when to swallow food material to avoid aspiration secondary to the ventilator providing a preset breath. The patient is asked to swallow just after a spontaneous breath or a breath from the ventilator. As with any patient with a tracheotomy, deep suctioning at the completion of the swallowing evaluation is required for signs of aspiration and the evaluation should be repeated in 24 hours and prior to clearance for oral feeding.

IV. SPECIAL CONSIDERATIONS

Nasogastric feeding is commonly used to provide short-term nutrition. Nasogastric tubes reduce pharyngeal sensitivity predisposes to gastroesophageal reflux (GER) and may produce inflammation and pain that interferes with laryngeal elevation, increasing the risk for swallowing difficulties. Large-bore, hard plastic nasogastric tubes predispose a patient to mucosal irrita-

tion and ulceration and contribute further to pain and dysphagia. Whenever possible, small-bore, soft feeding tubes should be used to minimize interference with the swallowing mechanism.

As patients in the intensive care unit are sometimes unable to be removed from monitors, transporting them off the floor for a modified barium swallow (MBS) is not always an option. For a more quantitative evaluation of the swallowing reflex when the videofluoroscopic swallow study cannot be obtained, one can utilize the fiberoptic endoscopic evaluation of the swallow (FEES) at the bedside for direct visualization of the pharynx and larynx before, during, and after the swallow[3] (see Chapter 12).

Many critically ill patients will require mechanical ventilation with or without tracheotomy. The effects of endotracheal intubation and tracheotomy on laryngotracheal structures is well documented in the literature; however, less attention has been paid to the concomitant swallowing difficulties that follow extubation. It is believed that the prolonged presence of an endotracheal tube can result in desensitization of the laryngotracheal mechanism, laryngeal trauma, and stenosis.[4] Suprisingly, few references to this relationship in the critically ill patient can be found in the literature. Alessi et al studied 29 ICU patients requiring intubation ranging from 17 hrs to 11 days. Aspiration occurred in 10 of 29 patients and 3 of these died from complications associated with aspiration pneumonia.[5] DeVita and Spierer-Rundback found that prolonged intubation and tracheotomy are associated with swallowing dysfunction and increased risk for aspiration in the absence of neurologic damage. The authors suggested that dysphagia may be associated with decreased sensitivity, decreased laryngeal coordination, and muscle atrophy from lack of use.[6] The presence of a tracheotomy tube or endotracheal tube also limits the efficiency of a cough in clearing material from the glottis or trachea. Lastly, respiration normally ceases during swallowing and continues at the completion of a swallow. This pattern is disrupted for patients on a ventilator, adding an additional complication to swallowing with a tracheotomy or endotracheal tube.

Patients can eat with a tracheotomy tube; however, the potential for difficulty in swallowing is heightened. This may occur secondary to poor closure of the vocal folds in the absence of subglottic pressure, tethering of the laryngotracheal complex with decreased vertical mobility, pain with tracheal movement, and increased cuff pressure. Additionally, disruption of the normal airway by tracheotomy decreases the feedback provided by pharyngeal pressure changes that occur with swallowing. These changes of pressure in the pharynx and trachea provide a form of proprioception that contributes to the coordination of swallowing.[7] Absence of this sensation of pressure change predisposes to dysphagia and aspiration.

Mental status changes frequently occur in the critically ill patient and must be taken into account during assessment. There are multiple reasons for a patient's mental acuity to decrease, including brain injury, altered nutritional status and alertness, and medications. Attention must be paid to evolving neurologic injury, improvement or worsening of nutritional status, and alterations in medication administration that could alter the level of arousal. Interaction with the physician caring for the patient may shed light on an evolving clinical course and alteration in the treatment plan that may influence the dysphagia evaluation.

Surgical intervention in the head, neck, or chest regions is more likely to directly affect swallow function. During head and neck surgery, structures in the oral cavity, larynx/pharynx, and upper esophagus may be modified or removed. This alteration in anatomy pertinent to swallowing will inevitably cause a change in the swallow function (see Chapters 21 and 22). The influence of head and neck surgery on swallowing are discussed in detail in a separate chapter devoted to that subject. As surgery in regions distant to the head and neck can also alter swallowing function, familiarity with interventions at other sites is important. Cardiothoracic surgery, for example, has been documented to cause difficulties in swallowing secondary to retraction trauma during routine procedures.[8]

V. TREATMENT OVERVIEW

Postural changes, compensatory strategies, and diet modification can be introduced during the swallowing evaluation and later continued as treatment procedures to reduce the risk for aspiration. Observation of the oral and pharyngeal phases of the swallow with a variety of textured material is required prior to diet recommendation[9] (Table 52-1). As the medical status of a critically ill patient will fluctuate, frequent reassessment of the swallow is recommended. Frequent observation of meals, reinforcement of recommendations for compensatory maneuvers or diet changes, and monitoring the patient for signs and symptoms of aspiration are necessary prior to upgrading diet textures (Table 52-2).

Treatment of patients in the intensive care unit presenting with dysphagia is similar to patients in other settings. The principle difference lies with the integra-

Table 52-1. *Differential Diagnosis of Dysphagia*

Type	Signs	Possible Cause	Treatment
Oral	Buccal pocketing, labial leakage	Facial weakness Surgical revision	Oral motor exercises, present food to stronger side
	Labored mastication	Lack of dentition, poor cognition	Modify food texture
	Premature spill	Lingual weakness	Chin tuck position, modify food texture
Pharyngeal	Delayed swallow initiation	Poor oral phase, vagus nerve dysfunction, prolonged intubation.	Thermal stimulation
	Decreased laryngeal elevation	Tracheotomy, NGT, suprahyoid muscle dysfunction, edema.	Tracheotomy cuff deflation, d/c NGT
	Multiple swallow pattern	Decreased pharyngeal peristalsis/contraction	Alternate liquid and solid swallows
	Cough/throat clear immediately after the swallow	Aspiration secondary to decreased epiglottic deflection, poor oral phase	Supraglottic swallow, modify food texture
	Delayed cough, throat clear	Aspiration after the swallow secondary to pooling in the pharynx	Utilize dry swallow, alternating liquid and more solid swallows
	Change in vocal quality	Penetration to the level of the vocal folds, vocal fold weakness.	NPL. Modify food texture
Esophageal	Significantly delayed aspiration	Reflux, stricture	Medication, modify foods, GI referral

Table 52-2. *Clinical Signs/Symptoms of Dysphagia*

- Coughing/choking
- Frequent throat clearing
- Multiple swallow pattern
- Wet vocal quality
- Drooling
- Increased pharyngeal secretions
- Fever
- Increased white blood count
- Pulmonary infiltrate

tion of the treatment of dysphagia with a patient's evolving disease state. The reader is referred to earlier chapters for specific treatment options.

VI. CONCLUSION

Swallowing is a protective mechanism against aspiration of material into the respiratory tract and a means for alimentation. Alterations in swallowing have been associated with an increased risk for aspiration pneumonia. Critically ill patients are at-risk for swallowing problems because of alterations in upper airway sensitivity secondary to prolonged intubation, the presence of a tracheotomy tube, the residual effects of pharmacological intervention, mental status changes, and surgical alteration of the oral and pharyngeal anatomy. Ongoing assessment of a patient's changing clinical picture is critical to allow for modifications in the treatment of dysphagia. Communication with physicians and other health professionals keeps the entire care team informed and coordinated. The need for early diagnosis and treatment is emphasized to maximize oral feeding and minimize the life-threatening consequences of aspiration pneumonia for the critically ill patient.

References

1. Logemann J. Swallowing physiology and pathophysiology. *Otolaryngolo Clin North Am*. 1988;21:613-623.
2. Dikeman K, Kazanjian M. *Communication and Swallowing Management of Tracheostomized and Ventilator Dependent Adults*. San Diego, Calif: Singular Publishing Group Inc; 1995.
3. Langmore S. Fiberoptic endoscopic examination of swallowing safety: a new procedure. *Dysphagia*. 1988;2:216-219.
4. Bishop M. Mechanisms of laryngotracheal injury following prolonged tracheal intubation. *Chest*. 1989;96:185-186.
5. Alessi D, Hanson D, Berci G. Bedside videolaryngoscopic assessments of intubation trauma. *Ann Otol Rhinol Laryngol*. 1989;98:586-590.
6. DeVita M, Spierer-Rundback L. Swallowing disorders in patients with prolonged orotracheal intubation or tracheostomy tubes. *Crit Care Med*. 1990;18:1328-1330.
7. Nash M. Swallowing problems in the tracheotomized patient. *Otolaryngol Clin North Am*. 1988;21:701-709.
8. Hogue C, Lappas G, Creswell L. et al. Swallowing dysfunction after cardiac operations. *J Thorac Cardiovasc Surg*. 1995;110:517-521.
9. Logemann, J. *Evaluation and Treatment of Swallowing Disorders*. Austin, Tex: Pro-Ed; 1983.

CHAPTER 53

Dysphagia in the Elderly

Joseph R. Spiegel, M.D.
Robert T. Sataloff, M.D., D.M.A.
Jesse Selber, B.A.

I. INTRODUCTION

The elderly population in the U.S. is at its largest and is growing faster than ever. Swallowing problems in the elderly are well documented. Difficulties during eating have greater prevalence in the elderly for a number of different reasons. Many have poor oral intake, posture problems, or display other behaviors that impede the ability to eat, some of which are of a cognitive nature. With age, there can also be significant decline in the neurologic pathways of swallowing. Many systemic diseases that are more prevalent in the elderly, such as blood and immunologic diseases, cardiac diseases, dermatologic diseases, diabetes, and gastroenterologic and pulmonary diseases can contribute to dysphagia.

II. PATHOPHYSIOLOGY

The loss of motor function in the oral cavity, pharynx, and larynx associated with increasing age is largely responsible for the prevalence of dysphagia in the elderly[1]. Neurogenic dysphagia can occur in the form of discrete brainstem cerebrovascular events, or small, undetectable periventricular infarcts invisible to MRI. Cadaveric studies of changes that take place in the ultrastructure of the human superior laryngeal nerve (SLN) during aging show that there is a statistically sig-

nificant decrease in the number of myelinated sensory fibers. In addition, a variety of medications required for the treatment of these and other major medical illnesses may cause or exacerbate neurogenic dysphagia[2]. Psychiatric disorders and other forms of cognitive impairment can also masquerade as swallowing problems. Whether punctuated by neurological events, naturally occurring processes of aging, or other systemic problems or external influences, swallowing function will tend to decline as one ages.

Swallowing can have particular implications in the elderly population due to increased use of medicine. Because of nutritional requirements and increased incidence of disease, the elderly must often consume more pills than other demographic groups. Dysphagia is already more common among the elderly, but pill dysphagia becomes amplified in this age group. Medications can injure the esophagus either by direct contact or through systemic action. Not surprisingly, the incidence of pill dysphagia is closely related to the diseases occurring more often in the elderly for which the medications are prescribed. Medicines also can induce slowed muscle function, or decreased pharyngeal sensation, thus adversely affecting the ability to swallow normally.

Nutritional problems commonly afflicting the elderly may be compounded by dysphagia[3]. For instance, a patient with diabetes may have existing diet restriction or have to eat more frequently. A patient with dysphagia suffering from high cholesterol may be at a health risk eating dairy foods such as pudding and thickened milk that would otherwise be a mainstay for the dysphagia diet. Similarly, a patient with congestive heart failure or renal or liver disease may have fluid restrictions and, in addition, suffer from solid food dysphagia, compounding his or her health problems. Patients who require higher fluid intake, such as those with diabetes, will encounter similar problems if dysphagic to liquids.

A more concentrated focus of life-threatening dysphagia occurs in the nursing home setting. Nearly 2 million Americans reside in 16700 nursing homes and other long-term-care facilities nationwide. The majority of these residents are elderly patients with chronic debilitating illnesses. Aspiration pneumonia is the leading cause of death in nursing homes and the leading cause of transfer of residents from nursing home to the hospital[4]. Among nursing home residents, swallowing dysfunction is manifest in two forms: aspiration and/or malnutrition. A patient's risk of aspiration and ability or inability to maintain an adequate oral diet provides the basis for nutritional decisions. Many nursing home residents lose the motivation and the physical ability to consume enough liquid and solid oral nutrition to sustain themselves. To avoid some combination of aspiration and malnutrition, patients and families must often be asked to make the difficult choice to accept limited oral feedings or NPO status and institute enteral tube feedings. These decisions not only affect a patient's care requirements and independence, but are also critical issues in the individual's quality of life.

The nursing home is a highly specialized health care environment because of the health problems that are specific to aging. The causes and complications of aspiration pneumonia are complex and often quite subtle. Aspiration pneumonia is rarely an isolated incident, more often it is a complication of one or several other medical conditions. There has been relatively little work done in examining its broad impact on the U.S. health care system.

Cerebrovascular disease (CVA) is a common admission diagnosis to nursing homes and many patients suffer recurrent CVAs. CVA is the second leading cause of death in the elderly, but strokes rarely result in sudden death[5]. Fatality is most often related to long-term complications from aspiration, urinary tract infections, decubitus ulcers, and other sequelae. The acute and long-term care of cerebrovascular disease has led to enormous monetary expenditures in our health care system, greater that $19.3 billion in 1993[4].

Stroke is probably the most common etiology of aspiration. Aspiration is common in stroke patients because of the combination of sensory and motor deficits that can lead to both swallowing dysfunction and a loss of laryngeal protection (see Chapters 15 and 16). Studies following stroke indicate that there is a 20% incidence of death due to aspiration pneumonia in the first year following stroke, and that 10% to 15% of deaths each subsequent year are from aspiration[3]. In the United States, those percentages represent a death rate of 40000 people per year because of poststroke aspiration.

Dysphagia is recorded in 30% of all stroke patients, but based on the authors' experience, the prevalence may actually be considerably higher. This is not surprising as the complications of dysphagia often become apparent only during the period of long-term rehabilitation. Dysphagia secondary to stroke may result in difficulty eating and/or inadequate oral nutrition, dehydration, or aspiration. Additionally patients unable to maintain an adequate oral diet, or who suffer from aspiration during their hospitalization for the acute stage of a CVA, may be quickly placed on alternative nutrition, thus deferring any evaluation of the swallowing mechanism until after they enter a chronic care facility. These patients may have much more functional ability than was appreciated during an initial evaluation or may have significant recovery in the weeks and months after a stroke. Thus, some patients are admitted to nursing homes with a tube in place for enteral nutrition, but may have the ability to safely resume an oral diet.

Nutritional deficiency is a far-reaching consequence of dysphagia and aspiration. It is often the underlying cause of many unwanted clinical outcomes and frequently is unappreciated. The factors affecting oral nutrition include taste, smell, desire, oral condition, oralpharyngeal transit, pharyngeal strength, cognitive ability, patient mood, and eating atmosphere. Recent studies have shown that 35% to 85% of the nursing home population are malnourished. An in-depth report on malnutrition in long-term-care settings found that the causes of malnutrition in nursing homes include inappropriate use of restricted diet, plus unmet needs for eating assistance, modified diet, and dysphagia workup[4].

Aspiration and malnutrition are further complicated in the elderly population because of nosocomial infections. Nosocomial infections in long-term-care residents have been reported to occur at an average of 4.6 infections per 1000 patient days[7]. Twenty-one percent of these infections occur in the respiratory tract and nosocomial pneumonia is the most frequent fatal infection. In a study of mostly neurologically disabled residents done by the Aspiration Pneumonia Task Force at Canandaigua Veterans Affairs Medical Center, 25% of a 257-person study group aspirated during an 8-month observation period. In 56% of the patients, aspiration progressed to nosocomial pneumonia. During the study period, patients who aspirated were at three times the risk of dying, compared with those who did not aspirate. In 3 years, only 17% of the patients who aspirated remained alive compared to 60% of those who did not aspirate.[7]

Dementia is a common sequela of cerebrovascular disease and a common diagnosis in patients suffering from malnutrition and dysphagia. Nationwide, according to the Nursing Home Survey of 1985, there were 974 300 nursing home residents with mental disorders and 45.4% required assistance eating.[4] This survey found that the predominant indication for a percutaneous endoscopic gastrostomy (PEG) tube was dementia (52%), followed by cerebrovascular accident (24%). Among the group with CVA, dysphagia was the indication for PEG in 30% of the patients.[7] Malnutrition secondary to swallowing difficulty is the most common sequela associated with dementia due to deterioration of higher cognitive functions.[8] Thus, those patients with both sequelae of stroke and dementia are at the highest risk to develop dysphagia and subsequent complications thereof.

III. DIAGNOSIS

The evaluation of a patient with symptoms of dysphagia involves two principal aspects: determination of the functional level of a patient's swallowing ability and the search for the etiology of the swallowing disorder. In an outpatient setting, acute hospitalization, or rehabilitation consultation, assessment of all possible underlying conditions responsible for a swallowing disorder is generally of the highest priority. Unearthing an etiologic diagnosis can supply a clinician with both diagnostic and prognostic information to coordinate treatment of both the dysphagia symptoms and related medical conditions.

In long-term-care facilities, however, patients customarily present with dysphagia symptoms related to established chronic medical conditions. The question of whether the new symptoms of a swallowing disorder are due to an additional medical problem or progression of a known disease process is a secondary priority. In the long-term-care environment, the crucial questions relate to quality of life, requirements for daily care, and establishing appropriate levels of medical intervention. The essential clinical issue for dysphagic patients in chronic care facilities is the level of swallowing ability balanced against the risk of aspiration and maintenance of adequate nutrition and hydration. Evaluation of swallowing competence is further, based on related or unrelated medical conditions, patient and family request, cognitive function, and patient cooperation. The swallowing evaluation, itself, and the impact

these other factors exert on decisions about a patient's swallowing safety will be defined as the functional diagnosis of swallowing.

Dysphagic patients in skilled nursing facilities often suffer from deteriorating swallowing function simply as a result of the aging process, as opposed to a single etiology. Loss of dentition, weakening of the oral and pharyngeal musculature, poor posture or positioning, and depression can all act on a patient's swallowing ability. Additionally, common chronic conditions such as arthritis, osteoporosis, senile dementia, and the loss of normal bowel function can influence oral intake and lead to relative or absolute malnutrition.[1] The clinician is obligated not only to make the crucial determination of the patient's swallowing competence, but to consider the fluctuation in medical status and the rate of deterioration of a patient's general condition.[9]

IV. FUNCTIONAL EVALUATION AND THERAPY

The initial evaluation of a dysphagic patient in a skilled nursing facility is made by the in-house speech-language pathologist (SLP) as a result of a referral from the primary physician or nursing staff. The referral may be made because of observation of clinical symptoms, an immediate medical history of aspiration or malnutrition, at the request of the patient or the patient's family, or due to a recent onset of a neurological condition that predisposes a patient to dysphagia or aspiration.

The speech-language pathologist performs a review of the medical and nutritional history and a bedside evaluation to determine the stage of dysphagia. Sometimes the dysphagia will be isolated to the oral stage. Patients lacking normal sensation, dentition and muscular coordination in the oral cavity may be inefficient in preparing the oral bolus, but swallow without difficulty after that. In such cases, the SLP can treat the oral dysphagia with the expectation that if oral management improves, so will swallowing ability. If pharyngeal dysphagia is suspected, further diagnostic investigation is indicated. Symptoms of pharyngeal dysphagia can include gurgling or wet voice, choking, regurgitation, chronic cough, decreased oral intake, watery eyes, slowed swallowing, and pneumonia.

At this point in the dysphagia evaluation, further, direct assessment of the pharyngeal stage of swallowing is often indicated. In long-term-care settings, a fiberoptic endoscopic evaluation of swallowing or videoendoscopic swallowing study (FEES or VESS) provides the information required to make a functional diagnosis.[10]

Videofluoroscopy has long been the preferred method for determining the etiology of a swallowing disorder, because of the comprehensive diagnostic information it provides. However, because it requires patient transport, it is comparatively unwieldy, expensive, and difficult to perform. Thus, it has been difficult to formulate a program to manage swallowing function in long-term-care settings based on fluoroscopic evaluation. In most cases, a videofluoroscopic swallow study provides more information than necessary to make a functional diagnosis. An efficient, bedside method of assessment is optimal for a program that manages swallowing disorders for the homebound or institution-bound elderly.

Utilizing FEES as part of a comprehensive swallowing management program in long-term-care facilities offers other significant advantages as well. The evaluation is performed in the presence of the treating speech-language pathologist who is responsible for carrying out the skilled training of the resident. This greatly improves the efficiency of the FEES both for tailoring the study and focusing the results toward future swallowing therapy. Nursing home patients sent to a hospital or radiology suite for tests are often unfamiliar to that clinical staff. Perception of a foreign situation can create fear and lack of cooperation that can affect test results. Without the presence of the treating SLP, there is no way to assess whether patient behavior during a study is typical or atypical. Working with the speech-language pathologist who knows the patient and how to maximize their swallowing ability helps to avoid unnecessary diet restrictions and consequent malnutrition. The presence of the treating speech-language pathologist during FEES helps ensure that a realistic diet level will be suggested based on everyday, empirical knowledge of a given patient's swallowing ability. Finally, as a participant in the initial diagnostic study, the treating SLP can best determine the patient's progress and the need for further or repeat evaluation by VESS or other methods.

To best determine the functional diagnosis, the in-house SLP and the clinician performing the FEES must define the purpose of the study prior to its execution. The swallowing evaluation provides the assessment of oral and pharyngeal swallowing function, but numerous external factors can also affect a patient's swallowing function. From a review of over 250 consecutive patients evaluated by the authors, we have found that there are four fundamental indications for FEES in the long-term-care setting: *documented aspiration event(s), suspected pharyngeal dysphagia or aspiration, inadequate oral intake,* and *request to upgrade oral diet.* Depending on which of the four indications is noted and the SLP's bedside assessment, the clinicians performing the VESS must prioritize the questions that the study is to answer and design the study to answer these questions in the safest and most effective manner.

The defining questions include: What is the patient's current level of swallowing function? This question,

which lies at the heart of the swallowing evaluation, is best answered by organized subsets of questions that define the quality and degree of swallowing dysfunction in relation to a patient's nutritional status.

The first subset of questions is geared toward establishing the nutritional status of the patient. How does the patient receive nutrition and hydration? If the patient receives his or her diet orally, is it restricted? Is the diet restriction limited to solid food, liquids, or some combination? The current nutritional status can be understood diagrammatically as a tree and the clinician should first find the terminal branch of the patient's diet level (Fig 53-1).

After the patient's dietary status is established, the consequent nutritional level must be determined. Is the nutrition adequate? If it is not, is it deficient calorically or is it insufficient to hydrate the patient? Is the patient maintaining his or her diet level safely and without difficulty? Is the target weight level being maintained?

Once the current diet level and its degree of adequacy are determined, the clinician faces the next set of questions: determining the goals of that particular evaluation. The initial evaluation is the starting point in developing these goals, but as alluded above, the patient's desires, lifestyle, general medical status, body positioning, and cognitive status can all alter the initial evaluation. The VESS will be geared to determining either adequacy or safety of the current diet level or some combination of the two.

Many times, a patient will be readmitted to a nursing home from a hospital with an enteral feeding tube or will have suffered a change in mental status that affects swallowing function while in the nursing home. In cases such as these, the adequacy of the oral diet often cannot be determined prior to the study. It is then necessary to determine during the course of the study on which level, if any, the patient can manage an oral diet. When the ability to manage an oral diet is at issue, the study is performed to determine the amount the patient can consume and the efficiency of consumption. For these patients, cognitive status must be considered carefully. For example, if a patient has undergone multiple cerebrovascular events or is suffering from progressive organic brain syndrome, the patient may have severe fluctuations in awareness and function. If the management of an oral diet is in question, then the patient's cognition must be consistent enough to maintain his or her oral diet at a nutritionally sufficient level. In cases of fluctuating cognition, it may be necessary to do a follow-up study within a month to ensure safety.

If the FEES is designed primarily to determine safety of a currently maintained diet level, then swallowing competence must be tested on all food consistencies to determine safety, rather than efficiency of swallowing. If a patient is tube dependent, a VESS is often indicated to determine whether a patient can tolerate a recre-

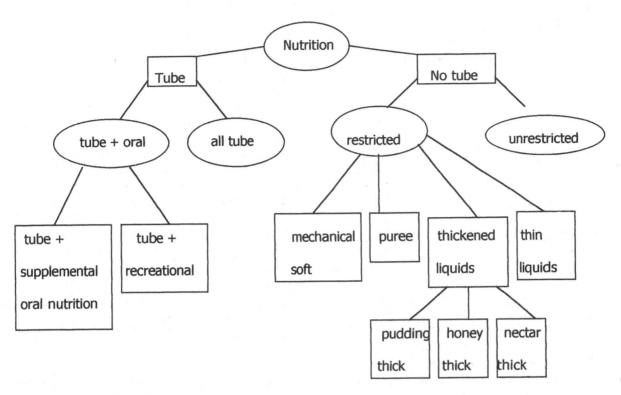

Fig 53-1. Decision tree for patient diet status.

ational oral diet or nutritionally supplemental oral feedings. For patients at this functional level, it is necessary to first observe how they manage their own secretions and to test for sensation. If secretions are pooled or passively aspirated or pharyngeal sensation is decreased, the examiner must proceed with extreme caution in feeding the patient. In patients with enteral feedings, issues of mental status and cognition are not quite as important as the patient who depends on oral intake for sustenance. When a tube is in place, if cognitive status wanes at any time, nutrition can be maintained well through the tube feedings.

Determination of the adequacy and safety of a patient's diet level can be complex. A number of other considerations deserve the attention of the clinician. One factor that can influence decision making is body position. If the patient is contracted or has a permanent lean to one side or the other, there may be a risk for aspiration because the patient may not have sufficient oral-motor compensatory abilities to manage the pharyngeal bolus under these circumstances. Sometimes it is helpful to try to adjust a patient's posture during a study to note the effect on swallowing competence, but it is important to be realistic about a patient's habits of position during consumption. Unless skilled speech-pathology assistance is recommended during all feedings, which is many times impossible, the patient may be fed in a position that compromises swallowing function. This should be taken into account. Patient cooperation can also compel clinical decision making. If a pa-

tient refuses to comply with compensatory swallowing maneuvers, or will not consume enough food to self-maintain nutrition, then appropriate diet restrictions or alternate feedings should be considered. Finally, ultimate prognosis can change the entire focus of a patient's swallowing problem. A patient might be at some risk to develop aspiration pneumonia, but in light of a diagnosis of a terminal disease, a continued oral diet may be quite reasonable to maintain a certain quality of life with known, established risks.

A team approach has several advantages when using VESS. An in-house speech-language pathologist knows the patient and is most aware of the current swallowing status and potential goals of a swallowing study. The patient may also be more willing to cooperate with the SLP who feeds or treats the patient regularly, resulting in a study that best represents the patients eating behavior. There is also significant benefit in having two sets of hands during a study. It is often necessary to control or calm the patient to some degree during placement of the endoscope, and, once the scope is placed, one person must operate it while the other feeds the patient the various food consistencies and perhaps guides compensatory maneuvers. Finally, having two evaluators rather than one reduces the risk of clinical error and increases the knowledge base for deciding appropriate dietary measures.

Patient cooperation may affect the way a study is performed. If a patient seems disturbed by the placement of the endoscope it may be useful to wait until the patient relaxes to get a study that reflects the patient's swallowing ability. Similarly, first trials are often not reflective of ability and multiple trials should always be employed when safety permits. If the patient becomes extremely uncooperative during a study, the clinician might be required to quickly assess the highest priority issue of the patient's swallowing function before the study must be aborted.

The most fundamental decision to make during FEES is the patient's risk of aspiration. Depending on the information provided by the in-house speech-language pathologist, the examiners should ascertain the approximate risk of aspiration prior to performance of a study. Determining the relative risk is important in guiding the path that the study will take. If the examiners conclude that the patient is at high risk for aspiration, the study should begin with feeding that person's lowest risk consistency, most often puree or thickened liquids. If the FEES begins with a consistency that the patient aspirates entirely, he or she is put at-risk for developing pneumonia from the study itself or, at the very least, an initial aspiration event can alter swallowing function in the remainder of the study. Sometimes a thorough examination of the patient's status regarding bronchopulmonary secretions and retention in the pyriform sinuses before the swallowing trials begin can provide more than enough information to terminate the study. If there is evidence of salivary aspiration with retained secretions, or passive salivary aspiration during the initial part of the study and there is deficient vocal fold sensation, the study should be discontinued and the patient designated or continued as NPO.

From the authors' experience, it is most effective to begin a study with solids and work through the progression of consistencies toward thin liquids. A patient at low risk for aspiration is most likely to aspirate thin liquids. If the study begins on thin liquids and the patient aspirates this consistency, the aspiration event can adversely alter or terminate the remainder of the study. The clinician might also keep in mind that the incidence of aspiration will increase as the patient tires over the course of the study. Similarly, when a patient's nutritional status is in question, the study should begin on solids and proceed to liquids, with the hope that liquid may wash down retained solid material in the tongue base, vallecula, and pyriform sinuses.

When the indication for the study is a request to upgrade the diet from a current level to another consistency, the examiner should start the patient on the consistency known to be tolerated well and either move up or down in consistency toward the desired level of consumption.

Because the nursing home environment implies such specific health care demands, it is only natural that a swallowing program in the nursing home environment would be tailored to deal specifically with those demands. A program that effectively evaluates and manages swallowing disorders in the elderly can limit the incidence of aspiration and, thus, reduce mortality, morbidity, and the costs of extensive medical evaluation and treatment.[11] Such a program can also provide accurate, timely information to guide the patient, family, and medical staff in the nutritional decisions critical to health and quality of life. The authors have developed a program that effectively handles swallowing concerns in the elderly.[12] The program is based on a team concept of evaluation by a speech-language pathologist, consulting otolaryngologist, and attending physician, as well as the other caretakers. It utilizes FEES on site to gain detailed diagnostic information about the swallowing mechanism.

Recently, the present authors conducted a pilot study of the first 122 subjects to be evaluated under the protocol. Examination of the cost-effectiveness of the available diagnostic protocols used to manage swallowing disorders in this population suggest that FEES should be considered routinely as an alternative to radiographic swallowing studies.[12]

All patients were referred for evaluation by their primary physician or by an in-house speech-language pathologist. The speech-language pathologist performed a bedside evaluation of each patient and made initial diagnoses of oral and/or pharyngeal impairment. In some cases, the results of other evaluations completed during recent hospital admissions, including videoendoscopic and videofluoroscopic studies, were also available.

All the evaluated patients underwent a videoendoscopic swallow study. Each study was performed by an otolaryngologist and a speech-language pathologist working as a team and viewing the studies as they were performed. The nursing home residents were studied either in a wheelchair or in a sitting or semisitting position in their beds. When indicated by the in-house speech-language pathologist, patients were reexamined at a later date for further evaluation. Indications for examination included coughing after meals, episodes of pneumonia of unknown etiology, a "wet" or gurgling sound in the voice, failure to maintain adequate oral nutrition, and choking. One year after the first swallowing evaluation was performed, the authors concluded the study period and recorded the diet level, aspiration status, and medical status of the patient group.

The average age of nursing home residents included in the study was 83 years with a range from 42 to 103 years. Seventy-two percent of the residents evaluated were female and 28% were male, the exact proportion reported by the National Nursing Home Survey in 1985 for nursing home patients across the United States.[8] Instead of reflecting a gender differential in swallowing disorder prevalence, these numbers are probably related to nursing home demographics, in general. The average age of evaluation in our study is greater than the average life span for a male in the U.S.

The average length of follow up was 5.3 months, with study periods ranging from 1 month to 1 year. Twenty-nine patients, or about 24%, died over the course of the study. The average age of the deceased group was 85 years and the age range at death was 69 to 102 years. There was no incidence of death by aspiration of oral feeding for the patients whose swallowing function was evaluated in this program. VESS was performed successfully on all patients for whom it was requested and there were no complications of VESS procedures. The population of this study was divided into four groups based on their dietary level at the time of the evaluation: residents with no oral feeding (NPO), those completely restricted from a liquid diet, those who tolerated thick liquids but were restricted from thin liquids, and residents who could swallow thin liquids (Table 53-1).

In the entire study population, 73% of the patients initiated and maintained suggested diet levels with good success over the course of the study. Of the 27% who did not tolerate diet recommendations, 32% had deteriorated in their medical status. As multiple studies were not performed on every patient with a change in medical status over the study period, it is difficult to quantify what effect these changes had on swallowing ability in that 32%.

Appropriate management and early intervention in nursing home patients with swallowing disorders provides benefits to the patients, their families, and to the physicians, nurses, and therapists involved in patient care. A protocol for evaluation and therapy based on videoendoscopic swallowing studies is convenient, cost-effective, and can improve the quality of life for residents.

References

1. Patterson WG. Dysphagia in the elderly. *Can Fam Physician*. 1996;42:925-932.
2. Stoschus B, Allescher HD. Drug-induced dysphagia. *Dysphagia*. 1993;8:154-159.
3. Sullivan DH, Walls RC. Impact of nutritional status on morbidity in a population of geriatric rehabilitation patients. *J Amer Geriatr Soc*. 1994:42:471-477.
4. National Nursing Home Survey. *J Vital Health Stat*. 1985; 1-18.
5. Horner J, Massey EW. Silent aspiration following stroke. *Neurology*. 1988;38:317-319.
6. Nelson KJ, Coulston AM, Sucher KP, Tseng RY. Prevalence of malnutrition in the elderly admitted to long-term-care facilities. *J Amer Diet Assoc*. 1993;93:459-461.
7. Pick N, McDonald A, Bennett N, et al. Pulmonary aspiration in a long term care setting: Clinical and laboratory observations and an analysis of risk factors. *J Amer Geriatr Soc*. 1996;44:763-768.
8. Robbins J, Hamilton JW, Lof GL, Kempster GB. Oropharyngeal swallowing in normal adults of different ages. *Gastroenterology*. 1992;103:823-829.
9. Gillen P, Spore D, Mor V, Freiberger W. Functional and residential status transitions among nursing home residents. *J Gerontol: Biol Sci and Med Sci*. 1996;51:M29-M36.
10. Aviv JE, Martin JH, Jones ME, et al. Age-related changes in pharyngeal and supraglottic sensation. *Ann Otol Rhinol Laryngol*. 1994;103:749-752.
11. Barker WH, Zimmer JG, Hall WJ, et al. Rates, patterns, causes and costs of hospitalization of nursing home residents: a population-based study. *Amer J Public Health*. 1994;84:1615-1620.
12. Spiegel J, Creed J, Sataloff RT. Evaluation and Management of Swallowing Disorders in Long Term Care Settings: A Program Utilizing Videoendoscopic Assessment. 1998. (in press)

Table 53-1. *Dietary Levels of Subjects*

Diet Level	No. Patients	Deceased	Patients Following Diet Suggestion	% Following Diet Suggestion	No. Not Following Diet Suggestion	No. Not Following Diet Suggestion with Change in Medical Status
NPO	24	4	16	80	4	2
Puree	13	5	4	50	4	0
Thick liquid	59	13	34	74	12	5
Thin liquid	26	7	14	74	5	1
All patients	122	29	68	73	25	8

CHAPTER 54

■ ■ ■

The Terminal Patient: Palliation of Dysphagia in Advanced Esophageal Cancer

Ninh T. Nguyen, M.D.
James D. Luketich, M.D.

I. INTRODUCTION

The number of new cases of esophageal cancer in 1996 was approximately 12 300, and 11 200 patients will likely die of their disease.[1] Up to 50% of patients diagnosed with esophageal carcinoma have advanced, inoperable disease at the time of presentation, which accounts in part for a dismal 5-year survival rate of only 5%-10%. In addition, esophageal cancer frequently occurs in elderly patients with associated poor medical conditions, prohibiting them from pursuing a surgical option.

The primary goals for these patients are to provide relief of dysphagia or odynophagia, to improve nutritional status, and consequently to improve the quality of life. Restoration of swallowing is an important determinant of overall quality of life in patients presenting with dysphagia caused by malignancies. Improvement of dysphagia correlates with an improvement in quality of life. The ideal palliative methods must be effective, have low morbidity, low mortality, require minimal or no hospital stay, be cost-effective, and be long lasting. Ideally, the palliative treatment should last until the patient succumbs to the cancer.

Multiple modalities are currently available for palliation of dysphagia. These modalities includes surgery, photodynamic therapy, expandable metal stents, Nd:YAG laser therapy, radiation therapy, and endoluminal brachytherapy.

II. PATHOPHYSIOLOGY

The most common manifestation of esophageal cancer is progressive dysphagia. Other symptoms include odynophagia, regurgitation, weight loss, and aspiration pneumonia. The elasticity of the esophagus allows swallowing even when it is partially obstructed. Thus, the majority of patients with esophageal cancer present at an advanced stage, only seeking treatment for dysphagia after the luminal diameter of the esophagus has been reduced by more than 50%.

III. DIAGNOSIS

The first diagnostic test in the evaluation of patients with dysphagia should be a barium swallow esophagogram. The barium swallow esophagogram provides a "road map" of the esophagus, providing information on the site of luminal narrowing, the degree and length of obstruction, and the presence of concomitant tracheoesophageal fistula. Fiberoptic flexible esophagoscopy with biopsy can be performed following the barium swallow to confirm the diagnosis of malignancy and further assess the extent of esophageal and gastric involvement. Bronchoscopy, in addition to esophagoscopy, is necessary to evaluate the trachea and left mainstem bronchus for possible transmural involvement in patients with cancer in the upper one third of the esophagus.

Once the diagnosis of esophageal cancer is established, a computed tomography (CT) scan of the chest and abdomen is helpful to evaluate the presence of loco-regional involvement or distant metastases. The role of positron emission tomography (PET) scan is currently being investigated for staging of esophageal cancer. In an initial study of 35 patients, PET improved the ability to identify unsuspected distant metastases in 20% of patients who had a negative survey by conventional imaging.[2] In addition, minimally invasive surgical staging using a combination of laparoscopy and thoracoscopy is under investigation for staging esophageal cancer at our institution.[3] Luketich et al, using minimally invasive surgical staging, identified distant metastases in 15% of patients with a negative CT of the chest and abdomen.[3] Thus, using more accurate staging protocols, patients who are determined to have limited disease may undergo surgical resection, patients with loco-regional disease undergo neoadjuvant chemotherapy, and patients with distant metastases are eligible for palliative therapies.

IV. TREATMENT

A. Surgical Palliation

Although surgery can provide excellent palliation for malignant dysphagia, it is rarely performed in patients with unresectable esophageal cancer because of the associated high morbidity, mortality, and the need for prolonged hospitalization in a category of patients with a life expectancy of less than 6 months. Surgical bypass, however, is an option for palliating dysphagia in a patient with good performance status for whom conventional palliative methods have been ineffective. The operative approach for palliation includes the conventional transhiatal esophagectomy, limited abdominal esophageal resection with low hiatus anastomosis, or, more recently, minimally invasive esophagectomy. Minimally invasive esophagectomy utilizes laparoscopic and/or thoracoscopic techniques to perform the esophagectomy.[4,5] Alternatively, a gastrostomy or jejunostomy tube can be surgically placed to provide enteral feedings, but the quality of life is diminished by depriving the patient of taking food by mouth (see Chapter 4.)

B. Endoscopic Palliation

The primary nonsurgical method for palliation of dysphagia is endoscopy. Endoscopic modalities include the ablation of tumor using Nd:YAG laser or bipolar electrocautery, photodynamic therapy, balloon dilation, placement of expandable metal stents, or endoesophageal brachytherapy.

1. Balloon Dilatation

One of the simplest, but least effective, methods of endoscopic palliation is balloon dilation (Fig 54-1). Hydrostatic balloon dilatation can be performed under conscious sedation with the use of fluoroscopy. The advantages of balloon dilatation are that it is simple, inexpensive, and easy to perform. The disadvantages are the risk of perforation and that the benefits are short-lived. This procedure is not recommended as the primary therapy for palliation of dysphagia as the duration of palliation may be as short as a few days.

2. Nd:YAG Laser Therapy

The Nd:YAG laser (neodymium yttrium aluminum garnet) has been used extensively for palliation of patients presenting with inoperable esophageal carcinoma. Nd:YAG laser therapy is performed through the endoscope, typically under intravenous sedation. The laser utilizes thermal energy (1064 nm) to cause tumor necrosis. In one large series, Nd:YAG was used as a palliative treatment for malignant dysphagia in 224 patients over a period of 8 years.[6] The esophageal lumen was successfully reopened in 98.2%, and 93.7% were able to ingest at least semisolids following the therapy.

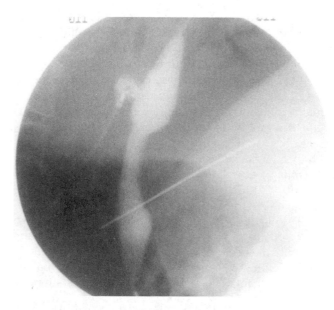

FIG 54-1. Balloon dilation of obstructing esophagus cancer under fluoroscopic guidance.

Esophageal perforation occurred in 2.7% in this series. Bourke et al also reported Nd:YAG laser therapy to be an effective initial palliation of inoperable malignant dysphagia in 70 consecutive patients.[7] Ninety-six percent of patients were palliated initially with one perforation (1.4%). The mean total number of laser treatment sessions was 3.4 with a mean interval of 27.2 days between each laser session.

3. Photodynamic Therapy

Photodynamic therapy (PDT) is a relatively new modality recently approved by the Food and Drug Administration for palliation of obstructive esophageal carcinoma. Using this method, a photosensitizing agent (Photofrin, Sanofi Winthrop, Inc., New York, NY) is injected intravenously. There is relative retention of this agent in tumor cell groups, compared to normal tissue. After a delay of 48 hours, endoscopy is performed and a red light (630 nm) is delivered through an optical quartz fiber to the site of the obstructing tumor. The 630 nm light activates Photofrin to an excited state that, in return, activates oxygen to produce singlet oxygen, hydroxy radical, and superoxide radicals. The propagation of these radicals results in endothelial damage, and vascular occlusion, with subsequent tumor necrosis (Fig 54-2). Lightdale et al reported results from a multi-center randomized trial evaluating 236 patients, in which PDT was compared to Nd:YAG laser for palliation of esophageal cancer.[8] The improvement of dysphagia was equivalent between the two groups, but PDT caused fewer acute perforations than Nd:YAG laser therapy (1% after PDT and 7% after Nd:YAG). The most common side effect is photosensitivity, which can last up to 6 weeks. Complications of PDT are minimal and may include nausea, fever, pleural effusion, and photosensitivity leading to sunburn.

At the University of Pittsburgh, 44 patients were treated with 75 courses of PDT for obstructing esophageal cancer over a single year period. There was a significant reduction in the mean preoperative dysphagia score (1 for no dysphagia to 5 for complete obstruction) from 3.2 to 1.9 postoperatively (p<0.05) (Table 54-1). Nineteen patients (43%) required more than one PDT course, and the mean time interval between PDT courses was 57 days. The 30-day mortality was 9%. In addition, PDT was used to treat 7 patients who initially achieved good palliation with an expandable metal stent, but who subsequently developed tumor ingrowth or spread of the tumor beyond the boundaries of the stent, leading to recurrent dysphagia. All patients reported improved dysphagia scores following PDT treatment.

4. Expandable Metal Stents

Deployment of esophageal stents has been a common method for palliation of malignant dysphagia. Until recently, most esophageal stents were plastic, difficult to place, and associated with a high complication rate. The introduction of expandable metal stents has essentially led to replacement of the use of the plastic endoprostheses. The expandable metal stents are placed with fluoroscopic guidance under conscious sedation. There are several different metal stents available. The esophageal Z stent (Wilson-Cook, Inc., Winston-Salem, NC) consists of a urethane-coated, steel wire mesh. In one study, the use of a 21 mm flanged Z stent resulted

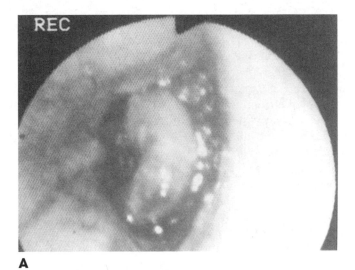

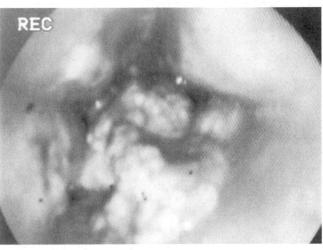

A **B**

Fɪɢ 54-2. A. Obstructing esophagus cancer prior to photodynamic therapy treatment. **B.** Endoscopic view of esophageal tumor showing tumor necrosis 48 hours following photodynamic therapy.

Table 54-1. *Dysphagia Score*

Grade 1 = No obstruction

Grade 2 = Difficulty with hard solids

Grade 3 = Difficulty with soft solids

Grade 4 = Difficulty with liquids

Grade 5 = Difficulty with liquids, including saliva

in excellent palliation of dysphagia but a high immediate complication rate (27% migration).[9] Recently, Kozarek and colleagues reported a decreased migration rate using a new 25 mm flanged Z stent.[10] Another commercially available stent is the EsophaCoil stent (InStent, Eden Prairie, MN). This prosthesis is composed of a flat nickel titanium alloy coil spring wrapped tightly on an introducer catheter that shortens and widens on release. Minimal clinical data are available regarding the use of this new prosthesis.[11]

In our experience, 64 expandable stents were placed in 50 patients for malignant esophageal obstruction (Fig 54-3). Either the Ultraflex stent (Boston Scientific Corp., Watertown, MA) or the Wallstent (Schneider Inc., Minneapolis, MN) were used. Immediate improvement in dysphagia score was reported in over 90% of patients. The mean dysphagia score decreased from 3.0 to 1.7 following stent placement (p = 0.001). There were no procedure-related mortalities. Early complications included chest pain, nausea, food impaction, stent dysfunction, stent migration, and perforation. Late complications were primarily tumor ingrowth and overgrowth.

C. Radiation Therapy

External beam radiation therapy (EBRT) has been one of the most common approaches in the management of obstructing esophageal cancer. EBRT can relieve dysphagia in 50%-70% of patients, using dosages ranging from 20 Gy-64 Gy delivered in varying fraction sizes.[12] Dysphagia may temporarily worsen during the course of therapy. Complications of radiation therapy includes esophagitis, stricture, and tracheoesophageal fistula. One of the major concerns of EBRT is the requirement for up to 4 weeks of outpatient treatment, with delays in improvement of dysphagia for several weeks. With the advent of expandable metal stents and photodynamic therapy, the role of EBRT for palliating dysphagia has been questioned. The SORTIE (stent versus radiation therapy) trial, sponsored by the Medical University of South Carolina, is currently underway to evaluate the efficacy of EBRT compared to expandable metal stents for palliation of esophageal obstruction.

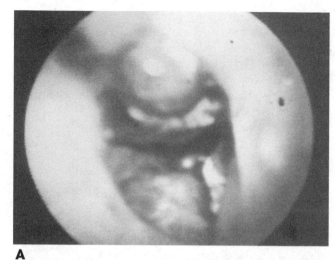

A

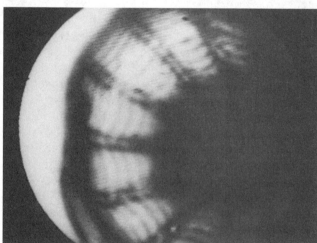

B

FIG 54-3. A. Bulky endoluminal obstructing esophagus cancer. **B.** Open esophageal lumen following deployment of an expandable metal stent.

The clinical endpoint in this randomized trial is improvement in dysphagia score.

Brachytherapy involves applying a radioactive source close to the tumor to maximize the delivery of radiation while minimizing its side effects. Palliation using brachytherapy involves an intensive short-course of intracavitary irradiation. The sources (cesium-137 or iridium-192) are placed through a nasogastric applicator. The treatment reported by Harvey and coworkers consisted of either a 1250 cGy given in a single fraction (high dose) or 2000 cGy in 3 fractions (low dose) given on alternating days.[13] Dysphagia was relieved in greater than 90% of patients. The duration of palliation was 4.5 months for those receiving the high dose and 5.1 months for the low dose group. The relief of dysphagia is faster with brachytherapy, but it carries a higher risk of esophagitis and expertise with endoesophageal brachytherapy is not universally available.

V. CONTROVERSIES

Palliation of dysphagia is the most important factor affecting the quality of life in the patients with malignant dysphagia. The ideal method for palliation of dysphagia should be safe, effective, low-cost, with minimal morbidity and mortality. Currently, there is no single preferred method of palliation. The availability of multiple palliative modalities indicates that the ideal treatment has not been established. One modality is often chosen over another based on the availability of instrumentation, characteristics of the tumor, the physician's expertise, the patient's preference and performance status, and patient participation in clinical trial. Therefore, it is important that the physician acquires knowledge and expertise in several different techniques to adequately treat malignant obstruction. At our institution, we are currently using PDT as the primary modality to treat malignant dysphagia. We have demonstrated that PDT is ideal for the palliation of dysphagia associated with a predominantly endoluminal obstruction, yielding a 85% success rate. Deployment of an expandable metal stent is effective to palliate patients with a significant extrinsic compression component.

References

1. Parker SL, Tong T, Bolden S, Wingo PA. Cancer statistics, 1996. *CA J Clin*. 1996;46:5-27.
2. Luketich JD, Schauer PR, Meltzer CC, et al. Role of positron emission tomography in staging the patient with esophageal cancer. *Ann Thorac Surg*. 1997;64:765-769.
3. Luketich JD, Schauer P, Landreneau R, et al. Minimally invasive surgical staging is superior to endoscopic ultrasound in detecting lymph node metastases in esophageal cancer. *J Thorac Cardiovasc Surg*. 1997;114:817-823.
4. Luketich JD, Nguyen NT, Schauer PR. Laparoscopic transhiatal esophagectomy for Barrett=s esophagus with high-grade dysplasia. *J Soc Laparoendosc Surg*. 1998;2:75-77.
5. DePaula A, Hashiba K, Ferreira EA, DePaula RA, Grecco E. Laparoscopic transhiatal esophagectomy with esophagogastroplasty. *Surg Laparosc Endosc*. 1995;5:1-5.
6. Maciel J, Barbosa J, Leal AS. Nd-YAG laser as a palliative treatment for malignant dysphagia. *Eur J Surg Oncol*. 1996;22:69-73.
7. Bourke MJ, Hope RL, Chu G, et al. Laser palliation of inoperable malignant dysphagia: initial and at death. *Gastrointest Endosc*. 1996;43:29-32.
8. Lightdale CJ, Heier SK, Marcon NE, et al. Photodynamic therapy with porfimer sodium versus thermal ablation therapy with Nd:YAG for palliation of esophageal cancer: a multicenter randomized trial. *Gastrointest Endosc*. 1995;42:507-512.
9. Kozarek RA, Raltz S, Brugge WR, et al. Prospective multicenter trial of esophageal Z stent placement for malignant dysphagia and tracheoesophageal fistula. *Gastrointest Endosc*. 1996;44:562-567.
10. Kozarek RA, Raltz S, Marcon N, et al. Use of the 25 mm flanged esophageal Z stent for malignant dysphagia: a prospective multicenter trial. *Gastrointest Endosc*. 1997;46: 156-160.
11. Goldin E, Beyar M, Safra T, et al. A new self-expandable, nickel-titanium coil stent for esophageal obstruction: a preliminary report. *Gastrointest Endosc*. 1994;40:64-68.
12. Reed CE. Comparison of different treatments for unresectable esophageal cancer. *World J Surg*. 1995;19:828-835.
13. Harvey JC, Fleischman EH, Bellotti JE, Kagan RA. Intracavitary radiation in the treatment of advanced esophageal carcinoma: a comparison of high dose rate vs. low dose rate brachytherapy. *J Surg Onc*. 1993;52:101-104.

CHAPTER 55

■ ■ ■

Aspiration Pneumonia

Magdy N. Falestiny, M.D.
Victor L. Yu, M.D.

I. INTRODUCTION

Aspiration may be acute or chronic. Although aspiration of oropharyngeal secretions is commonly seen in up to 45% of normal humans during sleep, the mucocilliary cellular lining of the tracheobronchial tree and the alveolar macrophages provide sufficient clearance to prevent infection.[1] Silent aspiration can occur especially in elderly patients as the protective closure reflex of the larynx becomes less dynamic and may represent up to 70% of community-acquired pneumonia in this group of patients.

II. ETIOLOGY

Aspiration syndromes can be divided into three forms distinguished on the basis of their pathophysiological characteristics: (a) chemical pneumonitis, (b) bacterial infection, and (c) acute airway obstruction.[2] The severity of aspiration depends on the amount, nature, consistency, and pH of the aspirate, cough reflex, and the host defense mechanisms. Aspiration of liquid material may disseminate in the lung fields by coughing or deep inspiration reaching to the peripheral alveoli. Moreover, aspiration of oropharyngeal or gastric secretion admixed with food may gravitate in the dependent parts of the lung, being the posterior segments of the upper or lower lobes in recumbent patients.

Aging causes a gradual increase in pharyngeal transit duration and a decrease in clearance of the laryngeal vestibule and esophageal motility (see Chapter 52). Several underlying diseases, shown in Table 55-1, predispose to aspiration. Nearly 70% of patients with altered mental status, regardless of the underlying disease, aspirate possibly because of the inability to protect the airways and the discoordination between breathing and swallowing. Dysphagia may result from several neuromuscular diseases. Conditions causing incompetency of the lower esophageal sphincter (LES) may promote gastroesophageal acid reflux (GER) and also predispose to aspiration. The frequent use of percutaneous or surgically placed gastrostomy feeding tubes in patients who fail to thrive may also cause aspiration of gastric contents and feeding formulas. Esophageal diseases and disorders of gastric motility may increase the risk of aspiration of gastric contents, especially if vomiting occurs frequently.

Patients with cerebrovascular accidents (CVA), multiple sclerosis (MS), and amyotrophic lateral sclerosis (ALS) are at increased risk for aspiration secondary to supraglottic and pharyngeal abnormalities. Aspiration is a common finding in cases with abrupt loss of consciousness, such as seizure disorders, because of lack of airway protection and frequent need for immediate tracheal intubation. Numerous pharmacologic agents affect the LES, leading to acid reflux and precipitate aspiration, especially anticholinergic and anesthetic agents.

Table 55–1. *Risk Factors for Aspiration*

Altered Level of Consciousness
Head trauma
Coma
Cerebrovascular accidents
Metabolic encephalopathy
Seizure disorders
General anesthesia
Drug/alcohol intoxication
Excessive sedation
Cardiopulmonary arrest

Neuromuscular Disorders
Parkinson's disease
Cranial neuropathy
Muscular dystrophy
Guillain-Barré syndrome
Myasthenia gravis
Polymyositis-dermatomyositis
Dysphagia
Vocal fold paralysis

Gastrointestinal Dysfunction
Scleroderma
Esophageal stricture
Gastroesophageal reflux
Erosive esophagitis
Zenker's diverticulum
Tracheoesophageal fistula
Esophageal cancer
Hiatal hernia
Pyloric stenosis/gastric outlet obstruction
Entral feeding
Pregnancy
Anorexia/bulimia

Iatrogenic
Prolonged mechanical ventilatory support
Tracheotomy
Anticholinergic drugs

Miscellaneous
Obesity
Neck malignancies

Although antacids and histamine type 2 (H2) receptors antagonists are used frequently in the prophylaxis against aspiration, both agents increase the gastric pH, but have no effect on the volume of gastric secretions. Even more, the higher pH induced by these agents may lead to colonization of the stomach by gram-negative organisms that are prevalent in the intensive care units.

Patients requiring prolonged mechanical ventilation and patients with a tracheostomy are especially at risk for aspiration.[3,4] Aspiration can occur after only 2 weeks on mechanical ventilation and nearly 85% of these patients fail modified barium swallow testing (MBS) with fluoroscopy for detection of aspiration. Many factors are implicated in swallowing dysfunction in these patients, including laryngeal edema, anatomic changes, cough impairment, esophageal compression, limitation of laryngeal elevation, decrease the sensitivity of the larynx, and the use of sedatives and neuro-

muscular blocking agents. Furthermore, deflation of the cuff may allow the migration of pooled oropharyngeal secretions to the lower airways. The risk of aspiration may persist after extubation, or decannulation, because of the delayed recovery or lack of treatment of the pharyngeal phase of swallowing.

III. CHEMICAL PNEUMONITIS

Instillation of acid into the tracheobronchial tree has been shown to cause profound bronchospasm and serious airway reaction in canine models. This type of pneumonitis was first described by Mendelson in obstetric patients aspirating gastric contents under general anesthesia. This condition is also seen in several medical and surgical conditions. The caustic effect of the gastric content on the tracheobronchial mucosa depends on the gastric pH. Serious mucosal damage occurs with pH less than 2.5, although aspiration of bile causes a similar degree of injury. Acute findings in acid aspiration-induced lung injury include mucosal edema, hemorrhage, and focal ulceration, followed by the development of focal necrosis and diffuse alveolar hyaline membrane formation. As bronchial mucosal cells endure the chemical insult, the surfactant production is greatly diminished, causing subsequent capillary leakage, bronchorrhea, decrease in lung compliance, and alteration in gas exchange. Aspiration of gastric contents mixed with food induces peribronchial inflammation and mononuclear granulomatous response. However, direct acid injury to the mucosal membrane is likely to be limited by the rapid neutralization by mucosal secretions. Aspiration of acidic material provokes the release of proinflammatory cytokines, promoting the recruitment and activation of polymorphonuclear neutrophils into the air spaces. When the amount of aspirated gastric content is small, resolution is usually rapid and repair of the injury is undertaken by alveolar macrophages and type II pneumocytes.

Aspiration of large volumes of gastric contents causes serious complications including respiratory failure and acute respiratory distress syndrome (ARDS), and nearly 20% of patients die secondary to the aspiration. For immunocompromised and chronically ill patients, this chemical insult is likely to be followed by infection as the aspirate is usually colonized by enteric bacteria, leading to direct inoculation to the damaged lung.

Finally, lipid (lipoid) pneumonia is aspiration of oil-based liquid such as mineral oil given as a laxative, oil-based nasal spray, or contrast material. Infiltrates seen on chest radiography predominantly involve the lower lobes. There is minimal acute inflammatory response and the alveolar air spaces are filled with lipid-laden macrophages that gradually coalesce, forming multinucleated giant cells surrounded by fibrous tissue bands, but true granulomas do not evolve.

IV. BACTERIAL INFECTION

Aspiration carries significant risk for pleuropulmonary infection. The development of pneumonia, necrotizing pneumonia, lung abscess, or empyema depends in part on the size of bacterial inoculum, the virulence of a specific organism, and the host defenses.[5] In ventilator-associated pneumonias in an ICU, aspiration of oropharyngeal bacteria is the primary pathogenic mechanism. The pathogens are polymicrobial, although anaerobes may dominate (Table 55-2). The major anaerobic isolates are *Fusobacterium nucleatum, Peptostreptococcccus,* and *Bacteroides* species. *Bacteroides fragilis* are not normal oral flora, although they have been isolated in some case series of aspiration pneumonia. Aerobic bacteria in the oropharyngeal secretions include microaerophilic streptococci, *Moraxella catarrhalis,* and *Eikenella corrodens.*

Colonization of the oropharynx with nosocomially acquired organisms is seen in several conditions such as periodontal diseases, alcoholism, and chronically debilitated and immunosuppressed hospitalized patients. In hospitalized patients, the alteration in gastric acidity by antacids and H-2 blockers also predispose to colonization of gram-negative enteric organisms in the gastric secretions. Acquired pathogens include *S. aureus,* Enterobacteriaceae (such as *E. coli, Klebsiella pneumoniae, Enterobacter* species, *Serratia marescens*) and *Pseudomonas aeruginosa.* Lung abscess and empyema are commonly seen in infection with *S. aureus, Klebsiella pneumoniae,* and *P. aeruginosa* and tend to pursue a rapid onset. Anaerobic necrotizing pneumonia usually follows a smoldering subacute course.

V. DIAGNOSIS

A. Clinical Evaluations

Aspiration of small amount of oropharyngeal secretions and gastric contents may go unnoticed by a patient or physician. In conscious patients, initial symptoms of aspiration may include cough, stridor, dyspnea, tachypnea, cyanosis, wheezing, weak voice, and palpitation. Aspiration of larger particulate material may cause sudden airway obstruction resulting in choking, apnea, cyanosis, and death. Aphonia occurs if the particulate material lodges at the level of the vocal folds. In unconscious patients, especially those requiring mechanical ventilation, fever, hypoxia, and excessive tracheal secretions may suggest pneumonia. The recovery of feeding formulas or emesis in the tracheal aspirate from these patients provides strong evidence of aspiration.

Findings on lung examination are nonspecific and may reveal wheezing, crackles, or bronchial or diminished breath sounds. Fever and foul-smelling sputum production can occur; the latter is a hallmark of anaerobic infection. The clinical course following aspiration is

Table 55-2. *Bacteriology of Aspiration Pneumonia*

Community Acquired	Nosocomial Acquired
Anaerobes	**Anaerobes**
Fusobacterium nucleatum	*Fusobacterium nucleatum*
Peptostreptococus spp	*Peptostreptococus* spp
Bacteroides melaninogenicus	*Bacteroids* spp
Other *Bacteroides* spp	
Aerobes	**Aerobes**
Microaerophilic streptococci	*Staphylococcus aureus*
Streptococcus viridans	Enterobacteriaceae
Moraxella catarrhalis	*Escherichia coli*
Eikenella corrodens	*Klebsiella* spp
Streptococcus pneumoniae	*Enterococcus* spp
Haemophilus influenzae	*Citrobacter freundii*
	Acinetobacter lwoffi
	Pseudomonas aeruginosa

variable: rapid improvement, transient improvement followed worsening clinical status, and rapid progression into pleuropulmonary complications including infection and ARDS.

Tests to assess the specific site and severity of a swallowing disorder are discussed in Chapters 11-14.

B. Chest Radiography

Radiographic infiltrates usually develop within few hours after aspiration and frequently progress for the first 24-48 hours. Although chest radiographic patterns post aspiration are variable, some degree of atelectasis exists in most of cases. Nearly 85% of patients with aspiration of gastric contents develop bilateral or asymmetrical pulmonary infiltrates on initial chest radiography depending on patient's position during aspiration. Interestingly, 10% of these patients may have a normal chest radiograph. The superior segments of the lower lobes or the posterior segments of the upper lobes are commonly involved (Figure 55–1). Diffuse bilateral alveolar infiltrates are seen in patients progressing into ARDS. Patients with recurrent aspiration may demonstrate fleeting pulmonary infiltrates in serial chest radiographs. The extent of the pulmonary infiltrates after aspiration does not necessarily correlate with the clinical outcome.

Complete resolution of infiltrates generally occurs within 1 week in uncomplicated cases; the chest radiograph usually lags behind symptomatic improvement. Worsening of chest radiography can include diffuse alveolar infiltrates, segmental air-space consolidation, cavitary lesions, and pleural effusion. A common radiographic manifestation of lipid pneumonia is poorly defined peripheral mass often mimicking neoplasm. A solid foreign body, depending on its size, may show complete or segmental atelectasis, particularly in the

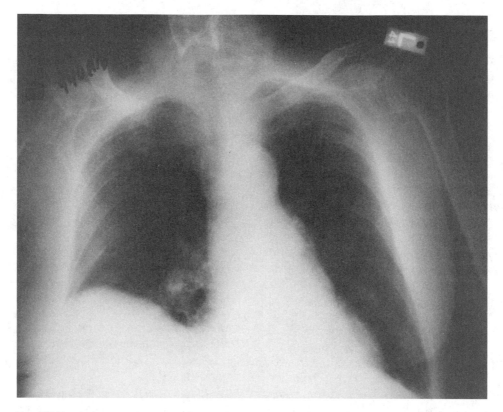

FIG 55-1. Anteroposterior chest radiogragh of a patient with a right lower lobe pneumonia. Notice the persistence of barium contrast in the pyriform sinuses and upper trachea.

lower lobes with contralateral shifting of the mediastinum. Air-trapping may be seen in expiratory films. Radiolucent foreign bodies such as coins and teeth can be identified on chest radiography.

C. Bacteriological Assessment

Methods used in obtaining specimens to diagnose infection include sputum culture, tracheal aspiration, protected brush bronchoscopy, and bronchoalveolar lavage. Expectorated sputum is contaminated with oropharyngeal flora and relying on culture results can be misleading. Diagnostic thoracentesis is indicated if pleural effusion is seen on chest radiography.

VI. MANAGEMENT

A. Swallowing Therapy/Diet Modification

Patients at-risk for aspiration should be identified and the reversal of the underlying cause(s) should be initiated. For patients requiring mechanical ventilation, placement in a semirecumbent position and active suction of the hypopharynx may reduce the risk of aspiration.[6] Continuous aspiration of subglottic secretions has been shown to be effective in minimizing ventilator-as-

sociated pneumonia by reducing the inoculum of oropharyngeal bacteria that might leak around the endotracheal tube cuff.[7]

In selected patients, feeding trials should be supervised by a speech pathologist with emphasis on techniques to stimulate pharyngeal swallow and vocal fold adduction. A Passy-Muir or other similar speaking valve may improve the swallowing ability and prevent aspiration when used in patients with tracheostomy undergoing oral feeding.[8] These issues are described in more detail in Chapters 34-37.

Patients receiving enteral feeding via nasogastric tubes should be monitored for possible migration of these tubes into the oropharynx or larynx. The migration of gastrostomy tube into the pylorus may cause pyloric stenosis, gastric distension, and protracted vomiting. An upper gastrointestinal radiographic series may detect patients with pyloric stenosis, acid reflux disease, and delayed gastric emptying. Gastrokinetic agents such as metoclopramide and cisapride increase the LES tone and promote gastric emptying.

B. Medical Treatment

Depending on the extent of lung injury in patients with aspiration, treatment may range from observation and intravenous hydration to mechanical ventilation and ICU monitoring.

The benefit of administration of prophylactic antibiotics is unclear and their use may even be harmful. Although prophylaxis initially reduces oropharyngeal colonization, which theoretically should minimize pneumonia secondary to these organisms, prolonged duration of broad-spectrum antibiotics clearly predisposes to the emergence of antibiotic resistant pathogens including *Pseudomonas aeruginosa*, *Enterobacter* spp, and *Acinetobacter* spp.[9,10]

Penicillin-G remains the antimicrobial agent of choice for treatment of aspiration-related infections in patients residing in the community. Penicillin-G can be administered intravenously in doses of 4-12 million U/d to an average-sized adult with normal renal function. Clindamycin or ampicillin-sulbactam are common alternatives. The polymicrobial nature of aspiration pneumonia limits the use of metronidazole as a sole therapy, as it does not provide coverage against streptococci. In chronically ill, hospitalized, and nursing home patients, a broader coverage with antimicrobial therapy is recommended to provide coverage for aerobic gram-negative organisms, *S. aureus*, as well as anaerobes. Ampicillin-sulbactam is ideal for nursing home patients, with ticarcillin-clavunate and piperacillin-tazobactam possibly preferred in ICU patients colonized with more resistant bacterial flora. Vancomycin can be administered, if methicillin-resistant *S. aureus* is consistently isolated from respiratory secretions. The duration of therapy should be 10-14 days; however, patients who develop lung abscess or empyema require up to 6 weeks of therapy or more. Thoracostomy tube drainage is indicated in empyema. Corticosteroids offer no benefit in treating chemical pneumonitis and are not routinely recommended.[11] Obstruction of the lower airways requires immediate intervention with flexible fiberoptic or rigid bronchoscopy to evaluate and remove foreign bodies. Finally, laryngeal framework surgery, including laryngeal diversion/separation, glottic and supraglottic closure, laryngeal stents and total laryngectomy, is an alternative approach for patients with intractable aspiration.

References

1. Huxley EJ, Viroslav J, Gray WR, Pierce AK. Pharyngeal aspiration in normal adults and patients with depressed consciousness. *Am J Med.*1978;64:564-568.
2. DePaso WJ. Aspiration pneumonia. *Clin Chest Med.* 1991; 12:269-284.
3. Tolep K, Getch CL, Criner GJ. Swallowing dysfunction in patients receiving prolonged mechanical ventilation. *Chest.* 1996;109:167-172.
4. Shifrin RY, Choplin RH. Aspiration in patients in critical care units. *Radiol Clin North Am.* 1996;34:83-96.
5. Finegold SM. Aspiration pneumonia. *Rev Infect Dis.* 1991; 13(suppl 9):S737-S742.
6. Rello J, Sonora Jubert P, Artigas A, Rue M, Valles J. Pneumonia in intubated patients: role of respiratory airway care. *Am J Respir Crit Care Med.* 1996;154:111-115.
7. Valles J, Artigas A, Rello J, et al. Continuous aspiration of subglottic secretions in preventing ventilator-associated pneumonia. *Ann Int Med.* 1995;122:179-186.
8. Dettelbach MA, Gross RD, Mahlmann J, Eibling DE. Effect of the Passy-Muir valve on aspiration in patients with tracheostomy. *Head Neck.* 1995;17:297-302.
9. Wunderink RG. Mortality and ventilator-associated pneumonia. The best antibiotics may be the least antibiotics. *Chest.*1993;104:993-994.
10. Goetz A, Yu VL. The intensive care unit: the hottest zone. *Curr Opinion Infect Dis.* 1997;10:319-323.
11. Wolfe JE, Bone RC, Ruth WE. Effects of corticosteroids in the treatment of patients with gastric aspiration. *Am J Med.* 1977;63:719-722.

INDEX